ROUTLEDGE HANDBOOK OF HEALTH AND MEDIA

The Routledge Handbook of Health and Media provides an extensive review and exploration of the myriad ways that health and media function as a symbiotic partnership that profoundly influences contemporary societies.

A unique and significant volume in an expanding pedagogical field, this diverse collection of international, original, and interdisciplinary essays goes beyond issues of representation to engage in scholarly conversations about the web of networks that inextricably bind media and health to each other. Divided into sections on film, television, photography, comics, advertising, social media, and print journalism, each chapter begins with a concrete text or texts, using it to raise more general and theoretical issues about the medium in question. As such, this Handbook defines, expands, and illuminates the role that the humanities and arts play in the education and practice of healthcare professionals and in our understanding of health, illness, and disability.

The Routledge Handbook of Health and Media is an invaluable reference for academics, students, and health professionals engaged with cultural issues in media and medicine, popular representations of disease and disability, and the patient/professional healthcare encounter.

Lester D. Friedman is Emeritus Professor of Media and Society from Hobart and William Smith Colleges. His publications include: *Cultural Sutures* editor, *Health Humanities Reader* (co-editor) and *The Picture of Health* (co-editor). He has also written books on Clint Eastwood, Steven Spielberg, *Frankenstein*, American Jewish Cinema, genre theory, and films of the 1970s. Currently, he is completing a book on Hollywood directors and composers.

Therese (Tess) Jones is Associate Director of the Center for Bioethics and Humanities; Director of the Arts and Humanities in Healthcare Program at the University of Colorado Anschutz Medical Campus; and Professor in the Department of Medicine. She has served as the editor of the *Journal of Medical Humanities*; lead editor of the *Health Humanities Reader;* and co-editor of the *Handbook on Health and Media*, and she has published and presented extensively on HIV/AIDS and the arts; literature, film, and medicine; and medical education.

ROUTLEDGE HANDBOOK OF HEALTH AND MEDIA

Edite[illegible]lman and Therese Jones

Routledge
Taylor & Francis Group
LONDON AND NEW YORK

Cover image: © Getty Images

First published 2022
by Routledge
2 Park Square, Milton Park, Abingdon, Oxon OX14 4RN

and by Routledge
605 Third Avenue, New York, NY 10158

Routledge is an imprint of the Taylor & Francis Group, an informa business

British Library Cataloguing-in-Publication Data
A catalogue record for this book is available from the British Library

Library of Congress Cataloging-in-Publication Data
Names: Friedman, Lester D., editor. | Jones, Therese, editor.
Title: Routledge handbook of health and media /
edited by Lester D. Friedman and Therese Jones.
Description: Abingdon, Oxon ; New York, NY : Routledge, 2022. |
Includes bibliographical references and index. |
Identifiers: LCCN 2022004983 (print) | LCCN 2022004984 (ebook) |
ISBN 9780367441081 (hardback) | ISBN 9781032309484 (paperback) |
ISBN 9781003007661 (ebook) |
Subjects: LCSH: Health in mass media. | Medicine in mass media. | Social medicine. |
Classification: LCC P96.H43 R68 2022 (print) |
LCC P96.H43 (ebook) | DDC 070.4/49613–dc23/eng/20220520 |
LC record available at https://lccn.loc.gov/2022004983 |
LC ebook record available at https://lccn.loc.gov/2022004984

ISBN: 978-0-367-44108-1 (hbk)
ISBN: 978-1-032-30948-4 (pbk)
ISBN: 978-1-003-00766-1 (ebk)

DOI: 10.4324/9781003007661

Typeset in Bembo
by Newgen Publishing UK

CONTENTS

FIGURES

ABOUT THE EDITORS

Lester D. Friedman, Ph.D., is Emeritus Professor and former chair of the Media and Society Program at Hobart and William Smith Colleges. Prior to his time at HWS, Professor Friedman taught cinema studies at Syracuse, Northwestern, and American Universities, as well as the Art Institute of Chicago. He also taught health humanities and bioethics at Upstate Medical Center (Syracuse) and the Feinberg School of Medicine at Northwestern University (Chicago). The author, co-author, and editor of over 20 books, he has written about Steven Spielberg, Arthur Penn, Peter Pan, Frankenstein, and Clint Eastwood, among others. He has authored two screenplays that have been the basis of independent films, been a winner of the National Jewish Book Award (Visual Arts), and is also a JEOPARDY! Champion.

Therese (Tess) Jones is Professor of Medicine, Associate Director of the Center for Bioethics and Humanities (CBH), and Director of the Arts and Humanities in Healthcare Program at the University of Colorado Anschutz Medical Campus. She received her Ph.D. in English from the University of Colorado, Boulder, with major emphases in American literature, modern and contemporary drama, and gender studies and completed a three-year postdoctoral fellowship in medical humanities. She has published and presented extensively on HIV/AIDS and the arts; literature, film and medicine; and medical education. She served as the editor of the *Journal of Medical Humanities* from 2003 – 2021 and was lead editor for the *Health Humanities Reader* (Rutgers University Press 2014).

CONTRIBUTORS

Gillian Andrews is a Ph.D. candidate in the English department at Lehigh University. Her publications include co-authoring "The Charlotte Smith Story Map" for *Romantic Circles* and a review of Lauro's *Zombie Theory* in *Science Fiction Film and Television*. Her primary research focuses on the interdisciplinary intersections between horror studies, bioethics, and health humanities. She is currently writing her dissertation, "Haunting Health: Disease, the Horror Genre, and Health Rhetoric."

Julie M. Aultman is a Professor of Medical Ethics and Humanities with the Department of Family and Community Medicine at Northeast Ohio Medical University, where she is also Vice Dean. Her publications include a recent article, "The Segregated Gun: Representations of the Gun in Film and Its Meaning and Impact on the Black Community", with Elizabeth and Jason Piatt. She has published a co-edited book, *Professionalism in Medicine: Critical Perspectives*. Currently, she is completing *Global Ethics and Social Justice for Refugees, Asylum Seekers, and Migrants*.

Olivia Banner is Associate Professor of Critical Media Studies at The University of Texas at Dallas. Her publications include: *Communicative Biocapitalism: The Voice of the Patient in Digital Health and the Health Humanities*; *Teaching Health Humanities* (co-editor); and numerous articles on digital health. She is working on a monograph, *Screening Madness, 1933–2020*, about the 20th-century genealogy of digital psychiatry in relation to racial capitalism, heteropatriarchy, and activist responses.

Catherine Belling is Associate Professor of Medical Education and graduate faculty in Medical Humanities and Bioethics at Northwestern University's Feinberg School of Medicine. Her book, *A Condition of Doubt: The Meanings of Hypochondria*, won the 2013 Kendrick Book Prize (Society for Literature, Science, and the Arts). She has published in journals such as *Narrative*, *Academic Medicine*, *Genre*, and *Perspectives in Biology and Medicine*, and was editor of *Literature and Medicine* (JHUP) from 2013 to 2018. Her current work explores the place of horror (as both affect and genre) in medicine.

Rebecca Burditt is an Assistant Professor of Media and Society at Hobart and William Smith Colleges. Her publications include "Reality TV, Genre Theory, and Shaping the Real," in *Teaching Media Quarterly* and "Death and Lipstick: Commercial Moments in Niagara," in *The Journal of American Culture*. She is currently working on a project about humor in American media and gag reels, as well as co-authoring *Fifty Years of Women Media Makers: From New Hollywood to You Tube*.

Tod Chambers is Associate Professor in the Center for Bioethics and Medical Humanities at Northwestern University's Feinberg School of Medicine. His publications include *The Fiction of Bioethics* and *Prozac as a Way of Life* (co-editor). He has also written on narrative and rhetoric in bioethics and cross-cultural issues in clinical ethics. Currently he is working on a second monograph on the poetics of bioethics arguments.

Andrea Charise is Associate Professor of Health and Society at the University of Toronto Scarborough, and the author or editor of the *Routledge Companion to Health Humanities* and *The Aesthetics of Senescence*, a finalist for the 2020 British Society for Literature and Science's Book Prize. She curates *The Resemblage Project*, an intergenerational digital storytelling initiative and is Principal Investigator of "Flourish: Community-Engaged Arts as a Method for Social Wellness," an interdisciplinary research cluster dedicated to advancing creative arts engagement across the life course.

Alicia Chester is Visiting Lecturer in the Department of Art and Art History at the University of Rochester. Her publications include: *Visual Studies: Writing Through the Discipline* (co-editor), "Outmoded Instant: From Instagram to Polaroid" in *Afterimage* and "Arcadia and Anxiety: Travel Trailers and Fallout Shelters in Midcentury America" in *Dialectic*. Her research takes an interdisciplinary approach to historical, medical, and vernacular photographic practices.

MK Czerwiec is a founding board member of the Graphic Medicine International Collective. Her publications include *Taking Turns: Stories from HIV/AIDS Care Unit 371*, *Graphic Medicine Manifesto* (co-author), and the Eisner Award-winning anthology, *Menopause: A Comic Treatment* (ed.). MK is the Comics Editor for *Literature & Medicine*. She regularly teaches graphic medicine at Northwestern Feinberg Medical School and the University of Chicago.

Lisa Diedrich is Professor and Department Chair of Women's, Gender, and Sexuality Studies at Stony Brook University. Her research and teaching interests are in critical medical studies, disability studies, feminist science studies, and graphic medicine. She is the author of *Indirect Action: Schizophrenia, Epilepsy, AIDS, and the Course of Health Activism* and *Treatments: Language, Politics, and the Culture of Illness*.

Carol-Ann Farkas is Professor of English at Massachusetts College of Pharmacy and Health Sciences (MCPHS) University, and the director of the University's undergraduate degree program in health humanities. She the editor of *Reading the Psychosomatic in Medical and Popular Culture: Something, Nothing, Everything*. Other publications include "The Blind Men and the Elephant: Mediating Conflicting Views of Controversial Diagnoses" in *Trespassing Journal*, and "What's the Difference?: Pathologizing Genius and Neurodiversity in Popular Television Series" in *Genius on Television: Essays on Small Screen Depictions of Big Minds*. Year."

Bianca C. Frazer is a Postdoctoral Research Associate at the University of Illinois Chicago. Her writing appears and is forthcoming in *(Un)Doing Diabetes: Representation, Disability, Culture, Metanarratives of Disability: Culture, Assumed Authority, and the Normative Social Order, ArtsPraxis,* and *Theatre Journal.* She has also written on diabetes and American drama. Currently, she researches the performance aesthetics of non-apparently disabled people, specifically those with any form of diabetes.

JV Fuqua is an associate professor in the Department of Media Studies and the director of the Women and Gender Studies Program at Queens College/City University of New York. Fuqua's publications include the monograph, *Prescription TV: Therapeutic Discourse in the Hospital and at Home.* Currently, Fuqua is writing on trans identity and environmental cultural studies.

Sander L. Gilman is a distinguished professor emeritus of the Liberal Arts and Sciences as well as emeritus Professor of Psychiatry at Emory University, and is the author or editor of over one hundred books, including *Stand Up Straight! A History of Posture*; his most recent edited volume is *The Oxford Handbook of Music and the Body* (with Youn Kim). His *"I Know Who Caused COVID-19": Pandemics and Xenophobia* is in press.

Barry Keith Grant is Emeritus Professor of Film Studies and Popular Culture at Brock University, Ontario, Canada, and an Elected Fellow of the Royal Society of Canada. His books as author include *Voyages of Discovery: The Cinema of Frederick Wiseman, 100 Science Fiction Films, Monster Cinema,* and *Shadows of Doubt: Negotiations of Masculinity in American Genre Films,* and as editor, *Five Films by Frederick Wiseman, The Dread of Difference: Gender and the Horror Film,* and four editions of *Film Genre Reader.*

Amanda K. Greene is an Andrew W. Mellon Postdoctoral Research Associate at Lehigh University's Humanities Lab. Greene's research operates at the nexus of feminist technoscience, media theory, visual culture, and disability studies, and her scholarship explores how everyday habits of visual media readership shape human bodies and embodied practices of sense-making. She has published in venues such as *Feminist Theory, Perspectives in Biology and Medicine, Psychology of Sexual Orientation and Gender Diversity, Feminist Media Studies,* and *Information, Communication, Society.*

Shoshannah Bryn Jones Square is a Research Affiliate with the University of Manitoba Institute for the Humanities (UMIH) and is currently co-editing the collection *Sex and Medicine: Intersex and the Health and Medical Humanities*; Bryn's chapter is "Occupying Spaces of Possibility: Intersex, Complexity, and Our Shared Multiplicity." She has had articles on Mary Shelley, Romanticism, hyper-empathy, suicide, emotional contagion, and social change published in *Essays in Romanticism* and *Studies in the Literary Imagination.*

Allison Kavey is Professor of History at CUNY John Jay College of Criminal Justice and CUNY Graduate Center. She is the author of *Books of Secrets: Popular Natural Philosophy in England (1550–1600).* She contributed to the *Health Humanities Reader* and the forthcoming *Routledge Guide to Health and Media* and was co-editor of the volume of *Literature and Medicine* devoted to *Frankenstein.* She has written and edited books on a variety of interdisciplinary topics, including books about alchemy, Peter Pan, and Frankenstein. She is currently working on a book about Agrippa von Nettesheim's magical cosmology.

Rae-Ellen W. Kavey is a retired Professor of Pediatric Cardiology from the University of Rochester School of Medicine. Her career in academic medicine focused on diagnosis and management of children with congenital heart disease and on the prevention of acquired atherosclerotic disease; she has more than a hundred publications on these subjects in the medical literature. She co-authored *Viral Pandemics: From Smallpox to COVID-19* and is currently working on a book on poverty and health in childhood.

Erik Larsen is Assistant Professor of Medical Humanities at the University of Rochester, and is the co-editor of *Tattooed Bodies: Theorizing Body Inscription Across Disciplines and Cultures*. His articles appear in *Nineteenth-Century Literature* and *Levinas Studies*. In 2019–2020 he was a contributing writer for *Synapsis: A Health Humanities Journal*. Currently, he is working on articles exploring the biopolitical assumptions informing popular horror media.

Marjorie Levine-Clark, Professor of History at the University of Colorado Denver, has published *Beyond the Reproductive Body: The Politics of Women's Health and Work in Early Victorian England* and *Unemployment, Welfare, and Masculine Citizenship: "So Much Honest Poverty" in Britain, 1870–1930*, as well as numerous articles and chapters on gender, health, poverty, and welfare. She recently completed *Work and Unemployment in Britain, 1834–1911*, and her current project is tentatively titled, "Unemployment, Health, and the Body in Britain from the New Poor Law to Thatcher."

Deborah Lupton is SHARP Professor and leader of the Vitalities Lab at the Centre for Social Research in Health and Social Policy Research Centre and leader of the UNSW Node of the Australian Research Council Centre of Excellence for Automated Decision-Making and Society, University of New South Wales. She is the author/co-author of 19 books and editor/co-editor of a further nine volumes, the latest of which are *The Face Mask in COVID Times* (co-author), *COVID Societies* (author) and *Creative Approaches to Health Education* (co-editor). She is currently completing a book on animals and digital media.

Nicole Matthews teaches media and cultural studies at Macquarie University, Sydney. Her most recent book (written with Naomi Sunderland) is *Digital Storytelling in Health and Social Policy* (2017). Her work on the convergence between mobile phones and hearing devices has been published in *Television & New Media*, *Media International Australia*, and *American Journal of Audiology*. She is currently working on a collaborative project around the barriers to health professionals listening to clients' account of lived experience.

Christie Milliken is an Associate Professor in the Department of Communication, Popular Culture and Film at Brock University, and is the co-author of *Reclaiming Popular Documentary* (2021), in addition to several journal and book chapters on sex education film, AIDS video activism and 1960s cinema. She is currently exploring issues related to environment, scale, magnitude, and drone photography in the film work of Edward Burtynsky and Ai Weiwei.

Nigel Morris is retired from the University of Lincoln, UK as Associate Professor of Media Theory. Author of *Empire of Light: The Cinema of Steven Spielberg*, he edited the Wiley-Blackwell *Companion to Steven Spielberg* and has published on other aspects of Hollywood cinema, British cinema, representations of science, television genre hybridity, adaptations, reality television, film and modernism, German expressionism, and Welsh cinema and broadcasting. Current projects include a monograph on realism in film and television.

Danielle Ofri is one of the foremost voices in the medical world today, shining an unflinching light on the realities of health care and speaking passionately about the doctor–patient relationship. Her writing appears regularly in the *New York Times*, as well as in the *New Yorker*, *Slate Magazine*, the *Lancet*, and the *New England Journal of Medicine*; she has written six books including *When We Do Harm: A Doctor Confronts Medical Error; What Doctors Feel: How Emotions Affect the Practice of Medicine;* and *Singular Intimacies: Becoming a Doctor at Bellevue.* She is a founder and Editor-in-Chief of the *Bellevue Literary Review.*

Kirsten Ostherr is the Gladys Louise Fox Professor and Chair of the Department of English and Director of the Medical Humanities program at Rice University. Her publications include *Medical Visions: Producing the Patient through Film, Television, and Imaging Technologies* and *Cinematic Prophylaxis: Globalization and Contagion in the Discourse of World Health*. She is editor of *Applied Media Studies* and co-editor of a special issue of the journal *Discourse*. She currently leads a digital health humanities project that identifies international humanities-based pandemic responses to document and build upon these creative efforts.

Tim Seiber is Associate Professor of Science and Media Studies and the Director of the Johnston Center for Integrative Studies at the University of Redlands. His publications include: "Ideal Positions: 3D Sonography, Medical Visuality, and Popular Culture" and "Playable Virus: HIV Molecular Aesthetics in Science and Popular Culture." Other publications discuss digital media, gossip, and higher education pedagogy. Currently, he is working on a book project about electronic music, public policy, and discourses about wellness.

Matt Selway is a Senior Lecturer in Media & Communication and Film Studies at York St John University. His primary research concerns the relationship between mental health, film, and media. His publications have been featured in journals such as *Sound Studies* and *The Journal for Cultural Research* as well as in edited collections such as *Narratives of Suffering: Meaning and Experience in a Transcultural Approach.*

Lorenzo Servitje is Associate Professor of Literature and Medicine, and has a dual appointment in the Department of English and the Health, Media, and Society Program at Lehigh University. His monograph, *Medicine Is War: The Martial Metaphor in Victorian Literature and Culture,* traces the metaphorical militarization of medicine in the 19th century. He has co-edited three collections: *The Walking Med: Zombies and the Medical Image* and *Endemic: Essays in Contagion Theory*, and *Syphilis and Subjectivity: From the Victorians to the Present*. Servitje's current book project is *The Science and Fiction of Antibiosis*.

Leah Shafer is an Associate Professor of Media and Society at Hobart and William Smith Colleges and has published essays in *Film Criticism; ReFocus: The Films of John Hughes; Feminist Interventions in Digital Pedagogy; The 25 Sitcoms that Changed Television: From I Love Lucy to Modern Family; and The Wiley-Blackwell Companion to the War Film.* Shafer is a scholar/artist whose experimental documentaries are in the permanent collection of national museums.

Agnese Sile is a Teaching Fellow in Design Cultures at the University of Edinburgh. Her recent publications include "Echo and the Failure of Knowing in Judith Fox's Photographic Project 'I Still Do: Loving and Living with Alzheimer's" in the *Journal of Medical Humanities* (2018); a book chapter "Gestures of care in Briony Campbell's photographic essay 'The Dad

Project'" in *Discourses of Care: Care in Media, Medicine and Society*; a journal article "Exploring Intimacy in Collaborative Photographic Narratives of Breast Cancer" in *Humanities* (2020).

Joseph G. Turow is the Robert Lewis Shayon Professor of Media Systems and Industries at the University of Pennsylvania's Annenberg School for Communication. Recent books include *The Voice Catchers*; *Media Today: Mass Communication in A Converging World* (7th edition), and *The Aisles Have Eyes*. His research and writing focus on the intersection of marketing, digital media, and society and explores the power dynamics that shape commercially-driven cultural materials.

Sathyaraj Venkatesan is Associate Professor of English in the Department of Humanities and Social Sciences at National Institute of Technology, Trichy (India). His research concentrates on graphic medicine and global health humanities. He is the author of six books and over 90 research publications; he most recently co-authored *Gender, Eating Disorders and Graphic Medicine* and *India Retold*. Currently, he is completing a book on "Pandemics and Epidemics in Cultural Representation."

Caroline Wellbery is Associate Deputy Editor of *American Family Physician* and Professor in the Department of Family Medicine in the Georgetown University School of Medicine. Her publications include: "Climate Change and the Local Environment: Communicating with Your Patients about Health Impacts"; "Art–Science Collaborations: Why Do They Matter to Medicine?": "Can We Make Empathy More Intelligent? Try Social Empathy!" (*Handbook of the Medical Humanities*). She has recently completed a memoir, *The Examining Room,* and is working on a coming-of-age novel about trauma and resiliency.

Ian Williams is a comics artist, writer, and family doctor in Brighton, UK. His publications include: *The Bad Doctor, The Lady Doctor, The Graphic Medicine Manifesto* (co-author) and *Sick Notes* – a weekly comic strip in *The Guardian*. He has been the recipient of several grants, has contributed to numerous medical, humanities, and comics publications, and has sat on the board of a number of arts and humanities organizations.

FOREWORD

Danielle Ofri

The progenitor of all health media is the medical chart. Long before anyone blogged, tweeted, posted, or podcasted, long before anyone published op-eds, documentaries, or memoirs, generations of doctors and nurses dutifully penned the stories of their patients in the lowly medical chart.

Originally long-hand on paper, later pecked out in the electronic medical record (EMR) or dictated on tape, the dramas, characters, conflicts, and denouements spooled across the chart, often over years and decades. The language has surely evolved, from the florid Victorians observing the musicality of murmurs to the acronym-laden, box-checking clicks of the EMR, but it still carves out a story that the writers seek to communicate to an audience of readers.

Up until recently, the audience for the medical chart was one and the same as its writers: the chart existed solely to communicate between members of the medical team. It consisted mainly of jargony acronyms that could compress an entire medical history with an efficiency that puts Twitter to shame.

But a growing democratization of the medical chart has expanded the audience, culminating in federal regulations in 2021 that made open notes mandatory. Patients have full access to everything in the chart from their uric acid levels to the nursing procedures to the doctors' diagnostic strategies. Few patients perusing their charts will stumble upon metaphorical musings worthy of Sir William Osler or expository emanations in the vein of Dr. Oliver Sacks, but the medical chart remains the Rosetta Stone of health media.

From this raw yet intimate accounting of disease has flowed all manner of media – illness narratives by patients, medical memoirs from doctors and nurses, scientific reporting in newspapers, disease-of the-week movies, impeccably coiffed television health correspondents, patient advocacy blogs, pharmaceutical ads sporting requisite golden retrievers, health policy op-eds, muckraking investigative documentaries, wellness podcasts, gritty graphics, medical education Tweetorials, anti-vax memes, GoFundMe campaigns for medical bills, and any number of TikTok videos belting out the fortes and foibles of our healthcare system in full Broadway timbre.

Judging whether this is a salutary development or a travesty depends on where in the media currents you find yourself swimming, as well as the very nature of those currents. The explosion of health media can overwhelm even the technologically facile and leaves many of us mortals with a dyspeptic cocktail of vertigo and migraine. Which is why a *Handbook on Health and Media* is so timely.

The Virgils of this handbook guide us through the full gamut of health media, starting with exploring the printed word, both on paper and online. We then move on to images – photography, fiction film, documentary film, and comics. The section on "Apps, Devices and Wearables" brings us into the world of artificial intelligence, big data, and phones that are smart but not necessarily wise. Last, but not least, we plunge into the roiling waters of the internet, podcasts, social media, and the various spinoffs thereof.

While these media vary widely in style, substance, reach, and credibility, they all retain the commonality of attempting to tell a story. More often than not, it is the story of a patient, even if not framed as such. In this regard, the wide-ranging health media of today retain the touchstone of the medical chart. It may not necessarily be obvious to the casual observer, but if you examine it carefully, it's there. So the next time you're perusing an Instagram story, or listening to a podcast while you chop onions, or digging through 3,000 comments on a post about vaccinations, imagine the patient grappling with that issue, the nurse observing the clinical course, the doctor scribbling notes.

The universality of the story is what unites not only the media, but all those who read/watch/listen/comment/digest it. The story is what keeps us coming back for more. The story is what keeps us connected. The story is what keeps us imagining.

The next chapter on health media hasn't been written yet because we don't yet know what it will be. It could involve nanoparticles, drone drops, or induced auditory hallucinations – who knows? But it will be a story. And we'll all tune in, because we always want to find out how the story ends.

ACKNOWLEDGMENTS

While most of the chapters in this handbook do not directly or explicitly reference our current pandemic, all of us engaged in the project have been influenced, impacted, and injured by it just as have our families, friends, colleagues, students, and neighbors. We are so grateful that our contributors stayed with us to produce an extraordinary collection of original work. Our own families have been, as always, supportive during this time as well, and we owe a special bouquet of gratitude to Rae-Ellen Kavey and Christopher Jones. At Routledge, we sincerely appreciate the patience, generosity, and kindness of our editor, Grace McInnes, and her assistant, Evie Lonsdale. When we began this project with them, we never imagined producing and completing it through a plague year, and their willingness to support us, our team, and our contributors was unwavering.

We are also deeply grateful to our resourceful and scrupulous assistant editor, Kathleen Pachucki, who has worked with Tess since 2009. To say that "we couldn't have done without her" is not hyperbole; without her we would still be trying to figure out how Dropbox works. Finally, we want to acknowledge and thank David Weil from the University of Colorado Anschutz Medical Campus whose technical savvy and upbeat attitude kept us afloat.

Les and Tess (the rhyming editors) have been friends for a long time, and this book is a testament to their affection and respect for each other.

INTRODUCTION

The stories of our lives: narrative, media, and health

Lester D. Friedman and Therese Jones

This book grew out of our belief that incorporating media knowledgeably and effectively within the healthcare matrix obliges us to grapple with the complex issues that bind stories and broadcasting systems together into a formidable and dynamic force within all our lives. Each chapter contains original essays that focus on a how a particular medium displays a specific healthcare issue; then, the author branches outward toward more broad, sometimes theoretical, concerns about the ways in which that medium – that particular communication system – transmits materials to a potentially large array of receivers (aka readers). By expanding their ideas from the concrete to the general, our contributors foreground the specific characteristics that denote the most prevalent channels of communication, analyzing an extensive range of healthcare topics transported across a broad spectrum of platforms. Our introduction contextualizes these wide-ranging essays by providing a general perspective for the intricate symbiosis between the cultures of health and media. To do so, we explore the societal roles, functions, and formats of narratives – be they textual, visual, auditory, or performative; the purposes and meanings of stories in healthcare culture; and the transmedia linkages that broadcast, shape, and render health narratives accessible.

As a whole, then, this collection of interdisciplinary essays, written by an international assemblage of scholars, scrutinizes how particular mediums mold and circulate health narratives, how they influence the education and practice of health professionals, how they shape the expectations and experiences of patients and their families, and how they play a substantial role in sculpting the culture of healthcare systems. We have structured the chapters in a loose chronological order to spotlight the flow of mediums over time, noting how their popularity waxes and wanes in our personal and public lives. That said, we recognize that each medium possesses its own culture of particular methodologies and distinctive features but that all share similar characteristics. It remains important, therefore, to keep in mind that every medium builds upon the ones that precede it, and because the antecedent platforms still exist, old and new formats continually intersect with each other in myriad ways to form linked networks. As Marshall McLuhan aptly notes: "all channels of communication remain in constant 'interplay with other media'" (26). Such interactions between mediums inevitably changes them in sometimes subtle, sometime profound ways. For example, print media, the oldest format in this book, has adapted to and taken advantage of social media, the newest format in this book, to

DOI: 10.4324/9781003007661-1

become as culturally relevant, if not more so, in the 21st century as it was when Guttenberg invented the printing press. Thus, one medium characteristically involves the incorporation of other mediums, an amalgamation of communication formats that necessarily provides receivers with a "multimedia" or "multimodal" process of reception.

Here we must pause to address some basic terminology in our discussion of the design and deployment of words, sounds, and images. For the sake of clarity, we define a *medium* or its plural form, *media,* as singular or multiple delivery systems that incorporate technological, semiotic, and cultural dimensions. Throughout this book, we also use the word *media* – as it is in general parlance – to refer to any form of communication that delivers information or entertainment. *Mass media,* again in general usage, denotes those mediums or platforms by which this information and/or entertainment reaches large numbers of people. Such widespread dispersal of these elements depends on technological emergences and industrial evolutions that consistently produce ever-faster conduits for materials to be sent to and modalities to be received by a sizeable audience. However, neither the materials distributed nor the methods by which we access them are ideologically neutral.

In their study of a media-conscious narratology, for example, Marie-Laure Ryan and Jan-Noel Thon note that the different degrees of prominence of technological, semiotic, and cultural dimensions differs "from medium to medium, but all three must be taken into consideration in the description of medium's narrative affordances and limitations" (5). Thus, every medium is composed with and through a technological means of production in order to construct meanings that reflect, reinforce, or disrupt social institutions and industrial practices. Combined, these three elements configure a channel for sharing narratives – among other things. In addition, most media are *multimodal,* meaning that they contain more than one mode of communication. A film's mise-en-scène, for example, intermingles visual elements such as shot construction with music, sound effects, and spoken words – all different systems for conveying narrative information. Thus, each medium offers its participants – both producers and receivers functioning as co-creators of meaning – a particular set of possibilities and restrictions that can determine how the narrative is sent, recognized, and understood.

Although narratologists deftly distinguish between *stories*, *texts*, *plots*, and *narratives*, we sidestep this intricate warren of theories by employing the common practice of using the terms synonymously. Furthermore, and following in the tradition of film scholars, we use *mise-en-scène* to designate all the elements that appear before the camera and thereby within the frame. But whatever terms we choose to explore the narrative world and all that transpires within its boundaries, theoreticians and practitioners fundamentally agree that human beings constantly function as active tellers, interpretive recipients, and dynamic re-constructors of stories. Narratives play an indispensable role in defining our personal and public worlds, possessing the potential to influence, prod, or even inspire us. At their most compelling, they persuade us to reconsider opinions, or alternatively, reinforce our foundational beliefs, sometimes prompting us to action. Literary scholar and science writer, Jonathan Gottschall, describes stories as "the grease and glue of society. . . the center without which the rest cannot hold" (135); he argues that we are naturally and intrinsically "story telling animals [who] hunger for meaningful patterns and that translates into hunger for stories" (104). True enough, but as historian Elizabeth Einstein notes: "When ideas are detached from the media used to transmit them, they are also cut off from the historical circumstances that shape them, and it becomes difficult to perceive the changing context within which they must be viewed" (24).

Moreover, at their core, the fundamental work of all formats of mass media is "not to elicit belief but to maintain the apparatus of addiction" (Lasch 521) – i.e., their first, and often primary, goal is to perpetually reinforce existing and constantly search for new methods of self-preservation. Because the majority of our mass media functions under the thumb of corporate entities, these communication systems aggressively strive to remain relevant and profitable by becoming indispensable parts of our lives and the foremost means by which we retrieve information and entertainment. And they often succeed. For example, reporters Sheera Frenkel and Cecilia Kang inform readers that "The 2016 U.S. presidential election would stamp out any doubts about the importance of social media in political campaigns. By early 2016, 44 percent of all Americans said they got their news about candidates from Facebook, Twitter, Instagram, and YouTube." (6). So, too, the *New York Times* described a recent outage of Facebook as a "planetary demonstration of how essential [it] has become to daily life," indicating a "kind of global dependency on it" (www.nytimes.com/2021/10/05). To illustrate this point, let's briefly consider the elephant who currently rules the lush and tangled jungle of social media.

In the global digital ecosphere, Facebook's world dominance is the result of commercializing (some might even call it weaponizing) "the apparatus of addiction" to ensure the self-preservation of the company. In particular, the "social validation feedback loop" of this multinational conglomerate illustrates two specific nodes of addiction: neurological damage and social isolation. Facebook's management team knew full well that its algorithms were dangerous. The social media behemoth's ($85.9 billion in revenue in 2020) former president, Sean Parker, publicly lamented that "God only knows what's it doing to our children's brains," while his vice president, Chamath Palihapitiya, added that the "...short-term dopamine-driven feedback loops we created are destroying how society works. . .. I feel tremendous guilt" (Sales 281). The practice of profit-obsessed industries who knowingly market addictive products that harm consumers permeated the remarks of whistleblower Frances Haugen (a former Facebook product manager) who, while testifying before the Senate Commerce Subcommittee on Consumer Protection on October 5, 2021, invoked comparisons between Facebook and Big Tobacco's concealment of the dangers of cigarettes as well as Big Pharma's denial of culpability in the opioid crisis (https://profglantz.com/2021/10/06/facebook-is-like-big-tobacco/). As these patterns of rapacious manipulation exercised by such corporations come to light, we should all heed musician Jim Morrison's now-famous assertion: "whoever controls the media controls the mind."

Once upon a narrative

How many stories did you hear today? How many did you tell? Consider for a moment how much time you spend each day watching, listening to, imagining, and telling stories? Our appetite for stories is hard-wired and to satiate our cravings, we routinely create, receive, decipher, and disperse cascades of stories. From the moment we heard our parents read "once upon a time" to us until we ourselves "rage against the dying of the light," we accumulate layer upon layer of stories from a proliferating variety of generative sources. Stories link us to the past and allow us to contemplate the future. They offer pathways to share the perspectives of others. Many of the narratives we encounter daily are not quarantined within those objects that society designates as art. To the contrary, a vast array of our narrative exchanges transpires outside of the boundaries of book pages or screen images. Even our conversational encounters contain many of the conventional narrative elements – characters, actions, settings – that artists traditionally employ to construct their fictional storied worlds. Not surprisingly, then, the desired effects of these conversational narratives replicate those of more formally structured productions: they entertain, enlighten, provoke, communicate, and persuade in one form or another through informal exchanges or mediated interactions.

The telling of stories precedes the written word. Unearthed in the artifacts of ancient cultures, they appear in the pre-historic figure drawings on the walls of France's Chauvet (some c. 32,000 to c. 30,000 years ago) and Lascaux (20,000 years old) Caves as well as the pictorial hieroglyphic symbols inscribed on papyrus scrolls from early Egypt. The Greek oral storytelling traditions of Aesop and Homer and the word-of-mouth passing of stories from one generation to the next in Native American tribes were integral components in their societies. Handwritten scrolls, codices, and illuminated manuscripts, first produced by monks and scribes on parchment sheets and then on paper during the Middle Ages, were supplanted by Johannes Gutenberg's revolutionary printing press (1440), leading to a slew of mechanical devices that reproduce stories and eventually create contemporary digital narratives. Some mediums, like music and the visual arts, impart their stories without spoken or written languages, although we usually employ words to describe and analyze them. Of course, different cultures have distinctive narrative traditions and even differing definitions of what constitutes art, but as Roland Barthes observes, "narrative is present in every age, in every place, in every society. . . it is simply like life itself" (251–2).

But what powers do narratives possess that grip us so intensely even when they detail violent, scary, or abhorrent events? Literary scholar Brian Boyd asks us to consider a fundamental question: "Why in a world of necessity, do we choose to spend so much time caught up in stories that both teller and told know never happened and never will?" (2). He contends that these mental playing fields generate creativity and imaginative exploration, that they provide "stimulus and training for a flexible mind" (86), helping to form social cohesiveness, strengthen cooperation and commitment to shared beliefs, arouse pleasure, and foster imaginative exploration. Philosopher Martha Nussbaum goes further by stressing that reading literature is a crucial activity because it amplifies our empathy and, thereby, enlarges our moral imagination: the ability to identify with the plights of others, for Nussbaum, is the wellspring of ethical action. Similarly, Jonathan Cohen talks about surrendering our own identity, about forgetting ourselves and "extending our emotional horizons and social perspectives" (249) through an imaginative identification with characters, a process Oakley labels as the mind's "flight simulator" (1). Such contentions designate a significant role for fictional scenarios within our decision-making matrix and a crucial component in the development of our moral sensibilities.

All of these commentators assert the widely accepted concept that engaging with narratives inevitably generates empathy and instills ethical reflection, but that engagement is not always a salutary activity. Nigerian writer Chimamanda Ngozi Adichie, for example, emphasizes both the destructive as well as the healing power of stories:

> Power is the ability not just to tell the story of another person, but to make it the definitive story of that person. ... Stories matter. Many stories matter. Stories have been used to dispossess and to malign, but stories can also be used to empower and to humanize. Stores can break the dignity of a people, but stories can also repair that broken dignity.
>
> *(www.facinghistory.org/holocaust-and-human-behavior/chapter-1/danger-single-story)*

Fictive narratives, especially, offer the potential for us to gain perspective about and compassion for others by vicariously experiencing events through the eyes of people different from themselves. But, "potential" remains the key word here and presupposes an uncontested reaction to a text, one affirming that most, if not all, readers, viewers, and listeners agree with the intentions of an artist (the infamous "intentional fallacy"). Do we all share the same responses to and opinions about Raskolnikov, Sethe, Gatsby, Florentino Ariza, Huckleberry Finn, Luke

Skywalker, or Kanji Watanabe? Today, for example, we read and view *Hamlet* far differently than did earlier audiences (and likely Shakespeare himself) who had no knowledge of Freud. It seems unsustainable, therefore, to lump all consumers of stories together – even those belonging to the same ethnic or gender groupings – as a homogeneous group confronting a text or performance. As is generally recognized, we bring our unique set of experiences into every interaction with a given work, a process that pretty much guarantees that some will "read against the grain." Ethnicity, life-experiences, cultural norms, gender, sexuality, and age – just to name the most obvious – differentiate us, and even within these subgroups, substantial variances will produce an assortment of approaches and responses to any shared narrative. We also have ample evidence that, although texts remain fixed, their meanings possess elasticity: the culture that surrounds them is always in flux, always prompting and providing new avenues of interpretation and new ways of constructing meaning that challenge canonical interpretations.

Such so-called "resistant readings" draw alternative, sometime starkly opposing, conclusions from what ostensibly seems to be the narrative thrust of the work. In addition, competing narratives can cover the same ground but arrive at totally divergent conclusions. For example, we can trace how fundamentally different MSNBC, CNN, FOX, and the BBC report and analyze the same story in a single twenty-four news cycle. On a bigger stage, narratives that encapsulate powerful religious doctrines have spawned generations of brutalities, wars, and deaths: "religious convictions derive less from doctrine than from story . . . religion consists less of a coherent body of dogmas or explanatory systems than of these memorably surprising stories" (Boyd 204). Gottschall puts it even stronger when he writes, "Religion is the ultimate expression of story's domination over our minds. . . people base life and actions on sacred stories" (119). Yet another dark side of narrative manipulation is the explosion of omnipresent conspiracy theories, often in the service of White Nationalism, Neo-Nazism, and other racist organizations. The alt-right's story, promulgated mainly on social media, that various legitimate businesses shielded covens of high-ranking Democrats engaging in human tracking and child sex rings dramatically illustrates how narratives that claim to provide adherents with a window into the nefarious activities of their opponents can exert a powerful, even deadly, influence.

Before leaving this intersection of narratives and empathy, we want to reference Molly Worthen's article in the *New York Times* (September 6, 2020), which foregrounds the delicate issues that arise when empathic responses conflict with identity boundaries. Worthen asks a common but still fundamental question: is it possible to teach empathy? The uncertainty around this question often pits those who believe that responding emotionally to suffering is instinctual – a person is either born with this quality or not – against those who assert that empathy can and should be taught, using a variety of tools including narratives. What stands out as new within her discussion, however, is that some scholars contend that, even if empathy can be learned, the attempt "to step into the shoes of those very different from us . . . (might) do more harm than good." Worthen notes how some skeptics allege that "empathy has to be considered in the context of institutions and power… . what seems like empathy often may be another form of presumption, condescension, or domination" (4). Such comments not only raise the complicated issue of how deeply we can ever immerse ourselves in narratives, particularly those stretching far from our own experiences, but also how much we should even attempt to do so. Can we really discard our own squint at the world and totally adopt, even during the time we engage with a given work, the perspective of a character totally different from ourselves? The best we can hope for is that, on some level, narratives emerge as persuasive tools that construct bridges to enable our understanding of the "common threads of human experience" (5).

Jonathan Gottschall observes that "We are a species addicted to story. Story is for a human a water is for a fish" (xiv). On the most basic level, narratives seem to perform significant functions in our personal and communal lives: "We do not have any mental record of who we are until narrative is present as a kind of armature, giving shape to that record" (Abbott 3). Put another way, "people create identities through narrative . . . personal myth brings together the different parts of ourselves in a purposeful whole . . . Stories create a shared history, linking people in time and event as actors, tellers, and audiences" (McAdams 12, 28). One might further suggest that we habitually reconstitute remembrances of things past by sculpting them into cause-and-effect narratives that usually cast us in a favorable light and, thereby, form a sense of the identities that define us – an ongoing process that Fulford calls "our negotiation with reality" (24). Thus, the lifelong manufacturing and renovating of our personal narratives, the weaving together of our memories of past actions and our present needs, creates a "patterned integration" that "brings together the different parts of ourselves and our lives into a purposeful and convincing whole" (McAdams 12). We chronicle our passage through life and interact with others by sharing self-composed narratives in which we are the lead character. To paraphrase T. S. Eliot: "We tell stories to meet the stories that we meet." Beyond the personal, the collective master narratives that we tell – those foundational stories that we internalize and reproduce to maintain a particular social order – form the bedrock of nationalistic pride, religious beliefs, communal values, and cultural practices. Every country, every culture, every religion, every group of people who band together have such storied language, such compulsory discourses that encapsulates their deeply held secular and spiritual beliefs, their highest goals and aspirations, and their darkest anxieties and fear.

"We are obliged by the deepest drives of the human spirit to make more than animate dust, and we must have a story to tell about where we came from and why we are here" (Wilson 6). Most of the authorities who write on narratives, be they personal histories or social tales, sacred or profane, ultimately conclude that the primary function of stories is to impose order on anarchic events, to construct a sense of meaning that will combat which might otherwise be seen as an unrelated series of arbitrary episodes that constitute our lives. From fairy tales to funeral eulogies, from personal memoires to cultural myths, narratives confer a sense of organization, provide some level of coherence, and offer varied explanations to make sense of the seemingly capricious incidents that characterize our hodgepodge existence. A human being is an organism, according to the anthropologist Clifford Geertz, which "cannot live in a world it is unable to understand." He continues by observing that "humans are symbolizing, conceptualizing, meaning-seeking animals. . .The drive to make sense out of experience, to give it form and order, is evidently as real and as pressing as the more familiar biological needs" (quoted in Fulford 15). It is this instinctual and insatiable drive, most of all, that bestows power upon narratives.

So, what's your story?

Narratives and the health humanities

The founding and growth of the medical/health humanities and bioethics programs became and continue to be sites where narratives play a crucial role in healthcare practice and education. Such programs were initiated and sustained primarily by academics who relocated from two well-established fields of study: the former from literature and the latter from philosophy. Today, researchers and teachers from a growing number of disciplines – such as media studies, history, sociology, anthropology, religion, gender and queer studies, psychology, cultural studies, disability studies, and other subject areas – dot the topography of an expansive and inclusive health humanities landscape on undergraduate, graduate, and post-graduate levels, but their subject matter often centers around an evolving variety of narratives. As a result, much has already been written about the formative and extensive role narratives assume within the intellectual fabric of the medical/health humanities and by extension the matrix of medical culture, so we feel no need to restate or summarize here. Nonetheless, a brief excursion into this realm forms a useful bridge between how narratives function in our daily/cultural lives, how they operate with the medical world, and how they interact with media.

In the introduction to the *Health Humanities Reader*, "The Why, the What, and the How of Medical/Health Humanities," we contend that the competencies fostered by the study of stories – specifically reading, writing and interpretation – enhance both health professional education and patient care. In particular, the interpretive skills necessarily employed in analyzing literary texts supply "specific intellectual tools to the multiple dimensions of medicine," while the moral reflection it inspires engages practitioners with "the cultural perspectives on health and illness, social justice, and the moral dimensions of patient encounters" (Jones, Wear, and Friedman 3). Citing Martha Nussbaum's work on empathy mentioned above, some health humanities scholars and educators argue that "the nuances and complexities of literature can sharpen and deepen moral sensibilities" (3), while others in the field have challenged this view. What is unassailable, however, is that in its engagement with a broad range of narratives from diverse sources of media, the health humanities re-present, re-describes, and re-contextualizes issues within health culture itself. Such a process questions representations of caregivers and patients, challenges abuses of power and authority, and refutes the traditional boundaries between biology and culture (Jones, Wear, and Friedman 4).

Disturbed by the increasingly dehumanizing effects of a technologically-dependent medical system, medical/health scholars have stressed how "cultural values and social relations shape how we perceive and . . . recognize bodily symptoms, interpret complaints in the particular context of our life situation" (Kleinman xiii). Thus, the experience of an illness is always culturally molded, and health (or its absence) a form of subjective experience. What is "feeling healthy" to one person can be "feeling unwell" to another. Given the recognition that the exchanges between patients and professionals are, fundamentally, structured as narratives, health humanities practitioners highlight the importance of gaining competence in how to read, analyze, and interpret stories. Such skills, they contend, should remain essential elements in the education of professionals and play a substantial role in the delivery of health care, positioning narratives at the fulcrum of the art and science of the healing encounter. Given this perspective, health humanities scholars have consistently advocated for the inclusion of narrative theories and practices within the various components of biomedical and healthcare culture, claiming: "there is little in the practice of medicine that does not have narrative features, because the clinical practice, the teaching, and the research are all indelibly stamped with the telling or receiving or creating of stories" (Charon vii). The infusion of literary methodologies into health professions curricula to create narrative competence, they claim, is clinically relevant and necessary to produce more efficient and empathic practitioners.

However, it is vital to recognize and emphasize our increasingly media-inundated, digitally sutured, highly portable screen culture that is characterized as much, if not more, by images rather than words. Our world of proliferating technologies, both inside and outside of the healthcare ecosystem, makes it important to recognize that, despite often being relegated to the margins, visual images play an ever-expanding role in development of health culture, particularly in the training and clinical practice of healthcare providers. On a practical and concrete level, we have just witnessed an astounding expansion of telemedicine during the Covid crisis, an unanticipated pattern of growth that has already altered the contours of the medical encounter. We fully endorse the aims of narrative competence achieved with and through the written word but want to underscore how visual narratives offer equally layered webs of elements and multiple interpretive possibilities. They bring features such as physical characteristics and environmental context, camera movement and sound (including dialogue), color and lighting into the narrative that demand focused attention. Indeed, it is our belief that the visual elements of narrative have been often overlooked in the health humanities and is one of the factors that generated our desire to construct this book.

The narrative interface with media

In the previous section, we stressed how narratives fulfill essential needs in our personal, professional, and communal lives and how they function within healthcare culture. Here we explore the relationships between the form and content of narratives, keeping in mind Baudrillard's warning that we are too often guilty of forgetting "a little too easily that the whole of our reality is filtered through the media" (90). In our brave new technological world, we transmit stories by means of an ever-expanding swarm of technologically driven communication outlets. "The medium is the message," Marshall McLuhan's famous phrase from *Understanding Media* (1964), encapsulates the concept that the possibilities and constraints of myriad communication channels fundamentally shape the creation, transmission, and reception of narratives. As McLuhan observes, it is "typical that the 'content' of any medium blinds us to the character of the medium" (9), and the narratives that we fashion and receive are actually "shaped by the affordances and limitations of the media in which they are realized" (Ryan and Thon 2). Thus, form is content, and content is form.

Take, for instance, the same narrative transmitted in a novel, film, television program, or video game. Because verbal and visual languages are not identical, analyzing a film by employing the same terminology used to discuss that novel or TV show or video game ignores how each format brings its unique features into play and sculpts the material as well as its reception. The adaption of narratives across media, therefore, is inevitably a transformation rather than merely a translation. Such abstract concerns may not trickle very deeply into classroom discussions concerned with health care subject matter, but learners need to be aware that the distinctive properties of each medium affects our interpretations because format and meaning remain organically conjoined. Such recognition is a key component in the expansion of "media literacy": the development of critical skills that allow us to analyze and to evaluate how different types of platforms – such as those described in this book – mold our culture by the ways they process and present information.

As a practical example of this process, consider how Mary Shelley's *Frankenstein* (1818) expanded beyond its original, linguistically defined boundaries. The fundamental story first reached audiences in the form of a three-volume novel, written words on pages, and in 1831 as a two-volume edition with a new preface that spoke about its creation. Then, it was adapted into a stage play, eventually migrating across media platforms into radio productions, a blizzard of movies, several television series, a barrage of comic books, musical numbers, video games for children and adults, and even pornographic books – not to mention a mashup of references found on toys, games, Halloween masks, cereal boxes, posters, and action figures. While these iterations sometimes have similar characters, the mediums in which they are presented strongly influence basic decisions, such as what parts of Shelley's plot to highlight or eliminate, what new elements or characters to add. As a result, the format changes how the narrative was perceived and interpreted. In the early-stage plays, for example, time was needed to rearrange the scenery, so playwrights added another character, Frankenstein's stunted assistant, to entertain the audience in front of the curtain while the stage crew repositioned the set behind it. From that point forward, most *Frankenstein* productions featured this figure whom Shelley never mentions in the novel. Most significantly, we all picture Boris Karloff's iconic representation of Shelley's creature when invoking *Frankenstein* in most any context although the silent, clumsy, neck-bolted movie character bears little resemblance to his urbane literary forebearer.

Equally significant is that the theatrical, film, and television adaptations, which compel us to see and hear rather than read about the Creature's murderous actions and to witness Frankenstein's cruel rejection of his "offspring" considerably alter our responses to the story and its characters. Watching the pain of those murdered and hearing the cries of their loved ones makes engaging with Shelley's narrative a different immersive experience than imagining the events from reading her words on the page and forming our own images. Similarly, in the novel, Shelley describes the "birth" of the creature with relatively few words. Because moviemakers immediately recognized the inherent visual opportunities of the scene, subsequent films elongate it and display a dazzling array of sputtering, whirling, sizzling, and electrifying special effects. A more "realistically" constructed "birth" would persuade skeptical audiences that the impossible occurrences depicted on the screen were potentially feasible. This expansion of the creation scene, not to mention the more hideous appearance of the creature and the increasingly bloody presentation of the violence he perpetuates, disrupts the balance and focus in Shelley's novel and, as a result, abruptly shifts a reader/viewer's emotional and intellectual reactions to the narrative and its characters. Thus, although Shelley's *ur* text gave birth to the *Frankenstein* narrative, subsequent media technologies spawned a vast and quite disparate brood of offspring. In swapping one media for another during the adaptation process, total fidelity to a primary source is not necessarily the goal, nor is it possible due to "medium specificity" – the elements unique to each media that "invite certain types of communications and obstruct others" (Mittell 30).

Frankenstein's migratory behavior exemplifies what Henry Jenkins calls "convergence culture" – the idea that a storyworld gets enlarged and altered by being told and retold across multiple media platforms. Thus, as Jason Mittell concludes, the format of a particular narrative becomes a type of "technological determinism" (32) that shapes the storytelling. Such transmedia excursions increasingly inhabit our labyrinthine media systems, and, as Jenkins writes, they transform the traditional interplay among author, text, and reader by creating a participatory culture that generates collective meaning-making within popular culture: "Media producers and consumers are transformed into participants who are expected to interact with each other. Yet, each of us constructs our own personal mythology from bits and fragments of information we have extracted from the ongoing flow of media around us and transformed into resources through which we make sense of our everyday lives" (Jenkins).

As we have emphasized, the way we construct and communicate the personal mythologies that make sense of our everyday lives most often occurs in the form of narratives, but the medium that transmits them can offer an interactive, rather than static, experience. In particular, the incorporation of hypertext into electronic narratives is an innovative element that can convert a reader into as much of an author as the person who generated the original text. Ryan and Thon describe hypertext as a "matrix that expands into a multitude of texts as readers unravel new strings of signs from its finite database of discrete lexia" (340). One example is Michael Joyce's hypertext novel, *afternoon* (1990 on diskette), currently available on a multimedia CD that produces interactive reading by incorporating variations on the same narrative event: a recently divorced man named Peter witnesses a car accident. However, hypertext gives readers the navigational freedom to move instantaneously from one subject to another and from one environment to another without a predetermined arrangement of events, granting readers an agency not possible in more traditional formats. Along with this agency, however, comes increased responsibility because hypertext demands a reader's active participation in co-creating the story's structure. Thus, the inclusion of hypertext, as Abbott notes, de-constructs the linearity of a narrative by defying "the notion of any single narrative order, much less one that starts at the beginning and moves forward to the end" (33).

A more recent example of a convergence of passive viewing and active participation through the deployment and layering of different kinds of mediums is Hulu's original teen drama streaming series, *East Los High* (2013 – 2017). The storylines revolve around the lives of mostly Latinx high schoolers in East Los Angeles, but as *NPR* reports, the show is not only a soapy teen drama but also a public health campaign and social science experiment (Singh). The producers of *East Los High* worked closely with local health organizations to provide accurate information that was relevant to an episode's plot line (teen pregnancy, single parenting, sexual practices, and sexual health). That information was delivered through the dramatic arc of the show; through accompanying vlogs featuring Ceci (Danielle Vega) who talks candidly about teen pregnancy and single parenting; and through PSAs explicitly connected to plotlines and characters. In addition, as viewers streamed the series, the nearest locations of accessible and Latinx-friendly clinics were sent in real time to their devices. Researchers then tracked public health data and conducted field interviews to determine if the series actually encouraged Latinx teens to make healthy life choices.

East Los High stands out in the way in which the studio executives, screenwriters, and public health educators collaborated in the creation of a web of entertainment and information to achieve a laudable goal. Bear in mind, however, that most channels of communication media, which more often seem like hollow tubes, are intrinsically part of a manipulative process generated by the mass marketing of the mediated sharing of thoughts, emotions, and ideas. Partisans of one stripe or another seek to use media effectively to prove their point of view, to sell a product, to disseminate what they consider important, to get votes, to share something, to make you pay to see or do something, or to replicate what they are feeling. They construct images to influence what they want you to do and send it into the world wrapped by media. In this sense, Da Vinci is as much a propagandist as Marx – or Ceci. Thus, the role of the mass media in our culture is a two-way street. The daily events of our lives form the foundation of narrative recreations of existence, while on the other hand, our daily existence is clearly influenced by the creations viewed on screens of one sort or another.

Narrative/health/media

In her introduction to the *Best Short Stories 2021,* Jesmyn Ward writes that the best fiction provides us with "a sense of repair". No better phrase so succinctly encapsulates the connections among narratives, health, and media. Thus far we have explored our personal and cultural enduring desire for narratives, how stories function, and the ways they figure prominently within both health and media cultures. To integrate these spheres, we turn to the intricate latticework created by the interplay of these three elements. Individually, they each wield a powerful degree of influence, but fused together and viewed on screens, visual medical narratives exert prodigious leverage in the decisions we make and how we live our lives. They also have a profound impact on both the delivery of health care and patients' expectations of their role in that process (Friedman 5). We should remember that visual imaging modalities have been part of the diagnostic routine since 1896, when x-rays were first introduced (see Chester, Chapter 5, this volume). Indeed, over the decades, technical advances in ultrasonography, tomography, and magnetic resonance imaging (MRI) have produced screen images that provide visual evidence that functions as valuable diagnostic information, thereby assuming an expanding role in medical care. As a result of the Covid-19 pandemic, the dramatic upsurge in telemedicine – a system that allows practitioners sitting in front of a screen to evaluate, diagnose, and treat patients at remote sites – has become a progressively more central and available tool within the healthcare infrastructure.

In light of these imaging developments, sociologist Karin Knorr Cetina's evocative phrase, "viscourse," seems appropriate: "integrating explicitly visual dimensions in the production, negotiation, documentation and display of results. . .. It includes interactions with technical objects, presentation of visual materials and not only verbal reports" (quoted in Roethe 150). As such, she and other scholars argue that "visual narratives of medical content, experience and practice" (141) reflected in patient narratives and showcased in popular culture and social media should receive as much attention as written reports within healthcare culture, thus expanding realms of knowledge and augmenting patient care. Recognizing "the complex mediated ways of seeing that shape the meaning of images, narrative, data, and technology within and beyond the clinic" (7), Kirstin Ostherr rejects the false dichotomy between medical fact and medical fiction texts, between what most would consider authentic and unreal stories, because both "borrow their visual aesthetic and mode of production from the world of fiction" (217). As a result, both types of narratives profoundly contour our perceptions about and decisions within health care's visual culture. Indeed, the depictions of medical technology in film, television, and digital networks interconnect with the history of scientific developments and acquire cultural meanings because they remain "embedded within a complex ecosystem shaped by feedback loops between clinical and popular representations and the interpretation of these visualizations impacts the behavior of physicians and patients alike" (Ostherr 21, 25).

However, we need to bear in mind that popular culture is neither a framework nor a rigid structure that exhibits only one set of "true" values. Antonio Gramsci's widely discussed concept of "hegemony" theorizes that the landscape of popular culture is the site of ongoing, often strident, ideological struggles that pit resistant readings against dominant group reinforcement. That said, visual fiction seems better suited to the representation of changing belief systems than is non-fiction. Moreover, on a general supply-and-demand level, the health culture provides environments, subjects, characters, and stories across multiple platforms that range from movies to comics, from computer games to television shows, all feeding the insatiable appetite of media consumers for drama, comedy, information, and suspense. In turn, these medicalized narratives can highlight various topics, make controversial issues palatable for mainstream audiences, and alert or educate the public about health issues. Medicalized narratives put a human face on complex physical and ethical issues that affect societal attitudes about the world of health care. Although such dramatic representations inevitably value entertainment over medical authenticity, thereby running the risk of providing audiences with misinformation that can yield detrimental consequences instead of enlightenment, organizations such as the National Academy of Sciences' Science and Entertainment Exchange and the University of Southern California's Hollywood Health and Society Program supply productions with a range of expert consultants to assist them in providing more accurate health information.

In his definitive study of prime-time dramas from the 1950s through the 1980s, Joseph Turow not only analyzes how television programs such as *Ben Casey, Dr. Kildare, Marcus Welby MD,* and *M*A*S*H** shaped public perceptions of doctors, biomedical technology, and health care but also how the medical dramas themselves exploited such perceptions. Turow writes about how production companies' reliance on the medical establishment to provide expert advice and authentic locations came at the cost of reifying the hegemonic power of said establishment. Kirsten Ostherr agrees, writing that the American Medical Association's Advisory

Committee for Television and Motion Pictures provided a "coherent, consistent approach to cultivating the image of organized medicine" across all broadcast media (149). Ostherr goes on to discuss in depth the growing demand in the late 1960s of the public for more relevant and more accurate programming, a demand that coincided with organized medicine's realization that it needed to "rethink its relationship with patients" and producers to "rewrite their social contract with viewers" (152–3). One result of these changes, she notes, is that physicians began to speak directly to viewers, and "the modern, mass-mediated consumer-patient was born" (153). The changes also created an opening for medical documentaries such as Frederick Wiseman's 1969 cinema verité film, *Hospital*, winner of two Emmy awards (see Grant in this volume), which signaled the appreciation for a highly critical and unusual representation of medicine and health care as well as more scientific and technologically driven medical dramas such as *Medical Center,* which debuted in 1970. But it would be digital media that not only closed the gap between reality and fiction but that also unlocked access to health information and incited patient empowerment.

Bearing witness/making change

In his groundbreaking book on pathography, *The Wounded Storyteller: Body, Illness, and Ethics* (1995), sociologist Arthur Frank writes about an "ethics of telling": the testimony of an ill, injured, or impaired person that can repair the damage wrought from the experience; that can reclaim a self which may have been silenced and made invisible through the experience; and that can recover a voice recognizable as one's own (64, 71). Frank pairs this act of testifying with an "ethics of listening," which he notes is "one of our most difficult duties as human beings" (25) because the voices of the ill, injured, or impaired are easy to ignore. These voices falter, meander, and make us feel vulnerable. They make us face the stark realities of suffering and death. However, Frank insists that bearing witness to illness stories is a "fundamental moral act; to realize the best potential in postmodern times requires listening" (25).

In the final section of this introduction, we turn to social media which has become the most accessible and pervasive communication method for sharing personal stories of health experiences and for creating patient communities and networks. Given the vast number of individual videos and health-related websites, our discussion is obviously limited in scope, so we will simply provide some general information on the stupefying number of creators and users of online platforms and sites as well as the distinct advantages and disadvantages of sharing and seeking out health information, personal testimony, and emotional support.

In 2021, the approximate number of people who will access YouTube is 1.3 billion; 300 hours of video are uploaded every minute; five billion videos are watched every day; and the platform has 30 million visitors per day ("YouTube by the Numbers"). How many of these videos are health- and illness-related is anyone's guess, but even the most cursory scroll tells us that the number of makers and viewers is impressive. For example, the 3.6 million viewers of "The Morning After I Killed Myself," a poetic video about teen suicidality, is outmatched by the nearly nine million viewers of "What Is Depression," an educational narrative. Mental health/illness videos are one of two predominate categories in the social media realm, the second being chronic illnesses including stories such as Sita Gaia's "The Hell of Chronic Illness," which boasts 137,000 viewers and "Chronic Illness TikTok Compilation" with nearly 300,000 viewers of teens explaining and exhibiting what it means to live with seizure disorders, feeding tubes, and visual impairments. Thus, the metrics tell us that everyday millions of health consumers and healthcare professionals consume the stories of patients who have shared their experiences and opinions on video platforms such as YouTube. But a study published in the *Journal of Medical*

Internet Research, research tell us why so many patients are motivated to create personal videos; what objectives they hope to achieve with them; their perception of what community means; and finally, the negative consequences of the experience (Gomez-Zuniga et al.).

Not surprisingly, the major motivations for people to create and post health-related videos are a perceived lack of information about how to navigate daily life with a specific condition, as well as the inability or unwillingness of contemporary medical practice to meet a patient's needs. Most video makers rely on conventional literary elements – chronological timelines; cause and effect; setting; characters – to construct first-person stories about their illness experiences. For example, a 2011 study on cancer survivor videos on YouTube found that the "diagnostic narrative" is the most common rhetorical framing device for such stories and often includes an emphasis on how ordinary life is completely upended; a preference for specifying the time and place of diagnoses; and linguistic signals such as passive voice or switching from first-person to second person "you" to indicate the absence of control (Chou et al. 3). Another common feature of this sub-genre of health videos is what researchers' term, "depersonalized references to medical personnel" – the prevalence of either neutral or antagonistic stances toward medical staff such as "the doctor" or "they" (6). Such elements illustrate why video makers post their stories – to tell others about their experiences – and who they think the audience may be: persons who can understand and affirm their feelings. This dynamic exemplifies Frank's insistence that it is not only the telling of the illness experience but also the active listening and responding to it that is critically important for restorative healing. For example, one video maker emphasizes the importance for him to reveal the mistakes that he made during the course of his illness in order to prevent others from repeating those mistakes and to help them make better decisions and better cope with the challenges that come with the disease (Gomez-Zuniga et al.).

According to researchers, a common theme among all such videos is the search for a community, a way to mitigate isolation ("I literally felt like the only diabetic on the planet"), to find support, and to socialize. Connectedness is especially important for individuals with either contested illnesses such as chronic fatigue syndrome, fibromyalgia, and Gulf War Syndrome (see Swoboda) or un- and under-diagnosed diseases such endometriosis (see Greene, Chapter 30, this volume). According to participants in the 2012 YouTube study, the most common negative consequences of posting their videos were loss of privacy, negative or rude feedback, and being targeted to promote certain health-related products (Gomez-Zuniga et al.). The emotional support and social connectedness that prompt many patients to create and distribute a video testimony or personal story also drive them to self-organizing online communities focused on a particular disease. According to a Pew Research Report in 2013, 61 percent of all adult users had already turned to online health platforms (Fox and Duggan), which have evolved outside of traditional healthcare institutions and health policy practices. Tech analysts Paul Hodgkin, Louis Horsley, and Ben Metz describe the emergence and growth of patient communities as a "new phenomenon" (2018) and identify four reasons why such communities are valuable and popular:

- They provide patients and caregivers with new resources.
- They offer new insights to non-patients.
- They form part of a growing trend in data collection.
- They challenge traditional power dynamics between patients and clinicians.

The phenomenon began with the launch of health community websites such as HealthBoards, which Charles Simmons, a software engineer, founded in 1998 when he himself was searching for information and support. HealthBoards now offers two hundred message boards with over ten million visitors every month and nearly 900,000 registered members (www.healthboards.com/). PatientsLikeMe, which launched in 2006 for people diagnosed with ALS, currently covers nearly 3,000 health conditions. The ALS community now includes the largest population of ALS patients in the world with 10 percent of newly diagnosed individuals registering every month (www.patientslikeme.com/). A more recent newcomer to patient networks is MyHealthTeams, which was founded in 2010. It addresses 41 chronic conditions; numbers over two million registered members; and is available in 13 countries (www.myhealthteams.com/).

All three of these expanding and empowering patient communities aspire to provide emotional validation for and practical advice from people who are facing similar health issues. However, all three explicitly state their intentions to challenge, by any means necessary, traditional hierarchies and established practices in biomedicine including unequal relationships between professionals and patients; privileging clinical over social outcomes; discounting patient feedback on the efficacy of therapies, side effects, and disease progression; and influencing policy and funding decisions (Hodgkin et al.). For instance, one patient quoted by Hodgkin, Horsley, and Metz writes: "We don't want to be 'consulted.' We want to park our tanks on the hospital's lawn." The banner on the MyHealthTeams site also reads much like an activist call to arms: "social networks for chronic communities to disrupt healthcare." That network is especially focused on improving outcomes and addressing gaps in care for persons with chronic conditions. Finally, online patient guerrilla movements such as #WeAreNotWaiting for people with diabetes support both innovations and hacks (Hoyos et al.).

Narrative is fundamental to all of these patient communities operating on a variety of niche digital platforms. Objective truth, central to the model of medical care, has traditionally existed independently of our storied experiences, those anecdotes which are fraught with personal biases, subjective impressions, and messy emotions. However, in the world of online groups, the personal narrative matters; it contributes to education and transformation: "Where health care has a low tolerance of failure due to the consequences that can follow, online health communities thrive on stories of what went wrong and how people battled the system (Hodgkin et al.). There is also a growing body of evidence that telling and listening to stories leads to improved outcomes and practices. For example, stories on PatientsLikeMe have prompted the creation of DIY seizure trackers for people with epilepsy, "mood maps" for patients with mood disorders, and better compliance to treatment regimens. The number of benefits that patients report from using the site is strongly associated with the number of social connections, dubbed the "dose effect of friendship." Another platform, United Kingdom's CareOpinion, invites visitors to share their experiences, good or bad, and promises to "pass your stories to the right people to make a difference" (www.careopinion.org.uk/). The site not only tracks the number of stories told but also the number of staff members reading them. A rudimentary infograph beside a patient's post, for instance, indicates if and when changes in healthcare delivery are made in response.

Concerns from users about online patient communities are similar to those who post videos on YouTube: privacy violations, inaccurate information, and attempts to monetize individuals and groups. In a 2000 Pew Report, Lee Rainie and Susannah Fox wrote that 89 percent of respondents surveyed about the internet had concerns about privacy, especially Black users and patients, and there was an even split among the entire sample group about whether they believed the information that they accessed was or was not trustworthy. Concerns about credibility and transparency are not exclusive, however, to patient-driven sites; they extend to highly visible and institutionally sanctioned online purveyors of health news and information like WebMD.

WebMD, launched in 1996, could 20 years later boast an average of 179.5 million unique viewers per month, making it the leading health publisher in the United States according to Comscore (2021). In the first quarter of 2020, which marked the beginning of the COVID19 pandemic, the site had approximately 127 million unique viewers. The portal is not just for patients, however. The WebMD Health Network offers services to physicians including training materials, drug databases, clinical information, and discussion boards. In a scathing article for *The New York Times Magazine* in 2011, which she titled, "A Prescription for Fear," journalist Virginia Heffernan took on WebMD, whose name, she argues, is "synonymous with Big Pharma Shilling." She describes the site as not only a waste of time but also one "that preys on the fear and vulnerability of its users to sell them half-truths and, eventually, pills" (Heffernan). Those half-truths include "so-called information about cancer and depression" posted among the clutter of banner ads for brands such as Crest, Bounce, and Clorox. However, Heffernan strikes a more serious note when she discusses the influence of medical information sites such as WebMD on how Americans think about their health and in public debates about health care. While readers and viewers expect that a patient narrator with a limited viewpoint (first-person) and rhetorical aim (to be seen and heard) might craft a story laden with dramatic effects, exaggerated characters, and convenient timelines – the stuff of fiction – people actively searching for information about symptoms, diagnoses, and treatments may not be so attuned to the mash up of medical fact and medical fabrication that Heffernan argues is the dominant style of WebMD.

Julia Belluz poses a simple question at the outset of her article for *Vox* in 2016: "Can I trust WebMD?" While there is a lack of independent information on that particular question, she notes that there is a lot on how revenue for the publication is raised through advertising, sponsored content from pharmaceutical, biotech, and medical device companies, not to mention hospitals, health insurance providers, and lifestyle brands. The physicians whom she interviewed describe a "lack of context" and a "smattering of misinformation" in regard to the site's content. Belluz argues that may be an okay starting point for Wikipedia, but unlike Wikipedia, WebMD's business model relies on the same industry it reports on. The difficulty in separating medical fact from medical fiction, science from art, in social media and on internet platforms is illustrated most imaginatively and comically with Justine Cooper's multimedia exhibit for Havidol, which treats "Dsyphoric Social Attention Consumption Deficit Anxiety Disorder (DSACDAD): When More Is Not Enough." The slick and fake marketing campaign for the non-existent drug, which includes a web site, mock television and print advertisements, and billboards has fooled thousands of people; it has also, as Reuters reported in 2007, been folded into medical web sites for panic and anxiety disorder as well as depression.

So, who can we trust when it comes to health information? Perhaps, at no time in modern history, have we posed and pondered that question more thoroughly than since the emergence of SARS-COv-2 in December 2019. Since then, mass, and social media have been and continue to be the major sources of information about Covid-19, but the spread of mis- and dis-information has proven to be as much a threat to global public health as the novel coronavirus itself (World Health Organization). The same technologies – from traditional print media to digital platforms – that the scholars in this volume explore have created unlimited opportunities to keep us informed, safe, healthy, and connected and to give us voice and visibility. However, those same technologies have also enabled and amplified our current "info-demic." During the 1980s and 1990s, cultural critics and academic scholars dubbed HIV/AIDS as the first "postmodern disease," referencing how the constructions and representations of that epidemic were not only biomedical but also linguistic. In a similar vein, we might call Covid-19 the first "multimedia disease" because so much we have learned about it has been influenced and impacted by social media from a wide variety of platforms and political ideologies.

In their study of public health communication (2020), Anwar et al. highlight the multiple social, cultural, and economic issues arising from mass media's role in the pandemic. They highlight the inflammatory circulation of racial bigotries, linked to the origin of the virus, which has prevented scientific collaborations; the extensive coverage during lockdowns and quarantines, which has induced fear and psychological stress; and the public endorsements of unscientific cures and unverified treatments. However, they note, mass media has also tracked disease outbreaks, allowing for timely interventions and widespread communications; reinforced illness-prevention practices such as hand washing, face coverings, and social distancing; and promoted equal access to health care as well as an end to social stigmatization (Anwar et al.). It is a delicate and dangerous balance as the diffusion of false information about the severity and spread of Covid, conspiracy theories, and other unverifiable claims from athletes, politicians, and pop culture "influencers" on social media constantly threaten to overtake and overwhelm any credible information disseminated by trustworthy sources such as public health organizations, biomedical scientists, and front-line professionals.

In the first sentence of this introduction, we said that the impetus for this book was "our belief that incorporating media knowledgeably and effectively within the healthcare matrix obliges us to grapple with the complex issues that bind stories and systems together into a formidable and dynamic force within all our lives." To help readers do that, the essays incorporated into this book represent our best attempt to draw together a wide swath of ideas from some of the most insightful scholars investigating the field of health and media. These researchers come from different disciplines and bring different perspectives to their explorations in this field. They participate in and advocate for different types of health care systems. Yet, each of them understands how crucial it is for health care students and practitioners to understand the complex interconnections that tie narrative, media, and health into an intricate symbiosis heavily influencing and being influenced by the surrounding culture, the evolution of industrial production, the battles of clashing ideologies, and the unpredictable winds of chance. We hope our book shines light into some murky corners of the healthcare culture, that it engages the imagination of our readers, that it helps teachers to more effectively present media materials, and that it encourages other scholars to delve more deeply into the fascinating subjects raised in these essays.

Works cited

Abbott, Porter H. *The Cambridge Introduction to Narrative.* Cambridge: Cambridge University Press, 2008.

Adichie, Chimamanda Ngozi. "Holocaust and Human Behavior." www.facinghistory.org/holocaust-and-human-behavior/chapter-1/danger-single-story.

Anwar, Ayesha, Meryem Malik, Vaneeza Raees, and Anjum Anwar. "The Role of Mass Media and Public Health Communication in the COVID-19 Pandemic." *Cureus*, vol. 12, no. 9, 2020, www.ncbi.nlm.nih.gov/pmc/articles/PMC7557800/.

Barthes, Roland. "Introduction to the Structural Analysis of Narratives." *A Barthes Reader*, edited by Susan Sontag, New York: Hill and Wang, 1982, pp. vii–xxxvii.

Baudrillard, Jean. *The Transparency of Evil: Essays on Extreme Phenomena.* Translated by James Benedict. London, Verso Books, 1993.

Belluz, Julia. "The Truth About WebMD, a Hypochondriac's Nightmare and Big Pharma's Dream." *Vox*, April 5, 2016, www.vox.com/2016/4/5/11358268/webmd-accuracy-trustworthy.

Boyd, Brian. *On the Origin of Stories: Evolution, Cognition, and Fiction.* Cambridge, MA: The Belknap Press of Harvard University Press, 2009.

Charon, Rita. *Narrative Medicine: Honoring the Stories of Illness.* Oxford: Oxford University Press, 2008.

Chou, Sylvia Wen-Ying, Yvonne Hunt, Anna Folkers, and Erik Auguston. "Cancer Survivorship in the Age of YouTube and Social Media: A Narrative Analysis." *Journal of Medical Internet Research*, vol. 13, no. 1, 2011, pp. 1–9.

Cohen, Jonathan. "Defining Identification: A Theoretical Look at the Identification of Audiences with Media Characters." *Mass Communication and Society*, vol. 4, no. 3, 2001, pp. 245–64.

Colt, Henri, Silvia Quadrelli, Lester D. Friedman. *The Picture of Health: Medical Ethics and the Movies*. New York: Oxford University Press, 2011.

Comscore. "Top 50 Multi-Platform Properties (Desk and Mobile)." September 2021, www.comscore.com/Insights/Rankings/.

Einstein, Elizabeth. *The Printing Press as an Agent of Change: Communications and Cultural Transformations in Early-modern Europe (Vols I and II)*. Cambridge: Cambridge University Press, 1979.

"Fake Drug, Fake Illness – and People Believe It!" *Reuters*, February 16, 2007, www.reuters.com/article/domesticNews/idUSL16511952007 0216?&src=021607_1724.

Fox, Susannah and Maeve Duggan. "Health Online 2013." Pew Research Center, 2013, www.pewresearch.org/internet/ 2013/01/15/health-online-2013/.

Frank, Arthur W. *The Wounded Storyteller: Body, Illness, and Ethics*. Chicago: University of Chicago Press, 1995.

Frenkel, Sheera and Cecilia Kang. *An Ugly Truth: Inside Facebook's Battle for Domination*. New York: Harper, 2021.

Friedman, Lester D. *Cultural Sutures: Medicine and Media*. Durham: Duke University Press, 2004.

Fulford, Robert. *The Triumph of the Narrative*. Toronto: House of Anansi Press, Ltd. 1999.

Gawande, Atul. *Being Moral: Medicine and What Matters in the End*. London: Picador, 2017.

Gomez-Zuniga, Beni, Luis Fernandez-Luque, Moesta Pousada, Eulalia Hernandez-Encuentra, and Manual Armayone. "ePatients on YouTube: Analysis of Four Experiences from the Patients' Perspective." *Journal of Medical Internet Research*, 2012. (www.ncbi.nlm.nih.gov/pmc/articles/PMC4084771/)

Gorgen, Arno, German AlfonsoNunez, Heiner Fangerau, eds. *Handbook of Popular Culture and Biomedicine: Knowledge in the Life Sciences as Cultural Artefact*. Switzerland: Springer International Publishing, 2019.

Gottschall, Jonathan. *The Storytelling Animal: How Stories Make Us Human*. Boston: Houghton Mifflin Harcourt, 2012.

Heffernan, Virginia. "A Prescription for Fear." *The New York Times Magazine*, February 4, 2011, www.nytimes.com/2011/02/06/magazine/06FOB-Medium-t.html.

Hodgkin, Paul, Louis Horsley, and Ben Metz. "The Emerging World of Online Health Communities." *Stanford Social Innovation Review*, April 10, 2018, https://ssir.org/articles/entry/the_emerging_world_of_online_health_communities#.

Hoyos, Michelle L., Heather R. Walker, Caroline Fitzgerald, Mariana Gomez Hoyos, Dana Lewis, and Perry M. Gee. "Patient-Driven Diabetes Technologies: Sentiment and Personas of the #WeAreNotWaiting and #OpenAPS Movements." *Journal of Diabetes Science and Technology*, vol. 14, no. 6, 2020, pp. 990–9.

Jenkins, Henry. "Welcome to Convergence Culture." Henry Jerkins Blog, June 19, 2006, http://henry jenkins.org/blog/2006/06/welcome to convergence culture.html.

Jones, Therese, Delese Wear, and Lester Friedman, eds. *Health Humanities Reader*. New Brunswick, NJ: Rutgers University Press, 2014.

Joyce, Michael. *afternoon*. Eastgate Systems Inc; Mac/Win Edition, 1999.

Kirby, D. A. *Lab Coats in Hollywood: Science, Scientists and Cinema*. Cambridge, MA: MIT Press, 2011.

Kleinman, Arthur. *The Illness Narratives: Suffering, Healing, and the Human Condition*. New York: Basic Books, Inc., 1988.

Lasch, Christopher. *The True and Only Heaven: Progress and Its Critics*. New York: W. W. Norton & Company, 1991.

McAdams, Dan P. *The Stories We Live By: Personal Myths and the Making of the Self*. New York: The Guilford Press, 1993.

McLuhan, Marshall. *Understanding Media: The Extensions of Man*. New York: McGraw Hill, 1964.

Mittell, Jason. *Narrative Theory and Adaptation*. New York: Bloomsbury Academic, 2017.

Nussbaum, Martha C. *Poetic Justice: The Literary Imagination and Public Life*. Boston: Beacon Press, 1995.

Oakley, Keith. "The Mind's Flight Simulator." *The British Psychological Society*, vol. 21, 2008, pp. 1030–3, https://thepsychologist.bps.org.uk/volume-21/edition-12/mind-s-flight-simulator.

Ostherr, Kirstin. *Medical Visions: Producing the Patient through Film, Television, and Imaging Technologies*. Oxford: Oxford University Press, 2013.

Pew Trust. "Most Americans Want to Share and Access More Digital Health Data."Issue Brief, July 24, 2021,www.pewtrusts.org/en/research-and-analysis/issue-briefs/2021/07/most-americans-want-to-share-and-access-more-digital-health-data.
Rainie, Lee and Susannah Fox. "The Online Health Care Revolution." Pew Research Center, November 26, 2000, www.pewresearch.org/internet/2000/11/26/the-online-health-care-revolution/.
Roethe, Anna L. "Insights into Insights: Visual Narratives of Medical Imaging and Intervention Technologies and the Popular Viscourse." *Handbook of Popular Culture and Biomedicine: Knowledge in the Life Sciences as Cultural Artefact*, edited by Arno Görgen, German Alfonso Nunez, and Heiner Fangerau, Springer Verlag,2019, pp. 139–156.
Ryan, Marie-Laure and Jan-Noel Thon, eds. *Storyworlds across Media: Toward a Media-Conscious Narratology*. Lincoln: University of Nebraska Press, 2014.
Sales, Nancy Jo. *Nothing Personal*. New York: Hachette Books, 2021.
Schroder, Angela. "The Visual Claim within Medical Science and Popular Culture." *Handbook of Popular Culture and Biomedicine*, edited by Andreas Görgen, Gabriel Nunez, and Heiner Fangerau, Springer, Cham., 2019, pp. 115–24.
Singh, Maanvi. "'East Los High' Isn't Just a Soapy Teen Drama – It's Also a Science Experiment." National Public Radio "Code Switch." January 11, 2016. www.npr.org/sections/codeswitch/2016/01/11/451940463/east-los-high-isnt-just-a-soapy-teen-drama-its-also-a-science-experiment.
Solberg, Lauren B. "The Benefits of Online Health Communities." (2014) *Virtual Mentor: American Medical Associations Journal of Ethics*, vol. 16, no. 4, 2014, pp. 270–4.
Solnit, Rebecca. *Men Explain Things to Me*. Chicago: Haymarket Books, 2015.
Swoboda, Diane A. "Negotiating the Diagnostic Uncertainty of Contested Illnesses: Physician Practices and Paradigms." *Health*, vol. 12, no. 4, 2008, pp. 453–78.
Turow, Joseph. *Playing Doctor: Television, Storytelling, and Medical Power*. New York: Oxford University Press, 1989.
Ward, Jesmyn. "Introduction." *The Best American Short Stories of 2021*, edited by Jesmyn Ward and Heidi Pitlor, Boston: Mariner Books, 2021, pp. x–xiii.
Wilson, Edward O. *Consilience: The Unity of Knowledge*. New York: Vintage Books, 1998.
World Health Organization. "Social Media & COVID: A Global Study of Digital Crisis Interaction among Gen Z and Millennials." March 26, 2021, www.who.int/news-room/feature-stories/detail/social-media-covid-19-a-global-study-of-digital-crisis-interaction-among-gen-z-and-millennials.
Worthen, Molly. "The Trouble with Empathy: Can We Be Taught How to Feel Someone Else's Pain?" *New York Times*, Sunday Review, September 6, 2020, pp. 1–4/5.
"YouTube By the Numbers: Stats, Demographics & Fun Facts." Omnicore Blog, January 3, 2021, www.omnicoreagency.com/youtube-statistics/.

PART I

Print media

The four chapters in this section span a period from Britain's "great depression" in the 1930s, to the hormone replacement therapy story in 1960s America, to Greta Thunberg's 2016 "school strike for the climate," to the proliferation of "quaranzines" – handmade publications that provide public health information and suggestions for self-care in the current Covid-19 crisis. Together they demonstrate the crucial importance of print – the written word in traditional *and* digital media – and how such discourse can promote or impede important health policy; shape (or distort) life-saving medical research findings; and develop and document community activism.

In the first chapter, **"'"Fish and chips' as an excellent food': newspapers, nutrition, and government neglect in 1930s Britain,'** historian Marjorie Levine-Clark focuses specifically on how newspapers fueled aspects of what became known as the "nutrition controversy." Then as now, people turned to newspapers for health advice and to understand health information. In this case, the reading public had to grapple with conflicting messages about diet and nutrition circulated by a government loath to address the risk of malnourishment in low-paid and unemployed people and differing information disseminated by public health doctors and social welfare reformers increasingly concerned and vocal about deteriorating working-class health.

Rae-Ellen Kavey foregrounds a clear connection to Levine-Clark's essay in **"Breaking news: medical research reporting and its consequences"**: the general public obtains important medical information from mass news media. It begins with the headline – the attention grabber on the front page of the newspaper or the scroll at the bottom of the television screen – but it requires clear and careful analysis of complex research data. In this chapter, Kavey explores how the American press covered the results of the hormone therapy arm of the Women's Health Initiative to illustrate both the critical intersections between medicine and media and the crucial consequences of inaccurate, incomplete reporting.

It used to be, Carol-Ann Farkas and Shoshannah Bryn Jones Square write, that sharing knowledge meant engaging with ink on paper. However, in **"Climate health is human health: working through eco-anxiety with the written word in print and digital media,"** they argue that the conventions of traditional print persist in the variety of digital forms we experience today. The authors examine how the written word helps us engage with

DOI: 10.4324/9781003007661-2

the climate emergency as a collective illness experience to treat, manage, and cope with our eco-anxiety and eco-grief as a community.

In Part I's final chapter, **"Health zines: hand-made and heart-felt,"** Deborah Lupton introduces readers to the history of zines: the low-tech, mixed-media, self-published creations that engage people across age groups, political views, and literacy levels. As a medium for representing, documenting, and communicating health-related topics and experiences, this genre of zines began with the early era of HIV/AIDS and is now flourishing during the Covid-19 era.

1

"'FISH AND CHIPS' AS AN EXCELLENT FOOD"

Newspapers, nutrition, and government neglect in 1930s Britain

Marjorie Levine-Clark

As Britain's Parliament was preparing to debate new scales for unemployment benefits in July 1936, the *Reading Standard* published a small article indicating that Members of Parliament had called on the well-known Medical Officer of Health G. C. M. McGonigle to educate them about the diets of the unemployed. The *Standard* let its readers know that "Dr. McGonigle said starvation did not now exist in England, but the dietaries of many families lacked essential minerals and vitamins. He went on to praise 'fish and chips' as an excellent food, to say that herrings, in regard to food value, were not cheap, that tinned vegetables and fruit were as good as fresh, and that tinned tomatoes were the best source of Vitamin D" ("Unemployment Assistance"). Here was nutritional information available to all who read the paper, but the circulation of details such as these served as a point of contention in discussions about what constituted a sufficient diet for the poor and unemployed and how much responsibility the government should take for its citizens' health.

Politics, poverty, public health, and the press

In the middle of Britain's great depression and in a context of anxiety about the strength of British military recruits, public health doctors and social welfare reformers became increasingly concerned about working-class health. Scientific research into "the nutritive value of diets" exploded in the interwar years (Hollingsworth qtd. in Mayhew 446) and produced new knowledge about dietary elements such as calories, proteins, carbohydrates, and vitamins. Public health advocates urged the government to implement this new scientific knowledge, but the Ministry of Health was loath to release information about nutrition, fearing (rightly so) that opposition politicians and the wider public would wonder why government spending on nutritional support for low-paid and unemployed workers was so meager. In 1931, the new coalition National Government, which had been formed to deal with the emergency of the economic crisis, cut unemployment benefits by ten per cent, and this put unemployed people at real risk of malnourishment. Much of the public attention on diets focused on the provision of milk and school meals for children, but a wider discourse about nutrition entered the public domain in the 1930s, in large part because of the press. Newspapers, as the primary form of public media

DOI: 10.4324/9781003007661-3

at the time, became engaged with questions about diets and nutrition and what the government was doing to ensure that its citizens did not go hungry. These questions shared columns with other significant news of the day, such as Hitler's rise to power and Indian nationalism.

While scholars have explored the "nutrition controversy" from a variety of perspectives (Mayhew; Vernon, *Hunger* 118–34; and Oddy 122–32), none have focused specifically on how newspapers fueled particular aspects of the controversy. Newspapers, like other media, provide people with health advice and help them understand health information (Briggs and Hallin; Cooper, et al. 664–73; Seale 513–31; McCaw et al.; Jamil and Evans). They also actively construct the discourses surrounding health in the public domain and communicate the power relations involved in the construction of those discourses. In the 1930s, when people started to receive health messages about nutrition, newspapers served as one of the central outlets of those messages. The publication of doctors' findings about nutrition and health in local papers, especially, gave working-class people the opportunity to measure their diets against those being prescribed in the press and opened a space for poor and unemployed people to engage with "scientific" knowledge. The debates about nutrition could prove confusing, as experts from different professional communities warred with one another over the meanings of health and nutrition. In this context, newspapers helped nutritionists articulate arguments against government claims about suitable unemployment benefit scales in relation to recommended diets, portraying the government as being more interested in purse tightening than in the people's health.

This chapter takes up two moments in which newspapers helped shape a discourse on nutritional expertise about the diets of the poor and unemployed: the dissemination of the British Medical Association's (BMA) *Report of Committee on Nutrition* of 1933 and the publication of G. C. M. McGonigle and J. Kirby's *Poverty and Public Health* in 1936.[1] My examination of the chronological development of this news coverage will highlight three particular points. First, journalists were successful in claiming neutral "facts" and "expertise" to make strong political points about health against the government in the economic climate that existed in the 1930s. Second, although the government and its experts tended to blame bad "housewifery" for the mismanagement of working-class diets, newspapers privileged the "scientific" studies of nutrition, which argued that the incomes of poor families were inadequate to purchase recommended diets. Finally, while most newspapers favored the nutritionist over the government stance, they also sometimes produced a narrative that experts in general were out of touch with the everyday lives and needs of the working classes. Another major part of the nutrition controversy focused on children, but I will not be addressing that issue in this essay (see Durbach; Vernon, "Ethics of Hunger" 693–725; Burnett and Oddy 55–69).

Government pushback against the recommendations of the 1933 *Report of Committee on Nutrition* and the 1936 *Poverty and Public Health* gave editors and reporters ample material to present their readers with multiple positions on nutrition, poverty, and social welfare more broadly. The publications spurred journalism that highlighted challenges to the government's approach to both unemployment and nutrition, while simultaneously giving "nutritionists unprecedented visibility" (Vernon, *Hunger* 119) and a new forum through which to express their scientific expertise. As a result, newspapers from all over Britain printed articles that allowed nutritionists to speak to the public about the dietary needs of the poor and unemployed.[2] Print journalists drew national attention to politicians' refusal to accept scientific facts and public health expertise, the partisanship that shaped positions on science, the deep connections between poverty and reduced health chances, and women's challenges to scientific claims about what was best for their families' health. These themes are shockingly similar to issues raised by the media during the Covid-19 pandemic in 2020-2021 and the vaccination roll out in 2021, to which I will return at the end of this chapter.

Scholars who have examined the release of the British Medical Association's *Report on Nutrition* have almost universally concentrated on the Ministry of Health's powerful resistance to the conclusions of the *Report*, which journalist Mayhew has stated "caused near panic at the ministry" (450). They have investigated what government documents reveal about Ministry anger at the BMA for going against the Ministry's own recommendations about appropriate diets. These studies explore individual personalities, and some analyze play-by-play developments of goings-on behind the scenes in correspondence and meetings within the Ministry of Health and between the Ministry and other government units. Their emphasis is on the ways the Ministry tried to underplay connections between poverty and malnourishment. As Mayhew puts it, studies done by the Ministry "remained confidential if their results tended to have any political, economic or social implications which might have compromised the government" (453). We see some of this in the newspaper reporting, but the news for the most part lacks the detailed stories of individual players and in-fighting about government food policy evident in government records.

While press coverage of the nutrition controversy has not been the main emphasis of scholarly work, almost all studies that have examined working-class diets in this period have cited the case published by the *Daily Herald* in January 1933, investigated further and concluded by the *Week-End Review* in April 1933, of the mother who starved herself to death so that she could feed her seven children (especially, Vernon, *Hunger* 118–19; Mayhew 447; Oddy 122). This news of the "Heroic Mother [who] Starves in Silence" broke open the story of "Hungry England" that the papers continued to cover throughout the thirties. It prepared British readers for the potentially sensational news that might arise concerning poverty, hunger, and nutrition. The *Week-End Review*'s investigative journalism determined that some families would not be able to meet the Ministry of Health's recommended diet on the unemployment benefits then provided by the government (Oddy 122). This theme would explode in the press in less than six months with the publication of the BMA's *Report on Nutrition.*

The facts of nutrition and the working man's diet

In April 1933, the British Medical Association appointed a committee of nine physicians, surgeons, medical officers of health, and professors "to determine the minimum weekly expenditure on foodstuffs which must be incurred by families of varying size if health and working capacity are to be maintained" (3). Their conclusions, *Report of Committee on Nutrition*, came out as a special supplement to the *British Medical Journal* on November 25, 1933, just as groups of unemployed workers were planning for a national hunger march ("Unemployed Workers" 6). The experts on the BMA Committee determined that "a man of average stature leading a healthy life with moderate muscular exertion" should have a diet consisting of 3,400 calories a day (8). Additionally, of these calories, the Committee recommended that "50 grams of first-class protein" would be "sufficient to maintain the health and working capacity of the average man" (12). The *Report* showed how the committee had calculated the "man-values" of children and wives so as to figure the total household needs for a family. It provided 16 very detailed "specimen" diets, indicating the strengths and weaknesses of each in terms of calories, vitamins and minerals, proteins, fats, and carbohydrates, and how they would affect men, women, and children. The *Report* concluded that a satisfactory diet for a working man could be purchased for five shillings, 11 pence a week, which the newspapers publicized as the more memorable "5s. 10d."

With the release of the British Medical Association *Report*, many provincial newspapers picked up a syndicated item originating from London's newspaper district, Fleet Street, discussing the bare bones of the *Report*'s findings. Stories relating the fundamentals of the *Report* continued to appear more than a month after its initial release. The key points in the sometimes very brief notices were that the BMA had appointed "nine eminent doctors" who found that, with the prices current in June 1933, "the average man doing muscular work can feed himself for 5s 10d a week. A man, wife, and one child between one and two years old can maintain health and working capacity on 13s 6d" (for example, "Cheap Living" 9; "Life on 5s 10d a Week," *Dundee* 6; "Doctors and Family" 11; "How a Man Can Live" 4). Some papers reported more details on dietaries for families of other sizes, such as the *Berks and Oxon Advertiser*, which noted, "It is stated that a family consisting of man, wife, and three children between the ages of 6 and 8, 10 and 12, and 12 and 14, would cost 22s. 6 ½ d. a week to feed" ("10d. a Day" 8). Most papers, however, fixated on the figure of 5s. 10d. as the amount necessary to feed a working man.

Many newspapers simply recounted the "facts" of the BMA *Report*, a recapitulation that was important in itself. Yet others editorialized on the impact of these facts and used the findings to criticize the government. The *Lancashire Evening Post*, for example, reprinted an item from the *Preston Post* on November 27, 1933, soon after the *Report*'s release. This item challenged the "reassuring official pronouncements" of the government that the poor and unemployed were not suffering nutritionally. The writer lamented that "The disparity between individual purchasing power and the bare nutritional cost of health … is greater and more frequent than most people realise." Relying on the evidence of authorities such as the BMA, therefore, was of the utmost importance. The item recommended that the *Report* "should be carefully studied by all administrators of the Unemployment Insurance Acts, members of Public Assistance Committees and other similar bodies, and by all employers who desire to take a real interest in the health and welfare of their workers." If the welfare bureaucracy truly cared about the working classes, the paper implied, it would pay attention to the doctors' expertise. The newspaper stressed to its readers how difficult it would be – almost "absolutely impossible" – for unemployed and very low-paid workers to meet the minimum nutritional standard advised by the BMA ("Poor Family's Budget" 4). The paper hinted that welfare workers might have some influence in pressing for an increase in benefits to assist the unemployed in reaching that standard.

The *Northampton Mercury* on December 8, 1933 was also inclined favorably toward the BMA *Report*, claiming "Instincts No Guide" in people's choices of food, especially when they were forced to "do without" when poverty and unemployment limited their purchasing power. The *Mercury*, like the *Post*, emphasized the need to trust the expertise of the *Report*, as "our food is sophisticated," and laypeople needed doctors to translate the language of proteins, fats, carbohydrates, and calories for the population at large, so that they, too, might become "sophisticated" ("What the Doctor Says" 11). Here the lesson was for the working classes themselves instead of welfare workers. Rather than choosing empty calories, everyday people needed to be taught by doctors how to opt for nutritious foods on their restricted budgets.

Some newspapers took the opportunity to criticize the 5s. 10d. diet itself and printed stories that called into question the BMA's expertise. *The Yorkshire Evening Post*, among a number of papers, published a piece on November 24 in which other types of "experts" challenged the doctors of the BMA in their dietary claims. The headline read, "Living on 5s 10d a Week. Doctors Say a Man Can Do It. But Woman Expert Says It Is Preposterous." The paper presented the knowledge of Mrs. Beatrice Drapper, a former Mayor of Deptford in London who worked with populations of the docklands. Dockers, she claimed, would need twice as much to stay healthy. "The doctors," Drapper argued, "doubtless have based their estimates on theory and not practice," questioning BMA members' acquaintance with working-class populations. Drapper, as a community servant, had lived among the men under scrutiny, while "doctors" had little face-to-face contact on which to base their so-called expertise. The article, however, also quoted Dr. J. Neil Leitch, president of the London School of Dietetics, who agreed with the BMA findings. Professor Samson Wright, "another expert on dietetics," had a different opinion, stating that "Only the unemployed man, or the man engaged on exceedingly light work, can manage to live on a 5s 10d diet . . . The manual labourer will have to pay considerably more for the food which is to keep him in health." Finally, the article looked to an East End housewife for an opinion: "5s 10d a week to feed my husband? And with a joint [of meat] for three of us costing 5s. Nonsense" (15). The paper here gave voice to a housewife who dismissed doctors' familiarity with the costs of managing a household. How were readers supposed to wade through these troubled waters of nutritional advice? This newspaper clearly fell out on the side of the women "experts" who gained their knowledge through experience of life among poor workers and families.

In early January 1934, the papers started to fuel a real controversy by covering the Ministry of Health's differences with the British Medical Association. The originating story in the London *Times* reminded its readers that, in 1932, the Ministry of Health had put together its own committee, the Advisory Committee on Nutrition (composed of six medical experts), to investigate how to improve diets among the poor ("Weekly Expenditure" 14). The press conveyed the release of this Committee's report in late March 1932. The Advisory Committee memorandum recommended minimums of 3,000 calories a day with 37 grams of first-class protein for a working man, while "women and children need proportionately less" ("Perfect Diet" 9).[3] The Ministry of Health worked hard to avoid associating a cost with this diet and did not want to release any studies that would have political implications (Mayhew 448).

In view of the BMA Committee's suggestions for increases in both calories and protein, the Advisory Committee met again in 1933 and came to the conclusion that their previous advice was sound, and they would not recommend any changes. According to the London *Times*, the Minister of Health then communicated the Advisory Committee's memo as a unanimous reaffirmation to all local councils and sanitary authorities (14). This news was printed across Britain with headlines much less sedate than the *Times*'s "Weekly Expenditures on Food." The *Dundee Courier* announced "Doctors' Food Feud: Ministry Rebuff for B.M.A," while *The Scotsman* wrote of the "Minimum Diet Dispute" (7, 6). London's leftist *Daily Herald* did its best to rile up the government with its front page headline, "Doctor's Name in Ministry a Mystery: Denies He Signed Low Diet Report." In a story that ran to a second page, the *Herald* called the Ministry of Health's decision to stick with the original 3,000 calorie recommendation "an amazing document . . . deliberately encouraging the underfeeding of unemployed men and their families." Emphasizing the expertise of the BMA's committee – "months of research by nine famous doctors" – the *Herald* expressed shock that the Ministry of Health could cling to 3,000 calories. The article also revealed to the public that two members of the Ministry's Advisory Committee on Nutrition were also on the BMA's Committee on Nutrition, and one of these, Professor Mottram, told a *Herald* reporter that he had not signed the Ministry's recent report endorsing the 3,000 calorie recommendation although the Ministry had presented the report as unanimous (1, 3).

Neither side's experts, however, were free from question. The *Liverpool Echo* reported on the basics of the controversy, but their story went further, challenging the expertise of the doctors involved in both sides of the dispute. Simply titled, "Food," the item accused both the Ministry and the BMA of operating on the level of theory: "Such a dispute may be of considerable interest and importance to the medical men who have signed the report but it does not interest the man in the street for whose benefit the investigations are supposed to have been made." According to the reporter, even the BMA's recommendations did not go far enough. A diet that would keep working men truly healthy would cost more than 5s 10d., as "any woman who has the task of catering for a working-class family knows." Again, working-class women's expertise counted more than that of distant doctors. The journalist pressed the issue, emphasizing that "It is possible to keep alive on less than the amount allowed by the British Medical Association," because many families could not afford the recommended diets, but "Such families are underfed and semi-starved." According to this writer, only those who had to budget carefully to prepare meals for the poor – women – would know how meager 5s. 10d. truly were. The *Echo* also situated British diets in a global context: "the West does not take its standards from the East. The scientific five and tenpenny diet would represent luxury in the East. In our surroundings we know it represents a very low standard, and one that a man in full work would not tolerate without strong protests" ("Food" 8). Here the writer assumed a hierarchy of bodily need, placing the British man at the top. The Orientalist presentation of this dietary information had the effect of feminizing the man of the East, suggesting a body like a woman's, whose nutritional needs were smaller (Said).[4]

A series of articles focused on the BMA Committee's response to the Ministry of Health's circular letter confirming the 3,000 calorie diet and advising local authorities essentially to ignore the BMA's recommendations. Some news items concentrated on an interview with Dr. George McGonigle, a member of the BMA Committee and Medical Officer of Stockton-on-Tees, the locality on which the Committee's investigations focused, and with whose recommendation of fish and chips I opened this chapter. The *Gloucestershire Echo* on January 5, 1934 quoted McGonigle stating, "'Although 3,000 calories is usually accepted as an adequate diet . . . we put 3,400 calories because the terms of our reference were to devise a minimum diet adequate to maintain health and working capacity'." McGonigle continued, "'If anyone tells me that a housewife can go and buy the equivalent of 3,000 calories in food, take it home, prepare it, cook it, and serve it up without there being some waste I should not believe it. . . . We put in that extra 400 calories, therefore, not only to maintain the working capacity, but also to allow some margin for wastage'" ("Food Calories" 1; see also "Living off 5/10 ½" 9; "Ministry's Report" 8; "Health Visitors' Conference" 7). The articles quoting McGonigle stressed that the BMA investigation "specif[ied] a minimum standard not for a mere existence level, but for the maintenance of health and working capacity" ("Medical Defence" 7), not-so-subtly accusing the government of promoting a diet inadequate for men to maintain their ability to work.

In a front page article on January 6, 1934, from its political correspondent, the *Daily Herald* provided an incendiary headline, "Doctors Challenge Minister's Callous Diet Scale," describing the differences between the two committees as a "bitter controversy" that "threatened" the position of the Minister of Health, Sir E. Hilton Young. The item called the BMA's recommendations "absolutely essential for a man's minimum diet" and indicated that the Minister's advice to disregard these standards was "callous and inhuman." To make its point clear, the *Herald* quoted McGonigle "that one of the most important factors in public health today is this question of nutrition," implying that the Minister of Health was ignoring this "important factor." Indeed, the paper noted, "Eminent doctors from all over the country joined yesterday in a wholesale condemnation of the Ministry of Health." Quoting Dr. Neil Leitch of the London School of Dietetics, the paper informed its readers that the 3,000-calorie diet was insufficient for both scientific and practical reasons: it "'does not allow . . . any margin of resistance to infection, for stress and strain and for the weather. No allowance . . . is made for the fact that the unemployed may have to walk miles every day in search of work: they may be poorly clad and because of insufficient food unable to generate body heat'" (1–2). The article also stressed that other doctors thought the BMA scale itself was too low. This article relied almost entirely on the expertise of doctors to attack the government's treatment of the poor and unemployed.

Many items covering the competing dietary recommendations focused directly on the question of nutrition in relation to unemployment benefits. The *Lincolnshire Echo* had one of its reporters "make inquiries on the subject" of the diet controversy and in a front-page article on January 8, 1934, emphasized that the BMA seemed to be paying attention to nutrition, while the Ministry was more concerned with cost. The reporter interviewed the secretary of the People's Service Club of Lincoln, who commented, "'I think this new dietary emphasises more and more the inadequacy of the present benefits to enable the unemployed to maintain a decent health standard. . . What is the use of these low tables of nutrition if the unemployed cannot even afford these things'" ("Opinions" 1)? The *Lancashire Evening Post* pronounced that "this controversy must not be allowed to divert or delay the serious attention that must be paid the actual physical state of many of the unemployed and their families" ("Minimum Diet Problem" 3). Reporters repeatedly communicated the gap between recommended dietary standards and the reality of the lives of the poor and unemployed.

The overtly partisan nature of the controversy became increasingly evident in the reporting. The editorial of the *Western Daily Press* on January 14, 1934, for example, suggested that the Ministry of Health and the BMA were not asking the same question and stressed the importance of coming to a consensus, for "the Ministry is concerned lest the impression should be created that the standard of nourishment which it recommends and which is presumably followed by public assistance committees is insufficient. Nothing would better suit the Socialists than to be able to represent the Government as responsible for the under-feeding of the unemployed." The editor concluded that the scientific importance of the debate was getting obscured by "political exploitation . . . [and] partisan tactics and recrimination" ("Diet and Health" 6). From a different perspective, in the *Leven Advertiser and Wemyss Gazette*, the reporter William Smart wrote that "The Report on Nutrition is overwhelming proof that it is impossible for the unemployed and their families to secure a reasonable standard of maintenance on the amounts received in unemployment benefit. . . .Many thousands of unemployed, under the means test, are receiving less than the maximum benefit scales," which in themselves were not sufficient. Smart accused the Minister of Health of allowing children to starve while the government continued the controversy (8). On one hand, papers supporting the government did not want the "facts" of nutrition to be used against existing policies. On the other, government critics read these "facts" as "overwhelming proof" that change had to happen.

On January 19, the press announced that representatives from the BMA Committee and the Ministry Committee were going to meet to discuss the discrepancies in their recommendations (for example, "Nutrition Dispute" 8; "Calories Dispute" 9; "To Decide Battle of Diets" 2; "The Diet Dispute" 7). While the initial news reports indicated that the "conference" between the two sides was going to take place in a few days, it was not until May that press coverage announced "Diet Experts Agree to Report at 'Peace' Conference." This item in the *Western Daily Press* on May 16, 1934 reported that the "peace" arrived at was a sliding scale, because "owing to individual difference in physique, personal habits, likes and dislikes, and the variations in the degree of muscular effort involved in different occupations, it was not only impossible to define, but there did not in fact exist, any standard of food requirement which should be rigidly applied to all men alike." The scale, printed along with the article, ranged from a man doing heavy work, who required 4,000 calories gross (3,400 net), to a housewife who required 2,800 calories gross (2,600 net) (12). The *Western Daily Press* also offered an editorial expressing relief that the two sides had come together, for "At a time of severe unemployment the consciences of a great number of people are made uneasy by any suggestion that the standard diet adopted by the public authorities may be inferior to that prescribed by the savants of the BMA as essential to maintain health and fitness." The editor stressed to his readers that "The real problem is not so much one of minimum calorie values, as of ensuring that those who have to be supported out of public funds are not under-nourished" ("Diet and Health" 6). Again, the press framed the issue at heart to be about insufficient unemployment benefits.

The National Coalition Government brought in the new Unemployment Act on June 28, 1934. While the Act restored the ten per cent cut of earlier in the decade, it reaffirmed means testing for eligibility for benefits. This caused new concerns for nutritionists regarding the ability of the unemployed to afford a satisfactory diet. The *Yorkshire Post and Leeds Intelligencer* reported in early August 1934 that "a number of dietetic experts and physiologists . . . have addressed a warning to the new Unemployment Assistance Board, which has just been set up." Because the Act held that benefits would be granted according to an applicant's needs, the dietitians and physiologists, according to the paper, argued that these needs should be determined "in consultation with medical and other expert opinion qualified to estimate the minimum requirements of healthy living." Referring back to the recent debate between the BMA and the Ministry of Health, the warning stressed that "scientific knowledge" was available to determine the minimum diets necessary to provide nutrition and "maintain health and working capacity" ("Deterioration" 2). Similarly, the *Burnley Express* on August 4 reported on the "distinguished physiologists and medical experts" who were pressing the new Unemployment Assistance Boards to consult them to "see that every man has sufficient food to make him 'fit for entry or return to regular employment.'" The item reminded readers that even the experts had disagreed about what counted as "adequate nutrition," so it was important to look at each case on its own merits to make sure unemployed men got "a full and proper diet" ("Local Notes" 9). Here was clear advice that the government should rely on outside medical experts to assist them on dietary issues for the unemployed. The seeming outcome of the British Medical Association's *Report on Nutrition* was the journalistic construction of doctors' expertise on diets and nutrition, in particular in relationship to feeding unemployed men. Newspapers urged the government to rely on experts distinct from the Ministry of Health to provide the newest and best nutritional knowledge.

Public health expertise versus "cold-blooded capitalism"

Even before the papers became wrapped up in the controversy between the Ministry and the BMA, news began to appear of McGonigle's study of Stockton-on-Tees, a community in north-east England with one of the worst unemployment rates in Britain. In April 1933, the *Times* reported McGonigle's counterintuitive findings that poor families who were forced to move because of slum clearances to new model homes were less healthy than those who remained in poor quality housing. The difference in their health and mortality rates was caused by the fact that the money they spent on higher rents was taken away from their food budgets. As the *Times* put it, there was "Better Health in the Slums" (4). While these findings would become front-page news with the publication of McGonigle and J. Kirby's *Poverty and Public Health* in 1936, McGonigle had published his research in the *Proceedings of the Royal Society of Medicine* in February 1933, and the press was already communicating his conclusions. *The Nottingham Journal*, for example, published the joint committee of Industrial Women's Organisations' report that rent payments and other "necessaries" did not leave enough money for "'food of nutritive value'." Additionally, the committee made McGonigle's exact point that " 'moving from a bad house to a good one, where incomes are at a low level, means a higher sickness and mortality rate and increased malnutrition'" ("Food Income" 7). The more families needed to spend on things like fuel and light, the less they spent on food.

McGonigle had long been a thorn in the government's side through his participation on the BMA's nutrition committee. In his role as Medical Officer of Health in Stockton-on-Tees, however, he provided strong evidence of the inadequacy of the budgets of low-paid and unemployed workers to supply nutritious diets (Bambra 475–6). McGonigle wrote an editorial to the *Times* in March 1936 arguing that clear data demonstrated that "nutritional factors" were central to "state of mass ill-health" present in the nation: "Investigations show that the physiological efficiency of family diets varies directly with income." McGonigle was also at pains to make the point that wives from poor households were not to blame for their families' ill health, and in fact, they possessed "sound practical knowledge of dietetic principles. The rule-of-thumb methods used by these women work well, . . . [and] I can state with knowledge that on the whole the working-class woman buys food, to the limit of her purse, wisely and well." Malnutrition resulted from restricted purchasing power, not from the choices made by housewives ("Poverty and Public Health" 10). The focus on housewives throughout these debates illustrates the gendered practice among the working classes that assigned the domestic tasks of the household, including food budgets and preparation, to women (Bourke 62–71).

The publication of *Poverty and Public Health* in early June 1936 drew more attention from journalists sympathetic to McGonigle's arguments and in opposition to the government's policies. In addition to a chapter that essentially replicated McGonigle's paper on rent and food costs, the book contained a variety of topics that would prove alarming to the government including a condemnation of the health of the population overall and of children specifically, a discussion of childhood diseases like rickets (caused by malnutrition), a chapter on "food requirements," and a comparison of the mortality of employed and unemployed workers. The *Left Book News* (the book was published by the Left Book Club) in July 1936 dedicated an article to "The Press Reception" of the book, reflecting that "newspapers from all over the country and of all political colours . . . came out with startled headlines concerning the shameful revelations of hunger and ill-health in England made in that book." The *Left Book News* declared that "no less than 40 papers had reviewed the book," and "the remarkable thing is that not one newspaper has levelled at the book any suggestion of unreliability, 'scare-mongering', or 'propaganda' such as one expects any record of shameful government to bring forth from some quarters. The authors' standing is too good, and the facts they have marshalled are too convincing." This reference to the authors' reputation and the unassailable facts would become common, and the article noted the value of the book because of these factors to leftist groups as a tool to counter arguments about the standard of living among the poor ("'Poverty and Public Health': The Press Reception" 43–4).

The majority of the reviews and articles about the book underscored the expertise of the authors and the legitimacy of the evidence upon which the claims rested. The *Sunderland Daily Echo and Shipping Gazette*, for example, pulled out a quote from the study to make the point that "'on the evidence so far available it appears not improbable that nearly one-half of the population of England and Wales subsists, to a greater or lesser extent, below the safety line of nutrition.'" The article then cited McGonigle's credentials as the recipient of Dickinson Scholarship and Gold Medal at Durham University College of Medicine and his stint as president of the northern branch of the Society for Medical Officers of Health ("Poverty and Public Health: North-East" 2). The following week, the *Echo* carried another article titled, "Health of the North-East," giving more detail about the book and repeating McGonigle's credentials (2). The *Leeds Mercury* referred to McGonigle's paper, which had been read before the Royal Society of Medicine, as providing "facts" demonstrating that higher rents meant lower expenditures on food, which led to increased death rates in the Stockton study ("Children's First Need" 6). *The Scotsman* quoted McGonigle as stating, "It has been shown almost beyond any shadow of a doubt . . . that this increased death-rate [from the move] is definitely correlated with a diminished expenditure on food consequent on the increase in rents." The article emphasized the certainty of the findings, quoting McGonigle, "It must be obvious to every thinking person" that an improvement in housing conditions should not be at the expense of a decline in nutrition ("Death-Rate" 11). In the *Birmingham Daily Gazette* on July 14, 1936, the lead editorial declared that McGonigle "has also combatted the excuse raised somewhere that a great deal of the evil is due to the domestic inefficiency of housewives." The problem was rather prolonged unemployment and the government's agricultural policy ("Food of the Poor" 8). By providing a forum to assert McGonigle's evidence as well as his claims to authority, these papers helped build up the status of the nutritionist argument while making it seem outlandish to contradict the findings.

The press used McGonigle and Kirby's book to put forward empirical evidence that was meant to challenge the government's claims that working-class diets were satisfactory. The *Daily Herald*, in a front-page headline on June 8, 1936, announced "Hundreds Killed by Poverty" to send readers further into the paper to a review of McGonigle and Kirby's book that marshalled science in just this way. The review's author, Mary Sunderland, Chief Woman Officer of the Labour Party, highlighted that McGonigle and Kirby "write with authority, for their knowledge is based on long experience of public health work in industrial areas." Sunderland related her "hope that this book will be read by those who use official statistics to prove that things are 'not so bad' with the unemployed and with the children in industrial areas. Here we are told very plainly that the official statistics which are the basis of so many complacent, soothing utterances reveal a very unsatisfactory state of affairs." The same thing had been said about the BMA nutrition report. Sunderland informed the paper's readers that "it is stated emphatically by [McGonigle and Kirby] that a considerable proportion of our population cannot get a right diet because of poverty, and they are impatient with the news that inefficient housekeeping rather than poverty is the cause of faulty diet and bad nutrition." She concluded that these "scientific investigators" provided a path forward with regard to diets and nutrition, and people needed to use their political and economic power to see that their knowledge was implemented (1,10). A review in the *Hartlepool Northern Daily Mail* regretted that the book painted such a miserable picture of northeast England but stressed the book's "exhaustive data – child welfare records, food and family budgets and relation between income and death-rate, for example," that supported that picture. While commenting on the authors' lack of solutions to the problems they identified, the review stated that "their indirect hints both to national and local authorities are plain," meaning they called for the government to change its policies ("Through an M.O.'s Eyes" 6).

Leftist newspapers, especially, continued their assault on government neglect by piling on the "facts" uncovered by McGonigle and Kirby's scientific inquiry. London's *Daily Worker* on June 25, 1936 led with the disturbing headline, "20 Out of 1,000 Unemployed Die of Starvation – Not Just of Overcrowding, Bad Conditions . . . or 'Wasteful Cooking'." The article stressed the scientific objectivity of McGonigle and Kirby's approach, calling the evidence "unassailable." Indeed, the expertise of the authors was proven, according to the reporter, because "There is not a word of political argument between the covers." The evidence spoke for itself. *Reynolds Illustrated News* called poverty "Britain's Real Enemy," lamenting the conditions revealed by McGonigle and Kirby's book, "which should swell the nation's soul to rage." The "facts" indicated by the study clearly demonstrated that "malnutrition is a symptom of low wages . . . [and that] higher wages and high consuming power are the one defence against mass murder." A week later, *Reynolds* again commented on *Poverty and Public Health,* emphasizing the importance of "the public service in giving publicity to the shameful facts about poverty and low wages" and hoping that the book would "shock" the better off into action "against cold-blooded capitalism" ("Shameful Facts"). Stressing facts, both the *Daily Worker* and *Reynolds* marshalled supposedly objective science to criticize "cold-blooded capitalism."

Clearly, the book and its headlines were having an uncomfortable effect on the other side. W. Faulkner wrote a letter to the editor of the *Birmingham Post* in June 1936, complaining that Socialists were misrepresenting the claims *Poverty and Public Health,* "alleg[ing] that about half the population is underfed and that this underfeeding is due to an insufficient income." According to Faulker's letter, "There is some evidence of malnutrition in some areas where unemployment has been severe, and there is also evidence where there is an excessive consumption, not due to poverty, of canned foods, fish and chips, &c. But there is no justification for the sweeping assertions of Socialists – assertions made for the sole purpose of discrediting capitalism and winning support for socialism." Indeed, if the "facts" the newspapers reported were true, it would have been hard to argue against additional government spending to support better nutrition for the poor and unemployed.

Conclusions

Whether they were original stories, syndicated items, editorials, or letters to the editor, print journalism on nutrition and poverty in the 1930s provided a public space to articulate claims for facts, science, and public health expertise as a means to improve the lives of poor and unemployed populations through enhanced diets. Even when headlines and the overall tone of items tended toward melodrama, writers still appealed to scientific evidence to challenge government positions that blamed housewives for poor diets or played down malnutrition altogether. They sometimes, however, disparaged or were suspicious of professional expertise overall, mocking the "scientific" 5s. 10d. diet as out of touch with working-class economic realities. As an alternative, journalists held up the knowledge of working-class housewives who intuited the nutritional needs of their working husbands from real-life experience rather than scientific theory. Yet in general, newspapers shaped a public discourse of nutritional expertise that became practically irrefutable, embarrassing the government and exposing its policies as unscientific and opposed to recommended best practices. Rather than looking to change the ways that women managed food, nutritionists argued that the government should focus on the purchasing power of poor families as the key factor in nutritional health. In this way, print journalism proved a powerful force in helping public health doctors criticize government parsimony with regard to working-class diets and health. By ignoring evidence of extreme deprivation and the new scientific knowledge of nutrition, the government was repeatedly taken to task by journalists who trusted the facts and constructed expertise, giving the public a language in which to resist government complacency and miserliness.

From my location as an author in the United States, the power of print journalism – and other media – to emphasize scientific facts and public health expertise over politicians' denial of science was only too evident during the Covid-19 pandemic. However, 2020–21 was a very different era than the 1930s, with people able to obtain their news from sources well beyond their local newspapers, although local news continues to be an important resource (Shearer; Jurkowitz and Mitchell). As the public searched for information on Covid-19, the vast majority of journalistic outlets promoted scientific messages about the spread of the virus and necessary public health measures, such as masking and social distancing, even as the Trump administration and many Republican politicians challenged the facts of the disease from its onset in January 2020 (Viglione; Relman). This continued with the vaccination roll out in 2021, as newspapers and network and cable television channels, in particular, were mostly reliable sources of the rapidly-changing knowledge about vaccine development and implementation. Yet powerful news outlets such as Fox News and sites on social media like Facebook and Instagram claimed "alternative facts" that supported unscientific "versions" of the coronavirus and vaccination, and these dangerous narratives spread rapidly in a way that simply would not have been possible in the 1930s (Hart, Chin, and Soroka; Cassata). Just as partisanship played a role in the nutrition controversy, partisanship also shaped the response to Covid-19, and, as in the 1930s, journalists during the pandemic reported on the dangers partisanship posed to the clear messaging of scientific information to the public (Rothwell and Desai). The significance of the mainstream news in both historical moments was communicating evidence-based science to challenge politicians' and others' false claims about the "facts" when the public health community was trying to present the most up-to-date scientific information.

As was the case in the newspaper reporting of the nutrition controversy, media coverage of Covid-19 and its vaccines exposed essential knowledge about the ways the politics of everyday experiences shape health chances, decisions, and outcomes. Class was the fundamental marker of experience in the nutrition controversy, as journalists in the 1930s wrote of the ways the government was to blame for the poor health and even deaths of working-class people denied proper nutrition. Reporting on Covid-19 revealed the ways that intersections of class, race, age, geographical location, and occupation had a tremendous impact on health chances (Wallis). Poor, Black, Indigenous, Pacific Islander, older, and rural populations were most likely to contract the virus, need hospitalization, and die (APM Research Lab Staff). Many "essential workers" also came from these groups, making them most at risk to exposure to the virus because of their jobs (Kinder and Stateler). This news coverage helped the public understand already-existing health inequities and the broader connections between socio-economic status, race, ethnicity, and health (Chotiner).

In another interesting parallel, in the battle over the cost of a working man's diet, newspapers in the 1930s reported on housewives whose expertise gained through the experience of making meals challenged scientific conclusions about the 5s. 10d. diet. Familiar with the prices of food and the amounts their husbands ate, these housewives found the 5s. 10d. diet unrealistic. In the battle over coronavirus protocols and vaccination, women also appealed to their experience, this time as mothers, to oppose vaccines and masking as damaging to their children's well-being. In this case, however, they often spread misinformation on social media sites directed to other mothers, using language such as "Un-mask our kids. Let's talk mom to mom" (Dickson). Media forums provided locations for women to promote alternative forms of expertise based on their own domestic experiences.

The nutrition controversy of the 1930s obviously impacted fewer people than the coronavirus pandemic, but newspapers, using the voices of public health experts, rightly argued that proper nutrition was a question of life or death. They pushed the government to act in order to prevent unemployed men and their families from dying from inadequate diets. Journalists chose to communicate scientific, evidence-based messages at a time when politicians challenged the facts as a way to justify limited spending on benefits. Journalism's power to expose government neglect of the people's health is clearly a public good, but, as we learned with the Covid-19 pandemic, newspapers and other media also have the power to spread unsafe misinformation about public health. Gleaning the scientific health information from the chaff of falsehoods is a major challenge of our times.

Acknowledgments

I would like to thank Isabel Levine-Clark for her research assistance with this chapter.

Notes

1 The publication of Orr's *Food, Health, and Income: Report on a Survey of Diet in Relation to Income* also generated tremendous press coverage.
2 The research for this essay is based primarily on the London *Times* digital archive (www.gale.com/c/the-times-digital-archive) and the newspapers digitized in the *British Newspaper Archive* (www.britishnewspaperarchive.co.uk/). I examined all articles that appeared in combined keyword and chronological searches on the publication events. Many of the articles were duplicative: they most likely originated in London and were syndicated throughout the United Kingdom.
3 The Advisory Committee on Nutrition received much more attention regarding their recommendations for children's diets.
4 There is a rich literature on the British feminization of India and Indian men, in particular. See, for example, Sinha.

Works cited

"10d. a Day to Feed a Man." *Berks and Oxon Advertiser*, Dec. 29, 1933, p. 8.
"20 out of 1,000 Unemployed Die of Starvation-Not Just of Overcrowding, Bad Conditions...or 'Wasteful' Cooking." *Daily Worker*, International Press Cuttings Bureau, June 25, 1936. *Presscuttings*, M'Gonigle Collection, Wellcome Library, PP/GMG/A/8.
APM Research Lab Staff. "The Color of Coronavirus: COVID-19 Deaths by Race and Ethnicity in the U.S." *APM Research Lab*, Mar. 5, 2021, www.apmresearchlab.org/covid/deaths-by-race. Accessed August 15, 2021.
Bambra, Clare. "Lessons from the Past: Celebrating the 75th Anniversary of Poverty and Public Health." *Journal of Public Health*, vol. 33, no. 4, 2011, pp. 475–476.
"Better Health in the Slums." *Times*, Apr. 8, 1933, p. 4.
Bourke, Joanna. *Working-Class Cultures in Britain, 1890–1960*. New York and Abingdon: Routledge, 1994.
Briggs, Charles L., and Daniel C. Hallin. *Making Health Public: How News Coverage is Remaking Media, Medicine, and Contemporary Life*. New York and Abingdon: Routledge, 2016.
"Britain's Real Enemy." *Reynolds Illustrated News*, International Press Cutting Bureau, June 7, 1936. *Presscuttings*, M'Gonigle Collection, Wellcome Library, PP/GMG/A/8.
British Medical Association (BMA). *Report of Committee on Nutrition*. London, British Medical Association, 1933.
Burnett, John, and Derek J. Oddy. *The Origins and Development of Food Policies in Europe*. Leicester: Leicester University Press, 1994.
"Calorie Requirements: Committee's Dispute Settled." *The Scotsman*, May 16, 1934, p. 14.
"Calories Dispute." *Birmingham Daily Gazette*, January 19, 1934, p. 9.
Cassata, Cathy. "People Less Likely to Be Vaccinated Against COVID-19 When Facebook Is Their Main News Source." *Healthline*, August 5, 2021, www.healthline.com/health-news/people-less-likely-to-be-vaccinated-against-covid-19-when-facebook-is-main-news-source. Accessed August 15, 2021.
"Cheap Living." *Yorkshire Post*, November 24, 1933, p. 9.
"The Children's First Need." *Leeds Mercury*, July 10, 1933, p. 6.
Chotiner, Isaac. "The Interwoven Threads of Inequality and Health." *The New Yorker*, April 14, 2020, www.newyorker.com/news/q-and-a/the-coronavirus-and-the-interwoven-threads-of-inequality-and-health. Accessed August 15, 2021.
Cooper, Benjamin E. J. et al. "The Quality of the Evidence for Dietary Advice Given in UK National Newspapers." *Public Understanding of Science*, vol. 21, no. 6, 2011, pp. 664–73. Accessed February 9, 2020.
"Death-Rate Up After Removal to New Houses." *The Scotsman*, July 14, 1933, p. 11.
"Deterioration of Physique." *Yorkshire Post and Leeds Intelligencer*, August 3, 1934, p. 2.
Dickson, E. J. "Mom Influencers on Instagram Are Spreading Anti-Mask Propaganda." *Rolling Stone*, July 24, 2020, www.rollingstone.com/culture/culture-features/mom-influencers-instagram-covid-19-coronavirus-mask-propaganda-misinformation-1033154/. Accessed August 15, 2021.

"Diet and Health." *Western Daily Press and Bristol Mirror*, January 13, 1934, p. 6.
"Diet and Health." *Western Daily Press and Bristol Mirror*, May 16, 1934, p. 6.
"The Diet Dispute." *Dundee Courier*, May 16, 1934, p. 7.
"Diet Experts Agree." *Belfast News-Letter*, May 16, 1934, p. 16.
"Diet Experts Agree to Report at 'Peace' Conference." *Western Daily Press and Bristol Mirror*, May 16, 1934, p. 12.
"Doctors and Family Food Budgets." *Western Gazette*, November 24, 1933, p. 11.
"Doctors Challenge Minister's Callous Diet Scale." *Daily Herald*, January 6, 1934, pp. 1–2.
"Doctor's Name in Ministry a Mystery." *Daily Herald*, January 5, 1934, pp. 1, 3.
"Doctors' Food Feud." *Dundee Courier*, January 5, 1934, p. 7.
Durbach, Nadja. "The Science of Selection: Malnutrition and School Meals in the Interwar Years." *Many Mouths: The Politics of Food in Britain from the Workhouse to the Welfare State*. New York, Cambridge University Press, 2020, pp. 146–77.
Faulkner, W. "Poverty and Malnutrition." *Birmingham Post,* International Press Cutting Bureau, June 20, 1936. *Presscuttings,* M'Gonigle Collection, Wellcome Library, PP/GMG/A/8.
"Food." *Liverpool Echo*, January 5, 1934, p. 8.
"Food Calories: Doctor Replies to Ministry's Repudiation." *Gloucestershire Echo*, January 5, 1934, p. 1.
"Food Experts Fall into Line." *Dundee Courier*, May 16, 1934, p. 7.
"Food Income Not Enough." *Nottingham Journal*, October 20, 1934, p. 7.
"The Food of the Poor." *Birmingham Daily Gazette*, July 9, 1936, p. 8.
Hart, P. Sol, Sedona Chinn, and Stuart Soroka. "Politicization and Polarization in COVID-19 News Coverage." *Science Communication*, vol. 42, no. 5, 2020, pp. 679–97.
"Health of the North-East." *Sunderland Daily Echo and Shipping Gazette*, June 16, 1936, p. 2.
"Health Visitors' Conference: Ministry Circular on Diet." *Dundee Evening Telegraph*, January 5, 1934, p. 7.
"How a Man Can Live on 5/10 a Week." *Leeds Mercury*, November 24, 1933, p. 4.
Jamil, Nafeesa, and Charlotte E. L. Evans. "Nutrition in the Media: A Cross-Sectional Analysis of Health and Nutrition Articles Reported in Five Popular UK Newspapers." *Proceedings of the Nutrition Society*, no. 75, OCE3, 2016, dx.doi.org.du.idm.oclc.org/10.1017/S0029665116002147. Accessed February 9, 2020.
Jurkowitz, Mark, and Amy Mitchell. "Cable TV and COVID-19: How Americans Perceive the Outbreak and View Media Coverage Differently by Main News Source." *Pew Research Center*, Apr. 1, 2020, www.amanewyork.org/wp-content/uploads/2020/04/20.04.01.PewResearch.CableTVAndCoronavirusHowAmericansPerceiveTheOutbreakAndViewMediaCoverageDifferByMainNewsSource.pdf. Accessed August 15, 2021.
Kinder, Molly, and Laura Stateler. "Essential Workers Comprise About Half of All Workers in Low-Paid Occupations. They Deserve a $15 Minimum Wage." *Brookings*, February 5, 2021, www.brookings.edu/blog/the-avenue/2021/02/05/essential-workers-deserve-minimum-wage-increase/. Accessed August 15, 2021.
"Life on 5s 10d a Week." *Dundee Courier and Advertiser*, November 24, 1933, p. 6.
"Life on 5s 10d a Week." *Gloucestershire Echo*, November 24, 1933, p. 8.
"Living off 5/10½: Doctor's Retort to Ministry." *Edinburgh Evening News*, January 5, 1934, p. 9.
"Living on 5s 10d a Week." *Yorkshire Evening Post*, November 24, 1933, p. 15.
"Local Notes: Feeding the Workless." *Burnley Express*, August 4, 1934, p. 9.
Mayhew, Madeleine. "The 1930s Nutrition Controversy." *Journal of Contemporary History*, vol. 23, no. 3, 1988, pp. 445–64.
McCaw, Brian et al. "Online Health Information – What the Newspapers Tell Their Readers: A Systematic Content Analysis." *BMC Public Health*, vol. 14 no. 1316, 2014, bmcpublichealth.biomedcentral.com/articles/10.1186/1471-2458-14-1316. Accessed February 9, 2020.
McGonigle, George Cuthbert Mura. "Poverty and Public Health." *Times*, March 26, 1936, p. 10.
"Medical Defence of the 5/10 Diet." *Leeds Mercury*, January 6, 1934, p. 7.
Memorandum to the Minister of Health on the Criticism and Improvement of Diets. Ministry of Health, Advisory Committee on Nutrition, London, HMSO, 1932.
"Minimum Diet Dispute." *The Scotsman*, January 5, 1934, p. 6.
"Minimum Diet Problem." *Lancashire Evening Post*, January 9, 1934, p. 3.
"Ministry's Report Discussed." *Shields Daily News*, January 5, 1934, p. 8.
"Now You Know How Much You Should Eat." *Leeds Mercury*, May 16, 1934, p. 7.
"Nutrition Dispute." *Sunderland Daily Echo and Shipping Gazette*, January 19, 1934, p. 8.

Oddy, Derek J. *From Plain Fare to Fusion Food: British Diet from the 1890s to the 1990s*. Rochester, Boydell Press, 2003.
"Opinions on Minimum Diet Controversy." *Lincolnshire Echo*, January 8, 1934, p. 1.
Orr, John Boyd. *Food, Health, and Income: Report on a Survey of Diet in Relation to Income*. London, Macmillan, 1936.
"The Perfect Diet." *Staffordshire Advertiser*, March 26, 1932, p. 9.
"Poor Family's Budget." *The Daily Post*, Preston, November 27, 1933. Rpt in *Lancashire Evening Post*, November 27, 1933, p. 4.
"Poverty and Public Health: North-East Material in New Book." *Sunderland Echo and Shipping Gazette*, June 7, 1936, p. 2.
"'Poverty and Public Health': The Press Reception." *Left Book News*, July 1936, pp. 43–4. *Presscuttings and Collected Publications*, McGonigle Collection, Welcome Library, PPGMG/F/3/15.
Relman, Eliza. "Just 45% of House Republicans Say They've Been Vaccinated While 100% of Congressional Democrats Say They've Gotten the Shot." *Insider*, May 14, 2021, www.businessinsider.com/just-45-of-house-republicans-say-theyve-gotten-a-covid-19-vaccine-2021-5. Accessed August 15, 2021.
Rothwell, Jonathan, and Sonal Desai. "How Misinformation Is Distorting COVID Policies and Behaviors." *Brookings*, December 22, 2020, www.brookings.edu/research/how-misinformation-is-distorting-covid-policies-and-behaviors/. Accessed August 15, 2021.
Said, Edward. *Orientalism*. New York: Vintage Books, 1979.
Seale, Clive. "Health and Media: An Overview." *Sociology of Health and Illness*, vol. 25, no. 6, 2003, pp. 513–31. Accessed February 9, 2020.
"Shameful Facts." *Reynolds Illustrated News*, International Press Cutting Bureau, June 7, 1936. *Presscuttings*, M'Gonigle Collection, Wellcome Library, PP/GMG/A/8.
Shearer, Elisa. "Local News is Playing an Important Role for Americans during COVID-19 Outbreak." *Pew Research Center*, July 2, 2020, www.pewresearch.org/fact-tank/2020/07/02/local-news-is-playing-an-important-role-for-americans-during-covid-19-outbreak/. Accessed August 15, 2021.
Sinha, Mrinalini. *Colonial Masculinity: The 'Manly Englishman' and the 'Effeminate Bengali' in the Late Nineteenth Century*. Manchester, Manchester University Press, 1995.
Smart, William. "Is It Starvation?" *Leven Advertiser and Wemyss Press*, Fife, Scotland, January 16, 1934, p. 8.
Sunderland, Mary. "Hundreds Killed by Poverty." *Daily Herald*, June 8, 1936, pp. 1,10.
"Through an M.O.'s Eyes." *Hartlepool Northern Daily Mail*, January 15, 1936, p. 6.
"To Decide Battle of Diets." *Nottingham Journal*, January 19, 1934, p. 2.
"Unemployed Workers and New Scheme." *Edinburgh Evening News*, November 23, 1933, p 6.
"Unemployment Assistance." July 17, 1936. *Reading Source*, International Press-Cutting Bureau. *Presscuttings*, M'Gonigle Collection, Wellcome Library, London. PP/GMG/A/8, wellcomelibrary.org/item/b19695949#?c=0&m=0&s=0&cv=565&z=,%20.2149%2C-0.204%2C0.9787%2C0.6148. Accessed March 12, 2020.
Vernon, James. "The Ethics of Hunger and the Assembly of Society: The Technopolitics of the School Meal in Modern Britain." *American Historical Review*, vol. 110, no. 3, 2005, pp. 693–725.
Vernon, James. *Hunger: A Modern History*. Cambridge, Harvard University Press, 2007.
Viglione, Giuliana. "Four Ways Trump Has Meddled in Pandemic Science – and Why It Matters." *Nature*, November 3, 2020, www.nature.com/articles/d41586-020-03035-4. Accessed August 15, 2021.
Wallis, Claudia. "Why Some People Get Terribly Sick from COVID-19." *Scientific American*, August 20, 2020, www.scientificamerican.com/article/why-some-people-get-terribly-sick-from-covid-19/. Accessed August 15, 2021.
"Weekly Expenditure on Food." *The Times*, January 5, 1934, p. 14.
"What the Doctor Says: Food, Health, and Poverty." *Northampton Mercury*, December 8, 1933, p. 11.

2
BREAKING NEWS
Medical research reporting and its consequences

Rae-Ellen W. Kavey

The connection is simple: medical research findings are important information, and mass news media are the primary source of that information for the general public. The North American public identify mass media as major providers of medical information, so accurate, timely delivery is essential (Hesse et al.). Although healthcare professionals are more knowledgeable and credible information sources for patients and families, medical encounters are infrequent and time-limited, but mass-media information – from print, television and the internet – is constant, accessible, and pervasive (Gallup).

Medicine and medical research are as old as humanity and as long as there has been recorded history, healers have shared their efforts. Records from the Egyptians and then the Greeks and Romans document diagnostic and treatment efforts shared as expert-to-expert communications, primarily as letters and hand-written books. After the invention of the printing press, newssheets, almanacs and 'books of secrets' in the 15th and 16th centuries, as well as newspapers and magazines from the 18th century on, contained medical articles directed primarily to the reading public. Following the publication of the first medical journal in the United Kingdom in Edinburgh in 1731 – *Medical Essays and Observations* – and the initial publication of *The New England Journal of Medicine* in the United States in 1797, medical journals became the primary source of information for subsequent dissemination in the lay press (Booth; Cassedy).

The accurate, efficient communication of medical research findings from such peer-reviewed journals is important to physicians, the scientific research community, and the public. To researchers, publication in a high profile, peer-reviewed journal is the critical format for research reporting but dissemination in the lay press has become increasingly important for them as well. To readers, accuracy of information and personal relevancy are the most critical factors. A fundamental question for medical journalists is how to highlight legitimate medical information to compete effectively against other compelling stories and to meet the major responsibility of providing accurate and straightforward news coverage of emerging research findings, while avoiding public confusion, doubt, and even panic. Accurate reporting of the original medical report is especially critical since most subsequent descriptions are derived from that report rather than from the research publication itself. With rapid, widespread online coverage of medical information on social media, inaccuracies in fact or inference can be

DOI: 10.4324/9781003007661-4

globally disseminated within seconds of the first report. When flawed science combines with uninformed reporting, the results can be devastating to millions of people.

In this chapter, I explore the transmission of medical research findings in the lay press through the press coverage of the results of the hormone therapy arm of the Women's Health Initiative. I highlight two critical areas in the medical reporting: the headline and the statistical analysis, each of which can dramatically affect a reader's perception of research results. My findings illustrate the critical intersections between medicine and media and highlight the importance of accurate, complete reporting.

The hormone replacement therapy saga

The hormone replacement story began in 1962. It was a different time in medicine: evidence-based research standards were decades away when Dr. Robert Wilson, a Brooklyn-based obstetrician-gynecologist, published his first paper addressing the roles of estrogen and progesterone in breast and genital cancer in the prestigious *Journal of the American Medical Association* (Wilson, "The Roles of Estrogen"). This was a selective review of the evidence that treatment with estrogens does not cause endometrial or ovarian cancer in cell preparations, animals, or human females. The paper included the author's own case series of 300 women ranging in age from 40 to 70 years who had been treated with long-term exogenous estrogens. Wilson does not provide his treatment results, but no cases of cancer developed when 18 cases were expected based on existing cancer incidence reports. Wilson concluded that, "Estrogen does not cause cancer" (Wilson 331). In an intimation of future publications, he also wrote, "It would seem advisable to keep women endocrine rich and, consequently, cancer poor throughout their lives… A consequence of this would be the elimination of the menopause" (Wilson 331).

Historically, a therapeutic approach to menopause was limited, focused on managing symptoms with psychotherapy and sedation; all previous reports of estrogen treatment for postmenopausal issues alluded to its cancerogenic properties (Stefanick). Given the increasing age of the North American population, the number of women with postmenopausal symptoms was steadily rising with no consensus approach to management. This was the atmosphere in which Wilson and his wife, Thelma, a registered nurse, published what would prove to be a landmark 1963 paper in the *Journal of the American Geriatrics Society*, arguing that "all postmenopausal women are castrates" and that untreated menopause robbed women of their femininity and ruined the quality of their lives (Wilson and Wilson 347). The paper describes the loss of estrogen at menopause as catastrophic, resulting in a suddenly accelerated aging process associated with osteoporosis, progressive atherosclerosis, atrophy of the breasts and genitalia, disturbing emotional lability, and depression – a chilling but not inaccurate description of menopause and its consequences at their worst. This rapid failure of gonadal function differs between women and men; while women effectively lose all estrogen secretion within two years of menopause, men undergo a gradual decline in sex hormones as age increases. Wilson and Wilson describe postmenopausal women as aged, pathetic creatures, with thinning skin, progressive back curvature, frequent fractures and chronic back pain due to osteoporosis with an aggressively negative view of life (355). By contrast, they describe their husbands as active and vigorous. The article strongly recommends estrogen therapy for menopausal ovarian failure for every woman, to be continued indefinitely.

The publication of this paper coincided with widespread adoption of the oral contraceptive pill, a combination of estrogen and progesterone, the two major ovarian steroids. The pill was first released in 1960, and by the time the Wilson paper was published, a quarter of all women of reproductive age were using oral contraceptives to prevent pregnancy: thus, a theoretical hormonal treatment model for 'ovarian failure' was readily available (Tyrer).

In 1966, Wilson published *Feminine Forever*, funded by Wyeth-Ayerst, the company that produced Premarin, a common form of estrogen replacement (Wilson, *Feminine Forever*). In the book, Wilson expanded on his position that menopause was an estrogen-deficiency disease, which should be treated with replacement therapy to prevent the otherwise inevitable "living decay" that occurred in all women at menopause (37). The book was an unqualified success, selling more than 100,000 copies in its first year. Through the tireless promotion of his Wilson Research Foundation – funded entirely by the pharmaceutical industry – Wilson continued to "educate" women about the ravages of menopause and the miracle of estrogen therapy. The media picked up Wilson's" message, prompting dozens of articles in magazines from *Vogue* and *Good Housekeeping* to *Newsweek* and *Science Digest* with titles like "A Pill that Prolongs the Prime of Life" (Locke) and "You Need Not Fear the Menopause" (Scott). Within only a few years, medical journals described the treatment of menopause with estrogen preparations as "therapeutic replacement of gonadal steroids after ovarian failure" (Graham; Greenblatt) and in the lay press as "the elixir of eternal femininity" (Locke) (Figure 2.1).

In a culture that values youth as the standard for beauty, estrogen quickly became an important component in the anti-aging arsenal. From 1966 to 1975, annual estrogen prescriptions almost doubled, the market value almost quadrupled, and Premarin, the most popular estrogen format, became one of the top five prescription medications in the United States (Watkins). However, in 1975, two important studies reported that estrogen therapy significantly increased the risk of endometrial cancer (Smith, D.C. et al.; Ziel and Finkle). The *New York Times* led the subsequent press coverage with its front page, the same day the studies were published in the *New England Journal of Medicine*, an important intimation of the major role that media reporting would play in the hormone treatment story ("Estrogen is Linked"). Estrogen prescribing dropped precipitously, but ultimately, the carcinogenic properties of replacement estrogen alone were resolved by replacement with estrogen/progesterone combinations, renamed 'hormone therapy (HT)' (Gambrell; "Hormonal Contraception"). The annual number of HT prescriptions increased from 58 million in 1995 to 90 million in 1999; estrogen/progesterone combinations became the largest selling prescription drugs in the U.S. At the peak, an estimated 40 percent of women aged 50 and older were using HT (Hersh, "National Use of Postmenopausal Hormone Therapy").

Important medical problems do follow menopause. Foremost among them are heart attacks and strokes due to accelerated atherosclerosis – the process of vascular aging – and development of osteoporosis with associated pathologic fractures. As HT became common-place, researchers reported its use was associated with a decrease in cardiovascular disease events and with reduced osteoporosis (Bush et al.; Stampfer, Willett et al.; Meema and Meema; Lindsay et al.; Ettinger, Genant et al.). In 1992, a landmark systematic review analyzed the results of observational studies of postmenopausal HT on heart disease, hip fracture, breast cancer, and uterine cancer. The authors concluded that the reduced risk of heart disease and osteoporotic hip fracture outweighed the reported cancer risks (Grady et al.). An important example evaluating HT was the 1991 follow-up of cardiovascular disease in the Nurses' Health Study (NHS), a cohort of registered nurses which began in 1976. The HT report included follow-up of 48,470 women 30–63 years old with no history of cardiovascular disease at baseline. Over ten years, the study showed an impressive 44 per cent reduction in cardiovascular disease events in those women who were taking estrogen (Grady et al.; Stampfer, Colditz et al.).

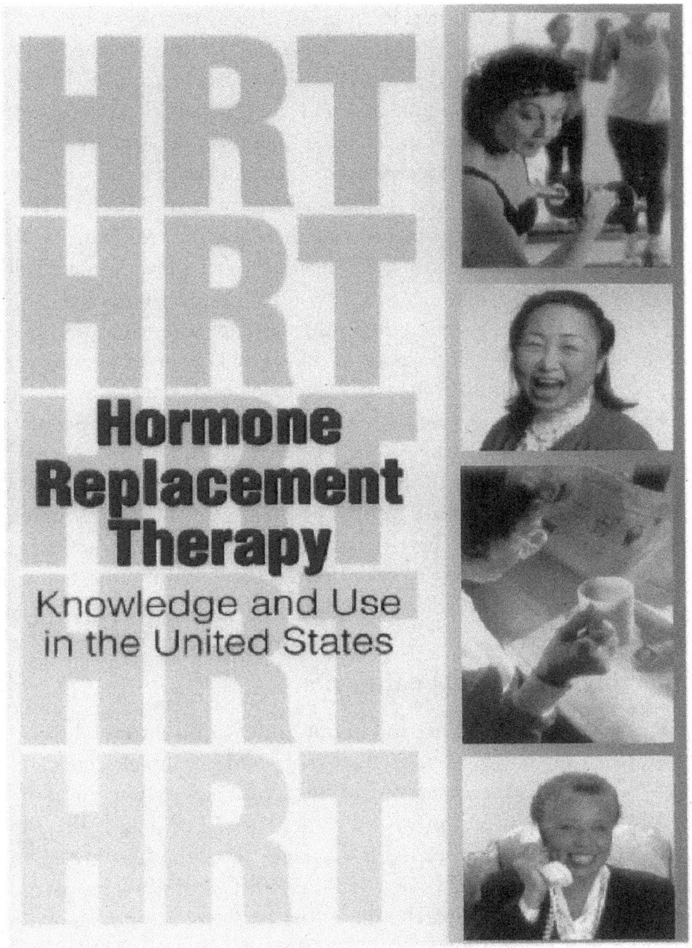

Figure 2.1 Cover of a chartbook entitled "Hormone Replacement Therapy: Knowledge and Use in the United States", published in 2001

Note: At the time of its preparation, half of all postmenopausal women in the U.S. reported having ever used hormone replacement therapy.

Source: Prepared by the National Center for Health Statistics, Centers for Disease Control and Prevention, National Institutes of Health and the Office of Research on Women's Health, the book documented the use of hormone replacement therapy in the United States from 1984 to 1998, using nationally representative data

This accumulating evidence of cardiovascular benefit led to recommendations that HT be considered for all menopausal women. By the mid-1990s in the U.S., HT became standard medical practice for women approaching menopause. The American College of Physicians, the American College of Obstetricians and Gynecologists, and the American Heart Association all endorsed prescription of HT for prevention of heart disease and osteoporosis in postmenopausal women. Wyeth, the leading manufacturer of estrogen preparations, even asked the US Food and Drug Agency (FDA) to include a statement on drug packaging that HT was protective against heart disease.

Although the reported findings were impressive, results from observational studies are inadequate to make evidence-based recommendations because an association between events is not proof of cause and effect. It is against this backdrop that the Women's Health Initiative (WHI), a randomized controlled trial of the effects of postmenopausal HT on the primary outcome of coronary heart disease (CHD, coronary artery disease, myocardial infarction [MI]/heart attack, coronary artery bypass grafting or percutaneous coronary intervention, cardiovascular deaths, and all-cause mortality) began in 1992, funded by the US National Institutes of Health (NIH). Women with a uterus were randomized to receive a placebo or an estrogen /progestin (E+P) combination, while women who were post hysterectomy received estrogen alone (E alone) or placebo. Secondary outcomes included invasive breast cancer, stroke, pulmonary embolus (PE), colorectal cancer, endometrial cancer and hip, vertebral, and other osteoporotic fractures. The study's stated intention was to address risks and benefits of initiating HT at older ages when these chronic disease outcomes typically manifest, so the trial staggered age at enrollment: only 10 percent of subjects were 50–54 years of age (the age when menopause usually occurs), 20 percent were 55–59 years old, and 70 percent were 60–79 years old. In addition to the primary outcome of time to first CHD event, analysis of the results included a global index based on time to diagnosis of the defined outcomes plus death from any other cause. The global index was intended to address simultaneous evidence of both risks and benefits (Women's Health Initiative Study Group). Reporting of the results of this massive trial gives us a unique opportunity to observe the impact of promoted medical research findings.

Reporting the WHI: headline news

The quest for good reporting begins with the headline; and in our information-saturated world where the headline is often the takeaway message, the effort to provide complete, accurate information can fail right there, before even the first word of the actual report. For the journalist, the headline is designed to grab the attention of the reader. Whether it is at the top of a newspaper article, on the scroll at the bottom of the TV screen, or as the heading of an online story, it is the intended equivalent of the flashing "BREAKING NEWS" that is the lead-in to almost every TV news report. Unfortunately, the effort to frame a report as critically important can mean the research information is exaggerated, distorted or misleading (Lomangino). Because of space requirements, headlines in any setting are abbreviated and often, the work of an editor rather than the author of the report. The saga of postmenopausal HT is a stunning example of the power of headlines in medical research reporting to influence cultural attitudes and medical decisions.

Researchers anticipated that the Women's Health Initiative – Hormone Therapy (WHI-HT) trial would require an average of nine years for heart disease outcomes to develop with a further five years to assess the incidence of breast and endometrial cancer – a total planned, initial follow-up of 14 years. It was a complete surprise even to the WHI investigators from the 40 individual trial sites when the Data and Safety Monitoring Committee, a routine part of all clinical trials, recommended stopping the trial after only 5.2 years. The findings which led to this dramatic move were small increases in the risk for breast cancer and for overall *combined* cardiovascular disease events (coronary artery disease, myocardial infarction [MI]/ heart attack, coronary artery bypass grafting or percutaneous coronary intervention, and cardiovascular deaths) *plus* small numbers of strokes and pulmonary emboli. The Committee felt these negative findings outweighed the evidence of benefit for fractures and possibly for colon cancer over the 5.2-year follow-up period ("Writing Group for the Women's Health Initiative"). The study researchers and the Data Safety Monitoring Committee interpreted the global risk/benefit index as indicating that there were more harmful than beneficial outcomes in the intervention E+P group than in the placebo group.

Rollout of the results could not have been more dramatic, with presentation at a highly publicized NIH press conference on July 7, 2002, several days before the hard copy of the journal containing the publication was distributed. The choice of headline for the press release was dramatic: "NHLBI Stops Trial of Estrogen Plus Progestin Due to Increased Breast Cancer Risk, Lack of Overall Benefit" (National Institutes of Health). At the press conference, Claude Lenfant, then Director of the National Heart, Lung and Blood Institute, made his own personal conclusions clear: "The cardiovascular and cancer risks of estrogen plus progestin outweigh any benefits – and a 26 percent increase in breast cancer risk is too high a price to pay, even if there were a heart benefit"("Hormone Replacement Study"). The press announcement from the *Journal of the American Medical Association (JAMA)* in which the article was to be published was equally dramatic, reading: "Hormone Therapy Study Stopped Due to Increased Breast Cancer Risk." The press release continued in almost breathless prose: 'major study ... stopped because of health safety concerns ... the importance of the researchers' findings' (Brown). In the largely pre-digital era of 2002, these press conference reports meant most physicians learned about the trial results when their patients did, from the media. The focus on reporting the breast cancer results was unusual since the primary outcome of the study was risk for coronary heart disease ("Writing Group for the Women's Health Initiative"). At that time, breast cancer was women's greatest health fear, ranked far ahead of the five other causes of death which exceeded it (Walsh-Childers et al.). Focusing publication of the study's findings on the breast cancer results guaranteed an enormous, highly concerned audience.

Newspaper coverage was immediate and intense. The *New York Times* placed their report on the front page of the paper, above the fold where the most important news events are positioned with the headline: "Study Is Halted Over Rise Seen In Cancer Risk" ("Study is Halted"). Their report stated that, "The directors of the study, known as the Women's Health Initiative, sent letters to the study's 16,000 participants...telling them to stop taking the medications." There is no doubt that women all over the world interpreted this as an emergency situation requiring immediate action. The global press reaction was enormous and equally dramatic: the results were front page news all over the world, exemplified by this headline from the *Sydney Morning Herald*: "Alarm over HRT Cancer Risk" ("Alarm over HRT"; "Hormone Treatment"). An independent analysis of newspaper coverage published in the *Journal of Internal Medicine* revealed an eight-fold increase in articles addressing HT in the month the WHI study was released, from 19 articles per month to 197 per month in July–August 2002; 40 percent of these reports were on the front page (Haas et al.).

TV news reporting was equally dramatic: from England, the BBC headline was "HRT Linked to Breast Cancer" and CNN's Headline News led with "Hormone Replacement Therapy Study Halted" ("Hormone Replacement"; "HRT Linked). Magazines followed. Less than two weeks after the WHI report, *Newsweek* magazine reported that the WHI announcement "caused a near panic among the more than 13 million American women now on HT" ("What's a Woman to do?"). Doctors' offices were overwhelmed by calls, and Wyeth Pharmaceuticals, the maker of Prem Pro (the E+P combination used in the trial) saw its stock price plunge by 25 percent overnight. By year's end, the Associated Press had named the WHI report the top medical story of 2002 (Brown).

There is no doubt that the headlines reporting the WHI results were initiated by the dramatic initial press releases from the NIH investigative team (Figure 2.2). In light of this reporting, it is not surprising that the overwhelming conclusion of the WHI-HT trial report was that HT caused breast cancer. Headline coverage of the early WHI results was an unnecessarily

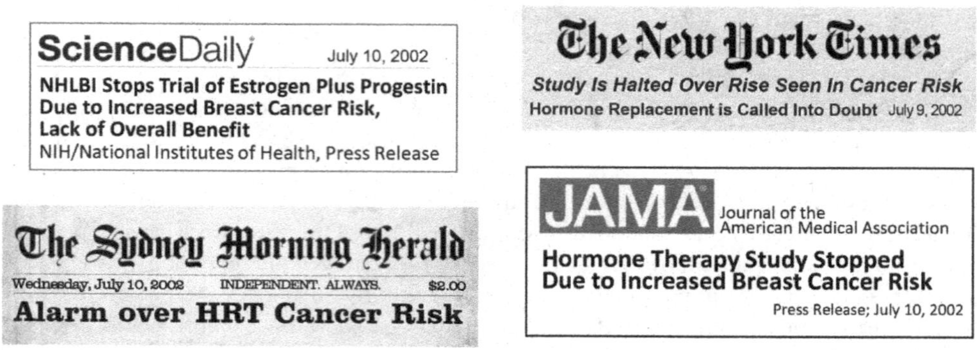

ScienceDaily July 10, 2002
NHLBI Stops Trial of Estrogen Plus Progestin Due to Increased Breast Cancer Risk, Lack of Overall Benefit
NIH/National Institutes of Health, Press Release

The New York Times
Study Is Halted Over Rise Seen In Cancer Risk
Hormone Replacement is Called Into Doubt July 9, 2002

The Sydney Morning Herald
Wednesday, July 10, 2002 INDEPENDENT. ALWAYS. $2.00
Alarm over HRT Cancer Risk

JAMA Journal of the American Medical Association
Hormone Therapy Study Stopped Due to Increased Breast Cancer Risk
Press Release; July 10, 2002

Figure 2.2 The anatomy of a health scare: headlines are not the place for nuanced reporting of complex results

Source: Clippings collected by the author.

sensational over-statement with important consequences. As this case amply demonstrates, reporters and editors need to carefully calibrate headlines in order to present medical research findings as an accurate, balanced message and to introduce a complete, nuanced report to follow, rather than following an "if it bleeds, it leads" mentality that stresses the sensational over the substantive.

The full report: statistical analysis

The headline is a critical introduction to any news story but reporting the results of the analysis of medical research data is an equally important part of medical journalism. Mathematical analyses of numerical data allow investigators to draw conclusions from often huge amounts of raw data. From the early 20th century when most medical research reports were descriptive and numerical analysis was rudimentary, use of interpretive statistical techniques progressively increased, and by the 1980s, sophisticated inferential mathematical analyses were increasingly common.

In terms of the WHI, one of the most disturbing things about the results described in the first report was the striking difference in the reported development of cardiovascular disease (CVD) compared with results from the reports of observational studies in which large numbers of women on hormone therapy (HT) followed over long periods of time showed major decreases in CVD. The statistical interpretation of observational studies can be compromised by a number of important concepts. Using the Nurses's Health Study (NHS) as an example, recall that this was a follow-up of postmenopausal HT in a large cohort of registered nurses with no baseline CVD. Over ten years, the study showed 44 percent fewer reported cases of CVD in women who were currently taking estrogen (Stampfer, Colditz et al.).

One problem which may have compromised interpretation of the NHS results was the assumption that women who took estrogen were the same as women who did not. Subsequent studies showed that wealthier and healthier women were more likely to be prescribed HT (Marks and Shinberg). Although the NHS corrected their results for many health-related factors, they made no correction for socioeconomic status. Another problem is compliance bias – the NHS identified a benefit to HT in women who were current users of the medication that was not apparent in women who had taken it in the past and stopped. And there is prescriber bias; an observational study cannot assess the often complex reasons why a physician prescribes a drug for one patient and not another. Another problem is potential extension of results from the trial participants to the general population. While nurses might be a healthier group than the general population and women who used HT were even healthier by a number of measures, direct extrapolation of the NHS results to the general population was difficult. Despite these limitations, the results of the NHS were strong and compelling and an explanation for the differences between studies like this and the WHI results should have been part of WHI reporting.

One major difference between these observational studies and the WHI lay in study design. In the WHI, researchers evaluated HT subjects prospectively, comparing women on HT with women on placebo; by contrast, in the NHS, HT information was recorded by survey at baseline and every two years subsequently, by the participants themselves. In the WHI, HT drugs were supplied to subjects by the WHI, and medication compliance was monitored by researchers as part of the study. In addition, the HT preparations in the two studies differed: NHS subjects were primarily taking unopposed estrogen compared with the E+P compound in the WHI study. Finally – subjects over sixty years of age were not included in the NHS analysis because there were too few in that age group. Given these issues, direct comparison of the results of these two studies would be difficult – but nonetheless, a discussion of these differences should have been part of the WHI report.

Statistical interpretation of randomized trial results for readers is equally challenging. The defined primary outcome of this trial was the effects of E+P on the incidence of coronary heart disease in postmenopausal women; monitoring for breast cancer was only a planned safety measure. Instead, the early release of the results of the WHI-HT study in 2002 focused on marginally increased risks for breast cancer and coronary heart disease, the latter only when all cardiovascular outcomes were combined – it was the results of this alternate analytic approach that led to widespread confusion, disbelief and anxiety. The focus was on the risk of breast cancer with no explanation for the change in the analysis that led to the cardiac results. For correct interpretation, researchers need to supply all the important statistical findings in a comprehensible format and journalists need to report these results accurately. In the absence of this information, it is easy to understand how women concluded that the only important finding of the WHI was that HT causes breast cancer.

One of the problems with complex statistical analyses is the inability of average readers to extrapolate the reported results to themselves. The original press releases reported only the hazard ratios for each outcome – these are a measure of relative risk, directly comparing the intervention group findings to those in the control group and these results led to the statements about percent increases in risk – a calculated result based on that statistical analysis. An emphasis on relative risk may incorrectly suggest a major hazard, frightening readers without giving any perspective on the underlying baseline risk. Not reported in the lay press were the calculated absolute excess risks for each outcome: over ten years, 1,000 women taking the E+P combination might experience seven more cardiovascular events and eight more breast cancers than a similar group of 1,000 women not taking these hormones. Looked at this way, conclusions were clearer, easier to understand and much less alarming – an example of the power of statistics to both confuse and to clarify. Finally, although the reported differences between the intervention and control groups were only marginally statistically significant, the report concluded with what reads as a powerful, definitive statement: "Overall health risks exceeded benefits from use of combined E+P for an average 5.2-year follow-up among healthy postmenopausal US women. **This regimen should not be initiated or**

continued for primary prevention ofcoronary heart disease" ("Writing Group for the Women's Health Initiative").

A critical part of the WHI study design received no attention when it was first reported: the pool of patients selected for evaluation (Reichel). Because the trial was designed to look at outcomes that increase with age, participation was limited to women over the age of 50, with 70 percent over 60 years of age – this meant the majority of study participants were far past menopause when HT began. The WHI study group was considerably older than participants in almost every observational study – for example, the average age of NHS participants was 52.5 years, with 80 percent between 43 and 62 years of age. In retrospect, the concept of initiating HT for the first time in older women more than a decade after menopause should have received much more attention when the trial was designed and when results were first analyzed and released ("Women's Health Initiative Study Group"). Enough younger subjects should have been included so that results could have been analyzed by age and by time since menopause. Failing this, identifying these limitations from the outset would have resulted in different conclusions – and likely a completely different response from women on HT. A major failing of the original interpretation and reporting of the data was the statement that these results of HT in older women should be extended to *all* women. The statement of the WHI project director Jacques Rossouw has had lasting resonance: "the adverse effects of estrogen plus progestin applied to all women, **irrespective of age, ethnicity or disease status"** (Roussouw et al.).

Repercussions

Within 18 months of the WHI report, between half and two-thirds of American women had stopped using HT (Ettinger, Grady et al.; Haas, Kaplan et al.; Kelly et al.; Hersh, "National Use of Postmenopausal Hormone Therapy: Annual Trends"). From telephone and office-based surveys, up to 57 percent of women had heard about the WHI study results from the media or from talking with others, and 74 percent were worried about HT use (Breslau et al.; Rolnick et al.; Ettinger, Grady et al.; Manson, Hsia et al.). And the impact of WHI reporting was sustained: from pharmacy data, the total number of hormone therapy claims dropped by a third by the end of 2002 and by more than 70 percent by 2009 (Ettinger, Wang et al.). (Figure 2.3)

Following the WHI report, professional societies completely reversed their previous position, with new guidelines recommending against HT for prevention of heart disease and advising current users to discontinue use. The U.S. Food and Drug Administration developed a new black box warning that postmenopausal HT should not be used for prevention of CHD and should be used at the lowest dose and the shortest duration for menopausal indications.

Newspaper articles reporting aspects of the WHI continued after the July 2002 report, tapering off over time from 149 major stories in 2002 to only 49 in 2003 (Brown). All this media coverage did a thorough and effective job of reporting the potential negative outcomes of HT use. Not measured or reported was the toll of untreated menopausal symptoms and osteoporosis that resulted from the reported conviction that HT is dangerous. The excessive conservatism engendered by the intense 2002 media presentation of the first WHI results disadvantaged decades of women who unnecessarily suffered severe menopausal symptoms and postmenopausal consequences.

WHI after 2002

After the enormous attention that followed release of the 2002 report, the WHI initiated an endless stream of analyses and re-analyses that continues to the present day. Many of these

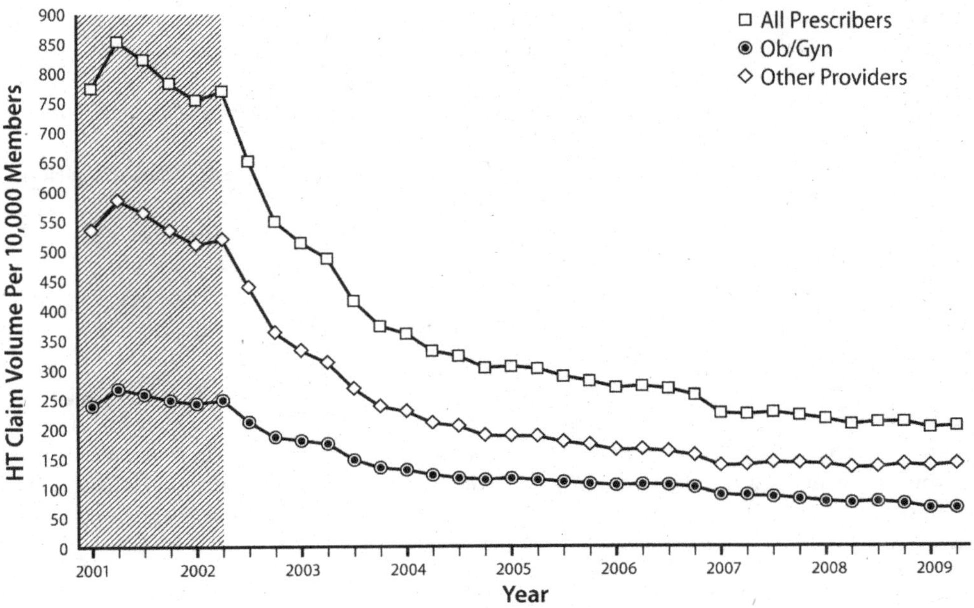

Figure 2.3 Quarterly claim volume per 10,000 covered members, overall by prescriber type. Shaded area indicates period before release of initial WHI results (Ettinger, Wang, et al.)

Source: Reprinted with permission from Wolters Kluwer Health, Inc.

results have important implications for the health and care of women, but no changes were ever made in the initial conservative recommendations to avoid HT. Any change would have required acknowledgement of the need for re-evaluation of the study design and analysis plan, and development of a new approach to information dissemination via a cooperative effort between the WHI team and the media. The review of WHI results which follows shows this never happened.

Hormone Therapy and Heart Disease

In 2003, final analysis of the combined E+P trial was released to little fanfare (Manson, Hsia et al.). Of note, the report was confined to analysis of the coronary heart disease results, and with this new analysis – using the original proposed analytic approach – there was **no** significant increase in CHD risk. The final conclusion was that, "Estrogen plus progestin does not confer cardiac protection and may increase the risk of CHD among healthy postmenopausal women..." No report of secondary outcomes like breast cancer – the stated cause for stopping the original trial and the focus of original reporting – was provided. These results are significantly different than the original 2002 report, but the differences were not addressed in the report and no headlines accompanied its release.

In February 2004, the "estrogen-alone" branch of the HT trial was stopped when estimated hazard ratios showed a small increased risk of stroke and pulmonary embolus but a decreased risk of CHD, breast cancer, and hip fracture. The study was terminated because "the burden of incident disease events was equivalent in the intervention and placebo groups," signaling no overall benefit to study continuation – an example of the application of the risk/benefit instrument (Women's Health Initiative Steering Committee). In striking contrast to the initial 2002 WHI report, response to the publication was muted. Given the hullabaloo that accompanied the original trial release, this was remarkable.

In 2008, the results of stratifying the patients by age and time since menopause were reported with the two HT groups combined in order to provide enough subjects for statistical analysis (Rossouw et al.). **With this pooled HT data, there was no excess absolute risk of CHD.** The small excess risk reported for combined E+P in 2002 was not validated for women below 70 years of age. In fact, CHD risk and total mortality were significantly reduced in women 50–59 years of age who received HT of either kind. Although this re-analysis produced important results supporting the safety and benefits of HT in terms of CHD risk when initiated in younger women, there was no change in recommendations from the study investigators and the response in the medical and lay press was minimal (Parker-Pope).

In 2013, the CHD results of extended follow-up of the WHI were reported. During cumulative follow-up of 13 years, there was no significant change in CHD risk in either the estrogen + progesterone (E+P) or estrogen alone (E) groups. In the E alone trial, lower CHD risk in younger women was suggested compared with the placebo group although this was not quite statistically significant. Again, there was no change in recommendations from the study investigators.

Hormone Therapy and Breast Cancer

In terms of breast cancer, the safety outcome that had received so much attention in 2002, re-analysis of the data showed varying results. With risk factor adjustment, the increased breast cancer risk was no longer statistically significant in a 2006 analysis (Anderson, Chlebowski, and Rossouw). The original finding of increased risk was found to be attributable to prior HT users with a greater cumulative exposure to HT; in younger women, there was no increased breast cancer risk, regardless of prior HT. Further analyses released in 2015 and 2020 showed that in fact, use of E alone was associated with significantly lower breast cancer incidence and lower breast cancer mortality. By contrast, use of combined E + P was associated with a small increase in breast cancer incidence but no significant difference in breast cancer mortality (Chlebowski, Anderson, et al.; Chlebowski, Rohan, et al.). Despite the striking difference between these results and the aggressive and alarming reports of breast cancer risk in 2002, lay press coverage of these reassuring results was virtually non-existent.

Hormone therapy and osteoporosis/fracture risk

The important, beneficial effects of E+P and E alone on fracture risk were reported in 2003 and 2006 (Cauley et al.; Jackson et al.). With both forms of HT, the risk of all fractures was significantly reduced by up to 24 percent, 33 percent for hip fractures. After three years of HT, bone mineral density had increased significantly at the lumbar spine and total hip. In the WHI extended follow-up published in 2013, a significant fracture benefit persisted after 13 years for combined E+P (Manson, Chlebowski et al.).

Hormone therapy: overall impact

In fact, an 18-year follow-up of the WHI study reported that across the board, the HT participants were less likely to die of heart disease, cancer of any kind, or of any other cause than were those in the no-HT control group. When younger women at study initiation – aged 50–59 years – were compared to women aged 70–79 years, all-cause mortality was 40 percent lower for the younger women during the intervention phase and 13 percent lower during 18-year follow-up (Manson, Aragaki, et al.).

In aggregate, these important results should have commanded attention by the media, practicing physicians and the general public, but this never happened. In defense of the WHI team, every publication attempted to balance overall risks and benefits for women but over almost 20 years of reporting, this resulted in over-generalized, conservative recommendations against use of HT in all women (Mooney). A more nuanced approach, matching study findings to individual patient requirements could have optimized application of WHI findings to the benefit of the health of postmenopausal women.

Pushback

Negative reaction to the early WHI reports began as early as 2004 with emphasis on the limitations of applying the results of a study of older postmenopausal women to all women (Goldman; Naftolin et al.). As subsequent analyses were reported, there was increasingly negative commentary on the changing results over time with no corresponding change in conclusions or recommendations. Particularly noted was the delayed reporting that in hysterectomized women treated with E alone, there was a significant reduction in breast cancer risk in all age groups and that re-analysis of the original E+P showed no significant increase in heart disease. Reviewers felt these results modified interpretation of the initial findings and should have revised the conclusions (Stevenson et al.; Rosano et al.; Maclaren and Stevenson). In 2007, a *Wall Street Journal* editorial reported that, "In the five years since federal researchers first unveiled their results, a series of follow-up studies calculated off the same government data found that many of the initial conclusions were premature, indefinite or just plain wrong" (Parker-Pope; Gottlieb). The reaction to the reporting of osteoporosis findings was especially critical since the WHI showed very significant reductions in total fracture risk with HT. A series of follow-up studies showed that women who discontinued postmenopausal HT had significantly increased risk of hip fracture and lower bone density compared with continuous users: women who discontinued HT were 58 percent more likely to have a hip fracture in the following year (Burger et al.; Lobo). Despite these findings, WHI researchers provided no recommendation for HT use to reduce fracture risk.

Beginning ten years after the early release of the WHI findings, evidence-based reviews reported the long-term negative impact of the global reduction in HT, asserting that no definitive reduction in breast cancer incidence after HT termination had been demonstrated, that no relationship with cardiovascular outcomes had been observed and that increases in osteoporotic fractures were definitive and serious (Sturdee and Pines; Shapiro et al.; Cagnacci and Vernier). Specific efforts were requested to reverse the pervasive, negative attitude toward HT that persisted in response to the excessive early media reports. A separate analysis addressed hysterectomized women post removal of the ovaries (Sarrel et al.). Premature onset of estrogen deficiency in this situation is associated with severe risk of bone loss, vasomotor symptoms, mood swings, coronary artery disease, dementia, strokes, and increased overall mortality. Post-ovariectomy status is considered a mandatory indication for hormone replacement therapy. Before the WHI 2002 report, these patients were prescribed HT as standard of care and 90 percent were receiving that treatment. After the WHI report, only one-third of these women were reported to use HT. An analysis of this population based on the WHI report of a 13 per 10,000-year mortality rate in 50–59–year-old hysterectomized and oophorectomized women assigned to placebo estimated that in the ten years after 2002, between 18,601 and 91,160 women died prematurely because of avoidance of estrogen therapy. These authors specifically address the persistent fears of women and their health care providers related to HT that followed the dramatic release of the WHI findings.

In summary, then, these writers contend that over-interpretation and misrepresentation of the WHI findings damaged the health of menopausal women by convincing them and their health care providers that the risks of HT always far exceed any benefits.

Conclusion

Reporting of the initial WHI HT results has had profound, negative impact on the management of women's health. The study was designed to critically evaluate the risks and benefits of HT in the prevention of coronary heart disease in postmenopausal women after multiple observational studies suggested strong potential benefits. The WHI results were the findings of a massive randomized, controlled trial, then and now the research gold standard for evaluating the risks and benefits of specific interventions. What went wrong?

Since the protocol was designed to evaluate primarily the older age group when coronary heart disease manifests in women, the study group of predominantly women over 60 years of age was theoretically appropriate. Unappreciated at the time was the critical importance of hormonal effects in the perimenopausal period so the study population was actually not appropriate to address the hypotheses of the study. This limitation and its impact on interpretation of the study results have never been clearly acknowledged. From the outset, the study relied on an internally created, unvalidated global measure to theoretically assess simultaneous evidence of risks and benefits. The E+P trial was stopped early because of a small measured increase in the incidence of all heart disease measures combined, and of breast cancer when all subjects were analyzed together. This minimal combined finding of lack of benefit and increased risk was determined to necessitate study termination (Mooney).

Results were rolled out in spectacular fashion in separate press conferences, headlined by selected fragments of the trial results. Prominent scientific figures from the WHI team and from the sponsoring National Institutes of Health were interviewed and their pronouncements lent weight to the reports. Media coverage in every setting was intense. All reports began with a headline declaration about increased risks for breast cancer, and this focus increased the impact of the original reporting because at that time, breast cancer was women's greatest health fear (Walsh-Childers, Edwards, and Grobmyer; "Socialstyren Statistic Database"; Velentzis et al.). The WHI team has continued this same analytic approach through now an additional 18 years of results and reporting, with sustained reliance on risks of CHD and breast cancer and the global risk/benefit measure, and limited emphasis on results associated with any other outcomes. Results attributed to the global index are especially concerning since this instrument was developed by the investigators and was never validated. Even when an 18-year follow-up reported that across the board, HT participants were less likely to die of any cause than no-HT controls, there was no WHI statement addressing this very important outcome in the context of the early result reports. Numerous evidence-based reviews and editorials in the medical literature have addressed these limitations, to no avail.

It is not surprising that media reporting of medical research influences popular opinion. We have convincing evidence of this in the persistent belief that vaccines cause autism, initiated by a single false report from a subsequently disbarred physician and sustained media reporting (Wakefield et al.; Smith, Ellenberg, et al.). Contemporaneously, we see daily the impact of media misinformation about Covid-19 (Evanga et al.). Less well appreciated is how distorted reporting of medical risks in the literature can induce persistent, inaccurate beliefs in healthcare providers and regulatory authorities as well as patients. With menopausal HT, the amplified reporting of exaggerated risks from the abbreviated WHI trial promoted major changes in all three spheres that persist to this time: HT decreased by as much as 80 percent with no identified rebound (Gartlehner et al.). Physicians from all medical specialties responded to the 2002 report with a sustained decrease in prescriptions for postmenopausal hormone therapy (Ettinger, Wang et al.). Professional organizations still recommend against the use of systemic HT for the primary prevention of chronic conditions in postmenopausal women, as concluded most recently in the 2017 statement from the USPSTF (Gartlehner et al.). While there is agreement that systemic HT is the most effective treatment for perimenopausal symptoms, recommended use even in this setting is limited (Manson and Kaunitz). All other major professional organizations including the American Heart Association, the American College of Obstetricians and Gynecologists, the Canadian Task Force on Preventive Health Care and the American Academy of Family Physicians still recommend against the use of postmenopausal hormone therapy for prevention of any chronic condition ("Hormone Therapy").

There has been ample opportunity for re-evaluation of this position. As described, subsequent WHI publications with more complete results, and independent analyses in the medical literature cast doubt on the initial narrow interpretation of the data. Imagine how the response by the public and by healthcare providers might differ if the WHI results of very significant decreases in osteoporotic fractures in HT women had been reported as breaking news, since an estimated 10.2 million US adults over 50 have osteoporosis and in women over 55, the hospitalization burden of osteoporotic fractures and related cost is greater than that of heart attack, stroke, or breast cancer (Wright et al.; Singer et al.). What if the results of the 18-year WHI follow-up had been introduced with extensively publicized press conferences and banner headlines (Manson, Aragaki et al.)? After all, the finding that on long-term follow-up, the HT participants were less likely to die of any cause than were no-HT controls is stunning news. At any time, introduction of a more nuanced approach, matching study results to individual patient risk assessments could have optimized application of study findings to the benefit of postmenopausal women. Equally, independent media reporting of the long-term findings of the WHI could have changed opinions and improved care (Russell).

The WHI story is compelling evidence of how distorted reporting of medical risks can promote persistent false information with sustained, negative impact on medical care and public health. Scientists and physicians can be overly committed to their research; with the WHI, a persistent attachment to the original study design substantially hindered dissemination of important positive study results. Members of the scientific community have an obligation to communicate accurately with the public through the news media. With the WHI, the enormous and sustained media response to preliminary, minimal study findings began with the investigators, who promoted their results as a research breakthrough with dire warnings whose impact persists to this day (Traish, Vance, and Morgentaler). Journalists often emphasize the dramatic over the ordinary when reporting medical research results (Moore). With the WHI, journalists relied on the information as it was presented by the investigators with little evidence that the actual findings of the research were ever explored or reported. The public relies on health-related information as reported in the media. The response to WHI reporting shows the importance of accuracy and integrity at every level of this process. Exaggerated reporting of medical risks as happened with the WHI has resulted in major, sustained damage to the health of menopausal women.

Works cited

"Alarm over HRT Cancer Risk." *Sydney Morning Herald*, September 10, 2002.

Allin, J. "Premarin Timeline 1686-1998." *Fund for Horses*, October 11, 2019, https://fundforhorses.org/2019/10/11/premarin-timeline-1686-1998/.

Anderson, G. L., R. T. Chlebowski, and J. E. Rossouw. "Prior Hormone Therapy and Breast Cancer Risk in the Women's Health Initiative Randomized Trial of Estrogen and Progestin." *Maturitas*, vol. 55, 2006, pp. 107–15.

Baber, R. "Hormone Alert for Cancer: How Not to Release Data from your RCT." *O&G Magazine*, vol. 18, no. 1, 2016, www.ogmagazine.org.au/18/1-18/hormone-alert-cancer-not-release-data-rct/.

Booth, C. C. "Medical Communication: The Old and the New. The Development of Medical Journals in Britain." *BMJ*, vol. 285, 1982, pp. 105–8.

Breslau, E. S., W. W. Davis, L. Doner, E. J. Eisner, N. R. Goodman, Meissner, et al. "The Hormone Therapy Dilemma: Women Respond." *J Am Med Women's Assoc*, vol. 58, 2003, pp. 33–43.

Brown, S. "Shock, Terror and Controversy: How the Media Reacted to the Women's Health Initiative." *Climacteric*, vol. 15, no. 3, 2012, pp. 275–80.

Burger, H. G., A. H. MacLennan, K.-E. Huang, et al. "Evidence-based Assessment of the Impact of the WHI on Women's Health." *Climacteric*, vol. 15, 2012, pp. 281–7.

Bush, T. L., E. Barrett-Connor, L. D. Cowan, et al. "Cardiovascular Mortality and Non-contraceptive Use of Estrogen in Women: Results from the Lipid Research Clinics Program Follow-Up Study." *Circulation*, vol. 75, 1987, pp. 1102–9.

Cagnacci, A., and M. Venier. "The Controversial History of Hormone Replacement Therapy." *Medicina*, vol. 55, no. 9, 2019, p. 602.

Cassedy, J. H. "The Flourishing and Character of Early American Medical Journalism, 1797-1860." *J Hist Med Allied Sciences*, vol. 38, no. 2, 1983, pp. 135–50.

Cauley, J. A., J. Robbins, Z. Chen, et al. "Effects of Estrogen plus Progestin on Risk of Fracture and Bone Mineral Density. The Women's Health Initiative Randomized Trial." *JAMA*, vol. 290, no. 13, 2003, pp. 1729–38.

Chlebowski, R. T., G. L. Anderson, A. K. Aragaki, et al. "Association of Menopausal Hormone Therapy with Breast Cancer Incidence and Mortality during Long-term Follow-up of the Women's Health Initiative Randomized Clinical Trials." *JAMA*, vol. 324, no. 4, 2020, pp. 369–80.

Chlebowski, R. T., T. E. Rohan, J. E. Manson, et al. "Breast Cancer after use of Estrogen Plus Progestin and Estrogen Alone: Analyses of Data from 2 Women's Health Initiative Randomized Clinical Trials." *JAMA Oncology*, vol. 1, no. 3, 2015, pp. 296–305.

"Estrogen Is Linked to Uterine Cancer." *The New York Times*, December 4, 1975, www.nytimes.com/1975/12/04/archives/new-jersey-pages-estrogen-is-linked-to-uterine-cancer-use-of.html.

Ettinger, B., H. K. Genant, C. E. Cann, et al. "Long-term Estrogen Replacement Therapy Prevents Bone Loss and Fractures." *Ann Inter Med*, vol. 102, 1985, pp. 319–24.

Ettinger, B., D. Grady, A. N. Tosteson, et al. "Effect of the Women's Health Initiative on Women's Decisions to Discontinue Postmenopausal Hormone Therapy." *Obstet Gynecol*, vol. 102, 2003, pp. 1225–32.

Ettinger, B., S. M. Wang, R. S. Leslie, et al. "Evolution of Postmenopausal Hormone Therapy between 2002 and 2009." *Menopause*, vol. 19, no 6, 2012, pp. 610–15.

Evanga, S., M. Lynas, S. Adams, et al. "Coronavirus Misinformation: Quantifying Sources and Themes in the COVID-19 'infodemic'." The Cornell Alliance for Science, Department of Global Development, Cornell University, Ithaca, N.Y.

Gallup. "Americans Rate Confidence in Doctors." December 10, 2002. www.gallup.com/poll/7369/Americans-Rate-Confidence-Doctors.aspx.

Gambrell, R. D. "Use of Progestogen Therapy." *Amer J Ob Gyn*, vol. 156, no. 5, 1987, pp. 1304–13.

Gartlehner, G., S. Patel, M. Viswanathan, et al. "Hormone Therapy for the Primary Prevention of Chronic Conditions in Postmenopausal Women." An Evidence Review for the U.S. Preventive Services Task Force. *Evidence Synthesis*, no. 155, 2017. AHRQ publication 15-05227-EF-1.

Goldman, J. A. "The Women's Health Initiative 2004 – Review and Critique." *MedGenMed*, vol. 6, no. 3, 2004, pp. 65–92.

Gottlieb, S. "Stop the War on Drugs." WSJ Updated17 December 2007. www.wsj.com › articles.

Grady, D., S. M. Rubin, D. B. Petitti, et al. "Hormone Therapy to Prevent Disease and Prolong Life in Postmenopausal Women." *Ann Intern Med*, vol. 117, 1992, pp. 1016–37.

Graham, D. C. "Ovarian Failure and the Menopause." *Can Med Assoc J*, vol. 92, 1965, pp. 982–3.
Greenblatt, R. B. "Estrogen Therapy for Postmenopausal Females." *N Eng J Med*, vol. 272, 1965, pp. 305–8.
Haas, J. S., B. Geller, D. L. Miglioretti, et al. "Changes in Newspaper Coverage about Hormone Therapy with the Release of new Medical Evidence." *J Gen Intern Med*, vol. 21, 2006, pp. 304–9.
Haas, J. S., C. P. Kaplan, E. P. Gerstenberger, and K. Kerlikowske. "Changes in the Use of Postmenopausal Hormone Therapy after the Publication of Clinical Trial Results." *Ann Intern Med*, vol. 140, no. 3, 2004, pp. 184–8.
Hersh, A. L., M. L. Stefanick, and R. S. Stafford. "National Use of Postmenopausal Hormone Therapy: Annual Trends and Response to Recent Evidence." *JAMA*, vol. 291, no. 1, 2004, pp. 47–53.
Hesse, B. W., D. E. Nelson, G. L. Kreps, et al. "Trust and Sources of Health Information: The Impact of the Internet and its Implications for Healthcare Providers: Findings from the First Health Information National Trends Survey." *Arch Intern Med*, vol. 165, 2005, pp. 2618–24. PMID:16344419.
"Hormonal Contraception and Post-menopausal Hormonal Therapy." International Agency for Research on Cancer (IARC). *IARC Monographs on the Evaluation of Carcinogenic Risks to Humans*, no. 72. IARC Working Group on the Evaluation of Carcinogenic Risks to Humans. Lyon (FR), 1999.
"Hormone Replacement Study Halted." CNN.com/HEALTH. August 14, 2002.
"Hormone Therapy for the Primary Prevention of Chronic Conditions in Postmenopausal Women." US Preventive Services Task Force Recommendation Statement. *JAMA*, vol. 318, no. 22, 2017, pp. 2224–33.
"Hormone Treatment Is Called Harmful: Menopause Study Cites Health Risks." *The Washington Post*, July 10, 2002, p. A1.
"HRT Linked to Breast Cancer." BBC News. Health. July 10, 2002.
Jackson, R. D., J. Wactawski-Wende, A. Z. LaCroix, et al. "Effects of Conjugated Equine Estrogen on Risk of Fractures and BMD in Postmenopausal Women with Hysterectomy: Results from the Women's Health Initiative Randomized Trial." *J Bone Miner Res*, vol. 21, no. 6, 2006, pp. 817–28.
Kelly, J. P., D. W. Kaufman, L. Rosenberg, et al. "Use of Postmenopausal Hormone Therapy since the Women's Health Initiative Findings." *Pharmacoepidemiology and Drug Safety*, vol. 14, 2005, pp. 837–42. PMID:15812877.
Lindsay, R., D. M. Hart, C. Forrest, et al. "Prevention of Spinal Osteoporosis in Oophorectomized Women." *Lancet*, vol. 2, 1980, pp. 1151–4.
Lobo, R. A. "Where Are We 10 Years after the Women's Health Initiative." *J Clin Endocrinol Metab*, vol. 98, 2013, pp. 1771–80.
Locke, J. "A Pill that Prolongs the Prime of Life." *Maclean's Magazine*, August 7, 1965.
Lomangino, K. "Headline vs. Study: A Battle Where Readers Often Lose." Health News Review.org. November 15, 2016,www. Healthnewsreview.org/2016/11/heath-news-headlines-vs-what-the-study-found/.
Maclaren, K. and J. C. Stevenson. "Primary Prevention of Cardiovascular Disease with HRT." *Women's Health*, vol. 8, 2012, pp. 63–74.
Manson, J. E, A. K. Aragaki, J. E. Rossouw, et al. "Menopausal Hormone Therapy and Long-term All-cause and Cause-specific Mortality: The Women's Health Initiative Randomized Trials." *JAMA*, vol. 318, no. 10, pp. 927–38.
Manson, J. E., R. T. Chlebowski, M. L. Stefanick, et al. "Menopausal Hormone Therapy and Health Outcomes during the Interventions and Postintervention and Extended Post-stopping Phases of the Women's Health Initiative Randomized Trials." *JAMA*, vol. 310, 2013, pp. 1353–68.
Manson, J. E., J. Hsia, et al. "Estrogen plus Progestin and the Risk of Coronary Heart Disease." *New England J Med*, vol. 349, 2003, pp. 523–34.
Manson, J. E. and A. M. Kaunitz. "Menopause Management-getting Clinical Care Back on Track." *New England J Med*, vol. 374, 2016, pp. 803–6.
Marks, N. E. and D. S. Shinberg. "Socioeconomic Status Differences in Hormone Therapy." *Amer J Epid*, vol. 148, 1998, pp. 581–93.
Meema, H. E. and S. Meema. "Prevention of Postmenopausal Osteoporosis by Hormone Treatment of the Menopause." *Canadian Med Assoc J*, vol. 99, 1968, pp. 248–51.
"Menopause, as Brought to You by Big Pharma." Natasha Singer and Duff Wilson, December 12, 2009, *The New York Times*, www.nytimes.com/2009/12/13/business/13drug.html?unlocked_article_code
Mooney, C. "Blinded by Science: How 'Balanced' Coverage Lets the Scientific Fringe Hijack Reality." *CJR*, vol. 43, no. 4, 2004, http://blogs.discovermagazine.com/intersection/2010/01/15/blinded-by-science-how-balanced-coverage-lets-the-scientific-fringe-hijack-reality/.

Moore, A. "Bad Science in the Headlines: Who Takes Responsibility when Science is Distorted in the Mass Media?" *EMBO Rep*, vol. 7, 2006, pp. 1193–5.

Naftolin, F., H. S. Taylor, R. Karas, et al. "The Women's Health Initiative Could Not Have Detected Cardioprotective Effects of Starting Hormone Therapy during the Menopausal Transition." *Fertil Steril*, vol. 81, no. 6, 2004, pp. 1498–1501.

National Institutes of Health. "NHLBI Stops Trial of Estrogen Plus Progestin Due to Increased Breast Cancer Risk, Lack of Overall Benefit." Press Release, July 10, 2002. www.sciencedaily.com/releases/2002/07/020710081413.htm.

Parker-Pope, T. "How NIH Misread Hormone Study in 2002." *Wall Street Journal*, July 9, 2007.

Reichel, C. "How to Spot Bias in Randomized Clinical Trials." *Journalist's Resource*, February 11, 2020, https://journalistsresource.org/politics-and-government/bias-clinical-trials-research/.

Rolnick, S. J., R. A. Kopher, T. A. DeFor, M. E. Kelley. "Hormone Use and Patient Concerns after the findings of the Women's Health Initiative." *Menopause*, vol. 12, no. 4, 2005, pp. 399–404. PMID: 16037754.

Rosano, G. M. C., S. Maffei, M. G. Andreassi, et al. "Hormone Replacement Therapy and Cardioprotection: A New Dawn?" A statement of the Study Group on Cardiovascular Disease in Women of the Italian Society of Cardiology. *J Cardiovasc Med* (Hagerstown), vol. 10, no. 1, 2009, 85–92.

Rossouw, J. E., R. L. Prentice, J. E. Manson, et al. "Postmenopausal Hormone Therapy and Risk of Cardiovascular Disease by Age and Years since Menopause." Published erratum appears in *JAMA* vol. 299, 2008, p. 1426. *JAMA*, vol. 297, 2007, pp. 1465–77.

Russell, C. "Covering Controversial Science: Improving Reporting on Science and Public Policy." *Science and the Media*, edited by D. Kennedy and G. Overholser, American Academy of Arts & Sciences, 2010, pp. 37–41.

Sarrel, P. M., V. Y. Njike, V. Vinante, D. L. Katz. "The Mortality Toll of Estrogen Avoidance: An Analysis of Excess Deaths among Hysterectomized Women aged 50 to 59 Years." *Amer J Public Health*, vol. 103, 2013, pp. 1583–8.

Scott, J. "You Need Not Fear the Menopause." *Ladies' Home Journal*, vol. 63, 1963, pp. 33–191.

Shapiro, S., T. J. de Villiers, A. Pines, et al. "Risk and Benefits of Hormone Therapy: Has Medical Dogma Now Been Overturned?" *Climacteric*, vol. 17, 2014, pp. 215–22.

Singer, A., A. Exuzides, L. Spangler, et al. "Burden of Illness for Osteoporotic Fractures Compared with other Serious Diseases among Postmenopausal Women in the United States." *Mayo Clin Proc*, vol. 90, no. 1, 2015, pp. 53–62.

Smith, M. J., S. S. Ellenberg, L. M. Bell, et al. "Media Coverage of the Measles-mumps-rubella Vaccine and Autism Controversy and its Relationship to MMR Immunization Rates in the United States." *Pediatrics*, vol. 121, no. 4, 2008, pp. e836-e843.

Smith, D. C., R. Prentice, D. J. Thompson, W. L. Herrmann. "Association of Exogenous Estrogen and Endometrial Carcinoma." *New England J Med*, vol. 293, 1975, pp. 1164–7.

"Socialstyrelsen Statistic Database for Drugs." 2010 and 2015, www.socialstyrelsen.se/statistik/statistikefteramne/lakemedel.

Stampfer, M. J., G. A. Colditz, W. C. Willett, et al. "Postmenopausal Estrogen Therapy and Cardiovascular Disease. Ten-year Follow-up from the Nurses' Health Study." *New England J Med*, vol. 325, 1991, pp. 756–62.

Stampfer, M. J., W. C. Willett, G. A. Colditz, et al. "A Prospective Study of Postmenopausal Estrogen Therapy and Coronary Heart Disease." *New England J Med*, vol. 313, 1985, pp. 1044–9.

Stefanick, M. I. "Estrogens and Progestins: Background and History, Trends in Use and Guidelines and Regimens Approved by the US Food and Drug Administration." *Amer J Med*, vol. 118, no. 12, 2005, pp. 64–73.

Stevenson, J. C., H. N. Hodis, J. H. Pickar, R. A. Lobo. "Coronary Heart Disease and Menopause Management. The Swinging Pendulum of HRT." *Athersclerosis*, vol. 207, 2009, pp. 336–40.

"Study is Halted Over Rise Seen in Cancer Risk." *The New York Times*, July 9, 2002, A-1.

Sturdee, D. W., A. Pines; IMS Writing Group. "Updated IMS Recommendations on Postmenopausal Hormone Therapy and Preventive Strategies for Midlife Health." *Climacteric*, vol. 14, 2011, pp. 302–20.

The Women's Health Initiative Steering Committee. "Effects of Conjugated Equine Estrogen in Postmenopausal Women with Hysterectomy: The Women's Health Initiative Randomized Controlled Trial." *JAMA*, vol. 291, 2004, pp. 1701–12.

The Women's Health Initiative Study Group. "Design of the Women's Health Initiative Clinical Trial and Observational Study." *Control Clin Trials*, vol. 19, 1998, pp. 61–109.

Traish, A. M., J. C. Vance, and A. Morgentaler. "Overselling Hysteria: The Role of the Media and Medical Journals in Promoting Questionable Risks – A Case Study of the Testosterone Controversy." *EMBO Report*, vol. 18, no. 1, 2017, pp. 11–17.

Tyrer, L. "Introduction of the Pill and its Impact." *Contraception*, vol. 59, suppl 1, 1999, pp. 11S–16S.

Velentzis, L. S., E. Banks, F. Sitas, et al. "Use of Menopausal Hormone Therapy and Bioidentical Hormone Therapy in Australian Women 50 to 69 Years of Age: Results from a National, Cross-sectional Study." *PLoS ONE*, vol. 11, no. 3, 2016, pp. e0146494.

Wakefield, A. J. "Autism, Inflammatory Bowel Disease and MMR Vaccine." *The Lancet*, vol. 351, no. 9106, 1998, p. 908.

Wakefield, A. J., S. H. Murch, A. Anthony, et al. "Ileal-lymphoid-nodular hyperplasia, non-specific Colitis, and Pervasive Developmental Disorder in Children." *The Lancet*, vol. 351, 1998, pp. 637–41 (retracted).

Walsh-Childers, K., H. Edwards, S. Grobmyer. "Covering Women's Greatest Health Fear." *Health Communications*, vol. 26, 2011, pp. 209–20.

Watkins, E. S. "Changing Rationales for Long-term Hormone Replacement Therapy in America, 1960-2000." *Health and History*, vol. 4, no. 1, 2002, pp. 20–36.

"What's a Woman to Do?" *Newsweek*, July 21, 2002.

Wilson, R. A. "The Roles of Estrogen and Progesterone in Breast and Genital Cancer." *JAMA*, vol. 182, 1962, pp. 327–31.

Wilson, R. A. *Feminine Forever*. 1st edition, M. Evans and Company, Inc., 1966.

Wilson, R. A. and T. A. Wilson. "The Fate of the Non-treated Postmenopausal Woman: A Plea for the Maintenance of Adequate Estrogen from Puberty to the Grave." *J Amer Geriatrics Soc*, vol. 11, 1963, pp. 347–62.

Wright, N. C., A. C. Looker, K. G. Saag, et al. "The Recent Prevalence of Osteoporosis and Low Bone Mass in the United States Based on Bone Mineral Density at the Femoral Neck or Lumbar Spine." *J Bone Miner Res*, vol. 29, no. 11, 2014, pp. 2520–2526.

"Writing Group for the Women's Health Initiative Investigators: Risks and Benefits of Estrogen plus Progestin in Healthy Postmenopausal Women: Principal Results from the Women's Health Initiative Randomized Controlled Trial." *JAMA*, vol. 288, 2002, pp. 321–33.

Ziel, H. K. and W.D. Finkle. "Increased Risk of Endometrial Carcinoma among Users of Conjugated Estrogens." *New England J Med*, vol. 293, 1975, pp. 1167–70.

3

CLIMATE HEALTH IS HUMAN HEALTH

Working through eco-anxiety with the written word in print and digital media

Carol-Ann Farkas and Shoshannah Bryn Jones Square

Coverage of climate change and environmental degradation has become inescapable in popular discourse. We are responding to the very real threat to our planet much as we do when confronted with terrifying illnesses: turning to our media to express our worry, our apprehension about potential loss and suffering – our *eco-anxiety*. In journalistic coverage and commentary, in print and online news, magazines, blogs, and social media, we struggle to understand our planet's condition: what must be done, how must it be done, and who is responsible for doing it? As with disease, we also use these media to share advice to promote wellness, to take action, to learn what to do, to heal what is sick and injured. In this chapter, we examine how the written word in print media, from traditional to digital, helps us engage with the climate emergency as a collective illness experience. We focus on how reading and writing create a shared discourse, a kind of large-scale support and activist group wherein we learn how to treat, manage, and cope with "landsickness" and eco-anxiety. This discursive space is also a communal space in which we can help one another understand our interconnectedness – that caring for the wellbeing of our imperiled planet is how we care for our own wellbeing, that we can (must) manage our eco-anxiety and eco-grief by changing how we live, advocating for political and economic change, and treating the natural world as an entity deserving of protection and compassion.

In this evolving discourse, writers and their audiences are engaged in a process of co-construction – going beyond a literal, concrete heuristic of problem/solution to a re-conceptualization of our identities and our relationships to one another and our planet. Sharing information and stories through the texts we read and write is a communicative, communal response that promotes healing care at the individual, community, and we hope, global level.

Print is dead, long live "print"!

It used to be that, in order to share knowledge and experience, to read or write about any issue, was to engage with ink on paper. That's what used to be. The development of digital media has made print historical; "print" is actual – what we can *do* with the written word *now* matters more than how, or whether, those words are materially bound. Technological innovation has

 DOI: 10.4324/9781003007661-5

driven a process of "*remediation*," whereby "traditional print genres have been imported into new media or [have evolved] into variants enabled by the affordances of new media" (Luzón and Pérez-Llantada 5). We have become used to the idea that making and sharing the written word is a process wherein varied "media are continually commenting on, reproducing, and replacing each other" (Bolter and Grusin 55). If the electronic version of a given written text hasn't entirely supplanted its print origins, it's becoming ever more rare to find such work *only* in print form. But the conventions of traditional print still persist in the digital forms of e-books, journal articles, and news "papers" even as our experience of those publications has become layered with images, video, music, and the constant chatter of social media.

We started this chapter in the spring of 2020 as our respective nations, Canada and the United States, were reeling under the onslaught of Covid-19. The role of print – as a technology of ink on paper – has been undergoing tremendous change in our culture in response to the rise of electronic media, but up until a few months ago, print was still a ubiquitous technology, especially in academic life. Then the surreal disruption of Covid, and so many of the habits and rituals that were benign and comforting suddenly became fraught with mortal peril. The immediate impact on this project was an ironic one: we're assigned a chapter on the physical medium of print just as the whole world has been mandated to Stop. Touching. Things. Bookstore, office copier, library, favorite cafe with just the right balance of people and noise, all shuttered; the articles we would have printed out and marked up, the books we would have bought or borrowed, suddenly inaccessible; the marginalia we would have scribbled, the pages we would have dog-eared and spilled tea and cookie crumbs on; the ink stains we would have had on fingers and clothes – our seemingly ingrained relationship to print as a physical, tactile, bodily experience situated within a network of spatial and social connections just had to *stop*.

In response to which, many of us concerned about climate change would shrug ruefully – what's bad for the medium of print is good news for the preservation of trees. That is, the modern environmental movement has always needed, and will continue to need, to make its case with *words*; but perhaps the days when those words needed to be printed on the dead residue of that which we've been trying to save are coming to an end. Our concern here is, therefore, to be as expansive as possible in our conceptualization of "print." Since both experts and lay people engage in environmental discourse as a discourse of care, the written word is indispensable to their efforts, and what drives their choice of technology is pragmatic consideration for access, timeliness, and availability, as much as (more so than) loyalty to, or idealism about, traditional print versus its digital manifestation.

At its origins in the early- to mid-20th century, the modern environmental movement had no option but to use print media – from books, newspapers, and magazines to newsletters, posters, and fundraising materials – as the conduits for translating analysis and theory into physical presence and action, providing the communicative means to teach and organize (Ogrodnik and Staggenborg). Now, in the contemporary media landscape of the early 21st century, "talking" about the climate emergency is a discursive process that unfolds across platforms and genres, and traditional hard-copy is usually found "remediated" (if not replaced) in a digital version, existing in a symbiotic tangle of links with TED talks, YouTube channels, and social media posts combining photos, links, commentary, and the telegraphy of hash-tagging. Of course, traditional print still has relevance. Readers of all ages continue to enjoy books and magazines printed on paper purchased at brick-and-mortar bookstores; older readers are more likely to pay for subscription to print news ("Print vs Digital Subscribers") but have come to favor e-readers, in no small part because of the adjustability of font size; Gen-Z or millennials might log a great deal of screen time, but if they want to read a book, they prefer it in print (Grady).

When it comes to the development and sharing of ideas about environmental issues, print still has a significant role to play, but as one vital media tool among many. This is especially the case in reaching younger audiences. The most compelling demands in the contemporary environmental movement are coming from teens and younger adults who are not only "deeply concerned with social, political, and environmental issues" but also "fully prepared to do something about them" (Day). Activists in their twenties, even their teens, are using every available platform to educate, "influence," and mobilize, from "Fridays for the Future" to the Slack group "Zero Hour," to social media, podcasts...and books (Jarvis). For example, Margolin's *Youth to Power*, "her instruction manual for young people who want to become activists" (Hurwitz), exists in print form and in the "remediated" form of an e-book. Choice of medium is not "either/or," it's "both/and": savvy youth activists understand that important messages must span *all* media. As Margolin's sister-activist Andrea Alejandra Gonzales observes, "The media – newspapers, magazines, TV shows, radio shows, blogs, online videos – shape the cultural narrative, the stories we tell, and the way we perceive the world around us...we as youth have the power to shape the media and, by default, the hearts and minds of millions of people... With media attention, one small action can spread into a worldwide movement that changes everything" (122–35).

Perhaps the most influential youth activist currently is Greta Thunberg, who embarked on her "skolstrejk för klimatet" (school strike for the climate) in 2018 when she was just 16. As Albrecht observes, Thunberg "represents all those of her generation [who] have no material stake in the present and can see with complete clarity that, with business as usual, they will have no stake in the future either" (28). Thunberg has rallied more than one million students to join her in protests "against climate change inaction" and is fearlessly outspoken in pointing out our failings as a society, and failures of leadership:

> Since our leaders are behaving like children, we will have to take the responsibility that they should have taken long ago. . . . We have to understand what the older generation has dealt to us, what mess they have created that we have to clean up and live with. We have to make our voices heard.
>
> *(qtd. in Day)*

A protest that began "analogue" soon went viral, thanks in large part to the passion and charismatic relentlessness with which Thunberg delivers her message across all possible media platforms.

At the same time, while Thunberg has been an instinctive adept with those digital media that privilege immediacy and impact, for more depth and thoroughness of an issue such as climate change activism, readers still rely on traditional journalism, even as that medium is forced to evolve beyond its print origins. For example, the United Kingdom's *Guardian* is currently one of the leaders in coverage of environmental issues; it has positioned itself as unabashedly biased in its commitment to addressing climate change, calling on both its readership and its competition to take immediate, drastic action (Hertsgaard and Pope). Its Environment section features ongoing, harrowing news coverage along with frequent, urgent editorials from activists such as writer George Monbiot and long-standing climate journalist Bill McKibben. *The Guardian*'s editors understand the power of the written word to reach readers; they also understand the value of combining remediated "print" with the expanded "affordances" of digital news, including gut wrenching photos, video, and podcasts, and abundant hyperlinks to additional sources. *The Guardian* had a print subscription of 138,000 per day in 2018 and was reporting a drop in print sales of as much as 39 percent at the height of the pandemic in May

2020 (Waterson; Sweney); however, as of June 2020, *The Guardian*'s digital edition reached 35.2 million readers per month (GNM Press Office). The lesson here is that the written word is indispensable in allowing a range of audiences to learn, and respond to, climate change, even as our means of disseminating those words is expanding to include, and exceed, the capacity of traditional print media.

Similar to journalistic and activist writing about environmental issues, writers in the relatively new fields of eco-literature and criticism reach their readership in the "pages" of literary magazines found both online and in hard copy (*Ecotone, Conjunction*, or *The Dark Mountain Project*). Print sources are our connection to the history of ideas and activism within the environmental movement: Rachel Carson's *Silent Spring, The Whole Earth Catalogue*, Al Gore's *Inconvenient Truth*, and *Adbusters*. That print history evokes the sensibility and values of a pre-digital age when our experience of place and time was more steady and present. It has become a common complaint that to engage with digital media is to be over-stimulated, to have our attention fractured. Our online discourse is now mediated by the very entities we hold responsible for environmental degradation, and even as we might use those entities to learn and communicate, we are being used in return – tracked, marketed to, branded, and, inevitably, distracted. Picking up a physical book or literary journal is a way to unplug from the machinery of digital media and engage with a legacy of like-minded artists and activists. Whether we are reading or writing about the environment, the act of sharing ideas in a non-electronic way is, in itself, an environmentalist practice, a practice of a certain kind of resistance (Odell).

And yet, as a technology for environmental discourse – the space wherein we learn, commiserate, and motivate one another to care for the planet – "print" has arguably become more useful, democratic, and hence more relevant than traditional print. The evocative, literary exploration of eco-grief motivating *The Dark Mountain Project* finds its ideal expression in the "uncivilized" medium of books, yet the Project's creators can't avoid the realities of trying to reach an anti-capitalist and anti-materialistic audience who can't, or won't, buy print ("About – Dark Mountain"). There must be a website with the Project's book and manifesto – rejecting the Anthropocene worldview – available online.

Take this chapter as another example. Due to the exigencies of the pandemic, this project would not have been feasible without digital media. At the same time, while most of our secondary, scholarly sources were journal articles that we accessed electronically, the conventions governing the publication of those sources are still rooted firmly in traditional print culture, as is the book in which this chapter currently appears. And in order to make or use such sources, one must have highly specialized training to navigate scholarly discourse – to write and read it and to know where to find it – and have an institutional affiliation to access specialized databases and get past prohibitively-expensive paywalls. Print culture in general, and academic print culture in particular, entails relationships to time, place, and status that bar entry for all but a privileged few.

Most pressingly, academic print publication is simply too slow to keep pace with climate change or the other drastic upheavals that characterize our historical moment. In just the past four years, the United States has been a morass of political divisiveness and social injustice; Brexit has upended the unity of the European Union; climate science has revealed that we are on the brink of environmental catastrophe, revivifying environmental activism while also provoking the new phenomena of eco-anxiety and eco-grief; and we are in the grip of a devastating global pandemic. Scholars write as thoughtfully and urgently as they can about these issues, but (1) what reaches the largest audiences *faster* is writing in the so-called "popular," non-academic press, and (2) increasingly, these audiences encounter written analysis and argument electronically as part of a highly textured, multi-genre environment of digital (online) media.

In the case of print as a medium for scholarly study of climate change, academic writers and readers have historically been privileged to experience time and urgency very differently from those experiencing immediate threat to their lived environment. The kind of scholarship that wends its stately way into print is that which values, and fetishizes, "systematic and rigorous articulation" even as it delicately avoids radical solutions (Boscov-Ellen 157, f6). As Boscov-Ellen points out in his critique of the discourse of climate ethics, it is not surprising that "activist knowledge is often ahead" of scholarly research: "[P]erhaps activists and front-line communities more accurately understand the dynamics involved in climate change, even if these understandings are not always systematically and rigorously articulated, because their lives [are affected] in ways rather remote" from most scholars (157). The same privileged conditions – of education, class, race, sex, and culture – that allow scholars to theorize social and environmental issues might also insulate them from the fullest grasp of the scope of those issues. The resulting analyses, as Boscov-Ellen drily observes, are not

> simply wrong, but… misleadingly incomplete and abstract; they fail both to interrogate the historical origins and ongoing systemic reinforcement of these disparities in wealth and power and to explore the complex ways in which these systemic processes are intrinsically intertwined with climate change. [Such] analytical blinders lead to inappropriate solutions.
>
> *(158–9)*

The tradition of print as *the* medium for scholarly publication has reified an epistemology that is oriented to the concerns of white, Western, patriarchal culture. It is a tradition of indifference (if not hostility) to other forms of creating and sharing knowledge, a tradition of exclusion of voices from Black, Brown, and Indigenous cultures (Hall and Tandon 6). At the time of writing this chapter, the Covid pandemic has underscored the pervasiveness of systemic inequality, especially along economic and racial lines; climate activists have, in turn, taken advantage of a growing concern for social justice by reminding us that the same conditions that drive inequality drive climate change, compounding the vulnerability of populations to oppression and deprivation (Watson et al.). These connections have been made in print and depend on print as the site of careful investigation and analysis. However, when we consider which media are mobilizing protest, especially among younger people, and which arguments have sparked outrage and a collective demand for change, we turn to journalistic coverage updated hourly, to cell-phone video footage taken by ordinary non-specialist people in the midst of confrontation, and to the rallying memes of activists posting on varied social media along with details of how and where we must show up to take action.

Obviously, online and social media create discursive problems even as they solve others. The ability to communicate obsessively, unreflectively, around the clock has made possible manipulative misinformation campaigns and conspiracy theories, which "pose a threat to democratic systems" (Sternisko et al. 4). If traditional media had a gate-keeping function that was also exclusionary, now digital media have become something of a free-for-all, and if social justice activists rely on social media to organize, so do white supremacists and fascists. But the near-ubiquity of digital media crucially allows voices to be heard in ways that would simply not be possible in print as a discursive space that is often barricaded explicitly (pay walls, institutional affiliation) and implicitly (the privilege of whiteness, wealth, and masculinity upon which those institutions are founded). Meanwhile, calls for activism and resistance in the social and environmental justice movements are coming from passionate, informed leaders who notably do *not* come from privileged groups (Watts and Vidal): "the challenge of climate change has so far largely been taken up by those least responsible for causing it – particularly indigenous groups and poor people in the South, many of them women" (Boscov-Ellen 167).

The leaders to watch now are not older white liberals critiquing from the safe remove of academic journals and monographs but grassroots activists – "BIPOC" (black, indigenous, people of color), queer, and *young* – and while their charisma and persuasiveness depends on eloquence in both speech and writing, they do not – cannot – rely on traditional print media to reach and inspire their audiences.

What are eco-anxiety and eco-grief, and how can "print" help us cope with these negative "earth emotions"?

While the recognition that "climate health is public health" has been "news" since *The Lancet*'s 2015 Report on Health and Climate Change, the connection has been integral to environmentalist thinking for much longer, acquiring greater urgency with the seemingly relentless rise in average global temperatures. As Horwitz and Parkes put it, "humans are 'part of,' and not 'apart from,'" the natural world. Consequently, our health depends on "landhealth" or "landsickness" (Leopold qtd. in Horwitz and Parkes). Landsickness will manifest as "somaterratic illness," harm to physical wellness caused by damage to the ecosystem. And beyond the effects of climate change that are most immediately experienced, our *awareness* of profound danger takes a toll on mental wellbeing, too, in the form of "psychoterratic illness." Albrecht coined the associated term "solastalgia" to describe "pain or distress" when there is the "lived experience of the physical desolation of home" (S95). As the *Lancet* Report put it, "solastalgia is connected to 'dis-ease,' or a lack of ease due to a hostile environment that a person is powerless to do anything about." Galway et al. add that, "[g]iven the speed and scale of climate change alongside biodiversity loss, pollution, deforestation, unbridled resource extraction, and other environmental challenges, more and more people will experience solastalgia" as we are forced to confront "the links between human and ecosystem health, specifically, the cumulative impacts of climatic and environmental change on mental, emotional, and spiritual health" (Galway et al.).

While the more poetic and evocative term, solastalgia, has not caught on in lay discourse, the more self-evident concept of "eco-anxiety" has. As Clayton explains, climate change "is a real threat, so it is rational to experience some worry; it is ongoing and developing, so simple adaptation to the change is not completely possible; it is uncertain, so anxiety may be a more and more common response than fear" (74). If the cause of eco-anxiety might be relatively novel, its effects on us are not; like anxiety as understood more generally, eco-anxiety affects our mood, energy levels, and cognition, all of which, in turn, affect our ability to cope with stressors. To be anxious is to be in a constant state of fight, flight, or freeze, our endorphins surging, our levels of stress ever-increasing.

Whatever the prompt (and the provocations of anxiety are innumerable), the condition of anxiety can uniformly be understood as "a *future-oriented mood state* in which one is ready or prepared to attempt to cope with upcoming events" (Barlow qtd. in Freeman and Freeman 11). The distress we might feel about events unfolding *now* is compounded by the irresistible specter of distressing events that could happen in the indefinite *then*. For example, even when we might be feeling well enough today, we might still experience health anxiety, a fear of what illness *might* do to our wellbeing (physical, emotional, mental, social) in the future. Similarly, building on Albrecht's neologism *solastalgia*, Moratis uses the term *anticipatory solastalgia* to describe our feelings of anxiety associated with "*expected* environmental change and its impacts" (1, our emphasis). "As such," Moratis writes, "anticipatory solastalgia captures the paradoxical situation of people intensely experiencing the pristine and immaculate, while simultaneously realizing its fragility and imminent loss" (1). One way to understand, and address, eco-anxiety and eco-grief, then, is to consider them as forms of health anxiety, experiences of stress and distress about the future of our own wellbeing or that of a loved one – in this case, our beleaguered planet.

Eco-anxiety and health anxiety are a lot alike: what we fear, and our response to that fear, is constituted through and plays a role in constituting a larger discourse of health, encompassing a variety of texts and communicative and relational practices. Whether that discourse relates *only* to our concern for our physical and mental wellbeing or extends to concern for the wellbeing of another, we might obsessively seek information in the belief that education about a problem is a means of controlling it. We acquire information and belief both deliberately and unconsciously from the people we know and from the media we consume; and we in turn share what we know, believe, and feel with others (Farkas). Reading and writing are a crucial part of this process: we consult self-help books and periodical articles in a fervent and reasonable desire to learn *more*; we join discussion threads and online support groups to learn, to share our fear and frustration, and to exchange strategies for coping (Barker); we read about the experience of others; we write our own experiences; we look to the written word, whether print or electronic, to make our feelings visible and to reassure us that our case is not an isolated one, that *we* are not isolated but part of a larger community.

Yet, while it may be true in a general way that "knowledge is power," when it comes to eco-anxiety provoked by a dire existential threat, "where ignorance is bliss, 'tis folly to be wise." A 2019 report from the Yale Program on Climate Change Communication explained that "[m]ore than half of Americans [surveyed] (56%) say they hear about global warming in the media at least once a month…66 percent of Americans surveyed said 'they were at least "somewhat worried" about climate change…' [and] 56 percent 'think extreme weather poses a risk to their community.'" Unsurprisingly, "as the environmental conditions around the world degenerate…we struggle to cope with unprecedented and deeply frightening crises and unsettling emotions" (Buzzell and Chalquist, *Ecotherapy* 1). Increased media coverage of climate change informs even as it "[assaults us] with news of deteriorating conditions around the planet." Whether we live through a flood (direct exposure) or read about someone living through a flood (indirect exposure), the mental health impacts are the same: "anxiety, depression, secondary trauma, and other psychological conditions" (Harrington). Popular media "messaging" emphasizing the threat of climate change – what Chapman, Lickel, and Markowitz refer to as "'doom and gloom' messaging" – can quickly overwhelm audiences with fear and pessimism; learning more about just how much danger we are in runs the risk of exacerbating eco-anxiety, "depress[ing] and demoraliz[ing] the public into further inaction" (850).

So how do we educate one another about the planet's health without being overwhelmed by crippling eco-anxiety? One answer is, paradoxically, to harness our fear of what might come, to "embrace the perceptual power of doubt" (Lotto 17). The deep and often debilitating state of uncertainty we are living can ignite our creative impulses, inspiring us to re-imagine how we live and act in our world. "Doubt," writes Lotto, "is the genesis of powerful, deviating possibilities" (12), requiring "the human brain … to shed constricting assumptions and see beyond the utility with which the past has trained it to see." That is, "[i]magined perceptions shape your future much like lived ones as both physically change your neural architecture" (136) – "[i]f you imagine complex, challenging possibilities, your brain will adapt to them" (137). Uncertainty gives us agency: we are led (willing or otherwise) to imagine the kind of world we want to live in, and we have the power to create it if we work together.

Indeed, reading and writing about new solutions to combating climate change, about the effectiveness of activism to change political and popular attention to the problem, and about the different ways we can be part of that movement ourselves all have the reassuring potential to help us feel that *we* have agency for change and that taking action is both urgent and imperative: "exposure to efficacy information indirectly increases participation via hope" (Feldman and Sol Hart 99). As Baden argues (2019), "A key challenge for climate change communication is to find ways to engage the wider public in pro-environmental behaviors and support for climate change mitigation policies . . . without triggering avoidance or reactive responses" (254). Stories matter as much as information. Seeing both expert and ordinary citizens acting as role models making an "easily imitable" difference helps us feel a greater sense of realistic, but ambitious, self-efficacy: "stories with a solution focus [are] more effective in motivating pro-environmental intentions than catastrophic stories" (254). In their study of climate change activism, Roser-Renouf, et al. have found that "efforts to increase citizen awareness should promote specific beliefs about climate change, build perceptions that political activism can be effective, and encourage interpersonal communication on the issue" (163), all of which can be facilitated through print and online media. Crucially, while McLuhan's dictum that "the medium is the message" still obtains, given the tools at our disposal and the peril we're in, the message matters more than the medium at this point. We must promote climate literacy by all means possible and with a focus on translating individual knowledge into cumulative action. According to Thunberg, "our actions are important not because they have a material effect on climate change, but because of the message they send to others" (qtd. in Rowlatt). Our actions matter: they influence and mobilize, and they can bring about radical and requisite change.

Vitally important is extending climate literacy to those with the greatest stake in it: younger rather than older audiences. Young people want to be included and know they can't afford to be sheltered from reality. According to Stevenson and Peterson, "climate literacy efforts designed for adolescents should emphasiz[e] that collective action does make a difference. Avoiding despair is important, but climate literacy efforts should not shy away from communicating the seriousness of climate change as adolescents are likely capable of productively responding to concern" (6). Again, these climate literacy efforts and initiatives must be promoted and enacted through the variety of media available to us, and even as traditional print loses its primacy, remediated "print" is indispensable for creating both the analysis and the narratives that harness the emotional impact of other media appeals and provide the coherence and purpose to make them *persuade*. Indeed, the variety of media available to the public now serve as " 'important arenas and important agents in the production, reproduction, and transformation of the meaning' of climate change" (Schäefer and Schlichting 143). This affirms the power and necessity of language and representation: print and online media can change minds and alter how we perceive the world and the way we live, behave, and act in it.

Moving beyond awareness to compassion and collective action

We are living in the Anthropocene; the fate of the planet is in our hands. Yet, as Rachel Hammonds points out, despite *decades* of warning, we refuse to face up to our Anthropocene catastrophe. Hammonds refers to a 2015 editorial in the *Health and Human Rights Journal* on climate justice and the right to health in which the authors ask whether "our era will be viewed as the era of the 'Great Procrastination'" guilty of " [s]quandering time, dithering on action, and engaging in half-measures woefully incapable of addressing a threat that our best science warns will be more catastrophic and less reversible each year'" (363). So why *do* we keep procrastinating? Although it's a common response to seemingly insurmountable obstacles – a common manifestation of anxiety, in fact – we are running out of time. It is time to act, to envision a better future through collective thinking and imagining and to then build it through collective action. The emphasis on the collective is key. We are part of an interconnected and interdependent system, "a living process" embedded "in a larger, living whole" (Macy and Brown 46). Planetary and personal health are thus inseparable; we are inextricably linked to our ecosystems. The antidote to our communal suffering, then, is the collective awakening of compassion for our planet and for all sentient beings. And as we exhort, encourage, and organize one another, we do so through language, through the written word in particular, whether as traditional print or remediated "print," playing its part in a network of discourse that becomes a part of us, embedded in our neural architecture, literally and physically transforming our perceptions and beliefs.

This is how climate-related messages have the potential to awaken our innate ability to identify and empathize with others and so to bring us together, and how our growing awareness (or recollection) of our interconnectedness may encourage collective eco-activism and inspire us to take the action necessary to save our planet and so ourselves. Buzzell and Chalquist refer to this emerging climate consciousness as an "eco-awakening," the experience of "awaken[ing] to the reality and enormity of the environmental threat to life on Earth" ("It's Not Eco-Anxiety"). Our media and social networks, whose structures mimic that of our hyper-connected brains and the universe itself, are critical to such an "eco-awakening." A pro-social discourse of climate activism can rouse us from inaction, galvanize and unite us to work as the superorganism we are to address one of the biggest crises our planet has ever faced.

Throughout this chapter, we have emphasized two assertions: (1) our inseparability from the living world means that we have an inescapable obligation to act, to care for it; (2) that we have learned that planetary health *is* human health is a consequence of a multitude of voices *reaching* us across disciplinary and genre boundaries, through the written word, through the medium of print (and "print"). Even as we are critical of the limitations of print, we are able to express those views to you here...through print. As we have discussed, the relationships that we establish through reading and writing play an invaluable role in our ability to learn about wellness, to commiserate, and to provide care in response to illness. In particular, the discourse of care provoked by the climate crisis has become a site of solace, as we express and share our eco-grief, and of inspiration, as we seek to translate our eco-anxiety into healing action. The role of print in this discursive process is undeniable.

And yet, could it be that the same features of print that we valorize for allowing us to develop and share knowledge are also contributing to the potentially fatal procrastination that Hammonds describes? After all, print is part of the same cultural and ideological system that has produced the Anthropocene...which is not an argument to jettison print; but it is a reason to un-sentimentally acknowledge it as one technology, one tool, among many, and the decision of which tool to use comes down to its potential to help or hinder in the effort to avert, or mitigate, the climate catastrophe. Reading and writing about the environment have to be part of the process of understanding and managing eco-anxiety...up to a point, beyond which, time spent reading and writing comes to provoke eco-anxiety, in part because it is time when we are not taking the action we know we must. If we can use print as a tool to promote care and healing – of one another, of the planet – then, ultimately, we must use that tool to communicate this to our readers:

It's time to put down this book, go outside, and *act*.

Works Cited

"About – Dark Mountain." *The Dark Mountain Project*. September 2020, https://dark-mountain.net/about/.

Albrecht, Glenn A. "Negating Solastalgia: An Emotional Revolution from the Anthropocene To the Symbiocene." *American Image*, vol. 77, no. 2, 2020, pp. 9–30.

Albrecht, Glenn A., et al. "Solastalgia: The Distress Caused by Environmental Change." *The Royal Australian and New Zealand College of Psychiatrists*, vol. 15, 2007, pp. 295–S98.

Baden, Denise. "Solution-Focused Stories Are More Effective than Catastrophic Stories in Motivating Proenvironmental Intentions." *Ecopsychology*, vol. 11, no. 4. 2019, pp. 254–63.

Barker, Kristen K. "Electronic Support Groups, Patient-Consumers, and Medicalization: The Case of Contested Illness." *Journal of Health and Social Behavior*, vol. 49, no.1, 2008, pp. 20–36.

Bolter, Jay David, and Richard Grusin. *Remediation: Understanding New Media*. Cambridge: MIT Press, 2000.

Boscov-Ellen, Dan. "A Responsibility to Revolt? Climate Ethics in the Real World." *Environmental Values*, vol. 29, no. 2, 2019, pp. 153–74.

Buglin, Ailise. "Popular Culture and the 'New Human Condition': Catastrophe Narratives and Climate Change," *Global and Planetary Change*, vol. 156, 2017, pp. 140–6.

Buzzell, Linda and Craig Chalquist, Eds. *Ecotherapy*. San Francisco, CA: Sierra Club Press, 2009.

Buzzell, Linda and Craig Chalquist, "It's Not Eco-Anxiety – It's Eco-Fear! A Survey of the Eco-Emotions." September 23, 2019, https://chalquist.com/its-not-eco-anxiety-its-eco-fear-a-survey-of-the-eco-emotions/.

Carson, Rachel. *Silent Spring: The Classic That Launched the Environmental Movement*. Mariner Books, Boston and New York, 1962.

Chapman, Daniel A., Brian Lickel, and Ezra M. Markowitz. "Reassessing Emotion in Climate Change Communication." *Nature Climate Change*, vol. 7, 2017, pp. 850–2.

Clayton, Susan. "Climate Anxiety: Psychological Responses to Climate Change." *Journal of Anxiety Disorders*, vol. 74, 2020.

Day, Harvey. "Five Teens Who Changed the World: These Young People Know How to Get Things Done." *BBC Future*, April 24, 2019, www.bbc.co.uk/bbcthree/article/0e9e80de-62cb-4782-a26f-1cd480d28f26.

Farkas, Carol-Ann. "The Bind Men and the Elephant: Mediating Conflicting Views of Controversial Diagnoses." *Trespassing Journal: An Online Journal of Trespassing Art, Science, and Philosophy*, vol. 4, 2014, http://trespassingjournal.org/Issue4/Abstracts/TPJ_I4_Farkas_Abstract.pdf.

Feldman, Laura and P. Sol Hart. "Using Political Efficacy Messages to Increase Climate Activism: The Mediating Role of Emotions." *Science Communication*, vol. 38, no. 1, 2015, pp. 99–127.

Freeman, Daniel and Jason Freeman. *Anxiety: A Very Short Introduction*. Oxford: Oxford University Press, 2012.

Galway, Lindsay P., et al. "Mapping the Solastalgia Literature: A Scoping Review Study." *International Journal of Environmental Research and Public Health*, vol. 16, no. 15, 2019, p. 2662.

Gonzales, Andrea Alejandra. "Don't Like the News: Become the News." *Youth to Power: Your Voice and How to Use It*, edited by Jamie Margolin. New York: Hachette Go, 2020, pp. 121–37.

Grady, Constance. "The 2010s Were Supposed to bring the eBook Revolution. It Never Quite Came." *Vox*, December 23, 2019, www.vox.com/culture/2019/12/23/20991659/ebook-amazon-kindle-ereader-department-of-justice-publishing-lawsuit-apple-ipad#.

GNM Press Office. "New Data Shows Guardian is the Top Quality and Most Trusted Newspaper in the UK." *The Guardian*, July 17, 2020,www.theguardian.com/gnm-press-office/2020/jun/17/new-data-shows-guardian-is-the-top-quality-and-most-trusted-newspaper-in-the-uk.

Hall, Budd L. and RajeshTandon. "Decolonization of Knowledge, Epistemicide, Participatory Research and Higher Education," *Research for All*, vol. 1, no. 1, 2017, pp. 6–19.

Hammonds, Rachel. "How Can We Respond to the Great Procrastination to Respond to the Climate Emergency?" *Health and Human Rights*, vol. 22, no. 1, 2020, pp. 363–6.

Harrington, Samantha. "How Climate Change Affects Mental Health: Experiencing Disaster – or Even Reading About It in the News – Can Be Stressful and Scary." *Yale Climate Connections*, February 4, 2020, https://yaleclimateconnections.org/2020/02/how-climate-change-affects-mental-health/.

Hertsgaard, Mark and Kyle Pope. "From the Climate Crisis to Covid-19: Can Journalism Focus On the Stories That Matter?" *The Guardian*, July 1, 2020, www.theguardian.com/commentisfree/2020/jul/01/climate-crisis-covid-19-journalism-newsrooms.

Horwitz, Pierre and Margot W. Parkes. "Intertwined Strands for Ecology in Planetary Health." *Challenges*, vol. 10, no. 20, March 2019,

Hurwitz, Sophie. "'Youth to Power' Offers Activism 101 for Students." *New Voices Magazine*, June 18, 2020, https://newvoices.org/2020/06/18/youth-to-power-offers-activism-101-for-students/.

Jarvis, Brooke. "The Teenagers at the End of the World." *The New York Times*, July 21, 2020, www.nytimes.com/interactive/2020/07/21/magazine/teenage-activist-climate-change.html.

Lotto, Beau. *Deviate: The Science of Seeing Differently*. Hatchett Books, 2017.

Luzón, María-José and Carmen Pérez-Llantada. "Connecting Traditional and New Genres." *Science Communication on the Internet: Old Genres Meet New Genres*, edited by Luzón and Pérez-Llantada, Amsterdam and Philadelphia: John Benjamin, 2019, pp. 1–18.

Macy, Joanna and Molly Brown. *The Updated Guide to the Work that Reconnects: Coming Back to Life*. Philadelphia: New Society Publishers, 2014.

Margolin, Jamie. *Youth to Power: Your Voice and How to Use It*, foreword by Greta Thuberg. New York: Hachette Books, 2020.

Moratis, Lars. "A New Form of Solastalgia?"*Australasian Psychiatry*, June 2020,

Odell, Jenny. "How to Do Nothing: Resisting the Attention Economy." *Talks at Google*, August 8, 2019, www.youtube.com/watch?v=izjlP9qtmBU.

Ogrodnik, Corinne and Suzanne Staggenborg. "The Ebb and Flow of Environmentalism." *Sociology Compass*, vol. 10, no. 3, 2016, pp. 218–29.

"Print vs Digital Subscribers: Demographic Differences and Paths to Subscription." *American Press Institute*, May 2, 2017, www.americanpressinstitute.org/publications/reports/survey-research/print-vs-digital/

Report on Health and Climate Change. *The Lancet*, June 2015, www.thelancet.com/commissions/climate-and-health-2015#:~:text=The%202015%20Lancet%20Commission%20on,of%20health%20for%20populations%20worldwide.

Roser-Renouf, et al. "The Genesis of Climate Change Activism: From Key Beliefs to Political Action." *Climatic Change*, vol. 125, no. 2, 2014, pp. 163–78.

Rowlatt, Justin. "Climate Change Action: We Can't All Be Greta, But Your Choices Have a Ripple Effect," *BBC*, September 20, 2019. www.bbc.com/news/science-environment-49756280#:~:text=Science-,Climate%20change%20action%3A%20We%20can't%20all%20be%20Greta%2C,choices%20have%20a%20ripple%20effect&text=Is%20individual%20action%20pointless%20in,has%20to%20be%20%22yes%22.

Schäefer, Mark S. and Inga Schlichting. "Media Representations of Climate Change: A Meta Analysis of the Research Field," *Environmental Communication*, 2014, vol. 8, no. 2, pp. 142–60.

Sternisko, Anni, et al. "The Dark Side of Social Movements: Social Identity, Non-Conformity, and the Lure of Conspiracy Theories." *Current Opinion in Psychology*, vol. 35, October 2020, pp. 1–6.

Stevenson, Kathryn and Nils Peterson. "Motivating Action through Fostering Climate Change Hope and Concern and Avoiding Despair among Adolescents," *Sustainability*, vol. 8, no. 1, 2015, p. 6.

Sweney, Mark. "UK National Newspaper Print Sales Plunge amid Coronavirus Lockdown." *The Guardian*, 21 May 2020, www.theguardian.com/media/2020/may/21/uk-national-newspaper-print-sales-plunge-amid-coronavirus-lockdown.

Thunberg, Greta. "Foreword: 'This Book Is Your Toolbox.'" *Youth to Power: Your Voice and How to Use It*, edited by Jamie Margolin, New York: Hachette Books, 2020, pp. xi–xii.

Waterson, Jim. "Guardian Media Group Digital Revenues Outstrip Print for First Time." *The Guardian*, July 24, 2020, www.theguardian.com/media/2018/jul/24/guardian-media-group-digital-revenues-outstrip-print-for-first-time.

Watson, Marlene F., et al. "COVID-19 Interconnectedness: Health Inequity, the Climate Crisis, and Collective Trauma." *Family Process*, vol. 59, no. 3, 2020, pp. 832–46.

Watts, Jonathan and John Vidal. "Environmental Defenders Being Killed in Record Numbers Globally." *The Guardian*, July 13, 2017, www.theguardian.com/environment/2017/jul/13/environmental-defenders-being-killed-in-record-numbers-globally-new-research-reveals.

4
HEALTH ZINES
Hand-made and heart-felt

Deborah Lupton

Introduction

A zine (short for "magazine") is a hand-made and self-published mini magazine or pamphlet that is traditionally produced as a form of small-run creative publication rather than for mass circulation and profit. The zine medium is a low-tech form of media production in which people can readily engage across age groups and literacy levels. Like blogging and other contemporary forms of self-publishing, zine making allows creators full control over the content, presentation, and distribution of their work (Stanley). What distinguishes zines from most other forms of self-publishing are their multi-modal dimensions, which in turn generate an expansive multiplicity of perspectives. Zine making builds on a body of work on art making, counter cultures, social activism, and storytelling. Zines are rich mixed-media creations, bringing together techniques and genres such as amateur journalism, self-help advice, painting, print making, photography, drawing, journaling, scrapbooking, political pamphlets and posters, collaging, graphic narratives, and creative writing. They can be one-off publications or part of a series, spanning years or even decades.

The history of zines has been closely associated with marginalized groups, progressive politics, punk culture, or niche interests (Duncombe). Zines have been described as contributing to the genre of alternative media – as "notes from underground" (Duncombe) or "media for the misbegotten" (15). As these descriptions suggest, zines often inhabit the role of "subversive media" (Desyllas and Sinclair). In recent times, however, the character of zines has changed, and they are now often used as an outlet for creative art making and writing beyond radical intentions or content. Zine making has become far more mainstream, with zine makers now able to promote and sell or distribute their zines on online platforms and social media. While political and fan zines are still popular types, the content of zines has diversified. Zine makers still tend to address niche subjects but not necessarily from an activist or alternative perspective. In the academic world, people are also experimenting with zine making as a pedagogical tool (Thomas), a research method (Lupton and Watson), or as a way to engage in open access translation of research findings (Merhar).

In this chapter, I discuss the role of zines as a medium for representing, documenting, and communicating health-related topics and experiences. The history of this genre of zines with a flowering of work in the early era of the HIV/AIDS epidemic and culminates in the Covid-19

DOI: 10.4324/9781003007661-6

era in a proliferation of "quaranzines," which provide public health information, suggestions for self-care, or recording everyday life during the pandemic. In what follows, I begin with an overview of the history of zines. I then provide examples of how zines have been used for health-related purposes: for expressing lived experiences of embodiment; political activism; therapy and self-care; pedagogical purposes; community building; and finally for research-creation activities.

Zines: an overview

Zines first emerged in the art and radical philosophy world of the 1920s, entered the fan culture (as "fanzines") and alternative political movements of the 1930s, burgeoned in the counter-culture political environment of the 1960s and the punk movement in the 1970s, and returned to their fan culture roots in the 1990s (Duncombe; Wan), becoming a growing avenue for creative explorations of lived experiences as well as social activism. Like traditional magazines, zines combine words and images and can be produced in both hard copy and digital versions. However, the do-it-yourself (DIY) approach to zines directly rejects the glossy, high-production look of mass-produced visual media as well as their commercialism. Zines can be sophisticated and complex in presentation, but they can also be very stripped down and simple. Indeed, it is this very hand-made, "amateur" style that promotes a visual appearance which works to convey the "realness" of the experiences and feelings portrayed by their creators (Piepmeier,"Why Zines Matter"; Sinor). Zine makers (sometimes referred to as "zinesters") typically employ visual approaches such as hand-drawn or re-purposed lettering and illustrations, sketching, painting, and collaging to make their zines look compelling and accessible. They often use short-form creative writing to express themselves, including genres such as poetry, fiction, diaries, and autobiographical writing. As White puts it, "The style is uniquely undesigned; it is a raw look that stands out in a polished digital world" (White). Figure 4.1 shows some examples of paper zines displayed at a zine workshop, demonstrating the multiplicity of formats and their hand-crafted appearance.

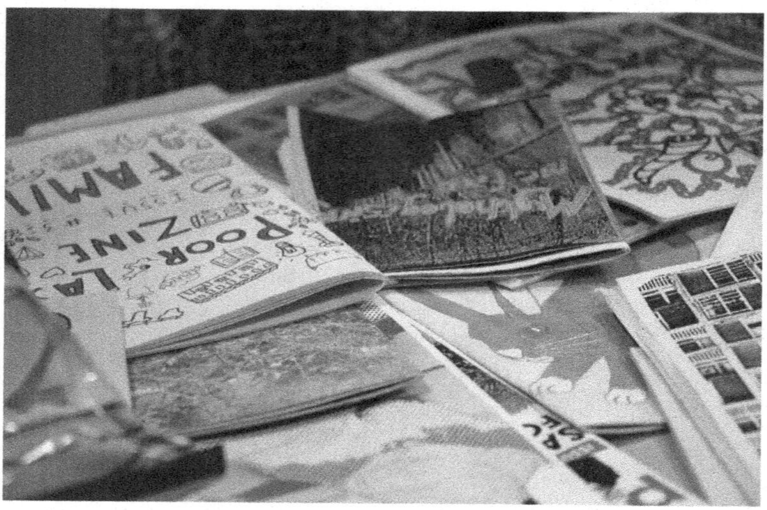

Figure 4.1 Zine display
Source: A Small Cinema, Flickr.

Zines are traditionally reproduced by photocopying or printing in small numbers, although these days they may be also or only made available in online formats or as PDFs to download. Some zines bring together analogue media with digitization in a hybrid format. While many zines these days may be offered solely online as digitized media, such zines often incorporate hand-made work that has been photographed for inclusion into a digital version. The proliferation on online platforms for self-publishing and vernacular content creation, such as blogs, YouTube and TikTok, has occurred at the same time that zine making has flourished, suggesting that zines retain a distinctive mode of publishing and media consumption. The move toward the digitization of zines has not been without controversy, with some zine creators insisting that zines by nature should be ephemeral media and that the tactile pleasures generated by handling paper zines is lost with digitization (Brouwer and Licona; Piepmeier, "Why Zines Matter").

Given this DIY approach, zine making is a highly democratic form of media production. Many zine makers work alone, but collective zine making events are also popular: particularly for political activism initiatives or as part of community art-making workshops (White). Zine making itself has become a focus for fan culture, supporting zine fairs, archived collections, and social media interest groups. Tumblr includes many accounts by zine makers displaying their publications, while the Zines Facebook group has tens of thousands of members. There are zines about zines and zines about how to make zines. Creators rarely make zines for profit: they are sold for small sums at zine fairs, specialized zine shops, bookshops or online (the arts and crafts platform Etsy features many zines for sale), given away for free or exchanged with other zine makers. Some public and university libraries have archived collections of zines, recognizing their importance as cultural artefacts (Stoddart and Kiser). There are zine exhibitions and even zine vending machines, such as the "zine-o-mat" machine at Auckland Central City Library, New Zealand, which offers zines for sale by New Zealand zinesters with a focus on marginalized, queer, and people of color creators.

Expressing lived experiences of embodiment

Authenticity and identity-work are key features of zine-making and consumption. Some zines include extremely personal content, adopting a confessional style to describe the creators' emotional struggles, deepest fears, traumatic events, and other raw thoughts and experiences that can be confronting or disturbing for the reader (Stanley). This style of zines is akin to "life writing" (Sinor). Such zines are sometimes referred to as "perzines" or personal zines (Nijsten). The hand-made, multi-modal, and democratic nature of the zine medium works both to encourage these kinds of disclosures and to render such writing as even more authentic than other modes of publishing. This type of content, together with the materiality of zines – their combination of visual and textual elements – can evoke powerful affective responses in both zine creators and their readers (Eisenhauer; Piepmeier "Why Zines Matter"; Stanley).

Making a zine can be an important way of safely exploring identity and embodiment (Eisenhauer; Sinor) and has constituted an important outlet for people of color, non-normative, gender diverse, and queer-identifying people (Boatwright; Bold). This is particularly the case for people who live in communities where they feel as if there is no one "like them." The autobiographical approach has been taken up by people living with mental health difficulties, experiences of abuse, self-harm or suicidal impulses, confronting bullying or homophobia, or living with chronic illness or disability (Eisenhauer). Zines about living with disability are readily found on platforms such as Etsy. When I searched Etsy for this topic in 2020, I found zines with titles such as *Ableist Practices*, *Disability is not a Burden – Ableism Is*, *Disability Manifesto*,

Existing Autistic, *Why Disabled People are Magic* and *Disability & Sexuality*. In one example, the *Existing Autistic* zine, published by Aven, is described by its creator as "a zine about being autistic, interacting with the world, and the difficulties this can pose" (Aven).

Along with other art making and crafting activities, zine making burgeoned during 2020, as many countries entered into months of Covid lockdowns. These zines were often shared on social media with the hashtag #quaranzine. Given the challenges that the Covid crisis – and particularly lockdown restrictions – posed to many people's mental health (Torales et al.), it is not surprising that during 2020, Etsy featured many zines that related the creators' experiences of struggling with depression, loneliness, and anxiety, including eatingkiwiskin's *Locked: Mental Illness Poems* (eatingkiwiskin). Community groups and libraries hosted online zine-making events or outlets for quaranzines (Stevens). For example, the Arlington Public Library, Vermont USA, initiated its online, *Quaranzine* series, inviting residents to contribute to a "weekly collection of creative works from the Arlington community that documents how we respond to this strange time we find ourselves in". (Arlington Public Library). Contributors could submit their work online for curation and incorporation in the series. One edition was entirely devoted to children's contributions. The series includes a wide array of artworks and short-form creative writing that depict Arlington residents' experiences during this phase of the Covid crisis in their area. The content in this series ranged from the whimsical (photographs of colorful balloons, captioned "These pictures are from a socially-distanced water balloon fight with friends who are moving out of the state") to the heart-rending (a mixed-media collage entitled "I Cry for the Lost Souls in This Time of the Covid-19 World Wide Pandemic" featuring images of dead bodies and sad faces).

More targeted zine-making activities also sprang up during the emergence of the Covid-19 crisis. The Queer Dot art collective, which aims to amplify the perspectives and voices of queer-identifying people, is based in Dundee, Scotland. In the spring of 2020, the collective called for contributions to its zine (the *Queer Dot Quaranzine*) about queer people's experiences during Covid lockdown. The zine included material on virtual dates, the video game Animal Crossing, Black Lives Matter, loneliness, the toilet paper shortage, rainbows to represent support for the UK National Health Service, growing plants, daily walking, and other ways that the lockdown had an impact on contributors' lives (The Queer Dot). The London-based small press, Bitter Melon, produced the *Stay Home Diary* zine project. Asian artists and writers from all over the world were invited to submit a short diary entry in any form to create an archive of their Covid experiences that were collected into a zine published in print and digital formats (Bitter Melon).

Political activism

Feminist zines have been made for decades (Boeckmann; Hays; Piepmeier, *Girl Zines: Making Media, Doing Feminism*), and other social justice issues have long received attention in zines (Guzzetti and Gamboa), including anti-racist and LGBTQ+ positive movements (Boatwright; Bold). When the HIV/AIDS pandemic emerged in the 1980s, activist movements sought to draw attention to the marginalization of and discrimination against at-risk groups such as gay men, sex workers, and injecting drug users. Zines played a role in these initiatives, constituting a grassroots "counterpublic" viewpoint in which opinions that challenge mainstream views could be published (Brouwer; Long).

The content of political zines directed toward highlighting social injustices related to health issues can often be deliberately transgressive and controversial (Brouwer and Licona; Long). In his analysis of two HIV/AIDS zines produced in the 1990s in the USA by and for gay men,

Brouwer noted that the contributors to the content of these zines sought to counter the portrayal of gay men as "deserving" of their HIV infection compared with the "innocent victims" trope (such as those infected through blood transfusions) that dominated mainstream culture during that decade. These zines sought to stridently eroticize gay sexuality. Their creators championed the idea that HIV positive gay men could still be sexually active, erotic subjects, as opposed to being portrayed as either desexualized due to severe AIDS illness or as sexually lethal and diseased objects of fear. The zines also published artwork depicting gay men with HIV/AIDS as grotesquely tortured by the neglect of the government, medical establishment, and mainstream society, attempting to draw attention to this neglect through these images of bodies *in extremis*.

Reproductive health and women's health are topics that have received a high level of attention from zine makers: particularly those adopting a feminist stance (Boeckmann; Nijsten). In her analysis of representations of the female body in feminist zines, Boeckmann shows that women have been able to use these media to portray their bodies as agential rather than as passive objects and promote the idea of "DIY healthcare" as a way for women to take control of their reproductive health (Boeckmann). One example is the *Thank God for Abortion* zine by artist and activist Viva Ruiz. Ruiz uses simple black-and-white images to document efforts from around the world to destigmatize women's access to abortion and their other reproduction rights. The zine is one medium used by Ruiz in her activism, inspired by the mass closing of abortion clinics across the USA, which includes t-shirts available for sale on her online shop and an Instagram account (Ruiz).

Feminist zines also often attempt to resist normative discourses and practices related to femininity and embodiment (Nijsten; Piepmeier, "Why Zines Matter"). Body positive and fat activists have sought to use the zine medium, for example, to counter anti-obesity and fat-shaming discourses and imagery (Piepmeier,"Why Zines Matter"). Examples I found on Etsy in 2020 include *Fat Kid Manifesto, Adipose Issue, Being Fat Means, Fat is Beautiful, No Guilt in Pleasure, Curvy Cuties,* and *I'm a Big Fat Body*. As these titles suggest, the content of such zines on fat bodies express counter-discourses to the dominant portrayals in popular media of fat bodies (and especially female fat bodies) as ugly, diseased, and shameful (Lupton, "Digital Media and Body Weight"). Instead, as part of broader fat activism efforts in other popular media platforms, these zine creators seek to make fat bodies visible in positive ways, adopting an "out and proud" portrayal that also works to personalize the experience of being fat in a world in which fat people are routinely marginalized and stigmatized (Lupton, *Fat*).

Therapy and self-care

Not all health zines these days are directed at collective action or challenges to mainstream ideas and practices in medicine, public health, and popular culture. Zinesters can view the process of zine making itself as a therapeutic activity, helping them process and recover from traumatic experiences or disturbing feelings or providing them with a creative outlet that helps distract them from negative thoughts and feelings (Stanley). Making zines can also give people a sense of purpose and identity (Boatwright; Nijsten).

Many contemporary zines engage with the "wellness" and "self-care" ethos that is currently a popular approach in both expert and lay portrayals of health promotion in popular literature and social media (Petrakaki et al.). When I reviewed zines available for sale on Etsy in 2020, I discovered examples such as the *So You're Anxious as Fuck* zine, which provides tips and tricks for dealing with anxiety (Menezes); *Trauma: How to Heal from Trauma and Feel Safe in the World* (Rad Cat), described by the creator as "an empowering DIY mental health mini zine" targeted at people "wanting to learn tools for self love and mental wellness"; and *The Sleep Zine* (Kajal K), described as a "carefully curated for those with sleep issues. Take it as a little paper friend on nights you feel alone and your anxiety is not letting you sleep." These types of zines have burgeoned in Covid times. For example, Clara Camm made *Isolation Nation: Entertainment in the Age of a Pandemic*, with "simple DIYs and distractions for those times you feel down in the dumps" (Camm). Even more targeted is *PhD Life in a Pandemic* zine, recounting how the author had dealt with the challenges of working on a doctoral thesis over eight weeks of lockdown (adisordered mind).

Some intriguing overlaps in the content and approach of these zines intersects with the growing sphere of wellness "influencers" or "micro-celebrities." These influencers constitute a group of highly-followed people on social media platforms (particularly YouTube, Instagram, and TikTok) who use their platforms to disseminate content that focuses on self-care, self-help and other personal health-promoting activities such as "fitspo" (fitness inspiration) and "clean eating" (Baker and Rojek; Lupton "Digital Media and Body Weight"). In their focus on wellness, self-help and self-care practices, this social media and zine content often reproduces the individualistic approach to health and health care that has been characterized as "healthism" (Crawford). The discourse of healthism, emerging with a focus on the contribution to "life-style"-related causes of illness and disease in the mid-20th century, assumes that people should take responsibility for protecting their own health and that "good citizens" should adopt this self-help approach to avoid using scarce health resources (Crawford). The broader sociocultural, political, and economic causes of ill-health and disease tend to be obviated in these approaches (Lupton, *The Imperative of Health: Public Health and the Regulated Body*). Rather than challenging the status quo or resisting bodily norms, therefore, such zines tend to reproduce and support them.

Pedagogies

There are various ways in which zines are used for pedagogical purposes. Zines expressing personal beliefs, ideas and experiences have been described as a form of "micropolitical pedagogy," as they can educate readers about the lived experiences of the author (Piepmeier, "Pedagogy of Hope"). Further, such zines have been described as offering a "pedagogy of hope" by demonstrating that hardships and barriers can be overcome (Piepmeier, "Pedagogy of Hope"). Zines have also often been produced as a way of engaging in public pedagogy, sharing information about health issues as a form of public health communication.

The makers of some Covid-themed zines have sought to engage with publics in this way by providing information about how the coronavirus is spread and what people can do to protect themselves and others from infection. One example is Katherine Liu's *Staying Home* zine, offered online. Illustrated with cheerful, colorful images, the zine provided details of Covid-19 symptoms and advice on what to do if a person has these symptoms, outlined hygiene and social distancing procedures, and gave suggestions for how to help others as well as giving instructions of breathing exercises to strengthen the lungs and how to remain mentally positive and connected to others (Liu). Other zinesters have offered tips on how to make fabric masks at home or cooking meals for quarantine times. On a less serious level, Zappix's *Things That Are Not Face Masks* zine depicted drawings of a series of incongruous objects worn on people's faces (a vacuum cleaner, a packet of seeds, a dog) as a light-hearted way of drawing attention to the importance of wearing the appropriate kind of mask for Covid protection (Zappix).

The process of zine making has been used as a pedagogical tool in classrooms as a way of inspiring political awareness, empowerment, and transformation (DeGravelles; Desyllas and

Sinclair; Way). In one example of such an approach, zine making related to social justice issues was used as a critical pedagogy activity for social work graduate-level university students at a university in the USA. The idea was to engage students in thinking through power relations, using zine making as an alternative form of knowledge production. Students were asked to respond to the prompt "social justice in action," synthesizing the key themes in the course they were taking on social justice in social work. Once the zines were individually created, students were asked to share and discuss their zines together (Desyllas and Sinclair). Another university-based zine workshop held in Vancouver, Canada, involved students making zines about the foodscapes of their university. They were provided with the definition of foodscapes: a concept from cultural geography that acknowledges the spatial, political, and cultural dimensions of food production and consumption. The students then worked in response to an assigned reading and a published zine made by food activists. The zine produced by the students adopted a decolonizing approach by highlighting the role of Indigenous peoples' food knowledges in the Vancouver area (Bagelman and Bagelman).

Community building

Collective zine-making activities are one way in which communities can engage with each other and form close ties through creative participation (Nijsten). The act of zine making as a group activity works to inspire discussion as people sit together and share materials and ideas in creating their zines. Simply sharing and reading zines can also contribute to feelings of shared community, even if people have never met face-to-face. Research on women's experiences of reading zines that question body norms has shown that the opportunity to gain insights into other people's struggles can help them to feel less alone (Nijsten). Indeed, zines can be characterized as a way of creating an "embodied community" that is built on human bodies' physical encounters with zines – making them and touching them as they are read (Piepmeier, "Why Zines Matter").

Writing in 2003, Sinor remarked on the ways that zinesters and their readers can form communities across geographical boundaries, building networks and connections through writing and reading, noting that they were "the precursors to virtual communities created in cyberspace" (Sinor 244). Since the early 2000s, there has been an explosion of blogs, online forums and social media groups where people share interests or experiences, connect with each other, and feel that they are not alone. People with similar health difficulties or diseases often use social media platforms such as Facebook groups to generate that sense of community (Maslen and Lupton). It is notable even in the face of the growing use of online forums and groups, zines have continued to maintain their niche as a form of community building. In light of the growing popularity of zine making and the use of social media to publicize and distribute zines, a "zine subculture" now exists (Wan), supported by zine fairs and online interest groups, and offering an alternative to mainstream approaches to digital publishing (White).

One example of using zine making to build a community is the development of the collectively created series of *Flux Zine* for queer people of color living in the USA. Working together on this zine series allowed participants to tell their stories while acknowledging the intersectionality of their experiences and identifying the social, political, and economic challenges they face (Boatwright). A zine-making project conducted in a US-based care home drew on the principles of art therapy to facilitate collaboration. The "Write for You" project began as a group for residents at the facility, all of whom were older people with restricted mobility, to engage in free-writing activities. The work that was generated was then collected into a series of zines shared with other residents and staff. The zine making gave the participants not only an outlet for creativity, self-expression and sociality with the group working together but also a way to communicate with others in their care home, work for change, and counteract the stigma with which residents of such facilities are often confronted. The group also visited a zine fair to display and sell their zines and were able to feel part of this larger zinester community (Houpt et al.)

Research-creation

Even though arts-based and other creative methods are burgeoning in social research (Lupton and Watson), thus far, few researchers have experimented with zine making as a method. One example is a workshop held by the Vitalities Lab, a research team that I lead. The zine making workshop was part of a series of creative research methods that we ran, which were designed to introduce other researchers to these methods. Led by Vitalities Team member Ash Watson, the workshop invited participants to reflect on the topic of "algorithmic micropolitics": lived experiences, feelings and imaginaries about the ways in which personal information is generated, collected and algorithmically processed during online activities. We worked with prompts provided by Ash to create pages for a collective zine that inspired us to consider the role of algorithmic manipulation of our personal digital data. We used excerpts from academic articles, magazines and children's picture books to create the zine, which was scanned and formatted as a PDF available for download (Vitalities Lab). Figure 4.2 shows the zine making in progress at this workshop.

In another example of a project involving zine making, my colleague Deana Leahy and I ran a zine-making workshop at a food festival for children in Melbourne. Using the prompt, "If you were the boss of food at your school," we asked children what kinds of food they would like to bring to school or that the school canteen would offer. We provided materials for participants to make a zine demonstrating their ideas (images of many kinds of food, plain paper, glue, and colored pens). Across this drop-in workshop running continuously across the day, over 50 children from preschool age to early high school level participated in this activity. They created imaginative and colorful zines containing many ideas (see Figure 4.3 for an example), some of which were quite unexpected. For example, one girl wrote that she would like to eat with

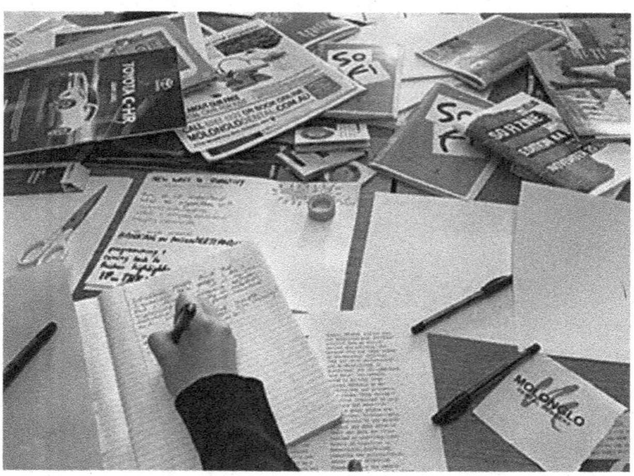

Figure 4.2 Zine making in progress at the 'Algorithmic Politics' workshop

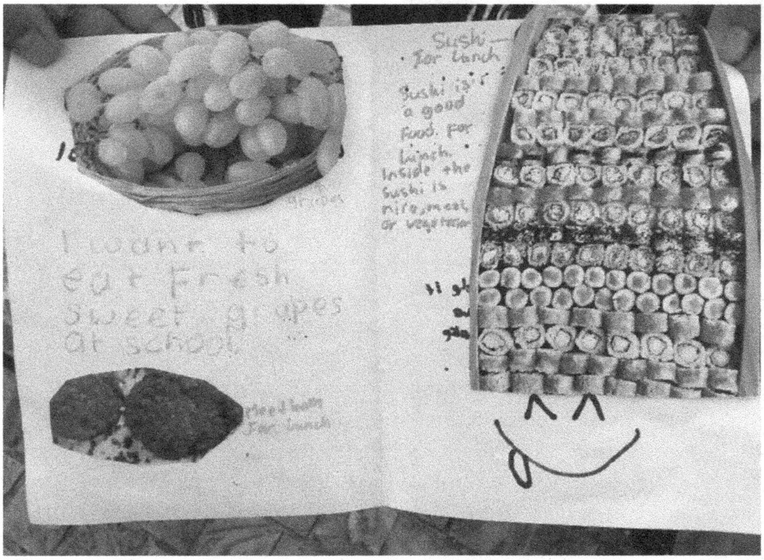
Sushi
for lunch
Sushi is a good food for lunch. Inside the sushi is rice, meat, or vegetarian
I want to eat fresh sweet grapes at school

Figure 4.3 Completed 'School food futures' zine by a high school student

her teachers for a more sociable experience. While some children included sugary foods such as sweets or cakes or "junk food" such as fries in their ideal school foods, most depicted foods such as sushi, stir-fried noodle dishes with meat and vegetables or a wide choice of fresh fruit as those they would like to eat at school. Other children wanted to see more environmentally sustainable or vegan food offered.

These types of "research-creations" can be used as materials for social inquiry. As the term "research-creation" suggests, arts-based materials generated as part of social inquiries blurs the boundaries between social research and creative activities (Springgay and Truman). Artefacts such as the zines made in these workshops can be analyzed for the ways they represent the makers' affective responses and imaginaries and also work well as stimuli for discussions about the topic (Lupton and Watson).

The participants' work in the "Algorithmic Micropolitics" zine-making workshop reflected on the ways that people's personal digitized information, including data about their bodies, was collected and algorithmically processed. The images and words used referred to feelings of being watched as part of the mundane routines of everyday life as well as ambivalence about wanting to be visible but also feeling uncertainty about data privacy and concerns about who owns and accesses personal data. For the children making their zines for the "School Food Futures" workshop, the activity gave them a voice in imagining how food provision in their school could be improved: a topic that children are rarely given an opportunity to consider or express their views about. For researchers, the zines created by the children allowed a better understanding of what kinds of food children valued and wanted in the context of the education system.

Like other arts-based methods of social inquiry, zine making can facilitate a more-than-representational approach, in which it is acknowledged that creative activity is highly generative and expressive of affective forces and sensory modes of knowing and doing beyond the spoken word (Springgay and Truman; Vannini). Participants in zine making and other research-creation workshops often express their appreciation at being able to participate in this kind of creative work, which can help them express ideas, imaginaries, or feelings that otherwise may be difficult to surface or put into words (Lupton and Watson). In this way, zine making as a research-creation mode of social inquiry is both a way of knowing and a way of showing (Foster).

Concluding comments

Contemporary zines dealing with health and medical issues are diverse. They span a range of political positions: from the traditionally activist approach characteristic of zines published last century to those engaging with an individualistic ethos of healthism, self-care and wellness. Zines can offer insights into the very personal dimensions of lived experiences of illness and health care and work well as a way of capturing collective experience. Zine making can be pedagogical at various levels of engagement: as a way of sharing personal experience, as a public health education medium, or as a consciousness-raising exercise.

Despite some changes in the format, presentation and distribution of zines and transformations in how they are made, used, and read, zines retain their original character as hand-made and heart-felt media. They remain a mode of self-publishing that enables zine creators to express raw thoughts and feelings and their readers to feel that they are not alone in dealing with and overcoming health challenges. As Piepmeier argues, zines can be considered as contributing to a "gift culture," in which ideas are exchanged and affective connections are built between creators and their readers via the unique sensory encounters and materialities configured by the zine format ("Why Zines Matter" 214). In the face of the socioeconomic and cultural changes wrought by the Covid-19 crisis, zine making as a form of self-expression, a way of passing time, distracting oneself and participating in a wider community has renewed interest and importance. For academics interested in the sociocultural, political and affective dimensions of health, illness, and healthcare, zines are valuable pedagogical resources and offer great potential as research-creation materials.

Works cited

adisordered mind. "Phd Life in a Pandemic." 2020, https://etsy.me/38pGWbf.

Arlington Public Library. "Quaranzine Series." 2020, https://library.arlingtonva.us/2020/04/03/quaranzine-issue-1/.

Aven. "Existing Autistic." 2020, https://etsy.me/3x8v4ok.

Bagelman, Jennifer Jean and Carly Bagelman. "Zines: Crafting Change and Repurposing the Neoliberal University." *ACME: An International Journal for Critical Geographies*, vol. 15, no. 2, 2016, pp. 365–92.

Baker, Stephanie Alice and Chris Rojek. "The Belle Gibson Scandal: The Rise of Lifestyle Gurus as Micro-Celebrities in Low-Trust Societies." *Journal of Sociology*, vol. 56, no. 3, 2020, pp. 388–404.

Bitter Melon. "Stay Home Diary." 2020, https://bittermelon.weebly.com/about-the-project.html.

Boatwright, Tomás. "Flux Zine: Black Queer Storytelling." *Equity & Excellence in Education*, vol. 52, no. 4, 2019, pp. 383–95.

Boeckmann, Melanie. "Representations of the Female Body in Feminist Zines." *Health, Culture and the Human Body: Epidemiology, Ethics and History of Medicine, Perspectives from Turkey and Central Europe*, edited by Hafo İlkılıç et al., BETIM Center Press, 2014, pp. 659–64.

Bold, Melanie Ramdarshan. "Why Diverse Zines Matter: A Case Study of the People of Color Zines Project." *Publishing Research Quarterly*, vol. 33, no. 3, 2017, pp. 215–28.

Brouwer, Daniel C. "Counterpublicity and Corporeality in HIV/AIDS Zines." *Critical Studies in Media Communication*, vol. 22, no. 5, 2005, pp. 351–71.

Brouwer, Daniel C. and Adela C. Licona. "Trans(Affective)Mediation: Feeling Our Way from Paper to Digitized Zines and Back Again." *Critical Studies in Media Communication*, vol. 33, no. 1, 2016, pp. 70–83.

Camm, Clara. "Isolation Nation." 2020, https://etsy.me/3u9RWSG.

Crawford, Robert. "Healthism and the Medicalization of Everyday Life." *International Journal of Health Care Services*, vol. 10, no. 3, 1980, pp. 365–88.

DeGravelles, Karin H. "In the Ruins of Zine Pedagogy: A Narrative Study of Teaching with Zines."Doctoral dissertation, Louisiana State University, https://digitalcommons.lsu.edu/gradschool_dissertations/1247/ 2011.

Desyllas, Moshoula Capous and Allison Sinclair. "Zine-Making as a Pedagogical Tool for Transformative Learning in Social Work Education." *Social Work Education*, vol. 33, no. 3, 2014, pp. 296–316.

Duncombe, Stephen. *Notes from Underground: Zines and the Politics of Alternative Culture.* Microcosm Publishing, 2014.

eatingkiwiskin. "Locked: Mental Illness Poems." 2020, https://etsy.me/3rsVWft.

Eisenhauer, Jennifer. "Writing Dora: Creating Community through Autobiographical Zines about Mental Illness." *Journal of Cultural Research in Art Education*, vol. 28, 2010, pp. 25–38.

Foster, Victoria. " 'Ways of Knowing and Showing': Imagination and Representation in Feminist Participatory Social Research." *Journal of Social Work Practice*, vol. 21, no. 3, 2007, pp. 361–76,

Guzzetti, Barbara J. and Margaret Gamboa. "Zines for Social Justice: Adolescent Girls Writing on Their Own." *Reading Research Quarterly*, vol. 39, no. 4, 2004, pp. 408–36.

Hays, Anne. "Reading the Margins: Embedded Narratives in Feminist Personal Zines." *The Journal of Popular Culture*, vol. 50, no. 1, 2017, pp. 86–108.

Houpt, Katharine et al. "Anti-Memoir: Creating Alternate Nursing Home Harratives through Zine Making." *Art Therapy*, vol. 33, no. 3, 2016, pp. 128–37.

Kajal, K. "The Sleep Zine." 2020, https://etsy.me/3vhLWqv.

Liu, Katherine. "Staying Home." 2020, www.dropbox.com/s/v1hlmkysslq522r/Staying%20Home%20-%20reading%20version.pdf?dl=0.

Long, Thomas L. "Plague of Pariahs: Aids 'Zines and the Rhetoric of Transgression." *Journal of Communication Inquiry*, vol. 24, no. 4, 2000, pp. 401–11.

Lupton, Deborah. *The Imperative of Health: Public Health and the Regulated Body.* Newbury Park, CA: Sage, 1995.

Lupton, Deborah. "Digital Media and Body Weight, Shape, and Size: An Introduction and Review." *Fat Studies*, vol. 6, no. 2, 2017, pp. 119–34.

Lupton, Deborah. *Fat.* 2nd edition. New York and Abingdon: Routledge, 2018.

Lupton, Deborah and Ash Watson. "Towards More-Than-Human Digital Data Studies: Developing Research-Creation Methods." *Qualitative Research*, vol. 21, no. 4, 2021, pp. 463–480.

Maslen, Sarah and Deborah Lupton. " 'Keeping It Real': Women's Enactments of Lay Health Knowledges and Expertise on Facebook." *Sociology of Health & Illness*, vol. 41, no. 8, 2019, pp. 1637–51.

Menezes, Sonali. "So You're Anxious as Fuck." 2020, https://etsy.me/3JdZVCx.

Merhar, Amelia. "Too Long; Didn't Read: The Case for Academic Zines." *Northern Review*, vol. 49, 2019.

Nijsten, Nina. "Unruly Booklets: Resisting Body Norms with Zines." *DiGeSt. Journal of Diversity and Gender Studies*, vol. 4, no. 2, 2017, pp. 75–88.

Petrakaki, Dimitra et al. "Between Empowerment and Self-Discipline: Governing Patients' Conduct through Technological Self-Care." *Social Science & Medicine*, vol. 213, 2018, pp. 146–153.

Piepmeier, Alison. "Why Zines Matter: Materiality and the Creation of Embodied Community." *American Periodicals*, vol. 18, no. 2, 2008, pp. 213–38.

Piepmeier, Alison. *Girl Zines: Making Media, Doing Feminism.* NYU Press, 2009.

Piepmeier, Alison. "Pedagogy of Hope: Feminist Zines." *Feminist Media: Participatory Spaces, Networks and Cultural Citizenship*, edited by E. Zobl and R. Drücke. Berlin: Transcript Verlag, 2014, pp. 250–63.

Rad Cat. "Trauma: How to Heal from Trauma and Feel Safe in the World." 2020, www.etsy.com/au/listing/577949008/diy-mental-health-trauma-zine-how-to.

Ruiz, Viva. "Thank God for Abortion." 2020, www.thankgodforabortion.com/about.

Sinor, Jennifer. "Another Form of Crying: Girl Zines as Life Writing." *Prose Studies*, vol. 26, no. 1–2, 2003, pp. 240–64.

Springgay, Stephanie and Sarah E Truman. "On the Need for Methods Beyond Proceduralism: Speculative Middles,(in) Tensions, and Response-Ability in Research." *Qualitative Inquiry*, vol. 24, no. 3, 2018, pp. 203–14.

Stanley, Phiona. "Writing the Phd Journey(s): An Autoethnography of Zine-Writing, Angst, Embodiment, and Backpacker Travels." *Journal of Contemporary Ethnography*, vol. 44, no. 2, 2014, pp. 143–68.

Stevens, Ashlie D. "Self-Published Zines Are Back as Artists Respond to Our Reality in Quarantine." *Salon*, 2020, https://bit.ly/3jcNUT8

Stoddart, Richard A. and Teresa Kiser. "Zines and the Library." *Library Resources & Technical Services*, vol. 48, no. 3, 2013, pp. 191–8.

The Queer Dot. "Quaranzine." 2020, www.etsy.com/uk/listing/839729645/the-queer-dot-quaranzine?ref=shop_home_active_1&crt=1.

Thomas, Susan. "Zines for Teaching: A Survey of Pedagogy and Implications for Academic Librarians." *Portal: Libraries and the Academy*, vol. 18, no. 4, 2018, pp. 737–58.

Torales, Julio et al. "The Outbreak of Covid-19 Coronavirus and Its Impact on Global Mental Health." *International Journal of Social Psychiatry*, vol. 66, no. 4, 2020, pp. 317–20.

Vannini, Phillip. "Non-Representational Research Methodologies: An Introduction." *Non-Representational Methodologies: Re-Envisioning Research*, edited by P. Vannini. New York and Abingdon: Routledge, 2015, pp. 1–18.

Vitalities Lab. "Algorithmic Micropolitics." 2019, https://livingwithpersonaldata.files.wordpress.com/2019/09/am-zine-print.pdf.

Wan, Amy J. "Not Just for Kids Anymore: Using Zines in the Classroom." *The Radical Teacher*, vol. 55, 1999, pp. 15–19.

Way, Laura. "Here's Some Scissors, Here's Some Glue, Now Go Make a Zine! A Teacher's Reflections on Zine-Making in the Classroom." *Punk Pedagogies*, edited by G. D. Smith et al. New York and Abingdon: Routledge, 2017, pp. 144–55.

White, Aaron. "Design Trends: An Introduction to the Return of Zine Culture." *Shutterstock Blog*, 2019, https://shutr.bz/3uURbw4.

Zappix. "Things That Are Not Facemasks." 2020, https://etsy.me/3x6ocYI.

PART II

Photography

The four chapters in this section explore the deep intersections between photographic technologies and biomedicine. From its advent in 1839, photography became a tool for physicians to visualize the previously invisible. In the 19th century, practitioners photographed the body to read internal states of mind through facial expressions or to ascertain moral rectitude through posture. By the 20th century, however, brain imaging fueled the desire to penetrate more deeply into the body to view the immaterial mind and fix the moment of death.

Alicia Chester's chapter, **"Photography on the brain,"** opens this section with a genealogy of photographic technology beginning with 19th-century portraits of psychiatric patients and concluding with 20th-century brain imaging. She explores how individual practitioners and imaging practices in psychiatry and neurology represent breakpoints in the changing conceptions of photography, the mind, and the brain.

Tim Sieber's chapter, **"Power and pictures on the threshold of life: brain death and visual culture,"** continues this exploration of the brain. Sieber describes the "braided histories" of brain imaging and the ethics of diagnosing brain death. Brain scans, available for medical use since the mid-1980s, have emerged as a tool to detect and depict less than fully conscious neurological states including brain death, a fraught medical, political, and cultural subject bound up with organ donation, law, religion, and bioethics.

In the third chapter, **"Military bodies, healthy bodies, damaged bodies in the photography of August Sander,"** Sander Gilman explores the life and art of the most esteemed social photographer of Weimer Germany, August Sander. Sander himself was molded by military service and his photographs of the soldier's healthy, manly, and disciplined bodily posture became recognizable and exemplary of masculinity during this era. Although Sander's early work displayed the typical rigidity and static quality of the military body, his portraiture after 1919 abruptly changes, linking his work to ideas of disability and health by representing an encoded iconography of vulnerability and fragility.

In the final chapter in this section, **"Entangled subjectivities in Lisa Lindvay's photographic project *Hold Together*,"** Agnese Sile focuses on the contemporary American photographer's intimate portraits of her family members, all of whom are affected by her

DOI: 10.4324/9781003007661-7

mother's deteriorating mental health and deepening depression. While Lindvay's mother is conspicuously absent from the photographs, the effects of her illness still dominate the scenes of daily life and the spaces of home. In this way, Lindsey represents illness not as a uniquely personal experience but rather as an interpersonal, psychosocial, and cultural matter that reverberates throughout a family.

5

PHOTOGRAPHY ON THE BRAIN

Alicia Chester

Psychiatry and neurology evolved into independent branches of study in the 19th and 20th centuries alongside rapidly changing photographic technologies. Soon after the advent of photography in 1839, medical professionals adopted photography as a tool for documenting studies and patient histories due to its perceived precision and speed of production. Most importantly, physicians conceptualized photographs as reproductions of reality rather than merely representations, attributing veracity to them and upholding them as evidence of their findings. Despite the need for case histories and captions to accompany images for contextualization, medical publications cited photographs as empirical evidence for positivist assertions. They proved useful to visualize not only illness but also theories of the mind and brain when such entities could not be seen directly. In other words, photography provided a means to visualize the invisible and, in doing so, influenced discourses on the mind and its presumed physical location, the brain (Foucault xii–xiii).

With Henry Fox Talbot's book of 1844–1846, *The Pencil of Nature*, as a touchstone to assert that photographs are not imitations of nature but nature themselves, photography put the mechanical laws of nature into play: "The plates of the present work are impressed by the agency of Light alone, without any aid whatever from the artist's pencil. They are the sun-pictures themselves, and not, as some persons have imagined, engravings in imitation" (enclosed notice). As Talbot succinctly summarized, photographs were automatic images created by the action of light through the means of optics and chemistry. Not classified as mere imitations of nature, like drawings or paintings, viewers accepted photographs as products of nature itself produced with the aid of a practitioner who knew how to harness nature's laws. From this perspective, it is clear why images "impressed by Nature's hand" were readily endowed with the power of objective truth and instrumentalized as empirical evidence in the service of science (Talbot 1).

This chapter follows a genealogy of photographic technology beginning with 19th-century portraits of psychiatric patients and concluding with 20th-century brain imaging. Such visualizations began with photographing the exterior of the body as a technique of reading internal states of the mind (such as portraits of psychiatric patients) and developed into imaging the interior of the body itself (such as x-rays and brain imaging). This technological development was tightly associated with an epistemological movement away from deciphering facial expressions for clues about the mind in the 19th century toward localizing specific areas inside

DOI: 10.4324/9781003007661-8

the brain as physical sites of psychological states in the 20th century. Photographic technologies were at the center of this shift from exterior to interior. In becoming the tool enabling the creation of psychiatric and neurological images, photographic technologies shaped the desire for vision to penetrate ever more deeply into the physical body to view something quite immaterial: the mind.

A cursory history of occidental concepts of the soul and mind will help to understand how the soul became the mind and how the mind came to be viewed as a product of the brain. An Aristotelian framework dominated the 13th through 17th centuries in which the soul was understood as connected to life functions (Vidal, "Soul" 105–6). All living matter possessed an "ensouled body" within a hierarchy, at the top of which were humans: "the soul was a principle of life, or that which animated potentially live matter…if the eye was an animal, then sight would be its soul. …All [living beings] were 'animals' or ensouled bodies, and that is why the word 'psychology' (in use by 1590) originally designated the generic science of living beings" (Vidal, "Brainhood" 11). In the 17th century, René Descartes equated the soul with the mind through dualistic philosophy in which the material body and immaterial soul were separate entities that coexisted. Cartesian dualism retained aspects of the humoral theory inherited from the second-century physician Galen, in which blood became fluids called 'spirits' or *pneumata* by moving through the body and among which "the animal spirits were believed to reside in and move among the brain ventricles, which thus operated as the seat of mental faculties" (ibid. 12). Both Galen and Descartes localized thought as residing in the brain and concurred that the brain itself, as merely physical matter, did not produce thought. In the case of Galen, it was the movements of the soul ("animal spirits") within the empty brain ventricles that produced thought; for Descartes, it was the soul's interaction with the brain (specifically, the pineal gland) that produced thought. By having thought result from this interaction of soul and brain, Descartes's theory took a step toward materialism even while maintaining mind-body dualism. Although still considered immaterial, the soul gained a specific, physical location where it interacted with the body.

The soul was no longer regarded as the cornerstone of all living matter but became "conflated with the rational soul (mind) as pure thinking substance" (Vidal, "Soul" 105). Cartesian philosophy was important to this conflation since the self was linked to thought in Descartes's assertion, "*cogito ergo sum*" (Descartes 14). Now a familiar platitude, "I think, therefore I am" neatly equated thought with the self and, by extension, the soul with the self, "since thought, memory, and consciousness were properties of soul" (Vidal, "Soul" 105). By virtue of the conflation of soul and mind, "I think, therefore I am" created a chain of associations in which thought, mind, soul, and brain (as the seat of the soul) may each be interchangeably equated with the self. To add to Descartes's assertion, John Locke defined "personal identity as a continuity of memory and consciousness" (ibid.). Along with thought, memory and consciousness were also properties of the soul, so Locke's notion of identity was rooted in the mind and its supposed physical location, the brain. In both Cartesian dualism and Lockean identity, the soul coexisted with the body but was also separate from it, with the soul taking precedence in terms of personal identity. Identity was, therefore, not dependent upon the body, as Locke demonstrated in thought experiments involving swapping brains and bodies (which has become a strange premise of many screwball-comedy movies). The body was merely the material to which consciousness – i.e., the soul and mind – was "annexed" (Locke qtd. in Vidal, "Brainhood" 13).

What remains important in this shift is that not only did the soul become conflated with the mind, but the concept of self also became conflated with the soul and, by extension, its organic seat, the brain. Locke's thought experiments were intended to demonstrate that personal identity was linked to the immaterial mind rather than the material body, but they did so by way of imagining the transfer of a material portion of the body, the brain. This seems to be a contradiction, but it does account for historian Fernando Vidal's tracing of a shift toward what he calls "brainhood": "Bodies become things we have, not things we are; personal identity becomes purely psychological, and distinct from bodily identity. From the standpoint of ontological theory, and in comparison with the earlier insistence on the essential corporality of the self, the Lockean theory implied a loss of body" (Vidal, "Brainhood" 14). Vidal acknowledges the contradiction of proving the immateriality of selfhood by way of the physical brain, saying that "in practice, however, disincarnation could not be complete" (ibid.). Even if selfhood may be considered separate from the body and compartmentalized within the soul or brain, the physical body is necessary for the brain to live and the mind to think.

The body is also necessary to gather sensory input for the brain to process. Nerves played a central role as a mode of connection: "The nerves linked the external world and the brain as much as they united the soul and the body; these functions explain their broad cultural significance during the Enlightenment and the fact that the nervous system became the common ontological matrix of the sciences of the body and the sciences of the mind" (ibid. 15). In other words, nerves not only connected the brain with bodily senses and, thus, the external world, but they also connected the soul with the body by way of the brain. Disincarnation could not be complete because the soul relied upon the nerves to connect it to the brain, upon the brain to interact with bodily senses, and upon bodily senses to interact with the world. Without incarnation, no connection between the soul and the external world would exist.

The 19th century inherited Cartesian dualism as well as the "science" of physiognomy or the study of facial features, bodily form, and external appearance as a means to discern a person's character. Physiognomy postulated that the movements of the soul left visible traces on the body, especially the face, which could be deciphered. The practice of physiognomy dates to ancient Greece, but it was revived and popularized in the late-18th century by the Swiss theologian Johann Kaspar Lavater:

> Does not reason tell us that everything in the world has an internal as well as an external aspect, which stand in direct relationship to each other?...Does this not tell us that an exact relationship exists between the soul and the body, between the internal and the external of man, that the infinite variety of the souls or the internal nature of man creates an infinite variety in his body or externality. ...If such differences exist then they must be recognizable; they must also be the basis for an exact science.
>
> *(Lavater qtd. in Gilman,* Seeing the Insane *62)*

Despite Lavater's insistence upon "the infinite variety" of souls and bodies, his mode of conducting physiognomic study focused upon identifying fixed and classifiable facial traits that, when properly analyzed, would reveal the moral, psychological, and intellectual character of a person. He described the influence of psychopathologies upon facial expression, but being a pastor rather than a physician, he was concerned with creating a comprehensive system to judge moral character rather than finding the etiology of mental illness.

In the mid-19th century, practitioners of psychiatric portraiture strove to fix the movements of the soul by photographing physiognomic indications of mental pathology visible on the surface of the body with the intention of revealing psychological states. The etymology of psychology is rooted in "the study of the soul," since by the 1640s *psyche* meant "animating spirit, the human spirit or mind" (Harper, "Psychology" and "Psyche"). Psychology started as "the generic science of living beings" in the Aristotelian framework referenced above but evolved into the study of the mind under the influence of Cartesian dualism. Psychiatry is the study and treatment of mental disorders with the word dating from 1846 and meaning "a healing of the soul" (ibid., "Psychiatry"). Nineteenth-century psychology and psychiatry thus considered the soul and mind to be one and the same and postulated the brain as the mind's physical location.

The last quarter of the 19th century marked a turn in psychiatry and the nascent field of neurology toward a purely materialist understanding of mind and body, which "reduced [the] soul to a neurophysiological effect" (Vidal, "Soul" 106). A reversal took place in which, instead of the movements of the soul causing visible changes in the body, "the psychological derive[d] causally from the physical" (ibid.). Physiognomic portraits of psychiatric patients gave way to the photographic documentation of symptomatology and autopsied brains. The mind became part of the body, explicable in physical terms given sufficient knowledge. An aberration of the mind such as mental illness could thus be treated like a broken arm or pulled muscle if the mechanical workings could be understood. Photography was an epistemological tool that, like the materialist conception of mind and body, operated mechanically and was considered to be transparently truthful due to its status as "the pencil of nature." In an effort to picture and understand the mind, psychiatry and neurology invested faith in photographic technologies as evidential media, but recording merely the surface of the body proved not to be informative enough. By the turn of the 19th century, x-rays penetrated the surface of the body to reveal interior structures, and by the mid-20th century, brain imaging technologies began using data rather than optics to construct visual representations of the structure and functioning of the brain.

Hugh Welch Diamond, known as "the father of psychiatric photography," was the first to use photography to systematically record, study, and diagnose mental illness during his tenure at the Surrey County Lunatic Asylum. Diamond became the resident superintendent of the Female Department of the Surrey County Lunatic Asylum in 1848, a position he held until 1858 when he opened a private asylum. During his decade in Surrey, Diamond's practice of clinical psychiatry and his interest in photography developed concurrently. He published numerous essays and notes on photography, including "The Simplicity of the Calotype Process" in 1853, in which he promoted Talbot's calotype for its reproducibility and relative simplicity in comparison to the daguerreotype and in which he published his improvements to the process. He was also among the first to experiment with the collodion wet plate process developed by Frederick Scott Archer in 1851, which resulted in a glass plate negative yielding a sharper image than the softer paper negative of the calotype (Marien 35).

In his photographic series of "the types of insanity," presented in London in 1852, Diamond created a visual taxonomy of mental illness by taking portraits of his patients. While this series was the "first systematic use of photography in the history of psychiatry," Diamond's work was not without precedent (Gilman, "Hugh W. Diamond" 7). He was indebted to Jean-Étienne Dominique Esquirol, a pupil and colleague of Phillipe Pinel at the Salpêtrière in Paris, who commissioned over 200 sketches of mentally ill patients. Such visual methods of studying mental illness were brought to Great Britain by Alexander Morison, Diamond's predecessor at the Surrey Asylum. Morison included thirteen plates based on Esquirol's commissioned sketches in a syllabus for his lectures, which he prefaced with a statement on the physiognomy of insanity:

> The appearance of the face, it is well known, is intimately connected with, and dependent upon, the state of the mind. The repetition of the same ideas and emotions, and the consequent repetition of the same movements of the muscles of the eyes, and of the face, give a peculiar expression, which, in the insane state, is a combination

of wildness, abstraction, or vacancy, and of those predominating ideas and emotions which characterize the different species of mental disorder, as pride, anger, suspicion, love, fear, grief, etc.

(Morison qtd. in Gilman, Seeing the Insane *92).*

As evident in this preface, the sketches commissioned by Esquirol stressed facial expression as key to reading states of mind, and deciphering medical portraiture became requisite for learning to differentially diagnose psychopathologies.

Diamond believed that the state of the soul changed like the weather and was reflected in what he called "moveable" physiognomy. His conception represented a break from previously held beliefs popularized by Lavater. Rather than the physiognomy of fixed facial structures employed to discover the essential character of a person, Diamond was interested in the moveable physiognomy of facial expressions corresponding to a person's emotions and state of mind (Figure 5.1). The difference is not insignificant. While Diamond still sought to create a systematic taxonomy based on external appearance, it was not the person herself who was categorized and stereotyped but the psychopathology afflicting her. Diamond intended to categorize external appearances with a diagnostic rather than moral aim, using photography to document visual indications of mental illness through capturing his patients' moveable physiognomy. His methodology was based in the dualistic separation of soul and body inherent to physiognomy, and his photographic portraits reflected his belief that the motions of the invisible soul manifested visible changes in physical appearance. His studies were intended to better understand psychological afflictions in order to find their causes and develop treatments that would restore a mentally ill patient to a healthy state.

Diamond and his colleagues partook in the 19th century's faith that photography was objective, truthful, and infallible. One colleague, John Conolly, wrote a series of essays in 1858

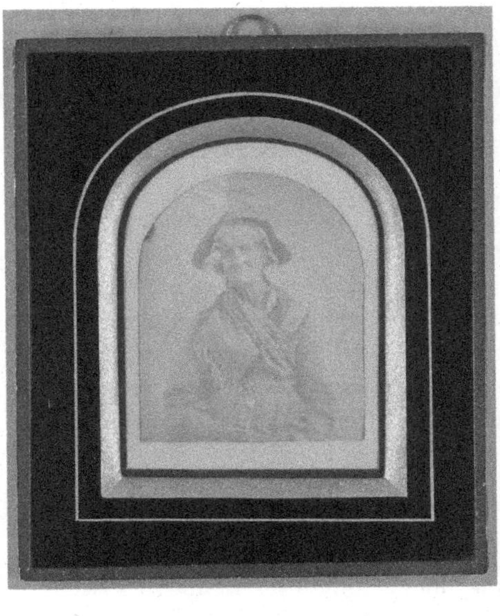

Figure 5.1 Hugh Welch Diamond, "Chronic Mania (Old woman in shawl and reversed straw bonnet)," c. 1852–1855, framed albumen print from collodion negative, 74mm x 62mm, catalogue number ETN 3/6/10/1, Norfolk Record Office, Norwich, U.K.

in which he referenced Diamond's photographic series of 1852 to describe "The Physiognomy of Insanity." Conolly wrote: "The modern artist and the photographer are enabled to represent true pictures of what is effected by mental malady, and to facilitate the knowledge of its association with bodily ailment or disturbance, capable of relief" (Conolly qtd. in Gilman, "Hugh W. Diamond" 12). Comparing Conolly's descriptions to Diamond's photographs, one physician praised "the great intrinsic value of photography in…reproducing minute characteristics of expression," in contrast to sketches or other means of representation (Wright qtd. in ibid. 11). In the first general history of photography, Ernst Lacan wrote that Diamond's "prints speak more than a whole book" (qtd. in ibid. 13). Such remarks indicate a hierarchical value to medical illustration, beginning with photography, proceeding to engravings based upon photographs, and ending with drawing.

What the medical community missed, however, was that photographs were not created in an aesthetic or cultural vacuum. Not only was Diamond's work indebted to the physiognomic tradition represented by the illustrations commissioned by Esquirol, but many of Diamond's photographs bear a striking resemblance to these illustrations, thus conforming to Pinel's categorizations of the insane that were "not inherent in the nature of the illness but rather stem from the posing of the patient, the concentration of the face, and the absence of background" (Gilman "Hugh W. Diamond" 8). Diamond's patients were pictorially isolated in front of a neutral backdrop, occasionally posed with props like books, a basket, or a crown of flowers, and his compositions adhered to contemporary conventions of portraiture. These observations are not to claim that Diamond feigned his patients' pathologies or meant to mislead his audience. Rather, Diamond inherited and employed preexisting aesthetic and representational structures as well as cultural and historical notions of mental illness in order to create images that were both aesthetically and medically interesting and intended to be clearly communicative (ibid. 8–9).

Diamond concluded his groundbreaking essay, "On the Application of Photography to the Physiognomic and Mental Phenomena of Insanity" (1856), with the utopian hope that photography, as "a perfect and faithful record," would record the truth of illness for study in the present and for posterity (24). He wrote in the belief that the means to understand and consequently cure psychopathology was in hand and that a well-executed photograph, as a "copy *drawn to life*," could stand in for "the original" to study and diagnose disease (ibid. 20). For Diamond, psychiatric photography evidenced the connection of the visible body and the invisible mind, literally exposing "the permanent cloud" or "the passing storm" afflicting the soul.

The French physician and physiologist G. B. Duchenne de Boulogne adhered to an understanding of physiognomy similar to Diamond's in that he studied how facial expressions revealed the movements of the soul. Concerned not with pathology but with understanding the physiological mechanisms responsible for translating states of the soul into facial expressions, Duchenne focused on the movement of facial muscles that create emotional expression. For his treatise *Mécanisme de la physionomie humaine, ou analyse électro-physiologique de l'expression des passions des arts plastiques* (1862), Duchenne experimented with electrical stimulation of facial muscles to simulate various expressions, thereby divorcing the appearance of emotion from the experience of emotion (Gilman, *Seeing the Insane* 194–5; Hustvedt 156–9):

> Using electrical currents, I have made the facial muscles contract to *speak* the language of the emotions and sentiments. …These lines and folds [of the moving face] are precise signs, which in their various combinations result in facial expression. Thus by proceeding from the expressive muscle to the spirit that set it in action, I have been able to study and discover the mechanism and laws of human facial expression. …In

> short, through electrophysiological analysis and with the aid of photography, I will demonstrate the art of correctly portraying the expressive lines of the human face, which I shall call the *orthography of facial expression in movement*.
>
> (Duchenne 1–2)

Still assuming the dualistic coexistence of the visible body and the invisible soul, he believed that emotions were closely tied to the movements of the soul from which they arise; the soul remained the cause and seat of emotion separate from the physical body, which operated mechanically at the behest to the immaterial soul. However, since he artificially simulated facial expressions in his subjects by electrically stimulating their muscles in the absence of genuine emotion, Duchenne represented the splitting of expression from emotion and inadvertently opened the way for the Cartesian mind-body dualism to collapse. Presenting photographs of synthetically induced expressions in the absence of real emotion as physiological evidence of how facial muscles produce expression would seem to be a contradiction. Reinforcing this contradiction was the fact that Duchenne rendered his subjects' bodies frozen in time in anticipation of photographing them when the object of his study was the movement of facial muscles. These were "expressions held in time," and the amount of time that Duchenne maintained the electrical stimulation of a subject's muscles was synchronized with the time required to expose a photograph (Pichel 33).

In the last quarter of the 19th century, Duchenne's student, the French neurologist Jean-Martin Charcot, represented the full abandonment of Cartesian dualism in favor of a materialist understanding of the mind as a product of the brain. He oversaw the production of the *Iconographie photographique de la Salpêtrière* (1875–1880) and the initial volumes of the *Nouvelle iconographie de la Salpêtrière* (1888–1918), which are the most extensive and well-known atlases of psychiatric photography from the turn of the century. They contain images produced in the same positivist spirit as Diamond's portraits, but rather than intending to construct a taxonomy of psychopathologies, the *Iconographie* was dedicated to documenting the various manifestations and cycles of neurological pathologies, most notably *hystéro-épilepsie*, an extreme form of hysteria with convulsive attacks resembling epilepsy. Charcot thought that hysteria had been misunderstood – importantly, he considered hysteria to be a neurological rather than psychological disorder – and that its plethora of confusing manifestations could be understood through meticulous observation, documentation, study, and classification aided by modern scientific methods and tools, not the least of which was photography.

Charcot privileged visual observation above other forms of empiricism. In perfect Foucauldian agreement, Charcot converted *voir* (seeing) into *savoir* (clinical knowledge), or, to collapse these together, he equated seeing with knowing (Gilman, *Seeing the Insane* xii). Working shortly before the advent of motion pictures, Charcot sequenced a large number of photographs documenting representative moments of hysterical attacks in order to form, literally, a clearer picture and description of the course of these attacks. Photography translated the three-dimensional space of hysterical attacks into the flattened two dimensions of photographic prints, and the temporal duration of these attacks was represented spatially through sequencing images for simultaneous contemplation. For Charcot, photography was a tool to sample time in the same way that histologic cross-sections (tissue samples mounted on glass slides for microscopic viewing) sampled diseased organs, with the part extracted in order to diagnose the whole. The photograph as histologic section formed a model for Charcot's approach to photography with each photograph representing a sample of hysteria. The compilations published in the *Iconographie* represented attempts to form a fuller picture of the disease, creating portraits of the illness rather than patients. Given the importance of visualization in Charcot's methodology, treating photographs as metaphorical histologic sections indicated a desire to penetrate the body of the patient to reveal the pathology within.

The final image in the first album of the *Iconographie* simply pictured a brain. It was common practice at the Salpêtrière to perform an autopsy upon a patient's death as a means to correlate brain lesions and abnormalities with symptoms recorded in life, given that the live patient could not be vivisected to view mental illness at work. The desire to visualize the interior of the body – to go so far as photographing an extracted brain – is realized in an attempt to grasp the organic seat of pathology. The body was like a machine, completely rational and explicable given sufficient knowledge, and the brain was not exempt from this model. Charcot did not find the organic etiology for hysteria, but he believed this was due to as yet insufficient knowledge and technology. Photography was a mechanical step toward more clearly visualizing pathology, literally and figuratively. By placing the once-hidden brain on visual display, the photograph at the end of the 1875 *Iconographie* album functions to reduce the immaterial mind to the physical organ, thus collapsing any distinction between mind and body. This photograph points to no internal reference of a soul. The brain is what remains of the mind once it is dislocated from its bodily housing and displayed for observation (Hustvedt 6).

In the paternal history of Western medicine, if Diamond is considered "the father of psychiatric photography" and Charcot the "father of neurology," then Harvey Cushing is "the father of neurosurgery" (Gavrus 324). He was known for meticulous methods of observation and documentation, including creating his own drawings of procedures immediately after surgery and preserving tumor and brain specimens for study. Most relevantly here, over the course of more than three decades as a practicing neurosurgeon, Cushing required that virtually every patient be photographed for his records (Wahl et al. xxi). He followed up with surviving patients for years, and "he often chronicled their clinic visits sending the patient down for a 'routine photo' as we would repeat an MRI scan today (Figure 5.2). This process apparently was so second nature to his patient care, like his operative sketches, that he never wrote about it" (ibid.). By the time of his death in 1939, the Harvey Cushing Brain Tumor Registry contained over 2,200 case studies, including preserved brains and tumors, microscopic slides, notes, and over 1,500 photographic negatives (Wahl 2).

Like his 19th-century predecessors, Cushing relied on portraiture for diagnostic and archival purposes, but he extensively employed other forms of visual imagery as well. Notably, he adopted radiology early on, that "next visual extension, peeling off one more layer between the viewer and the living brain," allowing the physician to view the interior of the body prior to surgery (Wahl et al. xxi). German physicist Wilhelm Conrad Röntgen announced the discovery of x-rays in 1895 when Cushing was a medical intern. Excited about the possibilities for medical applications, Cushing wrote to his mother: "Imagine taking photographs of gall stones in situ...foreign bodies anywhere – fracture... . Its [sic] fearfully uncanny. We won't be able to have any secrets if people can take photographs through stone walls" (qtd. in Bliss 89). Cushing soon procured a cathode-ray tube for Massachusetts General Hospital, hoping that the hospital would reimburse him. (It never did, so he took it with him when he moved to Johns Hopkins Hospital.) Despite his friend and colleague Amory Codman sustaining radiation burns, Cushing continued to act as the unofficial radiologist: "It is great sport, very useful in the out Patient to locate needles &c. We could look through the chest readily this morning – count the ribs – see the heart beat – the edge of the liver etc. It is positively uncanny" (ibid.).

The uncanniness of penetrative vision allowed Cushing to locate a bullet in the spine of a bartender's wife before operating to remove it, thereby taking the first radiograph at

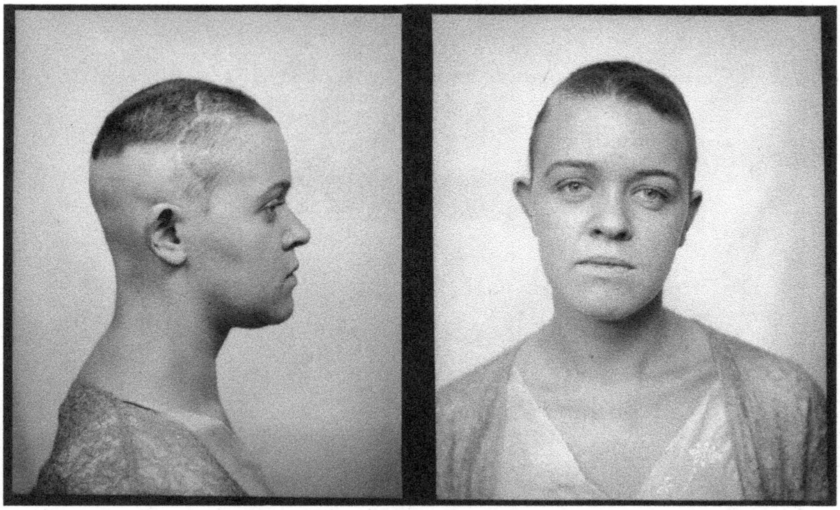

Figure 5.2 Unknown photographer, profile and frontal portraits of woman with scar on skull, March 8, 1932, digital scan of collodion glass plate negative, Cushing Tumor Registry: Medical Historical Library, Harvey Cushing/John Hay Whitney Medical Library, Yale University

Johns Hopkins Hospital (Wahl 16–17). X-rays became a principal method of visualization for Cushing although the technology remained too crude for a long time to detect anything in the brain other than abnormalities large enough to cause structural alterations (Aron 557). No single visual medium could encompass or reveal all the connections among symptomatology that Cushing sought, however. Another method valuable for diagnosing brain tumors was perimetry, the systematic measurement and representation of the patient's visual field, changes in which often indicated tumor placement and growth. With Clifford Walker, his ophthalmologist associate, Cushing studied pituitary disorders' effects on visual impairment, creating perimetric charts that plotted points and connected lines on a two-dimensional representation of human binocular vision, literally tracing the perimeter of a patient's visual field (Bliss 268). Cushing brought perimetry together with photographic portraits (including before-and-after surgery sequences), x-rays, photomicrographs, histologic tissue samples, and post-mortem photographic documentation of skulls, brains, and tumors to create composite charts resembling collages or photo album pages. The composites relied upon juxtapositions of imagery and text to create a story of diagnosis, treatment, and outcome for each patient. Like Diamond's physiognomic portraits and like the photographs of hysterical patients in the *Iconographie*, a main objective of these composites was to create taxonomies of illness, but unlike his predecessors, Cushing's composites told individual stories. Multiple forms of visualization attempted to create a more complete picture, and uncertainty of diagnosis and etiology was admitted in the notes with the seeming hope that the composites would prove useful for future study.

Twentieth-century medicine's dismantling of the interior/exterior dichotomy in which the body is still often conceptualized was dependent upon imaging technologies like radiography (Cartwright xiv). The "natural light" of x-rays enabled Cushing to employ radiography in tandem with photography to create a simultaneous visualization of the interior and exterior of a patient's body within the same medical chart (Figure 5.3). Through employing x-rays and photographs – and through shifting scales between portrayals of the full body

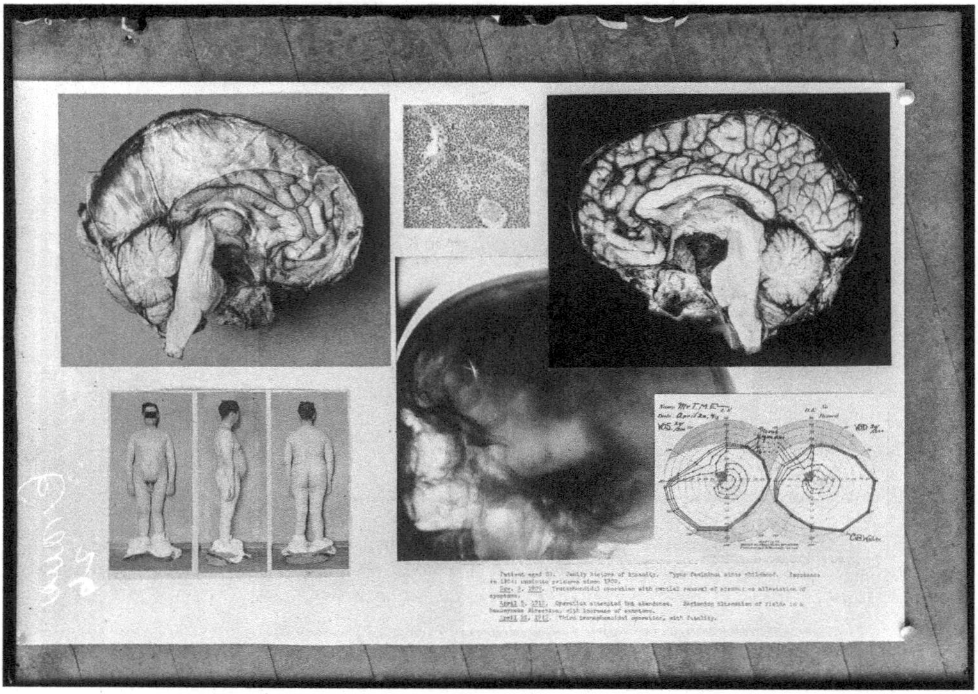

Figure 5.3 Composite chart with photographs of patient and brain, x-ray, histology, visual field, and case history, c. 1900, digital scan of collodion glass plate negative, Cushing Tumor Registry: Medical Historical Library, Harvey Cushing/John Hay Whitney Medical Library, Yale University

and slides of microscopic tissue samples – Cushing was reaching for a simultaneity of vision encompassing the entire living body that was unavailable within any single image or medium. The connections among internal and external, macro- and microscopic, and the phenomenological experiences of patients recorded using perimetry and patient histories strove for a comprehensive knowledge through visualization. In juxtaposing imagery of the interior and exterior of patients' bodies to gain a greater view of the whole, life and death were also juxtaposed – not only in the uncanny form of x-rays of living skeletons but also in the cases of patients who did not survive their conditions. Within a single chart, radiographs and pre- and post-mortem photographs collapsed spatial and temporal distinctions between inside and outside, life and death.

Transparency can be conceptualized as a window which visually connects two spaces while maintaining physical separation between inside and outside. As a literal and metaphorical ideal, transparency firmly linked visibility to rationality, knowledge, and progress (Rowe and Slutzky 45; Dijck 14). In the case of medical imaging, technology enables a metaphorical window through which the external viewer (usually, a physician) peers into the body's interior (of the patient), moving visually from surface to depth. However, in *The Transparent Body: A Cultural Analysis of Medical Imaging*, José van Dijck notes that "transparency…is a contradictory and layered concept": "Imaging technologies claim to make the body transparent, yet their ubiquitous use renders the interior body more technologically complex. The more we see through various camera lenses, the more complicated the visual information becomes" (3–4). The idea (or ideal) of a transparent living body is only possible through the mediation of technology. In the case of x-rays, electromagnetic radiation penetrates softer tissues and is blocked by denser materials like bones. In the cases of structural and functional magnetic resonance imaging (MRI and fMRI), magnetic fields are used in conjunction with radiofrequencies to measure water content and blood oxygenation and flow, respectively, to generate data used to create visualizations of interior bodily structures (MRI) and functions (fMRI). As technological complexity and mediation increase, so does the illusion of transparency. Even as contemporary medical imaging becomes increasingly removed from photography from technological and material standpoints, it has inherited the authority and reputation first garnered by photography in the 19th century as a "natural" technology – both "as technical transmitter of nature and as natural phenomenon itself" (Geimer 134) – that medicine continues to employ with the aim of achieving bodily transparency and knowledge (Wilder 352).

The MRI technique, dating from 1977, is analogous to still photography in that it focuses on brain anatomy while the fMRI technique, dating from 1990, is analogous to cinematography in that it follows neural activity. In other words, MRI studies static anatomy, while fMRI studies physiological function. MRI uses radio waves and magnetic fields to image the brain, while fMRI uses the same techniques to measure changes in oxygen in the blood, thus determining blood flow and, by extension, brain function. There are other brain imaging techniques, but MRI and fMRI are the safest methods and, therefore, are widely used not only for medical diagnosis but also research, including studies intended to visualize and understand how thought works. (Computed tomography (CT) or computed axial tomography (CAT) scans rely upon x-rays of the head from many angles, subjecting the patient to radiation, while positron emission tomography (PET) scans require radioactive material to be injected into the bloodstream.) Magnetic resonance imaging strays from traditional photography in a much greater way than x-rays do, but it is still subject to processes of collecting, processing, and interpreting data through systems comprising cultural biases just as older photographic techniques and practices do. On a basic level, MRI strives for the same thing that Diamond set out to accomplish using photography: to visualize the invisible workings of the mind.

The greatest difference between magnetic resonance imaging and photography (including photographically recorded x-rays) is that there is no necessary reason why MRI data are visualized as spatial representations of the brain. The data collected from the magnetic fields and radio waves could be (and sometimes is) visualized in any number of ways, but the most common way remains a topographical representation corresponding to the physical organ it is measuring. In "Are Neuroimages Like Photographs of the Brain?", Adina Roskies discusses the popular reception of MRI visualizations as being analogous to photographs and warns about the dangers of this comparison. MRI data could be translated into any type of visualization that proves to be useful, but most often the resulting images "look" like a brain. In other words, MRI data are most often visualized as topographical maps correlating data to the locations of structures or activity in the brain. A further effort to map the brain using MRI is made through tomography, which creates virtual histologic cross-sections of the brain. Reading topographical models of the brain can be reminiscent of viewing physiognomic portraits to decipher the state of patients' souls in that magnetic resonance images do not directly show their object of study (the brain) but represent data measured from it in an attempt to understand the still-invisible workings of the mind. "Neuro-realism" is the term for the widespread belief that brain scans are a direct index of brain activity despite the complexity of acquiring and interpreting data and despite subjective choices made in creating visualizations, like color and contrast. Asserted as representations of thought, pathology, or trauma, magnetic resonance images have inherited and superseded photography's historical claims to objectivity and realism, resulting in the belief that knowledge about the brain is generated through visualizing it.

Each practitioner or imaging practice in this essay represents a breakpoint where we can see changing and interrelated conceptions of photography, the mind, and the brain. How Diamond employed photography to create portraits of his psychiatric patients was predicated upon his understanding of the relationship of mind and body and what he believed photography could reveal. Duchenne relied upon the relatively brief exposure times of photography as a model for inducing similarly brief expressions on his subjects' faces in order to represent the appearance of emotion. Based upon the model of extracting tissue samples to view microscopic anatomy that otherwise remains invisible, Charcot treated photography as a method capable of excerpting samples of hysterical attacks by freezing details and moments that would otherwise escape his sight or memory. Cushing employed x-rays and traditional photographic media, including portraits of living patients and post-mortem photographs, to simultaneously visualize the interior and exterior of the body with the objective of creating a complete picture of the brain in life and death. MRI forgoes the exterior of the body altogether in favor of "transparently" imaging the brain, fulfilling the medical desire to visualize the living brain in situ while also pointing to the impossibility of seeing its structures and functions without technological mediation. Through exploring a genealogy of photography in psychiatry and neurology, we can better understand the role of photographic technologies in forming contemporary concepts of the mind and brain.

Works cited

Aron, David C. "The Path to the Soul: Harvey Cushing and Surgery on the Pituitary and its Environs in 1916." *Perspectives in Biology and Medicine*, vol. 37, no. 4, summer 1994, pp. 551–65.

Bliss, Michael. *Harvey Cushing: A Life in Surgery*. Oxford: Oxford University Press, 2005.

Cartwright, Lisa. *Screening the Body: Tracing Medicine's Visual Culture*. Minneapolis, MN: University of Minnesota Press, 1995.

Descartes, René. 1637. *Discourse on the Method of Rightly Conducting the Reason, and Seeking Truth in the Sciences*. Infomotions, Inc., 2000.

Diamond, Hugh Welch. "On the Application of Photography to the Physiognomic and Mental Phenomena of Insanity" (1856). *The Face of Madness: Hugh W. Diamond and the Origin of Psychiatric Photography*, edited by Sander Gilman. Brattleboro, VT: Echo Point Books & Media, 2014, pp. 17–24. [First published in 1976]

Dijck, José van. *The Transparent Body: A Cultural Analysis of Medical Imaging*. Seattle, WA: University of Washington Press, 2005.

Duchenne de Boulogne, Guillaume-Benjamin. 1862. *The Mechanism of Human Facial Expression*. Edited and translated by R. Andrew Cuthbertson, Cambridge: Cambridge University Press, 1990.

Foucault, Michel. 1963. *The Birth of the Clinic: An Archaeology of Medical Perception*. Translated by A. M. Sheridan Smith, 1973. New York: Vintage Books, 1994.

Gavrus, Delia Elena. *Men of Strong Opinions: Identity, Self-Representation, and the Performance of Neurosurgery, 1919–1950*. University of Toronto Ph.D. dissertation. 2011. https://tspace.library.utoronto.ca/bitstream/1807/32158/1/Gavrus_Delia_E_201111_PhD_thesis.pdf.

Geimer, Peter. "Noise or Nature? Photography of the Invisible Around 1900." *Shifting Boundaries of the Real: Making the Invisible Visible*, edited by Helga Nowotny and Martina Weiss, Verlag der Fachvereine Hochschulverlag AG an der ETH Zürich, 2000, pp. 119–35.

Gilman, Sander. 1976. "Hugh W. Diamond and Psychiatric Photography." *The Face of Madness: Hugh W. Diamond and the Origin of Psychiatric Photography*, edited by Sander Gilman. Brattleboro, VT: Echo Point Books & Media, 2014, pp. 5–16.

Gilman, Sander. *Seeing the Insane*. Hoboken, NJ: John Wiley & Sons, 1982.

Harper, Douglas. "Psyche (n.)." *Online Etymology Dictionary*, www.etymonline.com/word/psyche. Accessed July 28, 2021.

Harper, Douglas. "Psychiatry (n.)." *Online Etymology Dictionary*, www.etymonline.com/word/psychiatry. Accessed July 28, 2021.

Harper, Douglas. "Psychology (n.)." *Online Etymology Dictionary*, www.etymonline.com/word/psychology. Accessed July 28, 2021.

Hustvedt, Asti. *Medical Muses: Hysteria in Nineteenth-Century Paris*. New York: W. W. Norton & Company, 2011.

Marien, Mary Warner. *Photography: A Cultural History*. 4th ed. New York: Pearson, 2015.

Pichel, Beatriz. "From Facial Expressions to Bodily Gestures: Passions, Photography and Movement in French 19th-century Sciences." *History of the Human Sciences*, vol. 29, no. 1, 2016, pp. 27–48.

Roskies, Adina. "Are Neuroimages Like Photographs of the Brain?" *Philosophy of Science*, vol. 74, Dec. 2007, pp. 860–72.

Rowe, Colin, and Robert Slutzky. "Transparency: Literal and Phenomenal." *Perspecta*, vol. 8, 1963, pp. 45–54.

Talbot, William Henry Fox. 1844–1846. *The Pencil of Nature*. Burlington, VT: De Capo Press, 1969.

Vidal, Fernando. "Soul." *Encyclopedia of the Enlightenment*. Edited by Alan Charles Kors, vol. 4. Oxford: Oxford University Press, 2003, pp. 105–6.

Vidal, Fernando. "Brainhood, Anthropological Figure of Modernity." *History of the Human Sciences*, vol. 22, no. 1, 2009, pp. 5–36.

Wahl, Christopher John. *The Harvey Cushing Brain Tumor Registry: Changing Scientific and Philosophic Paradigms and the Study and Preservation of Archives*. 1996. Yale University School of Medicine, MD thesis. archive.org/details/39002086341949.med.yale.edu.

Wahl, Christopher J., Dennis D. Spencer, Aaron A. Cohen-Gadol, and Terry Dagradi. "Cushing Brain Tumor Registry: A Diary of Neurological Surgery during its Conception." *The Legacy of Harvey Cushing: Profiles of Patient Care*, edited by Aaron A. Cohen-Gadol and Dennis D. Spencer. Stuttgart: Thieme Medical Publishers and the American Association of Neurosurgeons, 2007, pp. xi–xxii.

Wilder, Kelley. "Visualizing Radiation: The Photographs of Henry Becquerel." *Histories of Scientific Observation*, edited by Lorraine Daston and Elizabeth Lunbeck. Chicago: University of Chicago Press, 2011, pp. 349–68.

6

POWER AND PICTURES ON THE THRESHOLD OF LIFE

Brain death and visual culture

Tim Seiber

August 2001 is a month easily forgotten in the minds of Americans. In September of that year, the death of thousands at the World Trade Center set off an endless war and continual renegotiations of what it means to be an American, a terrorist, alive. A renewed public debate about the coordinates of the treatment of humans – can they be humiliated? tortured? indefinitely detained? are some of them alive but outside the law? – was initiated. Today, these debates remain largely unresolved. As Thomas Stubblefield has argued, this event is marked by a particular kind of visual culture in which death and destruction are at once spectacularly visible and, at the same time, steeped in "absence, erasure, and invisibility" (3). In this case, death and new forms of mediation emerged simultaneously. Concurrently, another point of articulation between death and imagery was rapidly developing, in this case brain portraits of individuals in less-than-conscious states, made useful in determining if someone was brain dead. It is a similar complexity of both signification and death but on a much different scale, just as vivid but quieter.

Thus you might be forgiven for having missed or forgotten an article written by Gary Greenberg in the August 2001 issue of *The New Yorker* with a title that now sounds as prophetic as it is disturbing: "As Good as Dead." The essay tells the story of a young boy, Nicolas Breach, who at 14 was diagnosed with a fatal brain stem tumor (Greenberg). As his final wish, he wanted to be an organ donor. Complications arise from such lofty goals. In order to be a good match, donors must be alive right up until they are dead, their otherwise healthy organs fresh for transplantation. Thus, Nicolas would need to be dead, but alive enough that his organs still functioned. He would need to be brain dead.

Seventeen years later, *The New Yorker* returned to the topic of brain death, this time by introducing the story of Jahi McMath, a 14-year-old African American girl who suffered traumatic bleeding after a routine tonsillectomy (Aviv). As a result, she slipped into a subconscious state. Following guidance codified in law as the 1981 Uniform Determination of Death Act, which established national standards for the determination of "brain death," Jahi was declared dead by physicians at her hospital in Oakland, California. The family rejected this diagnosis, wanting to keep alive their daughter's body through artificial nutrition and hydration, two medical technologies widely available since World War II. Eventually Jahi was moved from California to New Jersey, one of only two states that allow families to reject the diagnosis of brain death on religious grounds. Legally dead in California, Jahi was legally alive in New Jersey.

 DOI: 10.4324/9781003007661-9

The complexity of these cases shows that we might not have clear, shared ideas about the purpose and consequences of a medical diagnosis of "brain death." As broader public debates about life – in the context of war, abortion, and global pandemics – become vectors for outrage and heated exchange, the topic of brain death provokes similar questions: do we know the difference between the living and the dead? Given the unique and special power of advanced medical imaging in the case of brain death, we might also ask, can we make visible the difference between the living and the dead?

In the United States, perhaps no greater pivot exists between Nicolas's case in 1984 and Jahi's in 2018 than the saga of Terri Schiavo, which was debated not just in Florida, where she lived and died, but also on the floors of Congress, in the White House, and at the Supreme Court. Schiavo's case was publicized partly due to the family drama around and through which her case was made public. A massive stroke left Schiavo in a vegetative state for nearly eighteen years, kept alive through artificial hydration and nutrition. A series of court battles hinging on visual evidence ranging from home movies to advanced brain scans resulted in Schiavo's life support systems being withdrawn in 2005. At that time, a final ruling of the court held that no further means of producing evidence – no means of making pictures of the brain, no family videos of Schiavo made by her family – would ever provide material evidence of the possibility of a recovery. The decision became yet another issue around which the concern about life's origins and ends catalyzed public discourse, crystallized political oppositions and became tangible through imagery. Here is, then, a case in which mediation and life-status became synonymous, in which how we demonstrate aliveness or deadness or brain-deadness is in part dependent on how images are made and framed, given context or ripped from it, made to mean or made to lack meaning. Since 1984, new imaging technologies have peered with ever more refined views into the brain and, we suppose, the mind. More broadly, medicine as media is everywhere in our society. Schiavo's case is a significant historical pivot point in which the mediation of life status through brain imagery shows how important the appeals to medical truth, made available to the public in the form of pictures, have become in widespread discussions of brain death.

In the four sections below, this chapter will pursue a critical analysis of the braided histories of brain imaging, debates about the ethics of a medical diagnosis of brain death, and the ways in which this braid is made possible through visual cultural. While brain images from drawings to photographs have a long history, it was not until the mid-1980s that scans of living brains could show structure and function in a medically useful way. Today, these scans are being asked to detect and depict less-than-fully-conscious brain states including brain death. Brain death is a fraught medical, political, and cultural subject bound up with the organ donation system, religious values, the law, and bioethics. First published in 1968, diagnostic standards for determining brain death were behavioral: persons could be declared brain dead if they did not respond to stimuli, breathe without a respirator, exhibit reflexes, or show electrical activity. Importantly, this declaration allowed for the harvesting of urgently needed healthy organs for donation. But today, with the advent of more powerful brain scanning tools, families, physicians, and the public are making increased demands not only to observe the brain dead body but also to show brain death itself. Schiavo's case gives these historical, medical, and cultural forces a specific context. Her case and others demonstrate how reliant we are on images to structure, narrate, and provide scientific backing to discussions about brain death. However, the promise that powerful images might dissolve ongoing dilemmas about the ethical principles, cultural rituals, religious values, and public policy intermingling in the zone between the living and the dead is overstated. While families and others may want these images to do the work of making brain death decisions more precise and certain, in fact current imaging cannot furnish visible evidence of brain death.

Getting there: death and the brain in visual media

Leading up to the final legal determination that Terri Schiavo was brain dead and that her artificial nutrition and hydration could be withdrawn was an excessively visual public battle about which pictures depicted the "real" woman who could not speak on her own behalf. Some images were produced by her parents, disability rights activists, and others who saw in the motion of arms and legs and in the perceived reactions to communication, an awake person who was simply trapped in a body that wouldn't cooperate – someone severely disabled but very clearly alive. These images took some familiar forms, including family photographs, home video, posed professional imagery, and documentary footage. However, a different image archive portrayed a different type of person. Medical images including positron-emission tomography (PET) scans showed a severely atrophied brain in which the location of consciousness had been destroyed through a massive stroke. In the image, a black irregular orb indicated that tissue had replaced with fluid in a place where a fully conscious person would have neurologically active gray matter. Clashing appeals to imagery were thus crucial in framing whether an individual was morally and medically alive or dead.

The family photographs and other associated imagery appealed to traditional interpretations of familiar genres. Their power derived from the everydayness of the framing and context and were easily relatable and highly emotional. The medical imagery, on the other hand, was persuasive in part because of the high-technology means of producing the pictures, which made possible new insights into brain function previously unobtainable. Although modes of peering beneath the skin into the tissues and surfaces of the inner body have been available since the late 19th century in the form of x-rays, it was not until the early 1980s that various modes of scanning, including MRI, PET, CT, and other methods were able to produce images of the brain at high enough resolutions to be diagnostically useful. While other means of making technological images of the brain including x-rays of the ventricular system and cerebral angioplasty are more than 100 years old, it wasn't until new techniques developed in the 1980s that "living images" could show structure and function allowing for medical interventions in living patients.

Still, we must be cautious about claims to the 'miracle' of modern image-making: a wealth of brain imagery has been produced from drawings of dissections in Ancient Greece to vascular drawings in 17th-century medicine to anatomical presentations produced by photographic dissections in the 19th century, including modern functional imaging. Photography was a crucial evolutionary step in this development, as it allowed brain maps to be made with exact mechanical vision and became increasingly necessary in the training of medical professionals (Hausman; Nolte).

Perhaps the most important source of information about this history and legacy is Edwin Clarke and Kenneth Dewhurst's *An Illustrated History of Brain Function*. Published first in 1972, the *Illustrated History* concluded its chronicle of the development of a concept called "functional localization" with modern imaging processes, including photographic images of dissected brains to in vivo computerized images made through X-ray (CT) and magnetic (MRI) visualizations. In the second edition, this section is extended to discuss the wide variety of technological advances made available through the 1980s and 1990s. Not surprisingly, the authors argue that future advances in neurology will be based on photographic and computational analysis of the human brain.

The *Illustrated History* organizes pictorial representations of the brain chronologically, beginning in antiquity and ending in the modern era. In the second edition, published in 1996, modern neurological medicine, aided in large part by CT and MRI imaging, associates behavior, attitude, self-awareness, motor skills, language, and myriad other aspects of human life with specific areas of brain activation. This now dominant theory of brain activity is called functional localization, an especially important development in attempts to establish relationships between images and medical diagnoses of brain death. If a picture can show that the areas of the brain associated with self-awareness and consciousness do not function or are entirely absent, then are we justified stating that a person is not present, even if other parts of the brain might still work? Crucially, brain images mediate not just medical knowledge, but also complex cultural ideas. This is accomplished aesthetically and these images become part of a public archive of pictures, which contain both medical and social information. Thus the authors state that, "although the main aim of the book is the portrayal of an idea, the techniques whereby anatomists and artists have attempted to achieve their purposes are also relevant and form a vital part of the history of art" (Clarke and Dewhurst 2). What I want to suggest here is that there is no history of the brain, and no kind of representation of the brain, that is not also essentially about the culture in which the image was made. This explains, in part, why representations of brain death, especially those of Terri Schiavo, produce such heated, politicized, and polemical arguments. Brain images are not just medical pictures but social ones as well.

In *Medical Visions*, media studies scholar Kirsten Ostherr analyzes a sweeping and comprehensive set of artifacts in which medical patients are "produced" through various forms of media, including film, television, and digital technologies. Discussing medical reality television, in which behind-the-scenes accounts of urgent medical procedures are edited to provide narrative, visual, and character continuity, Ostherr eventually turns to the role of medical imaging in such situations. In recounting one family's despair that their daughter, suffering from repeated seizures, had to wait in line for an MRI, she concludes that "within these storylines, medical imaging often plays a decisive narrative role by providing conclusive answers to diagnostic questions that had previously eluded comprehension" (195). Images play a crucial role in organizing expectations in many cases: "Good outcomes are presented as the result of following the course of treatment indicated by an imaging study," while bad outcomes are presented as patient's "bad decisions" (196). What is important to underscore here is the separation of the truth-generating power of medical technology from the decision-making power of the patient. In situations where peering into the body via technology becomes the basis of a diagnostic reality which cannot be experienced socially, the tense negotiations of medical and other kinds of truth are made apparent.

This is especially true of brain imagery and, increasingly, images that seek to "show" brain death. In part this is because for so long, personhood has been strongly linked with consciousness, which it often located in the brain. Recent studies of a myriad of advanced imaging techniques have begun the process of attempting to show brain death itself (Macdonald et al.; Gastala et al.). These studies hold out the promise, for physicians and for families, that images can describe a type of person, who is either alive or dead, with a type of visual certainty. In this way, these images become pictures of not just medical knowledge but of personhood. Scholars trained in film and media studies, aesthetic analysis, and medical anthropology have addressed the impact of brain scans on our thinking about what life is and how different types of life might be pictured. Joseph Dumit, in *Picturing Personhood*, traces the emergence of positron-emission tomography (PET) scans (9). His analysis of the links between medical imaging and personhood is instructive for any critical analysis of brain imaging. Dumit notes, for example, that "it is out of the busy intersection of technical, social, and cultural flows that scientists attempt to stabilize and conduct their experiments, and it is back into the intersection that their result must go" (9). Marking a distinct historical moment in which brain imaging is both circulated within and responsive to cultural modes of apprehending selfhood, Dumit argues that "there is an interplay between popularization processes and scientific inquiry … And we fashion our objective-selves with the fruit of this labor in the form of received-facts in our own continuously and often creative manner, no matter how skeptical we are. This way of living with and through scientific facts is our form of life" (9). Further, because the proliferation of brain types correlates to the construction of kinds of individuals and because brain scans "visually convey clear-cut graphical difference that can be easily read in some situations as referring to clear-cut statistical difference or even absolute differences in populations and brain types," they "can help produce, in some situations, the identification of groups as brain-types" (17).

Personhood as "seen" in medical imagery is coupled with the ability of these imaging processes such as functional MRI to produce medically useful information (Joyce 428). These ways of thinking and speaking about MRIs as a form of abstract and pure medical truth, however, obscure the aesthetic choices that are made by human agents. To make medical images of the brain, for example, technologists sit at computer screens; they use computer programs to decide the width of a particular picture, the total amount of the area being scanned, the resolution of the particular image, and so on. Like filmmakers or photographers, technologists have to frame the area and angle of representation that will be included in each picture. These decisions, or parameters, create the images, shaping the content in particular and significant ways (447). These images are, I am arguing, an attempt to stabilize in a visual artifact a set of potentially contested cultural values, presented as if they were the product of value-neutral machine vision. This is not, in fact, a correct interpretation. In the visual management of the brain through imaging processes, coupled with the historically-situated concept of functional localization, these pictures produce renderings of individuals – pictures of personhood – that mediate the medical as they are formed within social contexts.

One of the social functions, for example, is the management of ritual practices surrounding death. High-resolution imaging technologies have become increasingly important to doctors, patients, and families because of their aesthetic qualities, the status they are granted as "medical truths," and the belief that they are accurate depictions of certain types of persons. I have suggested that these properties become vexed and troubled in the context of brain death, which is a personhood status in which a body is both biologically alive and legally dead. In the next section, I will describe the history of the concept of brain death, how the role of image-making has intervened and dramatically changed the concept, and the ways in which this change has meaningful impacts not just within medicine but in the social understanding and management of death in general.

The temporal life of the dead in pictures and in practice

It can be very persuasive to see the relationship between the living and the dead of one of immediacy and certainty. A person is alive right up until she is dead. And once dead, there is no coming back. Of course, we know from our cultural stories of ghosts, spirits, vampires, and other figures, not to mention religious beliefs, that while we might think of biological death as an absolute, socially speaking we manage our relationship to the dead in much more complicated ways. American historian and anthropologist Thomas Lacqueur has investigated the cultural and historical coordinates of rituals surrounding death, positing that one crucial aspect about death and dying is that these processes unfold over time. What he means is that even though the standard model for establishing the physical death of the body, which occurs when it ceases to breathe, might occur at a specific time and place – a practice made famous by the innumerable statements of "time of death" in television and film – this isn't exactly the totality of a death. Rituals are performed. Memorials are staged. Physical objects are sorted;

some kept, others trashed. Thus, he concludes, "Becoming really dead … takes time" (Lacquer, "The Deep Time" 802). While much of his work deals with 19th-century burial and cultural practices, Lacqueur acknowledges that in its modern form, the temporality of death is given a new framework and new meaning in the context of brain death. The question "when is death" is now not just about social practices and biological determinations but also about technology, diagnostic criteria, family struggles, and today, images. On the topic of images, Lacqueur does not comment beyond noting that some hospitals use electroencephalography (EEG) "or other modern procedures to create a visually enduring and rhetorically more demanding high bar for taking the test that counts" (Lacquer, "Afterword" 148).

The "test that counts" is the apnea test in which physicians rule out other causes for a lack of response to stimulus and then demonstrate that the body cannot sustain breathing on its own. The battery of tests focuses on cranial nerves that test eye motion, gag reflex, blink reflex, inhalation reflex, pupillary photo reflex, and other stimulus reactions. If response is not observed, then the final stage of determining brain death is to remove artificial breathing supports and wait a minimum of three minutes to see if spontaneous breathing resumes (Lacquer, "Afterword" 148–50). While other test batteries, including the Glasgow Coma Scale developed in 1974, determine levels of responsiveness and can indicate degree of coma, only this comprehensive group of behavior tests can justify the classification of "brain death" (Teasdale et al.).

By "degree of coma," I am referring to the medical distinctiveness between various states of less-than-full-consciousness. In *Death and Donation*, philosopher D. Scott Henderson provides a nuanced account of the emergence of a concept of brain death. Established in 1968, an ad hoc committee at Harvard began to deliberate protocols for determining if a patient was brain dead. In part, this was due to the growing demand for donor organs, which had become a crucial piece of medical technology after the first successful heart transplant in 1967. Published in the *Journal of the American Medical Association*, this group argued that brain death was diagnosable if a patient did not respond to stimuli, did not spontaneously breath for three minutes after the removal of a respirator, did not exhibit reflexes, and had a flat EEG – indicating no electrical activity in the brain – for ten consecutive minutes (Henderson 8). These standards, though, had critics who argued that they were inhumane, arbitrary, untested, and medically unjustified. Some of these critics argued that if only some areas of the brain – those responsible for stimulus response and other functions – were inactive, yet others (such as the auditory system) were active, then in some way a person was still in the brain. In other words, he was not dead. Thus, the theory of functional localization became a topic of intense ethical disagreement in the context of brain death. This disagreement would ultimately become codified in often confusing and contradictory statutes and practices about the determination of death (Henderson). Scholars have noted, as well, that the brain dead body whose organs are harvested provoke "startling questions" regarding the "dynamic nature of self and personhood" (Sharp 304).

Some of the reasons why the concept of brain death produces such anxiety and heated debate is, certainly, that the medical perspective is not a diagnostically "pure" decision but rather a battery of behavioral tests that can be interpreted. In this way, brain death and the image are similar: while there may be an overriding collective sense of what we are looking at, there are counter-positions and different interpretations that throw into relief any universal perspective. Another reason, of course, is that we do not have well-established rituals and cultural codes related to how we treat bodies is a split state of aliveness. In the particular case of Terri Schiavo, the type of personhood under discussion is the persistent vegetative state (PVS.) Closely related to coma and the minimally conscious state (MCS), PVS patients remain bed-ridden with open eyes but without controlled response to stimuli. This situation can provoke in families, doctors, and researchers, the feeling that somewhere hidden deep in the brain, a person is trapped, looking out in the world and waiting to regain control of her body. This condition was first described in 1972, co-emergent with ideas about brain death, the Glasgow Coma Scale, and other advances in neurology (Jennett and Plum.) Based on a model of neurological medicine that required direct observation of patient behavior – which could indicate cognition – in order to determine the patient's brain state, the original article describing PVS does not once mentions brain imagery. There is, of course, a long history of the use of photography to establish medical truth through autopsy photographs. However, this was of no use in trying to determine brain states in living bodies – in 1972 brain death was impervious to pictorial representation. The behavioral model became increasingly refined throughout the 1970s and the 1980s. PVS, for example, was situated within a mosaic of other less-than-fully-conscious cognitive states; these standards are referred to as the Aspen Criteria (Fins Brain Injury).

But as with almost all areas of modern medicine, advanced computation and the proliferation of imaging technologies put pressure of the diagnostic mosaic around less-than-fully-conscious medicine to become more visible. Journals such as *Neurology* and *Neuroimage*, which began publishing in the early 1990s, showed neurological images with highly detailed portraits of the brain. Thus, some researchers and a great deal of the public sought to see an image to associate with each brain state – brain dead, PVS, MCS – each one picturing a different kind of person and, perhaps, different ethical status. While neurological images hold out the promise of more refined diagnostic claims, for now, consciousness cannot be imaged, only imagined, through brain scans. Even the most advanced research makes only cautious claims, arguing, for example, that, "we believe that the identification of positive results with fMRI using this simple task, may compliment the clinical assessment by helping attain a more precise diagnosis in patients with disorders of consciousness" (Beckenstein et al. 1).

Medical ethicist Joseph Fins argues that while neuroimaging can usefully differentiate between various brain states and physical responses to stimulus, it cannot conclusively determine whether someone is importantly and morally alive or dead. Like many ethical considerations of the brain, Fins equates biological status with ethical status, the physical activity of the brain as a metaphor for the affective activity of the human. In fact, the power of neuroimaging to disclose states of aliveness is often overstated for political or cultural purposes. As Fins notes regarding a *New York Times* article that described the "possibility" of new, advanced imaging techniques to provide "better pictures" of Schiavo's brain, "the utility of neuroimaging and its capabilities was at the center of the debate over whether she was or was not in a permanent vegetative state. The misappropriation of well-established diagnostic criteria … was an attempt to pursue a political agenda and what President Bush described as a 'culture of life' after Ms. Schiavo's death. But it was also a misrepresentation of the capabilities of current neuroimaging technologies" (Fins, "The Orwellian Threat" 56). In fact, as an overview article addressing the various states of compromised brain function suggests, even pictures produced from the express purpose of showing pain response in patients with MCS, PVS, and locked-in syndrome fail to differentiate clearly the anatomical and functional changes after severe brain injury (Laureys et al.).

In the case of brain death, with the advancement of pictorial technologies allowing physicians, families, and the public to peer into the brain of a living body, it was imagined that these pictures might picture personhood in the zone between the living and the dead, thereby informing ethical discussions related to end of life medical care, religious and cultural practices, and other important conversations. These images are not secondary to our primary cultural and social struggles but rather are structuring objects through and over which we struggle for interpretive, ethical, and political control of the ethical and biological thresholds separating the dead and living. In the next section, I will show how the case of Terri Schiavo, which began precisely in the midst of the increasing visualization of neurological medicine, shows how the framing, situating, and contesting of visual artifacts is at the heart of how we approach these debates.

Medical visuality and popular images: the case of Terri Schiavo

The Terry Schiavo Life & Hope Network became very involved in Jahi McMath's case. In part, they assisted the family in learning the visual techniques by which to show aliveness. The Network encouraged Jahi's mother to record "tests" on her cell phone in which she would give Jahi a command and then record the response. "Lift your right finger," her mother might say. A few seconds later a finger would lift; in some tests, the correct finger would slightly move. Skeptical of this evidence, a UCLA neurologist then investigated, looking at 49 videos made by Jahi's mom, suggesting then that Jahi may be in a relapsing/remitting state of awareness; another doctor, looking at the same footage, noted, "I'm always skeptical of videotapes, because of the videos of Terri Schiavo." This skepticism derives from the ways in which techniques of making persuasive imagery took on outstanding power in the social, medical, and legal proceedings of the end of Terri Schiavo's life. By the time her life became the subject of massive and politicized debate, various factors were at play framing and situating how the relationship between medicine and media would structure deliberations. The theory of functional localization and diagnostic criteria for establishing brain death allowed for a body to be physically alive while the person was declared legally dead; bioethics related to organ donation and healthcare costs was becoming an increasingly complicated analytical tradition; advanced imaging technologies made possible pictures of personhood of people, even if they could not speak for themselves; families and physicians frequently turned to images to share information and to provide vivid documents through which to narrate medical experience; faith in technological medicine to show us the truth was on the rise. All of these factors, and more, made possible and limited what could be said about Schiavo's case.

Within this context, visual media played a crucial role. In fact, so widespread was the mediation of Schiavo's medical situation that in the winter of 2006 a special section of the media studies journal, *Jump Cut,* was dedicated to the "emergency" of visual media produced about her. In her contribution, film scholar Diane Waldman notes that the use of home videos, excerpting and framing of family photographs, and presentation of serial imagery meant to imply movement suggested that Schiavo's parents, who wanted the Florida Supreme Court to rule that she was legally alive, "put their faith in the notion that the camera would provide direct access to truth otherwise kept hidden – by Michael Schiavo [her husband] … by the courts, and by the mainstream media." This faith was matched by a similar faith in the truth-producing capacities of medical imaging. Interestingly, this faith ran in two directions during the Schiavo court proceedings. When presented with an analysis of a CT scan of Schiavo's brain indicating massive atrophy in the areas of the brain responsible for consciousness, the family demanded a different type of scan, an MRI. When asked why an MRI was not produced, the chief medical expert in the case, Dr. Ronald Cranford, provided a detailed response. He noted, when asked by a blogger interested in the case, that "An MRI was never recommended because, in this case and other patients in a permanent vegetative state, the CT scans were more than adequate to demonstrate the extremely severe atrophy of the cerebral hemispheres, and an MRI could add nothing of significance … Plus the MRI is contraindicated because of the intrathalamic stimulators implanted in Terri's brain. A PET scan was never done in this case because it was never needed. The classic clinical signs on examination, the CT scans, and the flat EEG's were more than adequate to diagnose PVS to the highest medical certainty"

("Schiavo – Dr. Cranford"). Here, then, the family's appeal to powerful medical imagery, which is based in the popular belief that technology can help picture personhood, was countered by a medical expert who noted that this belief overestimates the power of visual images, which are aligned better with cultural desires to see truth and gain narrative control over medical situations than with diagnostic clarity.

Cranford, in his testimony before the court, summarized Schiavo's interactions with brain scanning. In 1990, 1996, and 2002, she underwent CT scans. Although appeals to more powerful technologies were made, they would not be medically useful. "The initial CT scan on the day of admission, February 25, 1990, was normal but further CT scans documented a progression of widespread cerebral hemisphere atrophy, eventually resulting in CT scans of 1996 and 2002 showing extreme atrophy" (Cranford 364). Almost all of the public commentary about these scans related to a side-by-side image showing two CT scans, one labeled, "Terri's Brain," and the other labeled, "Healthy Brain." The source of the "Terri's Brain" image is the 1996 CT scan. The scans, roughly similar in size, orientation, and shape, are presented to accentuate the contrast in the area of consciousness. Not only is the fluid in Schiavo's brain shown to occupy a large area, but the image itself is tinted blue set opposite a more "medical" image in grayscale. In Schiavo's brain scan, as well, the intrathalamic stimulator glows bright, indicating non-biological material. In 2005 as today, the internet was a crucial media space in which opinions and analysis – some from experts, some from the public – were forwarded and perhaps no more dramatically that in discussions of this image. One such string of commentary includes nearly 1,000 discrete observations, evincing remarkable and, at times, incredible variation. One commentator, a PhD neuroscientist, noted of the scans that "the large 'blue blobs' in the middle are ventricles … that have expanded to such a large size because overall brain volume is low." Another comment indicates that this medical description is inadequate: "For me, what it comes down to is this: If someone's body or brain lives, is it right to starve her to death? I don't believe so." A third focuses on technology. "Medical technology has blurred the boundary between life and death, causing us to make decisions we didn't use to have to make." Limiting the value of brain scans, another reader argues that "The brain scans and other diagnostic procedures performed on Terri tell us nothing we do will have any consequences for her, because she doesn't exist anymore as a conscious being" ("Regarding the CAT Scan.") (Figure 6.1).

Conclusion: now you see it?

In these competing and partial interpretations of these scans, viewers marshal their expert training, moral reasoning, and points of view to engage with an emergency taking place both in medicine and in visual media. It is tempting to respond to this in two ways. First one might want to develop some kind of principled analytical reading that sorts other's interpretations into categories – accurate or inaccurate, clear or clouded, expert or naïve. Second, we might try to assert some principle that suggests an interpretation that is most "medically accurate" is more true and thus better. But we are not just in the realm of medicine. We are also in the world of mediation. Scholars have noted that in the case of Terri Schiavo, corporate media, religious extremism, the willingness to ignore privacy concerns, and legal maneuvering inflamed passions and led to an excess of media production (Kellner). Given this, it is very tempting to produce corrective interpretations that fix spectacle against something we might want to call truth. But I want to point us in a different direction in which powerful imagery has its volume turned down, in which we do not interpret against emergency but rather slowly and quietly. I started this chapter by invoking both visual spectacle and forgotten tragedies experienced

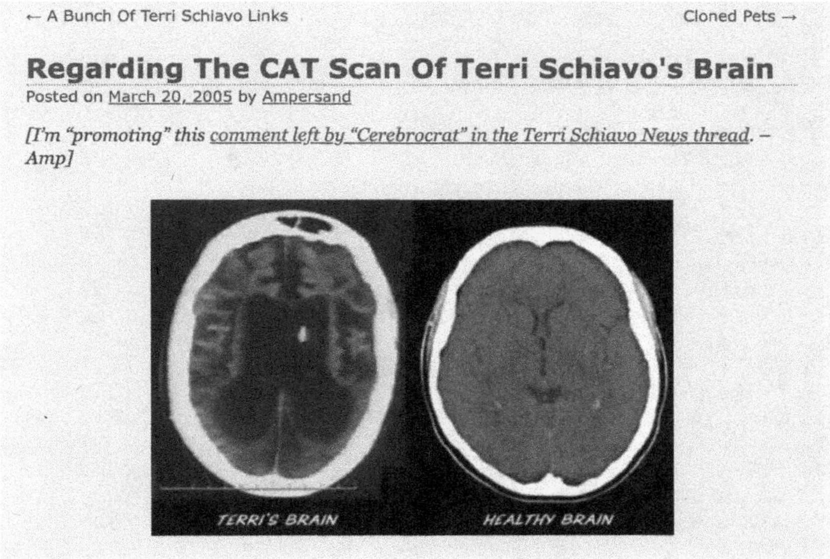
← A Bunch Of Terri Schiavo Links Cloned Pets →

Regarding The CAT Scan Of Terri Schiavo's Brain

Posted on March 20, 2005 by Ampersand

[I'm "promoting" this comment left by "Cerebrocrat" in the Terri Schiavo News thread. – Amp]

Figure 6.1 Still from "Regarding the CAT Scan"

socially, and I'll end by suggesting something about the future battles over life provoked by brain death: that in the new neurosciences of brain states, we will find ever more evocative pictures of our brains with increasingly refined resolutions. And that, as shown in the contested interpretations of Schiavo's brain images, the future technoportraits won't be able to help us at all, really, as we deliberate and determine matters of life and death.

Brain scans are small emergencies that conflate and unite medical dilemmas and visual interpretation. Emergent in the sense that they come forth within very specific and fraught medical situations; they are emergencies as well because while physicians, families, and the public may seek stability in the image; and they are equally capable of destabilizing our social conventions about care of the dead and near-dead. On one hand, these pictures organize a set of moments within an overall arc of medical care that can take amorphous guesses and suggestions – diagnostic ideas but also family investments – into something precise. Images can be looked at for guidance: here is where we might operate, that is where consciousness would be but it isn't. Peering beneath the skull is very powerful. On the other hand, the conflation of visual precision with medical precision is only ever suggested, but not accomplished, through brain imaging. Errors can be made by the technologist. Interpreters make assumptions that might or might not be accurate. Gaining narrative control over the emergency of brain death can be a very powerful way to confront a horrible situation, and images hold out the promise of gaining that control. For physicians, it is something to point to, a visual confirmation, something that can be described with clarity. For families making end-of-life decisions, these images can function as something like documentary proof, the "real" of the brain exposed with the powerful tools of medical truth-making. However, we should be careful not to overstate the power of these pictures, which are but one point of contact between the living and the dead. As we develop cultural rituals about how to incorporate an analysis of brain scans into our deliberations about who is alive, dead, or brain-dead, perhaps we will better understand our own investments in questions at the margins of life.

Works cited

Aviv, Rachel. "What Does It Mean to Die." *The New Yorker,* January 29, 2018, www.newyorker.com/magazine/2018/02/05/what-does-it-mean-to-die. Accessed December 30, 2020.

Beckenstein, Tristan, et al. "Functional Imaging Reveals Movement Prepratory Activity in the Vegetative State," *Frontiers in Human Neuroscience*, vol. 5, January, 2011, pp. 1–11.

Clarke, Edwin and Kenneth Dewhurst. *An Illustrated History of Brain Function: Imaging the Brain from Antiquity to the Present*, 2nd edition. Tampa, FL: Norman and Company, 1995.

Cranford, Ronald. "Facts, Lies, and Videotapes: The Permanent Vegetative State and the Sad Case of Terri Schiavo." *The Journal of Law, Medicine, and Ethics*, vol. 33, no. 2, 2005, pp. 363–71.

Dumit, Joseph. *Picturing Personhood: Brain Scans and Biomedical Identity*. Princeton , NJ: Princeton University Press, 2004.

Fins, Joseph. "The Orwellian Threat to Emerging Neurodiagnostic Technologies." *The American Journal of Bioethics*, vol. 5, no. 2, 2005, pp. 56–8.

Fins, Joseph. "Brain Injury: The Vegetative and Minimally Conscious States." *From Birth to Death and Bench to Clinic: The Hastings Center Bioethics Briefing Book for Journalists, Policymakers, and Campaigns*, edited by Mary Crowly, Garrison N.Y., Hastings Center, 2008, pp. 15–20.

Gastala, Joseph, et al. "Brain Death: Radiological Signs of a Non-Radiological Diagnosis." *Clinical Neurology and Neurosurgery*, vol. 185, October, 2019, pp. 1–11.

Greenberg, Gary. "As Good as Dead." *The New Yorker*, August 2, 2001, www.newyorker.com/magazine/2001/08/13/as-good-as-dead. Accessed December 30, 2020.

Hausman, Louis. *Photographs of Microscopic Serial Sections of the Human Spinal Cord and Brain*. Springfield: Charles C. Thomas Publishers, 1969.

Henderson, D. Scott. *Death and Donation: Rethinking Brain Death as a Means for Procuring Transplantable Organs*. Eugene: Pickwick Publications, 2011.

Jennett, Bryan and Fred Plum. "Persistent Vegetative State after Brain Damage." *The Lancet*, April, 1972, pp. 734–7.

Joyce, Kelly. "Appealing Images: Magnetic Resonance Imaging and the Production of Authoritative Knowledge." *Social Studies of Science*, vol. 35, no. 3, 2005, pp. 437–62.

Kellner, Douglas. "The Media and Death: The Case of Terri Schiavo and the Pope." *Flow*, April 25, 2005, www.flowjournal.org/2005/04/the-media-and-death-the-case-of-terri-schaivo-and-the-pope/. Accessed December 30, 2020.

Lacquer, Thomas. "The Deep Time of the Dead." *Social Research*, vol. 78, no. 3, 2011, pp. 799–820.

Lacquer, Thomas. "Afterword."*Interdisciplinary Perspectives on Mortality and its Timings*, edited by Shane McCorristine, London: Palgrave Macmillan, 2017, pp. 145–54.

Laureys, Steven, Adrian Owen, and Nicholas Schiff. "Brain Function in Coma, Vegetative State, and Related Disorders." *The Lancet Neurology*, vol. 3, September, 2004, pp. 537–45.

Macdonald, Derek, et al. "The Role of Neuroimaging in the Determination of Brain Death." *Journal of Neuroimaging*, vol. 28, no. 4, 2018, pp. 374–9.

Nolte, Josh. *The Human Brain in Photographs and Diagrams,* 5th edition. Philadelphia: Saunders, 2013.

Ostherr, Kirsten. *Medical Visions: Producing the Patient through Film, Television, and Imaging Technologies*. Oxford University Press, 2013.

"Regarding the CAT Scan of Terri Schiavo's Brain." Alas! – A Blog, March 20, 2005, https://amptoons.com/blog/?p=1423&cpage=4. Accessed November 11, 2009.

"Schiavo – Dr. Cranford Offers a Response." *Pekin Prattle*, March 18, 2005, www.pekinprattles.blogspot.com/2005/03/schiavo-dr-cranford-offers-reply.html. Accessed December 30, 2020.

Sharp, Lesley. "The Commodification of the Body and Its Parts." *Annual Review of Anthropology*, vol. 29, 2000, pp. 287–328.

Stubblefield, Thomas. *9/11 and the Visual Culture of Disaster*. Indiana University Press, 2015.

Teasdale, Graham, et al. "The Glasgow Coma Scale at 40 Years: Standing the Test of Time." *The Lancet*, vol. 13, no. 8, 2014, pp. 844–54.

Waldman, Diane. "Timely Triage." *Jump Cut: A Review of Contemporary Media*, vol. 48, Winter, 2006, http://ejumpcut.org/archive/jc48.2006/SchiavoWaldman/index.html. Accessed December 30, 2020.

7

MILITARY BODIES, HEALTHY BODIES, DAMAGED BODIES IN THE PHOTOGRAPHY OF AUGUST SANDER

Sander L. Gilman

When introduced to his future roommate by a common friend in *A Study in Scarlet* (1887), Sherlock Holmes immediately recognizes the physician, Dr. John Watson, as a former officer who had served in the second Anglo-Afghan campaign (1878–1880). Watson is puzzled by this revelation, and Holmes later explains that Watson had "the air of a military man" (Conan Doyle 14). Holmes' ability to see the soldier although clothed in mufti is a commonplace in the analysis of the modern soldier's body, visible even in civilian garb. We claim to recognize the modern soldier from afar – his (and they are always men) unconscious posture trained and shaped by the military. The rigid exterior of his frame mirrors, we imagine, the martial shaping of his soul.[1] We know that Holmes was not so loosely based on Arthur Conan Doyle's boss at the Edinburgh Royal Infirmary in 1877, Dr. Joseph Bell, the forensic pathologist and famed diagnostician. While we often dismiss, in both the medical and critical literature, the diagnostic gaze as biased or at least culturally determined, we are somehow lulled into imagining that this is a professional and not a human problem. As Carolyn Smith-Morris, in her introduction to *Diagnostic Controversy*, writes: "Diagnosis is among the first responses to suffering, the one that initiates and organizes all others" (1–2). She acknowledges its paradoxes, noting: "Diagnosis is a necessary and speculative tool for the identification of and response to suffering in any healing system. But it is also an expression and a vehicle of bio-medico-capitalist power" (19). Yet our assumptions about martial bodies seem to counter this. Modern critical discourse has reinforced our ability to "see" and therefore "know" the souls of soldiers even when their bodies are in disguise without framing this knowledge as fragmentary, contradictory, and always shaped by contingencies. Framing soldier's bodies in the world of health and illness means thinking beyond and with representations, for as we all know, "*Ceci n'est pas une pipe*" – but what are they in the end?

Military bodies seem to have been molded, according to Michel Foucault in *Discipline and Punish* (1975), "by the late eighteenth century … out of a formless clay, an inapt body, the machine required [to] be constructed; posture gradually corrected; a calculated constraint runs slowly through each part of the body, mastering it, making it pliable" in contrast to the self-shaped ancient warrior "who could be recognized from afar; he bore certain signs: the natural signs of his strength and his courage, the marks, too, of his pride; his body was the blazon of his

DOI: 10.4324/9781003007661-10

strength and valor" (135). Healthy and manly, the ancient warrior is born not made, his soul his own, not that shaped by the modern, militarized national state for its own interests.

Thus, the soldier's body seemed to have become, by World War I, even more a "stereometric figure," as the Nobel Prize winning thinker Elias Canetti observed, looking back in time from his exile in Britain during World War II, for "a soldier is like a prisoner who has adapted himself to the walls enclosing him and fights against his confinement so little that the prison walls actually affect his shape" (312). Canetti's view of the soldier's body sees this internalized rigidity as simply an expanded definition of the soldier, a body beyond history, indebted to the state's rules and orders that shout "stand up straight!" And these commands are heard not only by the soldier but also by every citizen.

August Sander in Weimar: a case study

Among those who shared in the experience of becoming a soldier in Wilhelmenian Germany was the young industrial photographer, August Sander (1876–1964), who became the most esteemed social photographer of Weimar Germany. Beginning as an itinerant portrait photographer in the Rhineland, having been apprenticed to an industrial photographer in the coalmines in the 1890s, he then spent his military service (1897–99) as a photographer's assistant. At the turn of the century, he worked at a portrait studio in Linz, Austria, and at the end of 1909, he returned to the Rhineland, to Cologne, to open his own studio. At the outbreak of the war, Sander was drafted into the *Landsturm* (territorial reserve) and his wife, Anna, maintained their Cologne studio by primarily photographing soldiers on home leave.

Even before the war, August Sander began to think of his commissioned as well as informal portraits as the core of a larger project on the state of Imperial Germany and its castes. In the early 1920s, Sander had come in contact with the radical, working-class "Cologne Progressives," who, as Wieland Schmied observed, "sought to combine constructivism and objectivity, geometry and object, the general and the particular, avant-garde conviction and political engagement, and which perhaps approximated most to the forward looking of the New Objectivity [*Neue Sachlichkeit*] …" (21). While Sander began as early as 1910 with the first series of portraits for his work, *The Face of Our Time* (*Antlitz der Zeit*), his broad physiognomy of the Weimar Republic was published in 1929. One of his social castes consisted of photographs from the Great War and Weimar under the rubric "The Soldier" (IV/23).

As noted, August Sander spent his military service (1897–99) as a photographer's assistant in Trier recording exactly the military bodies that came into the studio unformed and eventually left reshaped. Sander's curated images in his 1929 *Antlitz der Zeit* from the period of the Great War and its immediate aftermath reflect such presuppositions, even when the soldiers depicted as in his *Soldatische Größenunterschiede* (Height Differences in Soldiers, c. 1915) seem to stress humorous differences among such bodies. But most show how the military body is shaped and remains so, as in his *Oberst* (Colonel, c. 1916) as well as *Leutnant*, 1911–1914 (Second Lieutenant, 1911–1914). The military bodies as reflected by Sander in these images seem evocative of Holmes' seeing Watson's military posture even when he was in mufti. Being out of uniform or indeed, out of service, seems not to impact the soldier's body, if we accept the post-World War II expansion of his 1929 collection. Sander's photograph of a *Pensionierter Major* (Retired Major, c. 1930), included in the posthumous extended collection of images compiled after World War II, reflects the rigidity of the Imperial military body as imagined after the collapse of Nazi Germany.

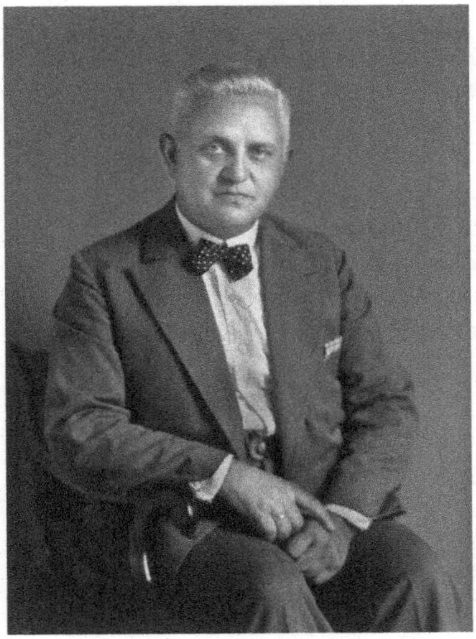

Figure 7.1 *Pensionierter Major*

The rigidity could be that of a posed portrait photograph of a middle-aged man, but in this context, we see, or at least believe we see, the rigidity of the military body (Figure 7.1). Would we see it this way if we did not know he was a "retired Major"? In other words, does the external "clue" of the title provide a lens though which we are encouraged to see and read the photo? Would we come to the same conclusion if the photo was labeled, "retired butcher" or "retired pastry chef"? (Gilman and Schmölders).

Sander's original volume of 1929, *Antlitz der Zeit*, was introduced by leftwing novelist, Alfred Döblin, whose bestselling novel of working-class life in Weimar Berlin, *Berlin Alexanderplatz*, appeared the same year to enormous praise. The protagonist of Döblin's novel, like the sitters in many of Sander's photographs, is a marginal member of the working class. Franz Biberkopf is mired in the economic collapse and political disarray of the times, damned to the eternal repetition of his marginality. As Döblin notes in his introduction to the photos, Sander, like himself, is aiming to create a cultural sociology of the present day with "superb material for the cultural, class, and economic history of the last thirty years" ("Faces, Images, and their Truth" 13). This view was echoed by Walter Benjamin in his classic 1931 essay on the nature of photography inspired to no little extent by Sander's photographs (Benjamin 520). The collapse of the German working as well as middle class in the inter-war years is mirrored in Döblin's insightful, innovative, and stylistically elegant montage mirrors much of Sander's work: brilliant, elegant, often beautiful, but always relentlessly brutal images of the marginal and those that believed themselves not to be marginal, but whom society damned any way.

For Döblin, the soldier's posture was problematic, as it was for most writers on the Left in the 1920s. In the novel, the narrative voice looks across the street at the stream of pedestrians, thinking that "they are as indistinguishable as those others sitting in trams and buses. They all sit in different postures, adding to the declared weight of the carriage. What is going on in them, who could write it, a monstrous chapter. And if someone did, then what? New books? The old ones don't sell..." (*Berlin Alexanderplatz* 158). No one, the author believes, can narrate the soul of those seen, no one can truly tell their inner story. Döblin's protagonist Franz Biberkopf thinks about his own posture in a conversation with a "stunted" friend on the street, who tells him:

> In our regiment we had an old reserve captain who was just forty, from Saarbrücken, lottery ticket seller – tobacconist to you, he says – he had arthritis at forty, in the lumbar region. He pretended it was his martial posture. He went around like a broom stick on wheels. He always had himself rubbed down with butter. And when there weren't no more butter, 1917 time, just Palmin, first-class vegetable oil, and rancid it were too, then he got himself shot."
>
> *(Berlin Alexanderplatz 160)*

Posture is imposture; martial posture can be read into pathology. You are what you see, maybe. And in the end, we are all dead, whether we know it or not, which seems to be the theme of Sander's work in the 1920s.

Sander's contemporary, the cultural commentator Oswald Spengler, observes in the *Decline of the West* (1922–23) that "the visible foreground of all history has the same significance as the external appearance of the human being, such as physique, facial expression, posture, gait; not what is spoken, but the speaking; not what is written, but the handwriting" (136). In the introduction to the 1980 revisionist edition of Sander's photographic project, undertaken with many of the additional photographs newly printed by his son Günther after World War II, the University of California art historian, Ulrich Keller, saw in Spengler the very conservative model, what has come to be called "reactionary modernism," defining Sander's work in the 1920s (Keller). Without agreeing with Spengler's pessimism, it is possible still to imagine understanding cultures from the representation of their postures (in all senses of that word) as being exceedingly problematic.

Yet Sander was understood in his time as a political figure of the Left, even though his own political ideology was much less rigid. He was considered by the Nazi state after 1933 and the post-war West German government after 1945 as a political opponent of the Nazis. After 1945, the category used to describe him was as a socially critical artist who, like Käthe Kollwitz, had created for the "desk drawer" during the Third Reich. Like Kollwitz, he was a pacificist, and while political in the broadest sense of the word, Sander claimed, at least in his 1927 advertisement for the book that "he has brought the task to completion with the fanaticism of a seeker of truth, and without prejudice either for or against any one party, tendency, class or society" (cited by Döblin, "Faces, Images and their Truth" 1).

Throughout Sander's work, especially after 1919, there is an engagement with re-reading images of militarism and the soldier's body. Given that this is linked to ideas of disability, health, and character throughout this period (on the Right as well as on the Left), Sander's project as well as the ancillary photographs made of soldiers during World War I and then again on leave during World War II, come to represent an encoded iconography concerning vulnerability and fragility in the guise of the rigid soldier's body. The program stressed by comparison the illusion of the rigid soldier's body to the human's vulnerability, both in physical and ideological terms of the lived experience of the Imperial and then, after 1933, the *Wehrmacht* (army) soldier. His project at its core was subversive but not because of any clear intention on his part. His work in the 1920s was clearly part of the employment of photography (directly or in the form of montage) as critiques from the Left and of the perceived reasons for German failure in World War I from the Right. What is most revealing is that the position of exposing the vulnerability of the soldier's body continues in his work after 1933, work that could not be as self-consciously political as in the 1920s.

Sander in the Third Reich

Elias Canetti evokes the stereometric soldier's body in his study of fascism and argues in his *Crowds and Power* (1960) that its rigidity of body and soul are both visible in the Nazi body after 1933. Canetti reflects the post-World War II obsession with flawed masculinity as a sign of or indeed as the source of fascism, as argued by Wilhelm Reich in 1933 (Reich). The image of the soldier's "muscle physis," as described in the same context by Klaus Theweleit, defines the proto-fascist body of the *Freikorp* soldier during the Weimar Republic soon to be in thrall to the *Führer.* For Theweleit, it is the internalization of a sense of rigid order, "wholeness," of the new "man of steel to pursue, to dam in, and to subdue any force that threatens to transform him back into the horribly disorganized jumble of flesh, hair, skin, bones, intestines, and feelings that calls itself human" (II, 160). This is part of the post-World War II world of imagining the Nazi soldier that included Foucault and Canetti as well as Theweleit.

After the 1933 "Enabling Act" and the seizure of power by the Nazis, Sander's work became unacceptable. His older son, Erich Sander (1903–1944), had been arrested in 1934 for political activity against the Reich as a member of the underground Socialist Workers Party (SAPD) and had documented his life in prison through a series of surreptitious photographs. He eventually died in a Nazi prison (Siegburg) in 1944 from an untreated, ruptured appendix. In 1933–1934, August Sander published five portfolios of landscapes and botanical photographs, some by Erich, entitled *German Land, German People* (*Deutsche Lande – Deutsche Volk*): *Die Eifel* (1933), *Bergisches Land* (1933), *Die Mosel* (1934), *Das Siebengebirge* (1934), *Die Saar* (1934) and *Am Niederrhein* (1935). However, this came to naught in establishing himself as a *völkisch* artist and his work was officially condemned by the Nazis in 1936. He was forbidden from publishing his photographs after 1938, when the printing plates for *Antlitz der Zeit* were seized and destroyed. After Erich's death, Sander had a death mask cast and photographed it in 1944. While his brother was imprisoned, the photographer Günther Sander (1907–1987), was drafted into the *Wehrmacht* in 1940, as were many of the men of his generation. He was captured by the American forces in France in 1944 and only returned to his photographic practice in Cologne after the war. Their father, August Sander, was able to earn his living as a portrait photographer under the Nazis until his studio was bombed in 1944, much of his archive destroyed subsequently in a fire in 1946.

In 1951, August Sander met Edward Steichen, then the director of MoMa's Department of Photography who subsquently included three of August Sander's photographs in the global "Family of Man" exhibit in 1955, along with works of the 273 most preeminent photographers of the day. Sander was well represented with three photos in the rubrics "Work," "Teens," and "Couples" from the 1920s. Sponsored by the United States Information Agency and Coca-Cola, it became a detailed counter to the claims of Sander's 1929 project. Central to this project was the universal nature of mankind subdivided into 32 themes, transcending race and cultural limitations; it was a project that responded to the rejection of fascist thought after Nazi racism and in light of nuclear disaster. It was shown throughout the world. In West Germany, it was displayed in West Berlin and Hamburg (1955) as well as in Munich (1958). Rather than social castes, as in *Antlitz der Zeit*, it covered the stages and ages of human life from "Loves" to "Work" to "Inhumanities," including some of the anonymous photographs from the Warsaw ghetto used in the Nuremberg trials. In the exhibit, a caption from George Sand, reading "Humanity is outraged in me and with me. We must not dissimulate…" was positioned above these horrific images. "Soldiers" needless to say was not a category. By 1966, the revision of the *Antlitz der Zeit* as an exhibition of photographs from the original collection augmented by photographs through the 1940s. This was brought to completion by August Sander's son Günther, following his father's post-war re-conception of the project, in his 1971 volume, *August Sander. Menschen ohne Maske* (August Sander: People without Masks).

In a talk at the Museum of Modern Art in 2019, I warned against our current tendency to lionize leftist struggles during the fascist era in Europe, while allowing instances of collaboration with or acquiescence to authoritarian regimes to disappear from scholarly view. My comments then focused specifically on Sander's sons: the radical affiliations of his eldest, Erich, are frequently invoked by critics praising his father, just as his younger son Günther's participation in the Wehrmacht is rarely mentioned. Thus, the standard entry for August Sander in the quasi-official *Neue Deutsche Biographie* from 2005 by Claudia Gabriele Philipp mentions Erich's political engagement, his imprisonment, and death, while only noting that his brother, who outlived him to 1987, was a "photographer" (417). But Sander's own career under National Socialism has also remained largely unexamined. The complexity of Sander's work before the rise of National Socialism likewise demands more detailed and nuanced examination.[2]

August Sander seems retrospectively to reflect on this notion of the transparency of the fascist soldier's posture during World War II as reflecting the remaking of the German soul. This has been often seen in his "*Soldat*, um 1940" (Soldier, c. 1940), an image which has become iconic in Sander's post-Weimar oeuvre.

One of the five soldiers, airmen, and sailors from World War II (Portfolio IV/23), printed by Günther Sander to be included in the post-World War II expansion of his father's earlier collection is often read as the rigid soldier reflecting a rigid ideology that destroyed the German soul, beginning with Imperial Germany and directly impacting the life of Sander and his family during the Third Reich (Figure 7.2).[3] And yet the face, if stripped of its helmet and uniform, for this is as much a commercial photograph as it is a social commentary, is that of a young man

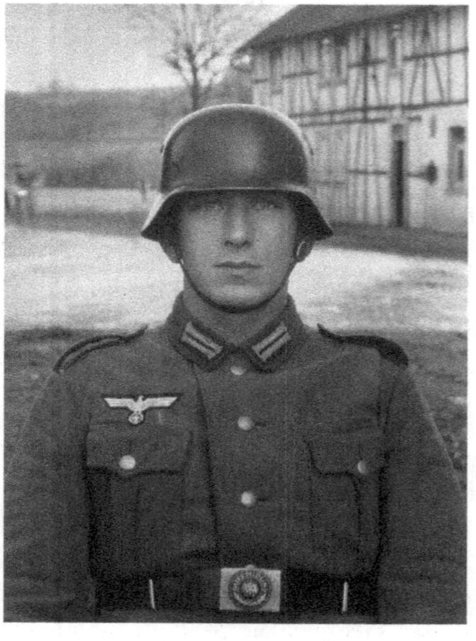

Figure 7.2 "*Soldat*, um 1940"

standing before his family's half-timbered farm house. It certainly was intended to be given to his family as a keepsake; Sander's commercial work from this period is full of such images of soldiers. The uniform may be rigid, but the face is not: the half-smile would not have been tolerated in ranks from the Enlightenment on. And indeed, the motto on his military belt, "Gott mit Uns" (God with Us), is a left-over employed by the Nazi Wehrmacht. It was first used by the Prussian king Frederick I in 1701 and then in Imperial iconography, adorning the spiked helmets of German officers during World War I. Anyone in 1940 seeing this would have known that this was a member of the Wehrmacht, the German army, and not the Waffen SS, the political units of Himmler's SS, who bore a belt with the motto "Meine Ehre heiße Treue" (My honor means fealty [to the Führer]). What this distinction meant up to 1945 we can only imagine but after Heinrich Himmler's suicide in May 1945 and the Nuremberg trial of major war criminals of 1945–46, the Waffen SS was intimately connected with atrocities throughout Europe. The Wehrmacht, composed of volunteers as well as draftees, seemed to be the antithesis, loyal soldiers of the state, not barbaric butchers.

Today we know that the Wehrmacht committed atrocities of extraordinary brutality, a fact driven home in 1995 by Hannes Heer's controversial and contested exhibit of over 1,000 amateur photographs of the atrocities committed by the Wehrmacht in the USSR and subsequent exhibitions in 2001 (Heer). One can add here that photographs from the concentration camps (but not the death camps) were regularly published in the German media during the war, and many others documenting the mass murders were used at the Nuremburg trials as evidence (Lower; Sachsse; Struk). A small selection of these reappeared in Edward Steichen's *The Family of Man*, as noted, and was prominent, especially in the reception of this exhibition in its European venues in the 1950s. The controversy in 1995 and thereafter emerged from a set of assumptions that isolated the often drafted soldiers in the "clean" army from those very charges against the butchers in the SS made after 1945. But this dichotomy was well known on the home front during the war, as documented in the official record of the time (Kulka et al.). Sander's photograph of the essential "soldier" stands very much in thrall to that assumption. Recall that the photographer who printed this image after the war was August Sander's younger son, Günther Sander, who had served in the *Wehrmacht* during his older sibling's imprisonment. The difficulty of such a role among those who after the war took positions that were highly critical of the Nazi period and those engaged in its atrocities can be measured by the utter horror of the German public in 2006 when it was revealed that the then 78-year-old Nobel Prize winner, Günther Grass, the fiercest critic of the Third Reich in West German letters, had long neglected to state that he, too, had been in the *Waffen SS* at the close of the war.

The post-war exhibits and eventual publication of the augmented *Antlitz der Zeit* in 1980 added to the corpus the images of Nazi soldiers as well as Jewish refugees. Sander began to rethink including such commercial photographs immediately after the war; this was very much in line with a number of artist and writers, the Nazi Emil Nolde immediately springs to mind, who needed to polish their anti-fascist credentials to be reintegrated into post-war society (Fulda). The noteworthy debate in May 1945 between Thomas Mann, living in California, and Frank Thiess centered on the culpability of those artists who remained in Germany for the horrors of what had not yet been called the "Holocaust." It was in July 1946 that Sander too began to look at the commercial images he took in a new light. Mann argued that no one who remained in Germany could shake off their responsibility; Thiess stated that those who lived in luxury abroad should not be the ones to cast the first stones. Out of this came the West Germany defensive position of these in the "inner emigration" who wrote (or photographed) for the "desk drawer" (*Schubladenliteratur*), which came to incorporate both conservative oppositional figures, such as Ernest Wiechert, as well as widely popular and politically honored writers of the Third Reich, such as Hans Carossa (Klieneberger). Sander's augmented collections appeared, well after his death, only in 1980. The passport photos of Jews applying for official permission to emigrate in the mid-1930s (portfolio VI/44: "The Persecuted") and "Political prisoners" (portfolio VI/44a: photographed by his son Erich at Siegburg) were paired self-consciously with those of Nazis (portfolio IV/23a: "Classes and Professions, The National Socialist"), as Sander had planned, but only after 1946. However, the juxtaposition is seen between the "Jews" and the "Nazis," the victims and the perpetrators. This has been a central problem of such photographs ever since the 1980s, when there was an attempt to restore Sander's socially critical reputation by pairing the images of Nazi soldiers in military dress with those of desperate Jews (Sekula). The solders play no role at all in this post-war reconstruction of the visual world of the immediate past. The Mémorial de la Shoah, the Holocaust Museum in Paris, stressed this with its exhibition in 2018 and a parallel volume of images printed by Günther Sander (Mémorial).

The Nazi images included in the post-war exhibits and folios are exemplified by his portrait of the young German soldier in 1940. Seemingly "informal" images, such as the "Family Portrait of the Sander Family, Hemmelzen, Westerwald 1943," don't make the cut in 1980 (Figure 7.3). The scribbled inscription on the reverse reads 'Kurt Sander, Hemmelzen." No portrait of son Günther in uniform is present in any of the public collections of August Sander's work. Now, if the portrait of the soldier taken in 1940, at the very beginning of the war, our

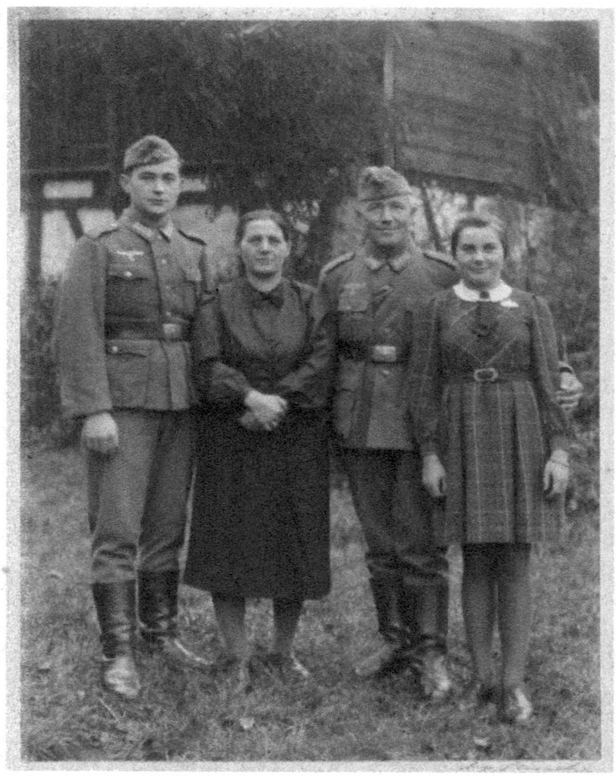

Figure 7.3 Family Portrait of the Sander Family, Hemmelzen, Westerwald 1943

projecting and accepting a notion of the rigid posture of the soldier as an index of the internal life of the citizen, explicitly of the soldier's soul, seems both easy to trace and to "see." The soldier as machine is an icon that disparages the modern soldier as a mindless cog in the wheel of war. In 1940, there is an attempt at the humanization of the solder's body and of his role. Yet this is a political interpretation that dominated Sander's world, the assumption that the Wehrmacht was composed of citizen-soldiers, free of the radical ideology of other military groups such as the SS. Historians, such as Christopher Browning, dismissed this notion in his work on *Ordinary Men,* his 1992 study of the war crimes committed by Unit 101 of Reserve Police Battalion in occupied Poland in 1942. The erect, perfect soldier's body, even in mufti, comes after World War I to represent the foolishness, indeed, the simple-minded destructiveness of the war. In a complex way, this infiltrated Sander's World War II images. In this photograph of the ordinariness of the Sander family in 1943, it is the age span of the two men, father and son, their relationship not only to the women in the family but also their clear discomfort in somewhat sloppy uniforms exemplified by the similarity in the posture of both the men and the women that draws our attention. In an odd way this does not occur even to the contemporary viewer: family photographs are supposed to look like this. But then the soldier's body does not, and that is the problem. For Sander, all his military photographs from 1914 to 1945 present to the viewer the "before" images of the soldier's body. It is the "after" photographs that are simultaneously denied by these images.

Wounded warriors

Sander's visual representation of the military, which we read as the intact, erect, perfect soldier's body across both wars, however, directly clashes with an equally powerful image: the mangled soldier's body that serves as icon for disability from the Weimar Republic to the Third Reich (Joshua and Schillmeier; Bösl et al.). Here the specificity of the public understanding of World War I among the inhabitants of what had been the "Central Powers" is vital. If there was a "lost cause" in the Confederacy after 1865, this was doubled after 1918. The Germans on the home front were totally unprepared for the devastating loss of World War I. Believing to the last month that they were winning the war, they were forced to come to terms not only with a lost cause but also with an overwhelming number of severely wounded ex-soldiers. It is the "after" image, of the horribly mutilated, blinded, amputated soldiers; of the solder from the trenches whose face has been reconstructed to appear now only vaguely human, that haunts all of Sander's images. Here we can mention the volume of photographs of facial reconstruction, Ernst Friedrich's 1924 pacifist book *War Against War,* which showed the state of the soldier's face and body "after" the bombast had passed (Gilman 1999, 159).

In work by left-wing artists such as Georg Grosz, Otto Dix, and Max Beckmann during the Weimar republic, these broken bodies came to represent visually the futile nature of the war itself (Poore 26–32). As we have seen with Alfred Döblin, such images permeated all cultural products at the time. In 1919, Beckmann published a series of lithographs entitled *Hölle* (Hell) in which the second, "Die Straße" (Street) showed a blind man and an amputee in a wheelchair in a chaotic street scene echoing the result of the war's sudden end. Dix in his 1920 *Die Skatspieler* (Men playing the card game Skat) presents three badly disabled officers, so badly disabled that they, as the Disability historian Carole Poore notes, could hardly have survived their wounds but are recognizable as German officers by the otherwise rigid posture and chest full of medals. Dix's cynical representation of "pompous military bearing" only highlights the horrors that they experienced (30), but this stance is not merely one of pacifism. The struggle against the war came to be defined by how one imagined the cause of the war: on the left, it was unbridled capitalism and the forces of imperial reaction; on the right the betrayal of the nation by the left (who called forth various instantiations of the Republic on November 9, 1918) and the Jews. Thus, disability becomes one with the struggle for political domination between the left and the right during the Weimar Republic. The politics of disability mirror the politics of the street. What is important is that while visual and literary representations of disability haunted the arts after 1919, it was the damaged bodies of the soldiers that were seen as the image of this struggle.

Does Sander simply buy into the ideology of the right in his selection of images of rigid, upright soldiers, visible even in mufti in 1929? The selection under the rubric for "Soldiers" in his 1929 *Antlitz der Zeit* collection seems to reflect this, yet it also signifies a self-reflexive questioning of the ideology within the totality of the piece. One image, echoing the varied images in the Weimar Republic of the damaged soldier's body, is present. In *Antlitz der Zeit*, the war wounded soldier does appear in one image: *Blinder Bergmann und blinder Soldat* (*Blind Miner and Blind Soldier*, 1930), taken in Düren, a small town near Cologne. This photograph is not to be found in the portfolio of the soldiers, even those in mufti, but in the section of *Antlitz der Zeit* entitled "The Last People: Idiots, the Sick, the Insane and Dying" (portfolio VII/45/7).

Sander seems to relegate the blind to the marginal world of the freak, the circus, the outsider, yet the blind soldier has a special meaning by the 1930s. By pairing the blind soldier (right) with a blind miner (left), Sander gestures not only to their marginal status, but, and this is a vital question in 1930, the role that the disabled citizen-soldier has in peacetime, where he can no longer be distinguished from other blind people. Indeed, had Sander not exhibited the "Blind Soldier" as a separate print in 1931, we could not know which of the *Kriegsblinden* was a soldier and which a miner (Figure 7.4).[4] In a sense he too is in mufti, but his civilian dress

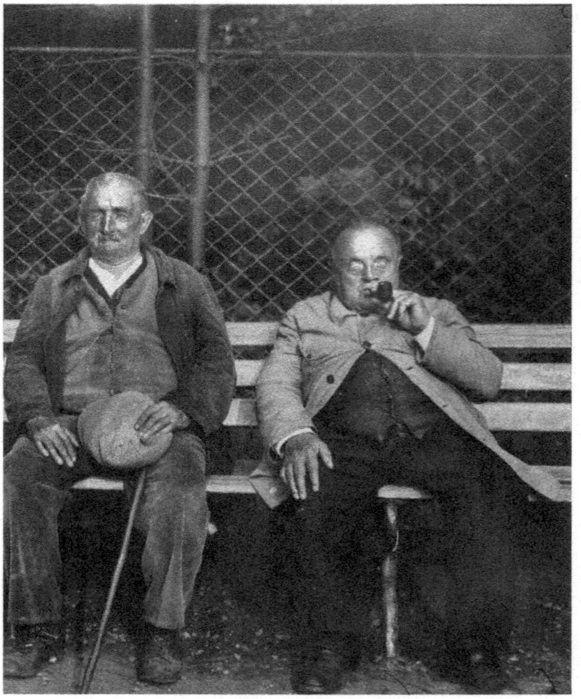

Figure 7.4 *Blinder Bergmann und blinder Soldat* (Blind Miner and Blind Soldier, 1930)

should be counted by some residual impression of the martial body. Here it clearly is not to be differentiated from any other blind man in mufti.

After January 1933 and overtly with the public degradation of "degenerate art" in 1937, even such an oblique reference to the military body as a critique of war vanished from within the Third Reich. In Nazi Germany, virtually everyone who was racially acceptable entered into fantasies of a rigid military body, including those otherwise labeled unfit for battle. For example, immediately after the Nazi's seizure of power, in February 1933, a Hitler Youth group of "genetically sound" (*erbgesund*) students was created at the State School for the Blind in Berlin-Steglitz (Degenhardt and Rath 125–32). In 1934, Eduard Bechthold, director of the Institute for the Blind in Halle and a member of the Nazi Party, created a "special section HJ-B" (*Sonderbann* HJ-B) for his "genetically sound" blind students. What had been for the left an image of the horrors of war, the blind and mutilated veteran, became for the right (and especially for the National Socialists) a need to have a soldier's body even when manifesting the disabilities often attributed to war. Blindness took on quite a different meaning, even in the early 1930s, with the accession of the Nazi Party and Adolf Hitler to political prominence.

One of the reasons it becomes relatively easy to recruit blind students for the HJ after 1933 is that the exemplary blind soldier (whom all of the blind HJ-members wish to emulate) is Adolf Hitler. Peter Plein, one of the leaders of the organization of blind veterans (*Verband der Kriegsblinde*), wrote at the time that:

> It is we, the blinded German veterans, who look to Reich Chancellor Adolf Hitler with particular trust; for, since he was deprived of his eyesight for several weeks because of a gas-related injury during that critical November of 1918, he, like no one else, will know how to show his appreciation for the heavy sacrifice that we blinded veterans have made for the fatherland, a sacrifice which we must bear for the rest of our lives.
>
> *(Richter 47)*

The blind soldier becomes the idealized type of the war wounded now in thrall to the new order. Blindness represented an acceptable form of difference, at least politically, if not in the lived reality of the Third Reich.

After 1945

In the 1920s, there had been those who had understood the horrors of trench warfare as a test of both bodies and souls, such as Ernest Jünger in his *Im Stahlgewitter* (Storm of Steel 1920). For Jünger, the erect body captures the very essence of *Kameradschaft* even in mufti. These were in the end, heroic bodies; answered then by Erich Maria Remarque's image of the soldier in his 1928 *Im Westen Nichts Neues* (*All Quiet on the Western Front*). The visual analog to Jünger would be the heroic bodies of the soldier in the massive public sculptures of Josef Thorak and Arno Breker, as well as the wide range of fascist and conservative artists working in the Weimar Republic represented in the Great German Art Exhibition of 1937. This was the parallel exhibit to the "Degenerate Art" exhibition of the same year, one of the rooms of which was dedicated to art that criticized the German soldier. The wide range of war art produced in the 1920s and even more extensively after the Nazi seizure of power certainly continues this image of the erect and rigid body as in Leni Riefenstahl's *Trumph des Willens* (*Triumph of the Will* 1935), the documentary film chronicling the 1934 Nazi Party Congress in Nuremberg. The rigid fascist body, the dominant images in film, circulated in the popular press of the time, such as a special edition of the *Illustrierter Film-Kurier*, found on every filmgoer's coffee table. In 1973, in an attempt to relabel herself as an "ethnographic" photographer rather than as a director, Riefenstahl's image of the superior posture of the Nazi body comes, in a bizarre way, to determine her view of the ideal Black African body in her *Die Nuba* (*The Last of the Nuba*) published in 1973 (Ludewig).

Riefenstahl's ideal bodies are, of course, in contrast to the round-shouldered images of the stereotyped Jew in the propaganda of the day, as in the work of the anthropologist Hans F. K. Günther (1891–1968), known at the time as *Rassen Günther* (Race Günther), who published pictures of characteristic Jewish posture in the Weimar Republic. He was one of the scientists who popularized *Rassenkunde* ("race science") and the idea of Nordic supremacy, and he was one of the few of the race scientists to have been a member of the Nazi party before 1933. Günther contributed to the new Nazi undertaking of identifying Jews by describing a pathological but "typical Jewish posture" (Kohn 36) and used posture as a sign of racial difference: "Günther believed that the virtues of the Nordic race were expressed in its male body type, with its straight posture, pronounced chest, and small abdomen. This posture (chest out and belly in) was alien to the Eastern man, whose appearance was a negation of the beauty ideal of the Occident . . ." (Hau 157). One can add that the ideal Nordic type for Günther was embodied in the soldier's body or perhaps that the soldier's body represented the ideal Nordic type. While such views had a place in the political spectrum until 1945, as with Riefensthal, Günther's views were unchanged after the war, even if in other contexts. For Günther in 1956 it was not the Nuba but the Greeks that the German soldiers "met" during World War II (his formulation for the brutal occupation of Greece after 1941) who formed an ideal (Günther, 283). Photography trumped all other proof of difference for those advocating for such differences before as well as after 1945 (Moses-Reich).

It is important to understand that distancing oneself from the Nazi horrors, especially if one had remained in Germany and especially if one had fought in the service of the regime was a central preoccupation of the generation both quietly before and then radically after 1968. No damaged bodies are present in the 1980 version of Sander's opus presented by his surviving son. It is not that such images were absent in the culture of post-war Germany. In immediate post-World War II German literature, the yellow armband with the three black dots signaling the blindness of the wearer seemed ubiquitous. In the Austrian novelist Ingeborg Bachmann's controversial Berlin speech, '*Ein Ort für Zufälle*' (A Place for Coincidences), given on the occasion of accepting the Georg Büchner prize in 1964,the armbands appear to signal the world in which the inhabitants are now thrust, a world of multiple war wounded. The narrator stands at the S-Bahn station Bellevue ('beautiful vista'), where the President of West Germany has his mansion and observes as the multitude of broken, crippled individuals spill out into the light with their yellow armbands with black circles and white canes (Bachmann). A world, however, which while overrun with such icons, seems not really to see the people attached to them. In the Swiss novelist Max Frisch's *Mein Name sei Gantenbein* (Let's assume my name is Gantenbein; translated as *A Wilderness of Mirrors*, 1964), perhaps they even include the narrator, who assumes new identities one after another beginning with that of Theo Gantenbein, a sighted person taking the role of a blind man wearing the yellow armband. "Even a blind man, he ought to have seen, is a member of society. Without the yellow armband he had no rights. . . . Don't they trust his official armband?" (Frisch 40, 45). The American novelist Kay Boyle, sitting in West Berlin, fills in the political "dots" for her American reader, which were quite obvious to the German of the post-World War II period. Her protagonist immediately thinks, "with some emotion that he could not name (bitterness, irritation, it may have been) that an entire division of men must have been blinded at the Russian front." This was the ubiquitous sign of the war, the destruction of Germany by the Nazis:

> the blind were everywhere; they sat in every streetcar, in every train, in every university hall. . . . even had they not carried canes and worn the yellow armbands, and even before the scarlet, empty button-holes of the eye sockets could be perceived, they were marked by their excessive cleanliness, their well-brushed clothing, their well-shined shoes, the hair so neatly trimmed and combed. . . . [T]he absence of vision making them, forever children for women to dress, and comb, and need, and bathe in the warm fluid of their love.
>
> *(Boyle 134–5)*

The yellow armband comes to be an icon for the dependent good Germans, clean, prosperous, but blinded to the reality of what had transpired.

We need then to rethink the idealized soldier's body. Central to our reading of Sander's blind World War I soldier is the simple observation that the blind, obese veteran is impossible to differentiate from his blind civilian companion. As with all of these images, it is unimportant whether the miner also served in the military or how the miner (or indeed how the soldier) was blinded. It is impossible to distinguish between these two men (and perhaps by implication, their souls); the reality is that we can never truly know the soul of those portrayed by their image. Thus, Sander relativizes the entire corpus of the "Soldier" through its implicative reflection of the role of ideology in shaping the modern martial body. Here too we need to rethink his visual vocabulary of the soldier's body in the Third Reich. These images were not as programmatic, as those collected by him in 1929 in his *Antlitz der Zeit*; those to be included in his post-World War II expansion were to be played off against "The Persecuted" with one section pitted against another. Yet the heighted expectation of the soldier's body is not parallel to the sight of the blind and maimed on the streets of post-war Cologne, creating a tension that undermines the notion of a martial body seen even in disguise. Rather these were commercial "snaps" taken for the healthy and intact subjects to send back to family as mementos before they were sent to the front, where... . and here we need to pause to ask ourselves whether Sander is indeed implicated in the creation of an image of the soldier's body, intact, functioning, visible, but also in thrall to the ideology of the state, "God is indeed with us." The photographs of atrocities that some of these Wehrmacht soldiers sent back from the Eastern front were part of the world that Sander inhabited.

We began with Michel Foucault, Elias Canetti, and Klaus Theweleit on the nature of the rigid soldier's body and have now come to the damaged and damaging body of the soldier in the context of 20th-century Germany. Tobin Siebers, writing from the point of view of contemporary Disability Studies, criticized Foucault's concept of the docile soldier's body as he conceived in the 18th century. Foucault distinguished between the pre-modern soldier, seen as healthy and erect, and the docile soldier, a body reshaped by the demands of the modern nation-state. Canetti very much follows this line of argument. According to Siebers, while Foucault was trying to demonstrate how the state gradually transformed the human body into a machine, he betrayed his own "purer and fitter conceptions of body and mind" in preferring what Foucault defined as the healthy, pre-modern soldier's body; for Foucault, docility begins to resemble disability, and the docile body is a faulty invention of modernity, just like the disabled body (Siebers 58). Our fantasy of a healthy body as the point of origin for medical humanities can follow this line of argument. The fact that "health" like "illness" is to be defined by the lived experience of the individual is central to Disability Studies. Sander's both draws this distinction into question after World War I and then is forced to rethink its implication during World War II. All such categories are contingent to our own manner of understanding ourselves in the world.

Notes

1 I am using "soul" [*Seele*] as Sigmund Freud does to reference the interiority of the individual. Many other terms including "character," "psyche," "spirit" were substituted for this in the course of the 19th and 20th centuries.
2 www.moma.org/calendar/programs/113.
3 These updated portfolios are available at the Museum of Modern Art (New York): www.moma.org/collection/works/portfolios/204751/.
4 Getty 84.XM.126.109.

Works cited

Bachmann, Ingeborg. *Eine Ort für Zufälle*. Berlin: Wagenbach, 1965.

Benjamin, Walter. "Little History of Photography." *Walter Benjamin, Selected Writings 1927–1934*, edited by Michael W. Jennings, Howard Eiland and Gary Smith, vol. 2. Cambridge, MA: Harvard University Press, 1999, pp. 507–30.

Bösl, Elsbeth, Anne Klein, Anne Waldschmidt, eds, *Disability History: Konstruktionen von Behinderung in der Geschichte: Eine Einführung*. Bielefeld, Germany: Transcript, 2010.

Boyle, Kay. *Generation without Farewell*. New York: Alfred A. Knopf, 1960.

Browning, Christopher. *Ordinary Men: Reserve Police Battalion 101 and the Final Solution in Poland*. New York: HarperCollins, 1992.

Canetti, Elias. *Crowds and Power*, translated by Carol Stewart. London: Victor Gollancz, 1962.

Conan Doyle, Arthur. *The Complete Sherlock Holmes*. New York: Doubleday, 1959.

Degenhardt, Sven and Waldraut Rath, eds. *Blinden- und Sehbehinderenpädagogik*. Weinheim: Beltz, 2009.

Döblin, Alfred. [1929]. "Faces, Images, and Their Truth." *Face of Our Time*, translated by Michael Robertson. Munich: Schirmer/Mosel, 2003.

Döblin, Alfred. [1929]. *Berlin Alexanderplatz*, translated by Michael Hofmann. New York: NYRB Classics, 2018.

Frisch, Max. *A Wilderness of Mirrors*, translated by Michael Bullock. New York: Random House, 1966.

Foucault. Michel. *Discipline and Punish: The Birth of the Prison*, translated by Alan Sheridan. Rochester, UK: Vintage, 1995.

Fulda, Bernhard. "Myth-making in Hitler's Shadow: The Transfiguration of Emil Nolde after 1945." *Rewriting German History: New Perspectives on Modern Germany*, edited by Jan Rüger and Nikolaus Wachsmann. London: Palgrave Macmillan, 2015, pp. 177–94.

Gilman, Sander L. *Making the Body Beautiful: A Cultural History of Aesthetic Surgery*. Princeton, NJ: Princeton University Press, 1999.

Gilman, Sander L. and Claudia Schmölders, eds. *Gesichter der Weimarer Republik: eine physiognomische Kulturgeschichte*. Cologne: Dumont, 2000.

Günther, Hans F. K. *Lebensgeschichte des hellenischen Volkes*. Pahl, Bavaria: Hohe Warte, 1956.

Hau, Michael. *The Cult of Health and Beauty in Germany: A Social History, 1890–1930*. Chicago: University of Chicago Press, 2003.

Heer, Hannes. *Tote Zonen. Die deutsche Wehrmacht an der Ostfront*. Hamburger Edition, 1999.

Joshua, Eleoma and Michael Schillmeier, eds. *Edinburgh German Yearbook*, vol. IV. Edinburgh: Boydell and Brewer, 2004.

Keller, Ulrich. "Sander and Portrait Photography," "August Sander: A German Biography," and "Conceptual and Stylistic Aspects of the Portraits." *August Sander: Citizens of the Twentieth Century*, edited by Günther Sander, translated by Linda Keller. Boston, MA: MIT Press, 1986, pp. 9, 15, 27.

Klieneberger, H. R. "The 'Innere Emigration': A Disputed Issue in Twentieth-Century German Literature." *Monatshefte*, vol. 57, 1965, pp. 171–80.

Kohn, Marek. *The Race Gallery: The Return of Racial Science*. Jonathan Cape, 1995.

Kulka, Otto Dov and Eberhard Jäckel, eds. *The Jews in the Secret Nazi Reports on Popular Opinion in Germany, 1933–1945*, translated by William Templer. New Haven: Yale University Press, 2010.
Lower, Wendy. The *Ravine: A Family, A Photfraph, a Holocaust Massacre Revealed.* Boston, MA: Houghton Mifflin, 2021.
Ludewig, Alexandra. "Leni Riefenstahl's Encounter with the Nuba." *Interventions: International Journal of Postcolonial Studies*, vol. 8, 2006, pp. 83–101.
Mémorial de la Shoah. *August Sander: Persecuted/Persecutors, People of the 20th Century*. Gottingen: Steidl, 2018.
Moses-Reich, Amos. *Race and Photography: Racial Photography as Scientific Evidence, 1876–1980.* Chicago: University of Chicago Press, 2016.
Philipp, Claudia Gabriele. "August Sander." *Neue Deutsche Biographie.* Berlin: Duncker & Humblot, vol. 22, 2005, p. 417.
Poore, Carol. *Disabilityin Twentieth-century German Culture.* Ann Arbor, MI: University of Michigan Press, 2007.
Reich, Wilhelm. *Massenpsychologie des Faschismus: zur Sexualökonomie der politischen Reaktion und zur proletarischen Sexualpolitik.* Berlin: Verlag für Sexualpolitik, 1933.
Richter, Gabriel. *Blindheit und Eugenik (1918–1945).* Idstein, Germany: Schulz Verlag, 1986.
Sachsse, Rolf. *Die Erziehung zum Wegsehen: Fotografie im NS-Staat.* Hamburg, Germany: Verlag der Kunst – Philo Fine Arts, 2003.
Sander, August. [1929], *Face of Our Time: Sixty Portraits of Twentieth-Century Germans*, with an Introduction by Alfred Döblin, trans. Michael Robertson. Munich: Schirmer/Mosel, 2003.
Schmied, Wieland. *"Neue Sachlichkeit – Der deutsche Realismus der zwanziger Jahre." Kritische Grafik in der Weimarer Zeit*, edited by Eberhard Kolb, Eberhard Roters, and Wieland Schmied. Stuttgart: Klett-Cotta, 1985, pp. 21–43.
Sekula, Allan. "The Traffic in Photographs."*Art Journal,* vol. 41, 1981, pp. 17–19.
Siebers, Tobin. *Disability Theory*. Ann Arbor, MI: University of Michigan Press, 2008.
Smith-Morris, Carolyn, ed. "Introduction: Diagnosis as the Threshold to 21st Century Health." *Diagnostic Controversy: Cultural Perspectives on Competing Knowledge in Healthcare*, edited by Carolyn Smith-Morris. New York and Abingdon: Routledge, 2016, pp. 1–26.
Spengler, Oswald. *Der Untergang des Abendlandes: Umrisse einer Morphologie der Weltgeschichte.* Munich: Beck, 1963.
Struk, Janina. *Photographing the Holocaust: Interpretations of the Evidence.* London: I. B. Tauris, 2004.
Theweleit, Klaus. *Male Fantasies*, translated by Erica Carter and Chris Turner. Minneapolis, MN: University of Minnesota Press, 1989.

PLATES

1. August Sander, *Pensionierter Major* (Retired Major, c. 1930). MOMA: 472.2015.305
2. August Sander, *Soldat*, um 1940 (Soldier, c. 1940). MOMA: 472.2015.309
3. August Sander, Family Portrait of the Sander Family, Hemmelzen, Westerwald 1943. Getty Museum: 85.XM.258.383
4. August Sander, *Blinder Bergmann und Blinder Soldat.* (Blind Miner and Blind Soldier, c. 1930). MOMA: 472.2015.610

8

ENTANGLED SUBJECTIVITIES IN LISA LINDVAY'S PHOTOGRAPHIC PROJECT *HOLD TOGETHER*

Agnese Sile

Introduction

In recent years, an unprecedented number of photographic essays depicting mental illness narratives have been published, both online and offline such as Arts website fragmentary.org established in 2015, that focuses on photography and mental health; Alejandro Kirchuk's *Never Let You Go* (2009), Joshua Lutz's *Hesitating Beauty* (2012), Melissa Spitz's *You Have Nothing to Worry About* ongoing series (2009–current), Christina Riley's *Back to Me* (2014), and Sohrab Hura's *Life Is Elsewhere* (2015). These photographic series are made not only by those who consider themselves as ill or sick but also by relatives and carers. This suggests an urgent need to find an expression by which to communicate such experiences as well as to seek a wider audience and recognition. This chapter focuses on the American photographer Lisa Lindvay's ongoing series, *Hold Together* (initiated in 2006), composed of intimate portraits of her family members, all affected by her mother's deteriorating mental health and depression. What makes *Hold Together* different from other photographic projects that portray mental illness and its effects on close family members, such as Léonie Hampton's *In the Shadow of Things* (2011); Lynne Warberg's *My Brain Is on Fire* (2012); Martha Fleming-Ives' *Red Parts Whole* (2015); and Louis Quail's *Big Brother* (2018) is that the person who is ill – in this project Lindvay's mother – is absent from the photographs. On being asked why she did not depict her mother in the photographic series, Lindvay stated: "It is easy to look at someone, classify, and judge. I chose not to photograph my mother because I believe that everyone deserves dignity. Outward appearances do not often reveal the complexity of a subject" (personal communication, July 26, 2021). Although Lindvay's mother is not portrayed in the photographs, she is also not excluded; her presence and the effects of her condition can be felt and observed. In this way, her mother's illness is not depicted as uniquely personal but rather as interpersonal, psychosocial, and as cultural matter that impacts and reverberates through the lives of those close to her (Kleinman and Seeman 231; Sile).

Lindvay's response quoted above resonates with medical historian Sander L. Gilman's assertion that the act of seeing the disease is socially coded, with the main aim being to differentiate the person who is ill from the viewer (*Disease and Representation* 3). In his seminal study, *Disease*

DOI: 10.4324/9781003007661-11

and Representation: Images of Illness from Madness to AIDS, he writes: "The examination of the image of the sufferer provides us with rigid structures of our definition of the boundaries of the disease, boundaries that are reified by the very limits inherent to the work of art" (2). Gilman refers here to a wide range of visual art forms, and he claims that the frame itself, including photograph, separates, alienates, and isolates the ill individual from others. By not depicting her mother in the images, Lindvay destabilizes and unsettles, rather than reifying the boundaries of mental illness. Although, as Gilman argues, the visual environment that surrounds those who are ill is in itself "the expression of an attempt to understand the insane" (*Seeing the Insane* xii), the photographs in this project often depict objects and scenes that viewers can easily identify with, thus denying any straightforward divisions. In this chapter, therefore, I am not concerned with photography's representational value, or even its narrative function, but rather its performative potential – what these photographs and texts do, not necessarily what they show and tell. This chapter will explore what kind of realities are disclosed in these photographic series, and how photography affords space for connection and transference between the participants in the photographic act.

My reading and analysis of Lindvay's project is informed by Julia Kristeva's text *Black Sun: Depression and Melancholia* and some of Roland Barthes's writings on photography, building upon a growing body of research on photography, feeling and performativity. In other words, I am interested in exploring how meanings emerge out of intersection or "intra-action," borrowing Karen Barad's term, between the participants in the photographic act, the camera, and the photographic image. For Barad, different materialities (human- and non-human entities, including apparatuses) function and exercise agency in a complex entanglement with one another, which means that agency is not pre-given but rather unfolds within this relationship and not outside it (214). Apparatuses, including photographic cameras, are not static and neutral; instead, as Barad argues, they are "open-ended practices" (170) and "dynamic (re) configurings of the world through which bodies are intra-actively materialized" (169–70). This materialization is a dynamic process that is "generative not merely in the sense of bringing new things into the world but in the sense of bringing forth new worlds, of engaging in an ongoing reconfiguring of the world" (170). In the *Hold Together* project, through photographs and text, Lindvay not only explores and questions mental health as a socially constructed category of difference but also challenges the norms and traditional roles of the nuclear family. I argue that whilst seeking the familiar and using photography to strengthen family bonds, Lindvay redefines expectations of the family and discloses intimacies that are usually hidden. In this way, the photographic act brings "forth new worlds" and engages "in an ongoing reconfiguring of the world."

Before engaging in deeper explorations and analyses of some of the images from Lindvay's *Hold Together* project, I will first briefly explore photography as performative practice.

Performing photography

The relationship between performance and photography has been explored from a range of perspectives by numerous theorists since the 1990s (Levin). Some thinkers have focused on the theatricality and artificiality of the pose and the ways the subject performs in front of and for the camera (Silverman; Jones). Since the early 2000s, the focus has shifted more toward the photographic act itself as performative process and how meanings are embedded in the act and communicated to viewers. In their essay, "From Presence to the Performative: Rethinking Photographic Indexicality," David Green and Joanna Lowry write that: "The very act of photography, as a kind of performative gesture which points to an event in the world, as a form of designation that draws reality into the image field, is thus itself a form of indexicality" (48). Each photograph not only effectively records traces of an event but also announces the presence and holds embodied affective histories of the photographer and the photographic subject(s). Green and Lowry point toward the similarities between photographic practice and performative speech acts. Speech act theory, developed by John Austin, is a proposition that language is a means of conveying information (for example, "The sky is blue"), as well as a mode of action ("I disown"). For Green and Lowry, the photograph communicates "the bodily presence of the photographer within a sensory field and to anchor a reading of the image in terms of an utterance designated by a first person pronoun" (58–9). Framing, angle, motion blur, lighting – each of these qualities expresses and embodies a particular position and being. The philosopher Richard Shusterman further develops the concept of photography as embodied practice. For Shusterman, performance starts before the shutter release – within the mise-en-scène, where multiple actions take place, such as the arrangement of the setting, and communicative interactions between the subject of the photograph and the photographer. As Shusterman claims, "photography's dimension of somatic, dramatic, performative process" (241) itself evokes certain emotions and the intensity of the experience can leave "its participants embarrassed once the drama of the shooting is over and they return to their everyday routine" (246). In his text, Shusterman describes a particular experience of creating experimental and artistic photographs; however, it cannot be denied that the photographic act can stimulate a strong emotional response from the participants and viewers.

In the past decade there has been increased interest in the intersection between photography, affect, emotions, and feeling (Brown and Phu; Phu, Brown and Noble) and the way images evoke and construct emotions. As such, photographs cannot be considered to be fixed and completed objects but, rather, affective agents. Photography is not a purely visual medium but rather a complex nexus that incorporates "the sonic, haptic, historical, and affective backgrounds and foregrounds through and against which we view photographs" (Campt 8). It is not only about what is visible, then, but also what is left outside the photographic frame and what can be "felt" during the process of looking through images. Therefore, viewing photographic images is not a passive act but an active engagement that evokes response.

In *Listening to Images*, Tina M. Campt proposes that instead of requiring a "looking at," photographs demand to be listened to: "listening to images is constituted as a practice of looking beyond what we see and attuning our senses to the other affective frequencies through which photographs register" (9). Listening involves being alert, "straining toward a possible meaning, and consequently one that is not immediately accessible" (Nancy 6). This resonates with Roland Barthes' notion of the "third meaning," or what he also refers to as the "obtuse meaning" (in the classical model of the five senses, the third sense is hearing or listening) ("The Third Meaning" 52–68). For Barthes, this third meaning is found outside the language-system; it is "an accent, the very form of an emergence, of a fold (a crease even) marking the heavy layer of informations and significations. [...] – anaphoric gesture without significant content, a sort of gash rased of meaning (of desire for meaning)" ("The Third Meaning" 53). I would argue that this "fold" or "gesture," which emerges in the act of viewing a photographic image is critical to engaging with lived illness accounts.

Some photographers have chosen to emphasize the performative potential and blur boundaries between photography and performance even further. In the context of health and illness, photography as affective and performative practice has been explored extensively by the British photographer Jo Spence in collaboration with Rosy Martin. In the series *The Picture of Health?* (1982–86), Jo Spence documented her experience living with breast cancer, and questioned how illness shapes identity. Spence writes: "Through photo therapy, I was able to explore how

I felt about my powerlessness as a patient, my relationship to doctors and nurses, my infantilisation whilst being managed and 'processed' within a state institution" (156). Re-enactment phototherapy allowed Spence to act out emotions and to express and recover a sense of agency. Similarly, the American artist and photographer Hannah Wilke took photographs of her mother who had cancer between 1978 and 1982 before documenting her own illness and changes in her body in the series, *Intra-Venus* (1992–93). Spence and Wilke created self-portraits, both staged and spontaneous, that involved dressing up, undressing, make-up, performing various roles in front of the camera and using props to explore identity with the potential of healing. These performances also aimed to challenge established conceptions of disease and illness. The two photographers predominantly focused on their bodies as the principal site on which social constructions of difference and trauma were inscribed, as well as how these constructions could be challenged and resisted. Although Lisa Lindvay also takes staged and spontaneous portraits of her siblings and father, the focus is more on the entanglements between them and their home environment. I will now turn to Lindvay's photo series and explore how it conveys and performs private expressions of mental health and intimacies between family members, whilst evoking change.

Hold Together

Lindvay notes that her mother had always wrestled with mental health difficulties, and in 2006, she sank into an episode of major depression (cited in Manning). She became unable to look after her two sons (aged 15 and 17) and daughter (age 14) from her second marriage. Lindvay's father, who had already been given custody of Lindvay after the divorce, assumed responsibility for her brothers, Ryan and Nicholas, neither of whom are his biological children. For Lindvay, taking photographs of her family was a reason to return to her home in Erie, Pennsylvania. It was "my way of understanding the complexities of our situation" (cited in Manning).

The feminist scholar Maria Tambokou foregrounds process over sequence as a necessary condition for making sense of narratives. She argues that "the attention to process brings in heterogeneous space/time configurations and invites the virtual to fill in the gaps and ruptures that appear in the sequential delineation of the actual" (284). In Tambokou's view, there is not one fixed and "true" reality but rather, a multitude of possibilities in which a narrative subject can emerge: "The stories of the narratable self can thus be seen as events, prisms refracting actual and virtual possibilities of becoming" (288). Thus, stories are not reflections or mirrors of experiences and events that took place but, rather, processes of self-making that allow new identities, affiliations and connections to be formed. The idea of refraction can be aligned closely with Karen Barad's theory of diffraction. In classical physics, the two concepts describe wave properties: refraction is the passing of a wave in a different direction that is provoked by a change of medium; diffraction is caused when a multitude of waves encounter an obstacle, which then causes the waves to overlap with one another or when the waves interfere themselves. This physical phenomenon is the foundation of Barad's theory of "intra-action" that "signifies the mutual constitution of entangled agencies" (33), unlike "interaction" that supposes pre-established identities. For Barad, agencies do not precede but emerge during their intra-action with one another. This theory is relevant in relation to Lindvay's series in which the sense of narrative emerges from connections and becomings. In addition, the photographic apparatus itself here is an active agent that plays a significant role in this process of intra-action. As of August 2020, 42 color photographs are presented on Lindvay's website. The images, displayed next to each other across eight rows, cluster around specific themes. For example, images of the house, interior spaces, and food are presented across three rows; photographs of

Lindvay's father and her siblings are each in a separate row. The project resists a straightforward linear narrative; instead, the images are decontextualized and recontextualized fragments, or an archive, of their daily lives. There are no clear beginnings, conclusions, or judgments but rather ambiguity, poignancy, and intimacy. The narrative is not complete; it evolves with every viewing. It is about "being-with" and being attuned to what each is becoming in the presence of the other. The subjects are carefully posed in contrast to their unposed surroundings. The camera, a familiar object within their shared space, does not intrude on the scenes of intimacy. Here, the photographic process itself represents the family's togetherness and reinforces their awkward bonding or holding together, as the title suggests.

No written accounts of the family's experiences or detailed descriptions of individual photographs are available on the photographer's website. The subject of Lindvay's work is her family and their shared home, yet language lacks to describe the project comprehensively. The titles in my analysis are taken from exhibition catalogues and online photography journals in which these photographs appear. In these publications, brief texts accompany the photographs and, in some cases, the year in which they were taken; for instance, "Nick in His Old Bedroom, 2007" (the same image on another site is entitled as "Bottles Under Bed"); "Ryan, 2007"; "T.V., 2007"; "Cheetos" and "Powdered Donuts." Instead of elaborating on what can be seen in the image or pointing toward the relation between the subject or object and a specific event or episode, the title simply repeats what is obvious. The verbal re-enactment of what can be seen calls attention to itself as lacking meaning or an explanation. The caption freezes the meaning and drains its significance; instead of allowing for a move away from what is shown in order to find a connection, or what Susan Sontag calls "the missing voice" that "is expected to speak for truth" (84), the text solidifies what can be seen in the image. It plainly points back to what is obvious.

This suggests a lack of language to describe the experiences that Lindvay and her family are going through. In *Black Sun: Depression and Melancholia*, the psychoanalyst Julia Kristeva proposes that depression is a "linguistic malady whose primary symptom is chronic asymbolia or loss of meaning" (Kritzman 144). Kristeva points out that depressed speech is "built up with absurd signs, slackened, scattered, checked sequences, conveys the collapse of meaning into the unnameable" (52). There is a certain resemblance in this to the uses of text in Lindvay's project – the captions, when included, are repetitive and empty, and the lack of text can be interpreted as an expression of silence or "the collapse of meaning into the unnameable." This absence of text also implies that language itself is to be mistrusted to represent lived experiences or "mirror preexisting phenomena" (Barad 133). "[A] performative account," as Barad claims, "insists on understanding thinking, observing, and theorizing as practices of engaging with, and as part of, the world in which we have our being" (133). Photography, as performative practice and embodied form of being, perhaps then contests "the excessive power granted to language to determine what is real" (133) and, instead, privileges a "felt sense" of experiences. This resonates with Kristeva's view, that when language fails, artistic image holds a promise of liberation and resurrection. She writes that:

> The work of art that insures the rebirth of its author and its reader or viewer is one that succeeds in integrating the artificial language it puts forward (new style, new composition, surprising imagination) and the unnamed agitations of an omnipotent self that ordinary social and linguistic usage always leave somewhat orphaned or plunged into mourning. Hence such a fiction, if it isn't an antidepressant, is at least a survival, resurrection...
>
> *(51)*

Kristeva suggests that artistic expression "repeats the initial creative act" and therefore can be likened to re-birth, a return to " 'mother' or origin through art" (Miller 7). This is particularly poignant in the context of Lindvay's project. The series not only provides hope for reinvention and survival but is also an attempt to rediscover her mother.

Maternal presence/absence

The question of maternity is spread across human and non-human relationships in Lindvay's photographs. All photographs in this project are taken within their home and courtyard. Gaston Bachelard's *The Poetics of Space* links the image of house and home to the maternal. The house in his texts stands as a protective and womblike space, which "shelters day-dreaming, the house protects the dreamer, the house allows one to dream in peace" (8). The psychologist and theorist Lisa Baraitser points out that from early childhood we are faced with an "ever present fantasy mother home" (4) in which mothers have to find a balance between being present and absent, caring whilst not appearing overly clingy. The absence of the mother and the silence of her voice "gives rise to the classic characterisation of the mother as the unthematizable, unrepresentable and unrecoverable presence that haunts each subject" (5). Lindvay's mother is carved out through the negative space of absence. As the British cultural theorist and philosopher Mark Fisher in his *Ghosts of My Life* states: "Everything that exists is possible only on the basis of a whole series of absences, which precede and surround it, allowing it to possess such consistency and intelligibility that it does" (17–18). Lindvay's mother here is a spectre that is simultaneously present and absent and acts without being physically present in the photographic frame. Through objects, scenes, and poses, Lindvay seems to attempt to recover and question the mother role. In a similar way to the "Winter Garden Photograph" that depicts Barthes's mother as a child and that is the central point of discussion in *Camera Lucida* yet is never shown, Lindvay's portraits and juxtaposition of objects also establish their own uneasy bond with the absent mother.

Images of junk food and unmade beds all signify the absence of a typical maternal presence in the photographs. Baraitser states that food is "one of the primary materials of motherhood" (130), and food is explored in great detail in the photographs of this project. Doritos, cheesy puffs, and pepperoni pizza appear almost as often as family members. Here, the respective food symbolizes not only its nutritional value or lack thereof but also questions of class and taste (Dluzen). A photograph entitled, "Dinner," depicts Lindvay's father in the center and her two brothers sitting on each side of him at a family dinner table (Figure 8.1). Her father's open arms, forward-leaning pose, and slightly tilted body remind the viewer of *The Last Supper* by Leonardo Da Vinci. The boys seated like his apostles and her father in the center recreate a holy scene. While their bodies create a triangular shape, their facial expressions are disconnected, each of them absorbed in his own thoughts. As in *The Last Supper*, they are sitting behind a table covered with drinks and bread, but this time their origins are given away by garish McDonald's packaging. The "Golden Arches" logo, which may be more globally recognizable than the Christian cross, here stands for fast, predictable, and cheap food ("McDonald's 'bigger than Jesus Christ'"). Notably, early McDonald's campaigns were purposely addressed to young families. Their slogan announced, "Give Mom a night off" (Cross 103), which in the context of Lindvay's photographs is particularly poignant. The McDonald's brand reflects the American Dream, rooted in capitalism and individuality as well as conservative, heteronormative and urban lifestyles. In Lindvay's image, however, family life is not romanticized or glamorized in any way. Lindvay uses parody through the appropriation and mockery of religious iconography to critique the American Dream of the idealized family and its values.

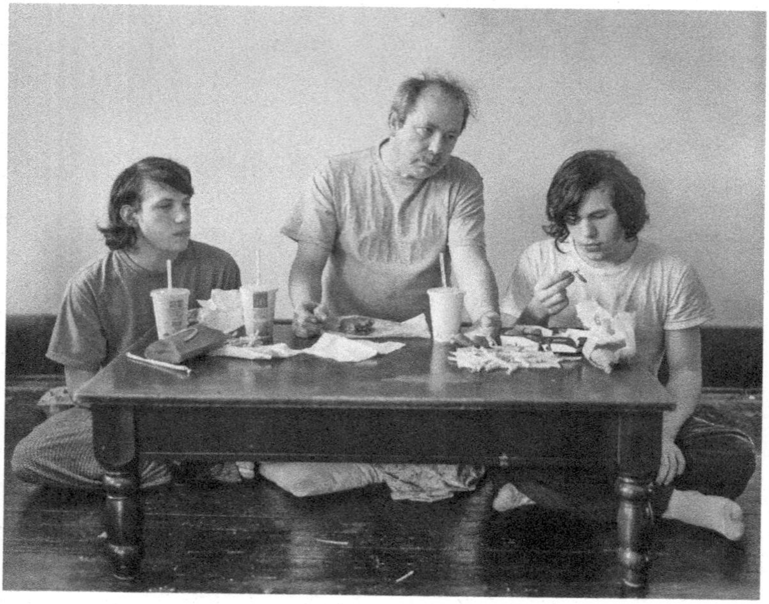

Figure 8.1 Lisa Lindvay, "Dinner"

Lindvay's photographic project unravels the idealized "fantasy" family and allows for the interrogation of the concept and significance of paternity and maternity within this union. The social and family expectations of the role of a mother – to teach, discipline, and provide emotional and physical support – are challenged here. The situation, as portrayed in Lindvay's project, opposes the general notion that children should be raised by their parents and particularly by their mothers. bell hooks argues that "Women and society as a whole often consider the father who does equal parenting unique and special rather than as a representative of what should be the norm" (138). In *Maternal Thinking,* Sara Ruddick proposes a rather romanticized vision of new ways of parenting:

> there will be no more "fathers," no more of either sex who have power over their children's lives and moral authority in their children's worlds, though they do the work of attentive love. There will be mothers of both sexes who live out a transformed maternal thought in communities that share parental care – practically, emotionally, economically, and socially. Such communities will have learned from their mothers how to value children's lives.
>
> *(227)*

Here, Ruddick suggests a move away from mother/father dualism toward "mothers of both sexes." Whilst still relying on the maternal to learn "attentive love," she associates parenting with ethical work. In her reading of Lévinas' texts, the philosopher Lisa Guenther argues that Lévinas denies any connection between motherhood and responsibility: "The maternity of Moses and of God suggests one is not born, but rather becomes like a mother" (138). She continues that "the biological fact of incarnation in a female body does not condemn me to the destiny of childbirth, nor does my incarnation in a male body free me from the responsibility of bearing

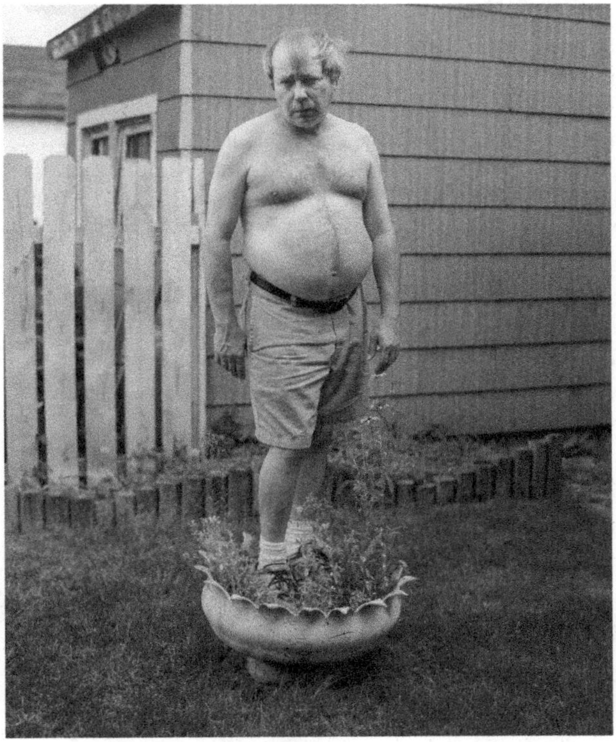

Figure 8.2 Lisa Lindvay, "My Dad Standing in the Flowerpot", 2009

the other 'like a maternal body'" (138). Rather, the other, who the person may or may not have "conceived and given birth to" (139), demands a response. Guenther here shifts the focus on the maternal "as a fixed biological or even social identity" (139) toward a more open interpretation of ethical response. Hélène Cixous questions: "Is maternal man a woman? Tell yourself rather: He is big enough and plural enough to be capable of maternal goodness" (50). In her fluid rhetoric on family roles that are undone and unfixed, however, Cixous emphasizes the function of, or rather necessity of, "maternal goodness."

In one photograph, Lindvay's father is standing in an ornamental garden planter, which is also the title of the photograph, "My Dad Standing in the Flowerpot," 2009 (Figure 8.2). The planter acts for a purpose of holding something together; furthermore, as Baraitser indicates, the garden planter as a receptacle and a container points toward the symbol of motherhood (24). The object and the setting's aesthetics convey a sentimental and melodramatic effect that is commonly associated with kitsch and lower-income American family home life. At the same time, her father's position, sideways pose and bare torso are reminiscent of *The Birth of Venus* painting by Sandro Botticelli. In Roman mythology, Venus represents love, sex, beauty, and fertility (Roman and Roman 71–3). According to legend, her extramarital activities with mortals and gods allowed her to produce numerous children. Lucretius begins *De rerum natura* (On the Nature of Things) with the words:

> Life-stirring Venus, Mother of Aeneas and of Rome,
> Pleasure of men and gods, you make all things beneath the dome

Of sliding constellations teem, you throng the fruited earth
And the ship-frightened sea – for every species comes to birth
Conceived through you, and rises forth and gazes on the light. (3)

The photograph and the legend of Venus resonate in several ways. Lindvay's father has also "fathered" several children, though not through the act of conceiving them. Venus, as a mother of Romans, produced children through extramarital affairs and the father figure in this does not seem to be of much importance. Although Lindvay's mother divorced and remarried, having more children in her second marriage, legal status does not matter here. Lindvay's father stands as a symbol of origin: by virtue of his guardianship, his children, whether conceived through him or not, can now rise "forth" and gaze "on the light." At the same time, her father's melancholic look, his round, protruding belly, like that of a pregnant woman, his feet on top of growing flowers, also suggest a regression: he is not depicted in the moment of birth like Venus but rather in a reversal. Here, birth, entropy and strict gender identities are deliberately confused. The image instead offers a liberation from pre-set roles and identities in the ageing figure of her father.

Repetition, boredom, and transgression

Hold Together, emphasizes spatial as well as temporal dynamics. The unfixed relationships and roles fulfilled by the siblings and Lindvay's father are played out in their home, in the back garden or their living space, a space that is similarly subject to change. In an e-mail Lindvay reflects: "Our domestic space is always changing. Things are added, rearranged, and removed; they build up, wear, and fall apart. I am interested in the ways our experiences are both reflected in and influenced by our environment" (personal communication, July 26, 2021). Peeling paint, damaged walls, textures, stains, plastic pop bottles, and food packaging provide not only a background against which the human subjects are posed but also the main focus point. One image depicts a line-up of worn, discolored, mismatched cotton socks that create a tonal rhythm pattern, entitled "The Boys' Mismatched Socks," 2011. Although the image depicts something that aesthetically is rather repugnant, it also has a heart-warming effect. These objects of intimate apparel are familiar; their protective, comforting qualities, showing the imprint of their wearer, become useless once the other is missing. The discolored, threadbare and holey fabric here signifies the passage of time.

Another photograph depicts a sink filled with cigarette butts, entitled "Cigarette Butts in My Mother's Sink" or "My Mother's Bathroom Sink" (Figure 8.3). In the subject matter, it resembles British artist Damien Hirst's ashtray sculptures, made between 1995 and 1997 – "Horror at Home," "Crematorium," "Necropolis," and "Party Time" – eight-foot diameter ashtrays filled with cigarette butts, cigarette packages, matches, ashes, and other paraphernalia.[1] For Hirst, cigarettes represent a fundamental metaphor for life – "beginning pure and white, burning down to ash and a crushed butt" (Vanderlip, cited in Zabel 77). This thought, also evident in the conflicting titles, simultaneously carries connotations of life and death. Smoking, as an action, represents immediate gratification and a working-class pleasure, as well as standing as a metaphor for passing or "killing" time. Similarly, in Lindvay's image, these remnants function as symbols of time gone, an accumulation of fleeting and perhaps mundane moments that took place in the past. In a way, the images of worn-out socks and cigarette butts in a sink evoke the tradition of the *memento mori*, which translates as "remember to die" or "remember death" ("memento mori, n."). The photographs act as a stark reminder of the ephemeral nature of human life, and time's effect on all matter and life. In her analysis of Tracey Emin's work, *My*

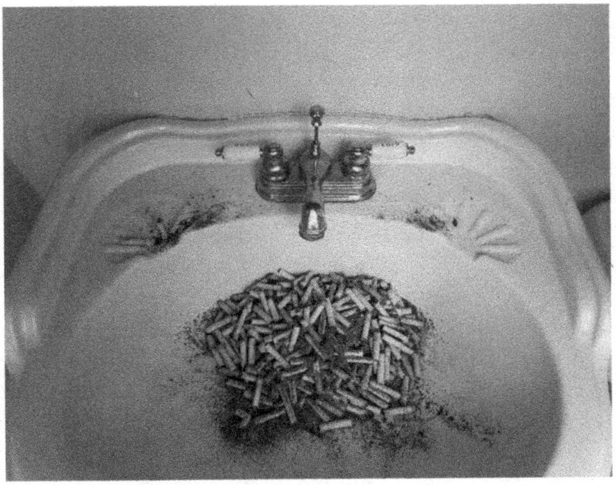

Figure 8.3 Lisa Lindvay, "My Mother's Bathroom Sink"

Bed (1998), Elizabeth Legge states that things presented as part of the artwork, such as cigarette butts, empty drink bottles, heaps of tissue paper and junk food packaging next to the artist's bed, "re-thought within the modern life of depression" act as "tokens of a kind of psychological repetitive action strain and cumulative tedium of life" (90).

Likewise, Lindvay's photographs of mundane objects represent exhaustion and reproduce tension and trauma. In *The Return of the Real,* Hal Foster analyzes the relationship between representation, trauma, and repetition in the context of Jacques Lacan's seminar, *The Unconscious and Repetition,* and Andy Warhol's *Death in America.* Foster writes:

> As missed, the real cannot be represented; it can only be repeated, indeed it must be repeated. [...] Repetition is not reproduction. [...] Rather, repetition serves to screen the real understood as traumatic. But this very need also points to the real, and at this point the real ruptures the screen of repetition.
>
> *(132)*

As Foster claims, the "real" and trauma cannot be directly represented; rather, it has to be performed or re-enacted. It is this "rupture" that occurs between "the perception and the consciousness of a subject *touched* by an image" that can reproduce the traumatic (132 original emphasis). This idea of "rapture" resonates with Barthes's description of the third meaning as "*an accent,* the very form of an emergence, [...] a sort of gash rased of meaning (of desire for meaning)" ("The Third Meaning" 62). For Barthes, this *accent* "carries a certain emotion" and can perhaps be likened to another concept that he develops later in his life – a *punctum*: "the word [...] also refers to the notion of punctuation, and because the photographs I am speaking of are in effect punctuated, sometimes even speckled with these sensitive points; precisely, these marks, these wounds are so many *points*" (*Camera Lucida* 26–7 original emphasis). The wounding in Lindvay's photographs becomes apparent in the deconstruction of time and space in assemblages of household waste. The punctum in these images are the multiplicity of the things represented.

In *Hold Together,* repetitions and play with temporality are evident not only in the composition but also in the poses of the subjects that echo religious iconography and mythology, as observed in the images discussed above in this essay – "Dinner" (Figure 8.1) and "My Dad Standing in the Flowerpot 2009" (Figure 8.2), and also between text and image. Repetitions within the images and recreations of iconography in *Hold Together* can be interpreted as a longing for the familiar, for the well-known, recognizable and, although not necessarily or as well as, in a sense of nostalgia, a desire for something that was never there in the first place. Mimicking of past styles and play with genres from other epochs are also characteristics of postmodernist pastiche and parody. In his book *Postmodernism, or, The Cultural Logic of Late Capitalism*, Fredric Jameson argues that fascination with recycling past images, which signifies "the desperate attempt to appropriate a missing past," leads to erasure of history (19). According to Mark Fisher, "Anachronism, the slippage of discrete time periods into one another [is] a major symptom of time breaking down" (5). This anachronism also brings about an inertia and paradox in which "life continues, but time has somehow stopped" (6).

The photographs in *Hold Together* represent a sense of meaninglessness, emptiness, and the alteration of time flow. This can be read as a mirroring or mimicking of Lindvay's mother's illness as well as an expression of boredom. As Barry Sandywell notes: "Descriptions of boredom and accounts of depression share the same semantic ground of devitalised inertia and existential dullness" (43). According to the American Psychiatric Association, symptoms of depression include sadness and/or irritable mood, social withdrawal, decreased energy, feelings of worthlessness, emptiness, loss of interest or pleasure and psychomotor disturbances, such as restlessness as well as slowed down thinking, speech, and movement. Similarly, boredom suggests "a temporal elongation" (Goodstein 107), a distorted experience of time that consists of "empty, inherently meaningless moments" (Goodstein 115). The sense of boredom in *Hold Together* is evident in the relentless attention to small details, as depicted in the photographs "Powdered Donuts," "Cheetos," and "The Boys' Mismatched Socks," 2011. The subject matter of these photographs revolves around scraps and fragments of the everyday, instead of pointing toward deeper meaning or expressing the banality of consumer culture. Here I borrow a question posed by Sandywell: "How to create values through intrinsically valueless acts?" (42). One possible answer here is that the photographic medium itself lends value to the seemingly meaningless acts. For Susan Sontag: "To photograph is to confer importance. There is probably no subject that cannot be beautified; moreover, there is no way to supress the tendency inherent in all photographs to accord value to their subjects" (22). The photography transforms unremarkable acts or objects into things worth being seen. Additionally, in the act of repetition, several contradictory actions take place, as Foster claims in the context of Warhol's images, "a warding away of traumatic significance and an opening out to it, a defending against traumatic affect and a producing of it" (132). Similarly, Lindvay's photographs are playful yet also open up to traumatic experiences that could not be otherwise accessed. These contradictory meanings are carefully balanced and coexist in uneasy accord.

As several theorists have argued, instead of "seeing boredom as incipient nihilism" (and this perhaps can also be extended to some forms of depression), it can also be regarded as resistance or "one phase of transgressive praxis [...] using the local paradigm of social withdrawal as a desire to reflect and renew self and community" (Sandywell 49; Haladyn). Exhausted elements, such as cigarette butts and worn socks here are re-energized by being assembled and presented in different contexts. Photography emerges reflectively as an embodied practice that, as Kristeva argues, "repeats the initial creative act" and in this process provides a possibility of reinvention.

Conclusion

The reading of these photographs is undoubtedly influenced by "middle-class values." The family's awkward poses and juxtaposition of fast food and their deteriorating surroundings function as critiques of the traditional family values depicted in family albums. Lindvay's photographs portray and communicate closeness and intimacy yet also show how these relationships and individuals' lives are affected by the "entropic state" of their matriarch. The idea of family as a foundation of privacy and protection here is fractured. The sense of failure and deficiency is reified in these photographs as the family fails to conform to the standards of a "normal family" life.

In this project, Lindvay seeks the familiar yet resists it and, in this process, re-invents it. Lindvay's photographs interrupt conventionality and question the norms and expectations of the family and the representation of mental illness as a socially constructed category of difference. In an e-mail, Lindvay disclosed that, "In the first year of working on this series I overheard someone asking in response to my work 'why would we want to look at this?'. After overhearing this statement it has been my goal to create points of connection between the viewer and my family's experience through seeking the familiar rather than othering" (personal communication, August 4, 2021). Lindvay here seeks an affective response, connection, or what Marianne Hirsch calls an "affiliative look" (xiii) from the viewers. Yet, the images resist assimilation and easy identification. As Hirsh states, "Familial looking is a powerful, if slippery and often deceptive, instrument of cultural dialogue and cultural memory" (xiii). The traditional, nuclear family reinforces its boundaries based on national, ethnic, and gendered borders. As Michael Hardt and Antonio Negri argue in their text *Commonwealth*, family, amongst other social constructs, such as the nation and the corporation, both "generates and corrupts the common" (175). They write that:

> The exclusive nature of the family model, which carries with it inevitably all of its internal hierarchies, gender norms, and heteronormativity, is evidence of not only a pathetic lack of social imagination to grasp other forms of intimacy and solidarity but also a lack of freedom to create and experiment with alternative social relationships and nonfamily kinship structures.
>
> *(176)*

Hold Together provides a model for interpersonal intimacies that are not based on sameness. By placing emphasis on performance, the photographs diminish the notion of the relationality of her father and siblings as static. The performance describes their relational link not as a thread, a linear reciprocity, or a pre-set order but rather as a process that takes place. References to religious iconography, mythology, and pop culture, with added humor, unsettle viewers' sense of reality, creating anxiety, and uncertainty. In this way Lindvay hopes to bring a new "vision of what the world might look like freed from societal assumptions that are circumscribed to my family – to all of us" (personal communication, August 4, 2021). Within this project, we drift between artificiality and authenticity, between performance and the exposure of vulnerability. Between powerful emotions and parody, grief and playfulness, these images try to articulate and express intimacies that are rarely given voice to. The contradiction and oscillation between familiar and unfamiliar bring to mind the experience of uncanny or the Freudian notion of the *unheimlich*. Freud concludes that "everything is uncanny that ought to have remained hidden and secret, and yet comes to light" (13). Yet, perhaps in this performative process of unveiling and revealing, repetition and play with temporality, new meanings can emerge and bring about renewal.

Note

1 The image can be seen here: www.damienhirst.com/crematorium.

Works cited

American Psychiatric Association. *Diagnostic and Statistical Manual of Mental Disorders*, 5th Edition: DSM-5, 2019.

Austin, John L. *How to Do Things with Words*. Cambridge, Mass: Harvard University Press, 1975.

Bachelard, Gaston. *The Poetics of Space*. Boston: Beacon Press, 1994.

Barad, Karen. *Meeting the Universe Halfway: Quantum Physics and the Entanglement of Matter and Meaning*. Durham, N.C.: Duke University Press, 2007.

Baraitser, Lisa. *Maternal Encounters: The Ethics of Interruption,* 1st. edition. New York and Abingdon: Routledge, 2008.

Barthes, Roland. "The Third Meaning." *Image, Music, Text*, translated and selected by Stephen Heath, London: Fontana Press, 1977, pp. 52–68.

Barthes, Roland. *Camera Lucida: Reflections on Photography*. London: Vintage Classics, 2000.

Brown, Elspeth H. and Thy Phu (editors). *Feeling Photography*. Duke University Press, 2014.

Campt, Tina M. *Listening to Images*. Durham: Duke University Press, 2017.

Cixous, Hélène. *"Coming to Writing" and Other Essays*. Cambridge, Mass.; London: Harvard University Press, 1991.

Cross, Gary. *An All-consuming Century: Why Commercialism Won in Modern America*. New York: Columbia University Press, 2000.

Dluzen, Robin. "Lisa Lindvay. Editorial Review." *Visual Art Source,* January 31, 2014, www.visualartsource.com/ index.php?page=editorial&pcID=27&aID=2644. Accessed September 30, 2020.

Fisher, Mark. *Ghosts of My Life: Writings on Depression, Hauntology and Lost Futures*. Winchester, UK; Washington, USA: Zero Books, 2013.

Foster, Hal. *The Return of the Real: Art and Theory at the End of the Century: Avant-garde at the End of the Century*. Cambridge, Mass: MIT Press, 1996.

Freud, Sigmund. *The Uncanny*. Penguin Classics, 2003.

Gilman, Sander L. *Disease and Representation: Images of Illness from Madness to AIDS*. Ithaca: Cornell University Press, 1988.

Gilman, Sander L. *Seeing the Insane: A Visual and Cultural History of Our Attitudes Toward the Mentally Ill*. Vermont: Echo Point Books & Media Brattleboro, 2014.

Goodstein, Elizabeth S. *Experience Without Qualities: Boredom and Modernity*. Stanford: Stanford University Press, 2005.

Green, David and Joanna Lowry. "From Presence to the Performative: Rethinking Photographic Indexicality." *Where is the Photograph?*, edited by David Green, Photoforum/Photoworks, 2003, pp. 47–60.

Guenther, Lisa. *The Gift of the Other: Levinas and the Politics of Reproduction*. Albany: State University of New York Press, 2006.

Haladyn, Julian J. *Boredom and Art: Passions of the Will to Boredom*. Winchester, UK; Washington, USA: Zero Books, 2015.

Hardt, Michael and Antonio Negri. *Commonwealth*. Cambridge, MA; London: Belknap Press/Harvard University Press, 2009.

Hirsch, Marianne. "Introduction: Familial Looking." *The Familial Gaze*, edited by Marianne Hirsch, Hanover; London: University Press of New England, 1999, pp. xi–xxv.

hooks, bell. *Feminist Theory: From Margin to Center*. New York and Abingdon: Routledge, 2014.

Jameson, Fredric. *Postmodernism, or, The Cultural Logic of Late Capitalism*. Durham: Duke University Press, 1992.

Jones, Amelia. "Performing the Other as Self: Cindy Sherman and Laura Aguilar Pose the Subject." *Interfaces: Women/Autobiography/Image/Performance,* edited by Sidonia Smith and Julia Watson, Ann Arbor, MI: University of Michigan Press, 2002, pp. 69–102.

Kleinman, Arthur and Don Seeman. "Personal Experience of Illness." *The Handbook of Social Studies in Health and Medicine*, edited by Gary L. Albrecht, Ray Fitzpatrick and Susan C. Scrimshaw, London: Sage Publications Ltd., 2000, pp. 230–42.

Kristeva, Julia. *Black Sun: Depression and Melancholia*. New York: Columbia University Press, 1989.

Kritzman, Lawrence D. "Melancholia Becomes the Subject: Kristeva's Invisible 'Thing' and the Making of Culture." *Paragraph*, vol. 14, no. 2, 1991, pp. 144–50. www.jstor.org/stable/43263369. Accessed September 30, 2020.

Legge, Elizabeth. "Boring Cool People: Some Cases of British Boredom." *Boredom Studies Reader*, edited by Michael E. Gardiner and Julian Jason Haladyn. New York and Abingdon: Routledge, 2017, pp. 81–98.

Levin, Laura. "The Performative Force of Photography, Photography and Culture." *Photography and Culture*, vol. 3, no. 2, 2009, pp. 327–36.

Lindvay, Lisa. *Hold Together*. 2020. https://lisalindvay.com/images.

Lucretius. *The Nature of Things*. London: Penguin Classics, 2007.

Manning, Lavonda. "Photographer of the Week #84: Lisa Lindvay." *Capricious*. June 10, 2015. https://becapricious.com/photographer-of-the-week-84-lisa-lindvay/. Accessed September 30, 2020.

"McDonald's 'Bigger than Jesus Christ'." *Marketing Week*. July 21, 1995. www.marketingweek.com/1995/07/21/mcdonalds-bigger-than-jesus-christ/. Accessed June 30, 2021.

"memento mori, n." OED Online. Oxford University Press, 2021. Accessed July 27, 2021.

Miller, Elaine P. *Head Cases: Julia Kristeva on Philosophy and Art in Depressed Times*. New York: Columbia University Press, 2014.

Nancy, Jean-Luc. *Listening*. New York: Fordham University Press, 2007.

Phu, Thy, Elspeth H. Brown, and Andrea Noble. "Feeling in Photography, the Affective Turn, and the History of Emotions." *The Routledge Companion to Photography Theory*, edited by Mark Durden and Jane Tormey. New York and Abingdon: Routledge, 2019, pp. 21–36.

Roman, Luke and Monica Roman. *Encyclopedia of Greek and Roman Mythology*. New York: Facts on File, Inc., 2010.

Ruddick, Sara. *Maternal Thinking: Toward a Politics of Peace*. Boston: Beacon Press, 1995.

Sandywell, Barry. "The Dialectic of Lassitude: A Reflexive Investigation." *Boredom Studies Reader*, edited by Michael E. Gardiner and Julian Jason Haladyn. New York and Abingdon: Routledge, 2017, pp. 38–52.

Shusterman, Richard. "Photography as Performative Process." *Thinking through the Body: Essays in Somaesthetics*, edited by Richard Shusterman, Cambridge: Cambridge University Press, 2012, pp. 239–61.

Sile, Agnese. "Mental Illness within Family Context: Visual Dialogues in Joshua Lutz's Photographic Essay *Hesitating Beauty*." *Arts and Humanities in Higher Education*, vol. 17, no. 1, 2018, pp. 84–103.

Silverman, Kaja. *Threshold of the Visible World*. New York and Abingdon: Routledge, 1995.

Sontag, Susan. *On Photography*. Electronic Edition, Rosetta Books, 2005.

Spence, Jo. *Putting Myself in the Picture: A Political, Personal, and Photographic Autobiography*. London: Camden Press, 1986.

Tamboukou, Maria. "Re-imagining the Narratable Subject." *Qualitative Research*, vol. 8, no. 3, 2008, pp. 283–92.

Zabel, Barbara B. *Assembling Art: The Machine and the American Avant-Garde*. Jackson: The University Press of Mississippi, 2004.

PART III

Fiction film

All four chapters in this section implicitly or explicitly wrestle with long-standing claims from scholars and clinicians of inaccurate portrayals and stigmatizing stereotypes in fiction films that feature stories about mental illness and characters with disabilities. The writers here provide nuanced and detailed readings of films to contextualize and complicate such assumptions.

The opening sentence of Matt Selway's contribution to this section, "**Brains For Hire: Exploring the Role of Psychiatric Consultancy in *The Aviator*,**" reads like a movie script: "Within twenty-four hours of taking a call from Leonardo DiCaprio's personal assistant, Dr. Jeffrey M. Schwartz, an expert in Obsessive Compulsive Disorder, found himself in the Hollywood superstar's living room." Selway argues that psychiatric expertise and its use in film productions are scarce and that we need scholarly critical and qualitative investigations to explore how filmmakers actually use such expertise. Drawing from interviews with Schwartz and one of his patients, both of whom helped craft DiCaprio's portrayal of Howard Hughes in *The Aviator* (2004), his chapter offers new insights into the role of psychiatric film consultancy.

In the second chapter, "**Recovering the Patient's Voice: The Diagnostic Process from Early Modern History to Oliver Sacks,**" Allison Kavey reminds us that the process of diagnosis, like the practice of medicine in general, is the product of history, and the position of personal medical narratives in that process has shifted over time. While she acknowledges that Michel Foucault's argument in *The Birth of the Clinic*—that patient voices have been lost and replaced by medical authority and technology—is universally accepted, historians of medicine have, nevertheless, corrected it, offering evidence of how socioeconomic status, time, and location determine the relative importance of patient voices in medical encounters. To illustrate, Kavey analyzes *Awakenings*, the 1990 film derived from Oliver Sacks' book of the same title and based on his case notes of treating patients who survived encephalitis lethargica.

In the third chapter, "**Beneath the Covers: The Illness of Sex as Depicted in Film,**" Julie Aultman analyzes three films—*Little Children* (2007); *The Sessions* (2012); and *The Nightingale* (2018)—to illustrates how fiction films often disembody persons as sexual beings because of dysfunction, disability, paraphilic deviancy, and disempowerment. Reading these cinematic texts as pathographies, Aultman argues that they speak to the multiple ways that "illness" is

DOI: 10.4324/9781003007661-12

understood in the context of sex including abnormal functioning, imbalance, immorality, and suffering.

In the final chapter of this section, "**'Stereotypes,' Focalization and Modality: Mainstream Cinematic Images of Disability**," Nigel Morris writes that the complex role of film in the evolving development of disability politics remains controversial and contentious. Many scholars and activists assert that disability is underrepresented in mainstream movies, which rely on and reinforce stereotypes. Morris contends that the most effective tactic to counter this entrenched notion of stereotyping is to scrutinize those films which do not represent disabilities in standardized ways and to demonstrate that these examples are not exceptional.

9

BRAINS FOR HIRE

Exploring the role of psychiatric consultancy in *The Aviator*

Matt Selway

Introduction: the accuracy fallacy

Within 24 hours of taking a call from Leonardo DiCaprio's personal assistant, Dr. Jeffrey M. Schwartz, MD., an expert in Obsessive Compulsive Disorder (OCD), found himself in the Hollywood superstar's living room. At the end of their conversation, it was agreed that Schwartz, a Research Psychiatrist from the University of Los Angeles California (UCLA), would take a role as psychiatric consultant to DiCaprio to advise him on how to craft his performance of notorious Hollywood director and aviator Howard Hughes. Over a number of weeks and lengthy pre-production meetings, Schwartz and DiCaprio extensively reviewed the first draft of John Logan's script for *The Aviator* (Scorsese 2004). Specifically, DiCaprio sought Schwartz's insight into the most effective ways to bring the symptoms and experiences of OCD to life on screen. As part of this arrangement, it was agreed that one of the film's production researchers would attend a session of Dr. Schwartz's weekly OCD support group to make notes about the members' lived experiences with the disorder. Due to the rich insights from Schwartz and the members of his group, the production then also employed the consultancy services of Edward (assumed name), one of the group's members, to provide a lived experience perspective alongside Schwartz's clinical research expertise.

Scholarly accounts and analyses of psychiatric expertise and its use in film productions are extremely thin on the ground. There is, however, a large body of scholarship that focuses upon the topic of media representations of mental illness. Through the majority of this work, some consistencies and trends warrant reconsideration and critical appraisal. First, research psychiatrists and psychiatric academics write the overwhelming majority of such texts. Consequently, the dominant critical rhetoric on representations of mental illness in media and film tends to be overly focussed upon notions of "inaccurate" portrayals and "stigmatizing" stereotypes being perpetuated by the mass media (cf. Wedding and Boyd; Byrne; Stuart; Wahl; Roberts; and Nairn, Coverdale, and Coverdale). This perspective will not come as much of a surprise, given that the majority of these writers have professional backgrounds in the discipline of psychiatry, and their clinical expertise usually leads them to a focus on the minutiae of symptomology and the representation of their profession in media imagery. However, what is surprising is the frequency with which these texts make broad claims about "media effects."

DOI: 10.4324/9781003007661-13

A small number of media studies scholars (cf. Philo; Blackman and Walkerdine; Cross, "Visualizing Madness," *Mediating Madness*; and Harper, "Media, Madness," *Madness, Power*) have challenged these over-simplified assertions whilst acknowledging the important need for advanced and nuanced study of the wider impacts and repercussions of mental health stigma perpetuated through the media. For instance, Stephen Harper ("Media, Madness" 479) points out that much of this psychiatry-based research seems to overlook the fact that 'the public does not always accept media disparagement of the mentally ill,' and audience responses to such imagery and stereotyping are almost certain to be varied and influenced by a wide range of demographic characteristics such as age, gender, race, and ethnicity, lived experiences of mental ill health, occupation, education, and other factors.

Another curiosity of this preoccupation with the perceived inaccurate portrayals of mental illness stems from a claim made by Emeritus Professor of Psychiatry Stephen Hyler in 1988. In *Comprehensive Psychiatry*, Hyler proclaimed that, in his estimation and experience of film and television depictions of mental illnesses, "a surprisingly large number of such portrayals are reasonably accurate" (205). Many, but by no means all, of these psychiatric forays into media representations of mental illness commonly overlook this point of view and persistently maintain that most media depictions are egregiously wide of the mark and therefore socially harmful. Even in cases of films that employed psychiatric experts as consultants, disagreements about the quality and convincing nature of the resultant depictions remain. For instance, the production team of *A Beautiful Mind* (Howard 2001) employed the services of Dr. Marianne Gillow, MD to act as a psychological consultant and gave a special thanks in the credits to Psychiatry and Neurology Professor Max Fink, MD for his advice. This inclusion of psychiatric expertise was one factor that led to Ben Green (2007) describing the film as "reasonably realistic,'" and Peter Remington stating that the film offered "a tidy representation of schizophrenia" (151). However, such praise did not prevent Russell Crowe's performance of the film's schizophrenic protagonist and the film's depiction of medication and psychiatric treatment from being sternly criticized by several other psychiatric writers. To take just one example, Ron Roberts criticizes *A Beautiful Mind* for its 'litany of lies and half-truths" (42) and for "promulgating psychiatric propaganda" (54).

Wedding, Boyd, and Niemiec state that "a mental health consultant may be used with certain films...particularly involving fine tuning the screenplay and helping the director and actors understand psychological phenomena; we believe mental health consultants should be sought out for *every* film portraying a psychological condition...Unfortunately, such consultants are sorely underutilized in cinema" (2, original italics). Whilst increased inclusion of psychiatric consultants would be welcomed by many, the disagreements among authors and experts in the fields of psychiatry about what constitutes "accuracy" and which portrayals satisfactorily match such criteria, highlights the limited use that such scrutiny can have both during the consultants' input, as well as in subsequent critiques of the texts they help to inform. Thus, a critical and qualitative investigation is needed to further explore and understand how psychiatric expertise is used in the context of film production and preparation. This chapter offers new critical insights and analysis into the role of psychiatric film consultancy, drawn from qualitative interviews with both Schwartz and Edward exploring their experiences in helping to craft DiCaprio's portrayal of Howard Hughes in *The Aviator*.[1]

Understanding symptomology and "finding the right feeling"

What spurred DiCaprio into seeking psychiatric consultation for the role in the first place was a segment of the screenplay that left the Hollywood star baffled. Over a section in which Hughes inspects in excruciating detail the steering wheel for a plane his company is building, Hughes's lines only read: "Show me all the blueprints." The five-word phrase is repeated more than a dozen times in succession. This is one of the story's key plot points, in which the severity of Hughes's OCD begins to envelop him and become apparent to others around him, including the audience. In Schwartz's recollections of his first meeting with DiCaprio he said:

> That line "Show me the blueprints," that was the initial thing that [DiCaprio] wanted my advice on… In the first ten minutes of me meeting him, that's what he wanted to know about. "What do I do with this?", [DiCaprio] said that himself. You know, here was a script just saying, "show me the blueprints" many times in a row, and he was kind of going "as an actor, what am I supposed to do with that?"
>
> *(Schwartz Part 1, 14:46–15:55)*

DiCaprio's uncertainty about how to approach the repetitive dialogue spoke to a need for having an appreciation and understanding of the minutiae of OCD's impact on the mind and the brain; how in the midst of severe episodes, these symptoms and mental rituals can become all-consuming to their subject. To guide DiCaprio on his approach bringing the dialogue to life Schwartz explained that:

> There would be two things going on, in a person with OCD, when they're saying the same thing again and again. Those two things would be basically some version of counting…where you would have some like magical number, like you have to say [it] a certain number of times and then, that gets coupled with a certain rhythm and a certain accentuation of the way the words come out.
>
> *(Schwartz Part 2: 1:03:08–1:06:27)*

Thus, DiCaprio's performance of the scene heavily leaned on the sense of rhythmical delivery and numerical repetition. His verbal delivery actually repeats the phrase, "show me all the blueprints," significantly more than the 13 times it is written in the script, accelerating and decelerating the delivery, at times coupling and overlapping the end and beginning of one repetition into another and in others distinctly separating the iterations with enunciated staccato. This is embellished with fluctuations in voice volume also, and extra depth and dimension are added by emphasizing Hughes's attempts to break the cycle of phrase repetition by inserting new phrases and mannerisms to try to disrupt the downward spiral. All these performative cadences and slight variations on the phrase that Hughes is stuck repeating were based on additional guidance and suggestions from Schwartz and Edward. The key aspect to both consultants' suggestions was to focus on how a person with OCD would at a moment like this try to find "the right feeling" (a common phrase that many people with OCD as well as clinicians use to describe colloquially the unexplainable trigger that finally satisfies and ends the cycle of OCD-related anxiety). In this case, it was emphasized by both consultants that the attempt to find the "right feeling" would be through variation in the verbal delivery, a form of experimentation with the stuck phraseology in order to discover and fulfil a mental sensation that ends the cycle.

Edward suggested a similar approach for a scene in which Hughes compulsively washes his hands in a restroom. For this, Edward reiterated to DiCaprio the importance of the fact that, in his experience, Hughes would likely feel it imperative to wash his hands until it "felt right," no matter how long that might take or how much consequential damage would be done to the skin on his hands. This recommendation stemmed from Edward's own personal lived experience of similar washing and hygiene routines based on a particular set of OCD triggers and symptoms connected to anxieties of contamination (something Edward insists was key to his selection to consult with DiCaprio above other members of the support group with lived experience of OCD). So too, Edward emphasized how precarious these rituals and routines can be, and how quickly they can become unsettled and thus need repeating. In his own words:

> [I said to DiCaprio] If you're washing your hands in the bathroom…and you go to dry them, and some water fell on your foot… [a person with OCD would think] "Oh shit! My hands aren't clean [I've] got to rewash them." Or, if you wash them and it didn't feel right, you know, there would have to be a certain feeling there, and if that feeling wasn't there you'd continue to wash until you get that feeling, but you can't explain what that feeling is, it just has to be the right feeling.
>
> *(Edward Part 1: 1:03:37–1:05:01)*

Indeed, this sense of "finding the right feeling" became a key component explored in a short info-film that was produced as a DVD extra for *The Aviator.* Titled *The Affliction of Howard Hughes*, it features excerpts of DiCaprio giving press interviews to promote the film in which he talks about the research that he did into Hughes's illness and the work he did with Dr. Schwartz. As well as these promotional materials, numerous talking head interviews with Dr. Schwartz, Edward (silhouetted out in order to maintain his anonymity), and several other members of Schwartz's OCD group at UCLA detail how they provided factual information about the condition. The inclusion of this film in the DVD extras came as a form of compromise to some suggestions made by Schwartz and Edward – to be discussed further in a later section of this chapter – and served as one of many "authenticating artefacts" used in the film's marketing to emphasize the sincerity, credibility, and legitimacy of the film's representation of mental illness.

"Authenticating artefacts"

Though critical arguments focusing on the perceived authenticity of representations of mental illness are, as outlined earlier, often quite limited, issues of accuracy and authenticity continue to have currency in popular discourse. Many film productions – especially those like *The Aviator,* which are based on real events or life stories – go to great lengths in their production and promotional strategies to emphasize the inclusion of what I call "authenticating artefacts." These artefacts, which can take many forms, seek to legitimize the credibility of the film's story by connecting the film's characterization and narration to relevant external artefacts or expertise that divert away from the film's narrative conceits and liberties in storytelling.

In many cases, certainly within the biopic genre, these authenticating artefacts may be historical or biographical, such as highlighting that the film is based on a real person's memoir or (auto)biography. There are numerous examples of biopics whose main subject experiences mental ill health – as well as a large range of other texts – that deploy this strategy, such as *Girl, Interrupted* (Mangold 1999), an adaptation of Susanna Kaysen's autobiography; *Prozac Nation* (Skjoldbjærg 2001), based on Elizabeth Wurtzel's memoir; or *Beautiful Boy* (van Groeningen 2018), developed from David Sheff's book recounting his son's troubles with drug addiction. In other cases, biographical films commonly show archival footage or photographs of the real-life subjects within the film or at the end in the final credits, emphasizing the physical likeness that the film's stars may have to their historical counterpart. As Dennis Bingham points out, this has almost become de rigueur for the genre and compels the audience into comparison (82). Some actors get the opportunity to meet the person they are portraying such as Jamie Foxx – despite already being a proficient piano player – taking lessons with Ray Charles as preparation for *Ray* (Hackford 2004) or Eddie Redmayne meeting with Stephen Hawking before shooting *The Theory of Everything* (Marsh 2014). Regardless of the specific form, these authenticators commonly constitute valuable promotional opportunities for studios, production companies and distributors to capitalize on the popularity of cinema's connection to "reality" so desirable in cinema culture. This perceived connection between cinema and reality often fares especially well during film awards season. As Robert Rosenstone notes, despite a seemingly poor reputation as a genre in public attention, a significant majority of Best Picture and Best Actor/Actress Academy Awards (Oscars) have gone to biopics over the last 45 plus years compared to other genres, in large part because of their apparent "worthiness" generated from a supposed connection to "real life" (101).

When it comes to films (whether biographical or not) that significantly focus on narratives of mental illness, the deployment and emphasis of authenticating artefacts continues to be an important feature. For instance, *The Three Faces of Eve* (Johnson 1957) opens with the film's narrator, real-life journalist Alistair Cooke, directly addressing the audience. Cooke proclaims that Eve's (Joanne Woodward) story presents a "true" account of Multiple Personality Disorder (MPD) made even more remarkable due to the large body of medical research that underpins the film. Cooke insists that the film does not resort to sensationalism and has not taken any creative liberties with the narrative, instead remarking that "the truth itself is fabulous enough." Cooke refers to the medical research as the authenticating artefact on which the film is based; a book of the same name by psychiatrists Corbett H. Thigpen, MD and Hervey M. Cleckley, MD about their experiences treating a patient with MPD. Cooke, a well-known journalist and broadcaster, adds an extra dimension of legitimacy by not depicting a character or absent narrator; instead, he functions as an omniscient narrator with real-life credibility, further codifying the film's content as ostensibly authentic by his professional status as a purveyor of facts. For a broadcaster of this stature to endorse and reify the medical research of Thigpen and Cleckley further enhances the sense of trustworthiness in the film's presentation of MPD.

Despite this emphasis on the psychiatric expertise reinforcing the film's credentials, Dr. Schwartz himself, when discussing the pervasive clichés of mental illness in the cinema, bemoaned the overly common presence of multiple personalities as a narrative trope and cinematic symptom presented for dramatic effect. Schwartz stated that, when he praised *The Aviator* as one of the best portrayals of mental illness in cinema at the premiere, one of the film's producers raised *The Three Faces of Eve* as part of that conversation. Schwartz dismissed it, stating:

> As far as [MPD in cinema] is concerned, I'm not going to waste my time, quite candidly. None of those films [depicting MPD] can possibly [compete with *The Aviator*] because, you know, multiple personality is such a bizarre thing and of all the things "psychiatric" that have been overdone in cinema, that's pretty clearly at the top… [when] it is not actually a well described syndrome. It's a very controversial mishmash of diagnostic entities.
>
> *(Schwartz Part 1: 39:49–44:02)*

In an effort to avoid many of the perceived mental illness clichés found elsewhere in cinema, Schwartz not only participated in extensive pre-production processes – such as vetting John Logan's screenplay and consulting with DiCaprio about particular mannerisms, symptoms, and underlying thought processes experienced by many people with OCD – but also framed his explanations by relating to other film representations. In their initial meetings, for example, Schwartz discussed the performances of "neurotic conflict'" and personality disorders by actors such as Robert De Niro in *Taxi Driver* (Scorsese 1976) and *Raging Bull* (Scorsese 1980), and Catherine Deneuve in *Belle De Jour* (Buñuel 1967). In doing so, and in primarily relating to Scorsese films, Schwartz also presented an authenticating artefact of his own by showing DiCaprio and Scorsese his level of cinema literacy, and as such, his ability to bridge the gap between his clinical psychiatric expertise and their cinematic production expertise. In a sense, we may interpret this as Schwartz informally auditioning for the role of advisor.

Schwartz insisted to DiCaprio and Scorsese that these previous film examples could be useful touchstones for crafting DiCaprio's performance of the more severe aspects of Hughes's condition. However, he also impressed upon them how *The Aviator* would benefit further as a result of being about a real-life subject who (retrospectively) had a real diagnosis. Thus, a blend of intertextual and clinical referents could be drawn on to inform and refine the performance of Hughes's OCD. In Schwartz's own words:

> I told [DiCaprio] that I thought [*Taxi Driver*] was an extremely good portrayal of what probably could be understood as paranoid schizophrenia, although it wasn't [specifically] a portrayal of paranoid schizophrenia in the sense that it was a fictional character…now, we're portraying a real person with a real diagnosis, so I mean, I think we're going to do considerably better than that in terms of portraying a psychiatric illness. And [DiCaprio] definitely got excited by that. So when I was framing what I was wanting to do with him, in terms of…using the portrayal of Travis Bickle, not as a kind of jumping off point in terms of what we're going to do because it's a different diagnosis, but saying "look, this is quite a realistic portrayal for a fictional character in a film that's not really about psychiatric disorder per se, and now with Hughes, it's a real person, with a real psychiatric disorder, and I'm an expert in that disorder, we're going to take this to the next level."
>
> *(Schwartz Part 1: 40:27–42:39)*

In order for Dr. Schwartz to get his points fully across and translate his clinical expertise into a form that effectively facilitates artistic expression, it was vital for him not just to recite and explain the intricacies of neurological and psychiatric knowledge to the performers and director but also to make this information tangible for the production personnel by connecting that knowledge to film discourse. As David Kirby explains in his account of scientific consultants working in Hollywood, "the goal for…consultants is to let filmmakers negotiate…accuracy within their own context of narrative, genre, and audiences" (8). Thus, expectations from external critics within the psychiatric discipline (or elsewhere outside of film and media studies and film production circles) about accuracy in representation is immediately diminished by the internal process of consulting, which inherently requires the traversing of clinical and artistic boundaries to effectively communicate knowledge in a meaningful way that enhances performance and representation.

The role(s) of psychiatric consultant

Initially, the input of psychiatric consultation in the film came in pre-production meetings between Dr. Schwartz, DiCaprio, and Scorsese and his personal researcher, Marianne Bower, in Los Angeles. As a group, they went through the whole script and discussed the intricacies of OCD symptomology and experiences as they arose. At this early stage, Schwartz said that they were primarily reviewing the descriptions of OCD in the stage directions and dialogue: "The corrections that were made [to the script] were all finer points of wording. The finer points of wording [...] about the way a person with OCD would actually think about what was going on [in that moment]."

One alteration that Schwartz felt was needed came in a scene where Hughes, usually very private and secretive about his OCD, confides to his lover Katharine Hepburn (Cate Blanchett) that he has experiences that he knows are irrational. Schwartz explained that in the first version of the script he felt the writing suggested that Hughes heard voices and that this needed to be addressed:

> We have no evidence to think that Hughes heard voices, and people with OCD do not hear voices. If they're hearing voices, then that throws the diagnosis into question [...] [The script] was written originally in a way too suggestive of a hallucination rather than a thought that was so bothersome that it felt like it was real without actually being a sensory hallucination; that I fixed.
>
> *(Schwartz Part 2: 1:06:43–1:09:13)*

This statement exemplifies how even minor imprecisions in the characterizations of mental ill health can feature incongruous symptomology. However, an illustration of just how difficult it can be for all parties involved in the process of psychiatric consultancy – in this case, Schwartz, DiCaprio, Scorsese, and Barrow – to come to the same wavelength about such details is exhibited in the director's commentary on the film's DVD, in which Scorsese claims:

> It was a long process. It's difficult to describe because people think "Oh, [DiCaprio] got it from a doctor, he got it from a guy who really had OCD," no, it's not that simple. It's based on what John Logan wrote, and Logan was able to layer it into the script in such a way that it withstood the scrutiny of the doctor(s) and the people who actually have OCD. It really withstood that, plus they helped us add to it. And when we added to it, we also realised that we were adding maybe too much, so we'd shoot, then do a version which had more, then less and that sort of thing.

In Schwartz's estimation, the original draft of the script was reasonably well-informed and sensitive to the symptoms and experiences of OCD. However, as the previous extract from our interview shows, imprecisions and anomalies needed adjusting. This was also true in Edward's view. As he explained:

> I spoke to [DiCaprio's] Personal Assistant [...] and she handed me a script. She said "We would like you to read through the script" [...] so I was just reading the script, and things just didn't sound right, in the script. I don't remember exactly what didn't sound right, but they just didn't sound right. I don't know how to explain it. [...] I spoke to [DiCaprio] and it ended up they gave me the wrong script. They gave me the first draft of the script.
>
> *(Edward Part 1: 19:38–21:52)*

Therefore, contrary to Scorsese's repeated claims that Logan's original script was approved by the consultants, both Schwartz and Edward independently expressed that aspects of the script's description of OCD could be refined to enhance the portrayal.

Once the cast and crew had flown out to their studio in Montreal, Canada, Schwartz's involvement was limited to infrequent phone calls to double check details or quick queries. However, it was at this stage of production that Edward's involvement became more pronounced. The production team invited Edward to Montreal for almost a week to help in the final preparations for DiCaprio's filming. However, despite having greater involvement at different points in the pre-production process – and both consultants having various different tasks based on their clinical and lived expertise – both Dr. Schwartz and Edward were also tasked with some similar responsibilities.

In both consultants' experiences, Scorsese requested that DiCaprio and Bower watch them "act out" moments of the script featuring Hughes having manifestations of OCD symptoms or an episode of obsessive thoughts leading to extreme compulsive behavior. In Schwartz's case, the acting out was part of vetting the screenplay and attempting to illustrate how the words on the page may look and sound when expressed by a person with OCD. Schwartz gave indications of the types of cadences typical in his experience of treating and working with patients who have excessive verbal repetition as a core symptom. These vignette performances were recorded by Bower to be referred back to in later stages of pre-production and filming.

Edward's experience of acting out scenes from the script were much nearer to the beginning of filming and involved the setting up of props and blocking. This approach was beneficial for two reasons. Firstly, it gave DiCaprio a sense of how a person with contamination obsessions and hygiene-focussed compulsive behaviors would likely behave in and embody the specific spaces within which the scenes would take place. Second, this more technical driven approach allowed the production crew to figure out lighting placement, camera positions, and the blocking of other actors present in the scene based on the ritualistic behaviors acted out by Edward. For instance, Edward spoke at length about his views on a key scene in which Hughes, attending a movie premiere, is washing his hands in a bathroom when another guest with polio (visible by his walking with the aid of crutches) asks Hughes to hand him a towel, something Hughes is unable to do on account of his contamination anxiety. In his reflections on this, Edward said:

> We practiced that scene in the bathroom, and he asked me "well why wouldn't you hand the guy the towel?" I said, "because with my contamination issues, it's my hands; [I worry about] my hands being exposed [...] it's not like the polio is going to jump on you or anything like that, you know? But still, just the idea of reaching over there [is too much]".
>
> *(Edward Part 1: 28:27–29:25)*

Following this insight from Edward, the cinematography of this scene – as well as a number of other bathroom scenes throughout the film – places great emphasis upon Hughes's hands. They are often closely framed and lingered upon as they are meticulously washed. When the towel is requested by the other guest, Scorsese's direction features a two-shot of the men facing the mirror as they wash at the basins. As Hughes glances to his side toward the stack of clean towels, the camera quickly cuts to a medium-close up of the towels and then another quick cut to a low angle shot from what Scorsese refers to in the DVD commentary as the "POV of the towel, looking back at him," emphasizing the irrational but powerful anxiety this moment causes Hughes: the towel almost intimidates and mocks Hughes by returning his gaze.

In a similar scene later in the film, Hughes scrubs his hands vigorously with his personal bar of abrasive soap. Exacerbated by the stress of having just been humiliated by Juan Tripp (Alec Baldwin), Hughes's greatest rival in the aviation industry, he cleans his hands to the point that he draws blood. After wiping the blood from his hand and discarding the towel, Hughes discovers a bloody spot on his shirt, which he then tries to wash out. The physical awkwardness of DiCaprio's movement emphasizes the extremity of the compulsive behavior and stubbornness of Hughes in his pursuit of total cleanliness, as he almost raises the shirt to his neck in an attempt to hunch over the basin and wash out the spot. These movements were taken from rehearsed recordings of Edward's acting out of the scene pre-filming. Once dry, Hughes approaches the door as a close up of his hand is shown, followed by an over the shoulder POV shot showing Hughes looking at the doorknob. Hughes slowly reaches out, his hand closely framed again as it trembles, before defeatedly putting his hand back by his side as he cannot bear to touch the knob. His anxiety is only worsened when he realizes that he has already soiled all the towels in the room and so cannot leave. Overwhelmed, he leans against the wall by the door until somebody enters the room and he is able to duck out without being seen or touching the door. Here, then, is a direct example of how Edward's input, as well as Schwartz's initial discussions of the screenplay, directly influenced the physical performance of this OCD episode. Edward explained to me that this concern about directly touching doorknobs was a prominent aspect of his own experience with OCD and that in his first meeting with DiCaprio he showed him his personal washing ritual:

> I said, "Do you want me to show you?" and he said "Sure." So, we went into the bathroom and I went through the compulsions I had for obsessions [...] I went through my washing ritual [and] when I was done washing my hands, I opened the door with a towel or a rag because I didn't want to touch the doorknob. Then I took the rag and threw it behind the door. That was one of the first things that we went over.
>
> *(Edward Part 1: 22:02–24:01)*

As a result of Schwartz and Edward's input, the production team came up with a comprehensive chart of Hughes's known OCD symptoms to be consulted during filming. This information was partially gathered from Schwartz and DiCaprio viewing archival footage of Hughes in public life to observe any moments where he exhibited tics that Schwartz felt would likely be linked to his OCD (such as his habitual tugging of his left trouser leg); the various notes and opinions given from the script vetting of both Schwartz and Edward; and Edward's demonstration of his washing rituals and associated obsessions and compulsions. Scorsese elaborated in the DVD commentary on using the chart:

> As [Hughes] gets older, in certain sequences...certainly in [DiCaprio's] perception of how to play the scene and also the different levels of manifestation of these obsessions, we had to have a chart of what manifestations could occur in the particular scene at that time in his life. Even though we shot out of continuity, we could always refer to the chart and play around with ideas [for what symptom/tic to use] – whether it was a nervous coughing or, the thing we noticed from footage of Hughes, he kept touching his pant leg this way – and when to introduce that.

Scorsese also said, whilst maintaining his view that the original script was approved by the consultants:

> We sort of had a chart of the whole movie and which aspect of OCD would be manifested in [a] scene; the one that's in the script, which passed the tests of all the experts, [or] we can add this, plus we can add a touch of that "left pant leg," he was always doing that. How many times shall we do that, and when we do it, when's the first time we should really see it? If it's the first time, should it be a little less, should it be something you hardly notice? ...Then we layer it in throughout the picture. So,

> we had a chart based on the research with Dr. Schwartz and [Edward] but, again, this is pretty well based upon what John [Logan] had in that script already.

What is important in these excerpts from Scorsese's commentary is the sense that much of the process of developing the sense of growing severity in Hughes's symptoms was done through the film's editing. Whilst this is unsurprising, considering the frequency with which feature films are shot out of continuity, what is surprising is that neither Schwartz nor Edward was involved in the editing in any way. Therefore, this highlights another area where the motivations and agendas of psychiatric consultants and filmmaking creative staff can lose synchronization in the balancing of "accuracy" and storytelling for entertainment purposes. Whilst Schwartz's and Edward's input, in both their views, were treated respectfully and appreciatively, they ultimately, and inevitably, relinquished control of how that information was put to use in the post-production stages.

Outcomes/conclusion

Despite not having any bearing on the postproduction process – which Scorsese insists is where the majority of the composition of Hughes's OCD characterization was achieved – Edward, and Dr. Schwartz especially, found themselves re-enlisted in their consultancy roles to assist in the film's marketing. It is in these moments that both Edward and Schwartz serve as "authenticating artefacts" for the film's portrayal of OCD. One of the compromises that needed to be made between Schwartz and Edward's input and the film's creative prerogatives came in discussion of the film's omittance of the actual term, "OCD." At no point in the film is the term Obsessive Compulsive Disorder used or referred to. Whilst that might seem problematic to some, Schwartz acknowledges that it is completely realistic that the film does not mention the name of Hughes's disorder because, in the period in which Hughes lived, the disorder was practically unknown compared to today. However, both Schwartz and Edward spoke to Scorsese and the producers at Miramax to request that, either at the beginning or end of the film, a digital on-screen graphic (DOG) appear on screen to explain that Howard Hughes suffered from what is now known to be OCD. These requests were not granted. Instead, a compromise was reached whereby Dr. Schwartz and Edward would participate in the making of a short info-film to feature in the DVD extras, which would directly address and explore the disorder. As such, this exemplifies the way that the insights of both consultants were only acted upon when the creative agents in the film production felt this contributed to the overall creative vision of the project. No graphic was included to contextualize Hughes's disorder because this was not seen as befitting to the creative style of the film.

Kirby explains that film studios "prominently feature their consultant's scientific expertise in publicity material. By hiring scientists, studios borrow their expertise to claim legitimacy for the science on screen" (9). This strategy is seen with the psychiatric consultancy services: *The Aviator* covers all bases by not only employing and broadcasting its inclusion of Dr. Schwartz's clinical and professional expertise but also Edward's lived experience of OCD as a means of further authenticating the film's depiction of the illness.

The DVD extras also include a recording of a round table discussion between Dr. Schwartz, Scorsese, DiCaprio, and Terry Moore (Hughes's ex-wife). In this recording, which preceded an advanced screening of the film for select Academy members in Hollywood, not only did DiCaprio pay tribute to Schwartz's expertise and contribution but also went as far as to say that in working with Schwartz he had retrained his brain to revisit and recenter neurological compulsions that he himself experienced as a child. In doing so, DiCaprio discursively aligned himself to Hughes and his condition, emphasizing a sense of shared experience between himself and his character in a manner similar to that which Bingham recognizes in film criticism and reception as descriptions of actors "channelling" specific real-life characters that they portray, evocating a sense of spiritual connection within the portrayal as opposed to a sense of sheer mimicry or impersonation (93).

There is also a sense of mutual benefit in the participation in psychiatric consultancy. Though both consultants had to make do with information about OCD being included in the DVD extras – which themselves perhaps only really came into being because of their value to the film's promotion and Miramax's aspirations for awards recognition – no doubt both consultants reaped benefits from this experience, a factor rarely acknowledged within psychiatric scholarship considering mental health expertise and media representation. On a professional level, Dr. Schwartz benefitted from DiCaprio's mentions in interviews that he had read Schwartz's book, *Brain Lock* (1997), before meeting Schwartz and was then able to include a testimonial from DiCaprio on the cover of his next book, *You Are Not Your Brain* (2011). Indeed, a later edition of *Brain Lock* released in 2017 began with a foreword based on an anecdote of one of Howard Hughes's compulsions. Schwartz includes publicity stills from the film premiere on his personal website and embedded a YouTube video of one of the DVD extras info-films on the site also, representing a reciprocal benefit whereby the film benefits from his clinical expertise whilst the film's status, publicity, and visibility enhances his professional endeavors. This culminated in Schwartz being invited to address the United Nations (UN) in 2008 to discuss advances in the use of mindful awareness as a means to treat OCD and other mental health issues. In doing so, Schwartz recounted a similar anecdote to that of DiCaprio in the info-film, in which he claimed to experience compulsive behaviors as a result of the work he had done with Schwartz in preparing to play Hughes.

For Edward, who had no professional stake in this process but instead one directly based on lived experience, the primary benefit was perhaps an unexpected one. In his own words:

> After I got back from Montreal, going through the script, discussing all the scenes, I became a lot better with my OCD. My OCD was really in check...Since Montreal I've been pretty damn good. What I got out of it was that I felt a lot better and I think I made a big improvement [with OCD].

In participating in consultation on the film, Edward felt an improvement in his wellbeing and a decrease in the severity of his obsessions and compulsions. I am in no way suggesting here that Edward's improved sense of wellbeing was not due to proper medical and psychiatric treatment but instead highlighting that undeniably both Schwartz and Edward were able to reap benefits from the process of consulting on film production beyond monetary compensation. This adds extra dimension and complexity to evaluating the role and input of psychiatric expertise and opens up additional avenues for critical exploration. As Stephen Crawford and Henri Colt state, "Through fiction and true-life stories, medical movies depict larger-than-life characters and situations that entertain, educate, infuriate, and illuminate us about the human condition" (30). This is certainly true with Howard Hughes and DiCaprio's performance of the eccentric billionaire. By employing varied psychiatric expertise, the characterization and representation of Hughes had greater dimension and attention to detail than it might have otherwise. However, in ways that would be hard to fathom without further qualitative exploration of the role of psychiatric consultant, the benefits of such expert contributions that extend outside the frame – such as Dr. Schwartz benefitting from the increased public attention in his work to advocate for meaningful changes in treatment to a broader audience and for Edward experiencing improvement in his personal wellbeing as a result of using his difficult challenges to benefit the film's portrayal of OCD – might go unrecognized as a form of social good that emerges from the process of psychiatric film consultancy.

Note

1 This interview research was carried out in 2014 with the ethical approval of the University of East Anglia's Research Office.

Works cited

A Beautiful Mind. Directed by Ron Howard, 2001.
Aviator, The. Directed by Martin Scorsese, 2004.
Beautiful Boy. Directed by Felixvan Groeningen, 2018.
Belle De Jour. Directed by Luis Buñuel, 1967.
Bingham, D. "Living Stories: Performance in the Contemporary Biopic." *Genre and Performance: Film and Television*, edited by C. Cornea, Manchester: Manchester University Press, 2010, pp. 76–95.
Blackman, L., and V. Walkerdine. *Mass Hysteria: Critical Psychology and Media Studies*. Hampshire: Palgrave, 2001.
Byrne, P. "Stigma of Mental Illness and Ways of Diminishing It." *Advances in Psychiatric Treatment*. Vol. 6, 2000, pp. 65–72.
Crawford, S., and H. Colt. "Visions of Reality, Sometimes Larger than Life." *The Picture of Health: Medical Ethics and the Movies*, edited by H. Colt, S. Quadrelli, and L. D. Friedman, Oxford: Oxford University Press, 2011, pp. 29–38.
Cross, S. "Visualising Madness: Mental Illness and Public Representation." *Television and New Media*, vol. 5, no. 3, 2004, pp. 197–216.
Cross, S. *Mediating Madness: Mental Distress and Cultural Representation*. London: Palgrave, 2010.
Girl, Interrupted. Directed by James Mangold, 1999.
Green, B. "Psychiatry in the Cinema." 2007, www.priory.com/psych/psycinema.htm. Accessed August 13, 2020.
Harper, S. "Media, Madness & Misrepresentation: Critical Reflections on Anti-Stigma Discourse." *European Journal of Communication*, vol. 20, no. 4, 2005, pp. 460–83.
Harper, S. *Madness, Power and the Media*. London: Palgrave Macmillan, 2009.
Hyler, S. "DSM-III at the Cinema: Madness in the Movies." *Comprehensive Psychiatry*, vol. 29, no. 2, 1988, pp. 195–206.
Kirby, D. *Lab Coats in Hollywood: Science, Scientists, and Hollywood*. Massachusetts: MIT Press, 2010.
Nairn, R., S. Coverdale, and J. Coverdale. (2011) "A Framework for Understanding Media Depictions of Mental Illness." *Academic Psychiatry*, vol. 35, no. 3, 2011, pp. 202–6.
Philo, G. *Media and Mental Distress*. London: Longman, 1996.
Prozac Nation. Directed by Eric Skjoldbjærg, 2001.
Raging Bull. Directed by Martin Scorsese, 1980.
Ray. Directed by Taylor Hackford, 2004.
Remington, P. "Twelve Pages of Madness: Development of Cinema's Narration of Insanity." *Promoting and Producing Evil*, edited by N.Billias, Amsterdam: Rodopi, 2010, pp. 143–60.
Roberts, R. *Real to Reel: Psychiatry at the Cinema*. Herefordshire: PCCS Books, 2011.
Rosenstone, R. *History on Film, Film on History*. 2nd Edition. New York and Abingdon: Routledge, 2012.
Schwartz, J. M. *You Are Not Your Brain: The 4-Step Solution for Changing Bad Habits, Ending Unhealthy Thinking, and Taking Control of Your Life*. New York: Avery, 2011.
Schwartz, J. M., and B. Beyette. *Brain Lock: Free Yourselffrom Obsessive-Compulsive Behavior*. New York: Regan Books, 1997.
Stuart, H. "Media Portrayals of Mental Illness and its Treatments: What Effect does it have on People with Mental Illness?" *CNS Drugs*, vol. 20, no. 2, 2006, pp. 99–106.
Taxi Driver. Directed by Martin Scorsese, 1976.
Theory of Everything, The. Directed by James Marsh, 2014.
Three Faces of Eve, The. Directed by Nunally Johnson, 1957.

Wahl, O. *Media Madness: Public Images of Mental Illness*. 3rd Edition, New Brunswick, NJ: Rutgers University Press, 2006.

Wedding, D., and M. Boyd. *Movies and Mental Illness: Using Films to Understand Psychopathology*. London: McGraw-Hill College, 1999.

Wedding, D., M. A. Boyd, and R. M. Niemiec. *Movies and Mental Illness: Using Films to Understand Psychopathology*. 3rd Edition. Gottingen: Hogrefe Publishing, 2006.

10

RECOVERING THE PATIENT'S VOICE

The diagnostic process from early modern history to Oliver Sacks

Allison Kavey

The process of diagnosis, like the practice of medicine, is undoubtedly the product of history, and the position of personal medical narratives in that process has shifted over time. In particular, many medical historians comfortably accept Foucault's argument: Patient voices have lost their place in medicine, replaced by rising medical authority and technology. Foucault's paraphrased thesis about the clinical gaze from his groundbreaking *Birth of the Clinic* (1963) remains one of the most compelling and universally accepted arguments in the history of medicine. Ironically, however, even those historians most committed to his argument have written corrections to it, offering useful evidence that socioeconomic status, time, and location play critical roles in determining the relative importance of patient voice in medical encounters.

This chapter contends that the patient's voice has not been steadily and universally displaced by medical authority, the physician's "gaze," and technology. A more nuanced reading of the classic Foucauldian argument, incorporating the role of socioeconomic status in maintaining patient narrative as part of diagnosis, provides a stronger sense of the patient's voice in the early modern medical marketplace, including the 18th century in which Foucault grounds his thesis. A review of existing scholarship demonstrates that those able to access private physicians and those who relied on informal or non-professional heath care kept their voices in medical exchanges. That scholarship also challenges the paradigm shift that was supposed to occur between in the clinic in the late 18th century, when patient voices – which had previously dominated medical exchanges – were silenced. In fact, different kinds of medical encounters from the 16th century forward possessed differing levels of patient engagement and medical authority. The idea that patients always controlled their medical care before the "birth of the clinic" and the rise of medical technology is as inaccurate as the argument that they lost all control after the rise of institutional medicine. This chapter also makes an effort to spell out the ways in which various factors determined the ratio of patient to practitioner voice at different historical moments preceding and after the rise of institutionalized medicine. It then takes a giant historical leap forward to consider these issues in a modern outlet that is more complicated than what we are usually able to resurrect from writing by early modern patients and doctors. I analyze *Awakenings* (Penny Marshall, 1990) derived from Oliver Sacks' book of the same title and based on his case notes as well as his memories of treating patients who

 DOI: 10.4324/9781003007661-14

survived encephalitis lethargica. This source is not an identical match, of course, as it is not Oliver Sacks' memoir. It is a popular culture interpretation of a physician's published professional memoirs, which were themselves produced for popular consumption. The argument for making this comparison comes from the fact that the early modern section of this paper includes Simon Napier, a 17th- century medical practitioner, whose casebooks were produced so that they could be published later. Moreover, patient voices in sources from earlier historical periods were often interpreted by medical professionals.

This analysis offers two small correctives to the Foucauldian argument. First, case notes are not the opaque tools of a profession removed from "normal" human speech by vocabulary and training but instead the narrative that physicians write based on their interactions with patients. They reflect medical practitioners' attempts to integrate patient voices, clinical observation, and technologically obtained data into a single narrative of health and disease. These comments are necessarily communicated in the words of physicians/practitioners, and this has been true for centuries. But they reflect an incorporation of the patient into the medical narrative, not patient deletion. As Kathryn Montgomery notes, physicians begin and end their presentations – at conferences and at ground rounds, on daily ward rounds and in MMRs – with a case narrative. "They were stories, narrative accounts of the action and motives of individual human beings, physicians and patients, who, variously, were frustrated by circumstance, rewarded for effort, and plagued by fate" (Montgomery, xiii). The second correction is perhaps even smaller: that medical practitioners in the early modern period were no less constrained by their professional and personal assumptions than modern physicians. Their ideas about the causes of health and disease, whether humoral, astrological, or sympathetic, shaped their reactions to patients' presentations and undoubtedly shaped how they heard patient narratives. Many early modern historians of medicine point to the "medical marketplace" of the 16th and 17th centuries as a place where patients' voices had more power. This might have been true for wealthier patients who, then as now, had a stronger role in determining their care, but for the majority of people hiring medical advice, their treatment was as determined by their practitioners' social and intellectual frameworks as it is now. Separating institutional history from medical history might provide a means of assessing the relative power dynamics experienced by hospital and private patients, but it seems critically important not to repeat the Foucauldian experiment: late-18th-century medicine at the largest poor hospital in Paris should not be thoughtlessly generalized.

The early modern historiographic corrections to Foucault's theses come from a variety of sources, including letters to physicians from patients and physicians' case notes. Sources shift toward the patient and physician duet in hospitals' clinical notes from the late 18th century onward. These sources offer a tiny correction that many physicians who worked in hospitals in the 19th and early 20th century also saw private patients and that their interactions with private patients were likely different – and included more patient accommodation – than their hospital interactions. A close reading of a modern medical film dramatizes the puzzle solving and humanizing aspects of diagnosis-driven patient interaction. While it might seem ahistorical to include film in this analysis, I contend that it is a legitimate source of evidence. Early modern medical practitioners frequently used patient narratives to advertise their services, indicating that these stories were intended for popular consumption. Physicians continue to present their case notes as evidence in articles and in grand rounds, demonstrating that they too were written for audiences other than the author. The stretch to a film built on a physician's case notes and recollections is not an epic leap, or even a dramatic extension of the word "audience" as it might have been imagined by early modern medical practitioners. *Awakenings* is an autobiographical account of Sacks' work with encephalitis lethargica patients in a Bronx hospital in the late 1960s and 1970s. This makes it similar, if not identical, in imagined audience to the case narratives used by early modern practitioners to demonstrate their competency and the intrinsic value of their approach. Dr. Sacks, and by extension the fictionalized Dr. Malcolm Sayer, saw his approach to psychiatric diagnosis as an important corrective to the broadly accepted one of institutionalization, insisting that his patients' voices form a critical role in their diagnosis and treatment.

Modern media, particularly television and film, has turned the hunt for a diagnosis into a Sherlockian drama complete with human heroes defined by their talent for deductive reasoning. Although much of the recent attention on diagnosis as a deductive process in modern media has been on the television show, *House*, this chapter focuses on *Awakenings*. It, like some of the powerful memoirs and novels to have been penned by modern physicians, provides a strong counter-argument to Foucault. Ironically, Foucault and those who followed his lead to use case histories as their sole insight into patient experiences in late 18th and 19th century hospitals made a crucial mistake; they did not talk to the physicians themselves. I understand that case notes can be read as a direct echo of physicians' voices, but, a more nuanced argument respects existing scholarship and recognizes that the same format said to have eliminated patients' from the narrative also erased physicians. With the clear understanding that we cannot consult early modern physicians and that it is always an error to read modern subjectivity back several centuries, I offer a limited argument that the evidence does seem to support. Practitioners' motivations and voices are important in understanding patient histories and experiences, and it is an error to assume that case notes obscure the humanity of only one side of the medical interaction.

Professionalization has many advantages for the professionals it benefits, but it also has costs: the hands that held stethoscopes to chests and wrote the case notes we now read were human hands. Recovering their interest in medical practice and their relationship with their patients deserves the same attention as patients' histories because it provides us with critical insight into the humanity behind medical practice. These are not the connections of equals – anyone can see that Sayer gets to leave the hospital at night, while the patients are left behind locked doors, and that Sayer can pursue his life as he wishes while the patients cannot. But equal status should not be required to justify an analysis of physicians' engagement with their patients. The film, clearly designed to demonstrate the idea of a medical duet rather than a physician directed narrative gives Leonard Lowe (Robert De Niro) – who begins and ends the film without a voice – the last word. He appears through the lens of the physician's camera and his introduction demonstrates that he owes his consciousness to his physician – his voice has newly emerged from the body Dr. Sayers helped him to escape. "My name is Leonard Lowe, and it has come to my attention that I have been away for some time. I'm back." His image is much larger than Sayer's, as it is broadcast behind the physician while he speaks to a gathering of hospital supporters. In this case, the patient's presence clearly outshines his physician, who is left behind to remind his audience of the importance of human connection – a skill he learned from his patients.

Diagnosis in early modern medicine

Foucault's thesis is based on the treatment of poor people admitted to Paris's giant charity hospital, l'Hotel Dieu, in the late 18th century during the tuberculosis epidemic, when diagnostic instruments such as the stethoscope and the ability to autopsy many patients presenting with similar clinical symptoms first permitted the formalization of disease categories and the emergence of the links between physical signs of disease (symptoms) and lesions within the body. This formal alliance of symptoms and lesions, strengthened by understandings of which microbes caused which symptoms and then diagnostic tests that permitted the diagnosis of some common diseases before death rather than only at autopsy, allowed patients' bodies to speak directly to physicians. The desire to construct a historical narrative of disease based entirely on symptoms and matched to lesions within the body discovered post-mortem drove this effort, which increasingly permitted the formalization of disease categories, a stronger connection between specific symptoms and the position the patient occupied within her disease's progression, and the slow erasure of the patient's voice from medical encounters. For Foucault, the construction of a clear disease progression was perhaps the dominant motivation behind the obsession with symptom-lesion based medical thought. "It is no longer a question of giving that *by which* the disease can be recognized, but of restoring, at the level of words, a history that covers its total being" (Foucault 95). Ironically this emphasis on learning the signs of disease progression as reconstructed through symptoms and lesions resulted in the displacement of patients' individual accounts of their disease progression. Partially, this results from an early modern understanding of disease that was not progressive but instead determined by individual constitution and a reiteration of congenital imbalance. We frequently locate that understanding in humoral medicine and often discard it as equally impractical, but it instead reflects a different understanding of health and disease, the body, and its progression through time that is more early modern than specifically humoral. Sympathetic systems of medicine shared this with antipathetic systems, so Paracelsian medicine, in which the body matches the outer world through shared elements and disease is treated through sympathetic application of those elements, sympathetic magic, and humoralism all consistently reflect this early modern understanding of health and disease.

Early modern medicine must be understood within the context of the medical marketplace, not just imagined encounters between university trained humoral physicians and their wealthy patients. In the hurly burly of the early modern medical landscape, university trained physicians competed with surgeons, barber surgeons, apothecaries, midwives, local women, and traveling remedy salesmen. The variety of medical practitioners allowed patients to dictate the kind of medical interaction they desired, as well as limiting them to what they could afford. This meant that the majority of early modern people never saw a university- trained physician and instead had their health managed by those who lacked formal training and came from a variety of theoretical approaches to disease, not solely the humoral (and later chemical) models favored by the universities. This suggests that there were many more available approaches to disease than those offered by the universities, as is demonstrated by a perusal of personal remedy collections or the recipes in books of secrets. That does not mean, however, that medical practitioners always saw their patients as equals or that they valued patient narratives above their own observations and ideas about disease causation and progression. Patient narratives from this period exist because they were either part of a letter intended to obtaining an appointment with a practitioner or because of clinical notes.

Two astrologers who practiced medicine in London, Simon Forman (casebooks available from 1596 to 1603) and Richard Napier (casebooks available from 1597 to 1634), have attracted Lauren Kassell's scholarly attention, particularly for their use of casebooks. She reminds us that astrologers – like every medical practitioner at the time – needed to demonstrate the value of their knowledge and establish their authority to patients. Casebooks were an integral part of that effort, establishing their literacy and numerancy and demonstrating their fluency in astrological symbols and chart casting. Patients initiated their medical interactions with both practitioners in two ways: either by writing a letter describing their problem or by coming in to their office hours and offering a verbal description. The casebooks consistently record the moment the message arrived or consultation started; the client's name, age, and gender; whether the encounter was in person or by message; and the question posed. They then drew an astrological chart providing the precise location of the stars at the moment the question was asked and used it to draw their conclusions, determine a remedy, and provide advice. Note that as both Forman and Napier were astrologers, not solely astrological physicians, not all of their consultations were medical. But their casebooks indicate a systematization that establishes their authority and provides a certain level of uniformity across cases that is not usually considered part of high end early modern medicine. Kassell's analysis of the professionalizing purpose of casebooks suggests that patient narratives and expectations actually motivated the keeping of records and the concomitant demonstration of the medical authority that they provided. She reminds us: "The patient did not necessarily believe in astrology; rather, the astrologer had to establish his authority and to negotiate a judgment about the nature of the disease and the possible therapies for it" (598). She also addresses the role of the astrologer in negotiating women's health care, a critical part of her analysis since women were a majority of these two male practitioners' cases. "The astrologer and his patient negotiated an exchange of trust for true judgments." (599). While she is addressing the trust women placed in astrologers, who were believed to be capable of divining not only their sexual secrets but their emotional ones, I want to extend her beautiful phrase to encompass early modern medical encounters that included an exchange of information: from the market stall where a patient might be given a patent remedy to cure a described ailment to the physicians' consulting rooms or the patients' sick room, the exchange of health or disease narrative for medical advice always constituted an arrangement of trust. It also reflected two individuals meeting with their own agendas, and while Kassell imagines perfect honesty in these exchanges, I would imagine that assumptions based on class, education, and gender informed both sides of these interactions.

The level of honesty achieved on both sides might depend on the nature of the medical relationship. It could be short-term, defined only by the efficacy of the treatment for the named complaint, or extended over the course of multiple medical interactions – or even the term of the patient's life. Gianna Pomata has written about the importance of contracts in further defining patient–practitioner relationships in early modern Italy, and like the casebooks, these contracts defined and professionalized the encounter while also enshrining the centrality of the patient's voice in medical encounters. She contends that these contracts, which guaranteed payment only if the physician actually cured the patient, provided a substantial amount of power to the patient in medical transactions. This is obvious, but what it can obscure is the fact that patients and physicians maintained their own perspectives on what constituted health, disease, and cure. These contracts were a means of defining such terms to both parties' satisfaction, and disagreements arose when their definitions did not match. While I obviously disagree here with her conclusion that "horizontal" relationships, in which patient and practitioner had equal power, were replaced by "vertical" ones empowering the physician as the early modern period and contracts for cures were supplanted by fees for service, these encounters certainly demonstrate the contractual and thereby temporally defined nature of these early modern medical encounters.

Late-18th-century hospital medicine, the foundation for Foucault's observations, did not occur in such a free market. Patients who came to Paris' hospital for the poor frequently lacked access to all resources, including family, that would have helped them secure care at home. The majority of patients were extremely poor, frequently migrants who came to the city for employment, and very sick. Prospective patients knew that, should they die there, their bodies would be autopsied, and many feared that fate and resisted it until there were no other options. The extremely high mortality rate at Paris's l'Hotel Dieu – 25 percent of those who entered there died – was certainly not a secret, so anyone who could evade its doors did so. There were two types of hospitals in 18th century France: general hospitals, or *hopitaux generaux*, which attempted to serve the dual purpose of acting as workhouses to discipline the able-bodied poor and return them to the economy while also caring for the "deserving poor": orphans and the elderly. Poor hospitals, or *Les Hotels Dieu,* solely catered to the sick, serving both the poor and, as finances dipped and the teaching function of hospitals increased, soldiers funded by the central government. These institutions were chartered by the government, headed by a local bishop, and supported by a board of important lay officials who contributed time and funds. They were also in charge of investing the bequests that formed the biggest source of funding for the hospital. Nursing sisters provided the majority of the labor, and over time, medical students joined them in providing some care for patients. While Paris' l'Hotel Dieu was notable for its vile conditions and the poverty and misery of its patients, other provincial hospitals in France provided better conditions and medical care with only about a 10 percent mortality rate for civilians and a markedly lower one for soldiers. Case records for these hospitals are not the opaque, limited notes described by Foucault that reduce the patient to a collection of clinical signs and symptoms. The case records from l'Hotel Dieu at Nimes, for example, included name, sex, age, marital status for women, occupation or husband's/father's occupation (for women), date of entry, date of exit or death, and a full complement of clinical notes. From these, narratives of the long-dead poor can be resurrected, and it is possible to locate a second voice contributing to the physicians' medical narrative. There is also no coherent medical voice but instead a clear sense of competing priorities and interests that makes these hospitals seem more dysfunctional institutions governed by competing priorities and personalities than single-minded clinical machines occupied by a clearly defined group of single-minded professionals.

Clearly 18th-century French hospitals were not all like the Parisian l'Hotel Dieu, and it is important to extend that analysis to conclude that not all 18th-century hospitals were like those in France. Mary Fissell's analysis of case records from the Bristol infirmary (founded 1737) provides some important reminders about 18th-century hospitals that are critical to properly contextualizing and understanding them. Hospitals began as charitable institutions where the poor or travelers who lacked family and support could go for spiritual and medical care. Hospitals also raised orphans, sheltered the homeless, and provided hospitality for those passing through a region in which they lacked connections or the funds to care for themselves. Secularization and medicalization occurred simultaneously, as did the increasingly class-defined nature of hospital care in the 18th century. Patrons, whose subscriptions earned them the right to name patients to be cared for by the hospital, replaced religious orders as hospitals' governing bodies, and Fissell contends that the formalization of hospital medical practice must be read parallel to a trend among the wealthy to reject and isolate popular medicine (2). She also sees the infirmary as a site where the elite used medical knowledge and institutionalization to gain control over the bodies of the working poor, arguing that physical control was more important than medicalization in determining patients' subject status (12). She goes on to assert, however, that "Infirmary surgeons granted the inmates of hospitals peculiarly opaque bodies that only the powerful could read, and robbed the patient of his or her understanding of illness" (15).

The direct patronage required to enter the Bristol Infirmary certainly differentiates it from Paris's Hotel Dieu. It also demonstrates a closer and more powerful connection between patrons and patients than was possible in larger urban hospitals and reiterates the notion of the "deserving poor," defined by those willing to cooperate with the hospitals' moral and behavioral regulations. Finally, it adds to the category of "deserving poor" not those too young, elderly, frail, or injured to care for themselves but instead those whose laboring bodies were required to keep the city functioning (Fissell 77). Hospitals paralleled workhouses in their emphasis on providing work or the means to return to it for family heads, while other institutions were left to care for the rest of the poor population. The trajectory of the Bristol Infirmary would have remained much like the history of the Bristol workhouse, Fissell argues, but the governors slowly abdicated control, and the surgeons took over, locating both a position of power and a source of income through the admission of paying students. By the final decade of the 18th century, surgical students comprised a significant part of the medical population, case notes were increasingly regularized and reflected a great deal of focus on the signs and symptoms of disease and very little room for patient voices, and surgical cases outnumbered medical cases because of their potential to bring in more income. But the case notes of physicians reflect that even under these increasingly formal and medicalized conditions, patients' voices did not disappear from all medical exchanges; they remained more powerfully present in private cases.

Two examples from 19th-century American medicine will provide the last pieces of evidence required to understand the limits of Foucault's thesis. Perhaps one of the most painful and egregious examples of this comes from the mid-19th century gynecological surgical experiments J. Marion Sims performed on slaves whose masters donated the women to his experiments because they were too affected by vesico-vaginal fistulae to work and had no value as "breeders." Three significant arguments define Sims' surgical experimentation on humans who had no legal control over their own bodies – doubly so, as they were slaves and female – as ethically bankrupt. The first is that he chose not to use anesthesia when it was available. His apologists, like L. L. Wall, contend that he joined other physicians of his time, such as Sir James Young Simpson who discovered chloroform and apparently was not popular with women, in denying anesthesia to women undergoing fistula repair because "the walls of the vesicovaginal septum are far less sensitive than you might a priori imagine" (Wall 348). This reinforces the idea that women, especially black women and even more especially enslaved women, lacked the voices to bring their embodied experiences to the attention of male medical authority.

The second argument L. L. Wall makes in support of Sims also highlights the lack of the patients' voices in these experiments. He contends that Sims did not operate on the enslaved women without consent because he obtained their owners' consent and legally that was all that was required. No statement better illustrates the complete absence of these women's voices from their own medical treatment. The third argument Wall proposes is the most pertinent to the question of whether women's voices – especially slave women's voices – ever entered male physicians' consciousness. He contends, in opposition to Ojanuga, that these women would certainly have consented to any operation to fix their vesico-vaginal fistula. He bases his determination on the words of a white male physician presenting about this condition at the April 1857 meeting of the Georgia State Medical Society: "The poor woman [with a vesicovaginal fistula] is now reduced to a condition of the most piteous description, compared with which, most of the other physical evils of life sink into utter significance." He goes on to describe the smell which drives others away, the pain from destroyed tissue, and the constant stream of urine that plagues the patient's existence (Ojanuga 19). This physician, who would never experience a vesicovaginal fistula himself, deems these women pitiful and disgusting and determines, on their behalf, that they must wish to undergo painful, humiliating, and repetitive experimental procedures in hopes of being returned to polite society and reproductive capability. He denies that their voices matter enough to enter the conversation, privileging his own judgment far above theirs. From his lofty perspective, the male guess at female embodied experience suffices to ensure their cooperation as experimental subjects. He fails to recognize, of course, that this is the same argument white slaveowners used to defend the institution of slavery itself. Given the terrible conditions in which Africans found themselves under their own oversight, they argued, slavery provided better conditions for which they should be grateful. Apparently Anarcha, Lucy, and Betsy were also supposed to be grateful for the opportunity to be experimental subjects. We do not know what Anarcha and Lucy and their co-sufferers said to Sims about their humiliating personal conditions, or if they spoke to him at all. We do know they suffered his invasive examinations and, after being diagnosed, his repeated attempts to correct their problems without anesthesia. But their voices – their understandings of their bodies and what happened to bring them to his backyard surgical "laboratory" – are lost.

Just as largely missing from the record are the voices of the white immigrant women Sims treated in his charity hospital in New York City. We know he found them to have lower pain tolerance than the slave women on whom he experimented, but their voiced experiences of their bodies and their pathologies do not seem to have entered the historical record. But does the lack of a record reflect a lack of interest? Because in the early 20th century, patient records of children taken from Tangier Island to be treated for tuberculosis and other ailments at Johns Hopkins reflect extensive case histories along with a great deal of laboratory work. Their voices are missing from these records, but their stories are not. These highly professionalized records, full of medical terminology and the assumptions that plagued physicians of the period, cannot hide the stories that these children brought across the Chesapeake Bay to Baltimore. And while they make fascinating reading, they are a double-edged sword. Those histories could as easily be used to empower patients as employed against them, used to support eugenics theories that justified keeping them away from their families in an effort to determine the effects of nature versus nurture. From 2021, it seems like this medical history narrative needs some clarifying. We perhaps mean that poor, Catholic, immigrant, black or brown, female patients were often used as medical subjects and their bodies employed, often without their knowledge, to support medical research, and their narratives were joined with technological and scientific ones to produce case histories that captured their subject status. Their voices joined a chorus of information provided by their bodies and interpreted by white men and machines, but they were certainly not a privileged part of the chorus. Race and social class always determine the kinds of treatment individuals receive and the level of respect they are accorded by their physicians. These categories also frequently determine how likely an individual is to become an experimental or teaching subject, as has been amply demonstrated by the story of Henrietta Lacks. But these generalizations, while true, are not the sole means by which we can assess the level of patients' voices in individual medical interactions.

Of course, the transition from medical marketplace to professionalized medical care coincided with the rise of science and technology in medicine. Historians of medicine contend that the slow erasure of the patient to be eclipsed first by his disease, then by the marks left in the body by it, and finally by the pathogen that caused it, can be traced to the late 8th century. The history of diseases penned by English physician Thomas Sydenham reveals a practitioners' shift in interest from patients and their individual narratives about their disease to an interest in the disease itself (or from groups of symptoms believed to be specific to each individual to constellations of symptoms experienced across individuals that could be collected into the definition of a specific disease) (Akernecht 122). Perhaps the loci of that transition, poor urban hospitals, which are the focus of Foucault's *Birth of the Clinic* and the site in which most medical research occurred beginning in the late 18th century, saw more focus on using autopsy to connect symptoms to lesions and then increasing interest in identifying lesions while patients were still alive. It certainly seems likely that physicians in those teaching and charity hospitals tended not to privilege the voices of their patients, whose socioeconomic status, especially their lack of education, would have made them "unreliable narrators." Nicholas Jewson argues that the shift in medical practice from the home to the hospital accompanied a shift in medical focus from the patient to the constellation of patients experiencing a disease or "cases." He takes his argument further, contending that the humans who became cases in hospital medicine lost their humanity as well as their individuality in laboratory medicine, becoming only constellations of cells. As Kassell so cleverly reprises Jewson, "the place of the patient shifts as the medical cosmology changes. Bedside medicine produces narratives about individuals; hospital medicine produces cases, which constitute collections of observable data" (Kassell 604).

For the tuberculosis patients who crowded urban European hospitals and provided the post-mortem proof of symptom-lesion correlation that comprise our first "modern" understanding of disease progression from cough, weakness, and shortness of breath to cyanosis and death, their stories of being embodied and growing sick – beyond perhaps their first symptom presentation – were eclipsed by the sounds physicians heard through stethoscopes pressed to their chests and the lesions marring their lung tissue. Some of their stories might still be recoverable through the kind of research Kassell has done on medical casebooks, but as Jewson and Fissell contend, the rise of hospital medicine brought with it a rise in professionalized record keeping that tended to obscure patient individuality through consistency in structure and content. For Foucault, that consistency was critical to creating disease categories out of individual cases and taking medicine from an individualized art to a categorizable epistemology of health and disease: "This conceptual transformation was decisive: it opened up to investigation a domain in which each fact, observed, isolated, then compared with a set of facts, could take its place in a whole series of events whose convergence or divergence were in principle measurable." He goes on to assert: "It gave to the clinical field a new structure in which the individual in question was not so much a sick person as the endlessly reproducible pathological fact to be found in all patients suffering in a similar way; in which the plurality of observations was no longer simply a contradiction orconfirmation, but a progressive, theoretically endless convergence… ." (Foucault 970). This convergence into a set of disease categories that exist beyond individual bodies produced modern medicine, which depends upon symptoms matching to diseases that are caused by known pathogens (viruses, bacteria, fungi) and can thus be treated pharmaceutically.

Foucault, Fissell, Jewson, and Kassell saw the rise of the clinic as a fundamentally paradigm altering occurrence, but they are wrong to assume that this paradigm shift was any more complete than any of the others historians have identified. The 16th- and 17th-century medical marketplaces, as Katherine Park, William Eamon, and Gianna Pomata so ably demonstrate, were complex, messy, and allowed patients to navigate among different kinds of practitioners to determine the kind of medical interaction they preferred. Of course, race, gender, and financial status also played a role in determining patient-practitioner exchanges, but it is impossible to deny that patient choice of practitioners ran the show, and thus patients frequently were able to dictate the narratives of their encounters. As hospitals shifted from sites of palliative and spiritual care to increasingly medicalized and experimental ones, the narrative space allotted to patients necessarily grew smaller and less individual. The voices of patients were condensed into shorter spaces and placed alongside anatomical and laboratory data, making a different kind of narrative authored by multiple individuals and written in the language of professional physicians. Foucault would contend that upon entering the medical space and time of the clinic and becoming the subject of the clinical gaze, patients became unmoored from their biographies and their own understandings of their bodies, their health, and their disease. But many patients never entered a clinic. Wealthier patients controlled their medical interactions by employing private physicians who met them at home, accepted their narratives, and kept their secrets. This did not end in the 19th century, or even the early 20th. Paul Monette reminds us, in *Borrowed Time: An AIDS Memoir*, that wealthier gay men controlled their medical interactions by visiting physicians they knew to be comfortable with homosexuality and the risks that came with it. And while it would be both historically ignorant and willfully ridiculous to contend that people who lacked wealth, y chromosomes, and white skin were equally powerful in keeping their voices at the center of medical interactions, it would be just as ludicrous to contend that no patient voices survived the rise of the clinic. The rest of this chapter uses modern media depictions of patient-physician interactions to suggest that the act of diagnosis and the place of patient narratives in it remains an integral and humanizing force in medicine. Romanticized and manipulated those modern media may be, the moments in which patients voices combines with physicians' voices to produce an accurate diagnosis and an effective course of treatment is the scientific equivalent of an operatic chorus.

Awakenings

No film better illustrates the importance of multiple voices in a diagnosis encounter than *Awakenings*. (Marshall 1990) Malcolm Sayer (Robin Williams) begins a new job in a long-term psychiatric institution, Bainbridge, located in the Bronx in 1969. He has previously only done research neurology, has neither interest nor experience with patients, and is clearly desperate for a job. The institution is characterized by locked doors and barred windows, patients doomed to live out the most practical definition of their name by waiting for nothing, loud intermittent noises made by patients, harsh fluorescent lighting glaring off white floors, and ongoing interruptions of the loudspeaker paging physicians. It is perhaps the most institutional institution that film could create. Sayer is not, however, an institutional man. He has resorted to working at Bainbridge only after years of non-patient based neurological research, reduced to patient care by the lack of scientific funding and the overall weak economy. His outstanding credentials earn him the position, but even in a top down, traditional place like Bainbridge, his lack of patient experience after residency gives the hiring committee pause. His career is about to take a dramatic turn toward patient care, but his background in research shapes his patient interactions and provides a great deal of the motivation he brings to his early interactions. The scientific method provides the map he uses to navigate his strange new world.

The first patient to attract Sayer's interest, Lucy (Alice Drummond), appears in his office on the morning of his second day, wheelchair bound, head lolling, affectless, and characterized by a vacant stare that does not appear to follow speech or movement. Her appearance is heralded by the nurse announcing her recent arrival and presenting her chart. Sayer turns to Lucy, introduces himself and attempts to determine if she is deaf by clapping his hands. She does not respond. He notices that her glasses are dirty, removes them from her face, cleans them, and replaces them; she does not respond. He turns back to this typewriter to write her intake clinical evaluation notes, settling on a diagnosis of dementia of unknown origin, and is startled by a change in the presence behind him. Lucy is bent over at the waist in her wheelchair, frozen with her arm extended and her hand wrapped around her glasses. He clearly believes at first that she has collapsed, but upon noting the glasses in her hand, he is driven to experiment. Note here the critical importance of a scientific background in driving his patient interactions – he wants to know what happened, and he turns to the first pillar of scientific methodology, reproducibility, to see if he experienced a fluke or a valuable phenomenon. He carefully brings Alice's body back upright, then places the glasses on the floor in front of her and turns away, mimicking the conditions under which he imagines the first movement occurred. Nothing happens. Rather than giving up, and even while visually acknowledging with a slight smile and shake of his head that this could be madness, he adopts a second experimental approach: he drops the glasses. And Alice catches them. This movement, her first deliberate attempt to interact with the world, signals Sayer's first foray into institutional medical practice and research. He immediately presents her to his physician peers, perhaps just fascinated by her and perhaps to gain support for his new interest. Their reaction demonstrates the lack of respect for patients in this institution that defines those who spend years there as "chronic" inmates of a "garden" where they are to be "fed and watered."

Lucy, still in her wheelchair and evidently non-responsive, head lolling, with a fixed unfocused gaze, is brought to the center of a group of doctors. She and Dr. Sayer's nurse, Evelyn Costello, (Julie Kavner) are the only women, and in comparison to the medical caregivers' white starched uniforms, Lucy wears a faded and shapeless housedress. The medical staff stands while she sits in her wheelchair in front of them. Her case history has grown in the interlude since she first appeared in Sayer's office: she has gained a last name and a story. She was found in a house with her several-days dead sister, she has no living relatives, and her current non-responsive state is, according to the neighbors, how she has always been. Sayer demonstrates her ability to catch a moving object, despite her overall lack of responsiveness. His colleagues scoff, dismissing her reaction as a reflex. Reflexes are very quick nerve-driven reactions that occur solely along neural pathways and do not reach the brain. Thus, even brain dead individuals can have reflexes, and current neurological research indicates that they cannot be used as proof of brain activity. The other physicians' categorization of Lucy's movement as a reflex reflects their determination that she is beyond medical help. They file out, leaving the nurse to wheel Lucy away and Sayer with his chief of staff. The chief asserts that this is an attempt to gain professional status, urging him with a humorous line to "let us know if she catches anything else." Of course, he means something that actually warrants medical attention because it fits into a recognizable disease category and can be treated. The prospect of doing research to better understand this patient and perhaps help her and push forward the practice of neurology does not seem to appeal to him.

Sayer's experimental approach allows him to locate a group of patients who share important similarities: their ability to catch moving things or otherwise develop independent motion in reaction to an external form of movement, lack of affect, near immobility, and records defined by a dizzying array of "atypical" diagnoses with no recommendations for treatment. Sayer searches for voices to help him turn "all these atypical somethings into a typical something." The first voice he finds belongs to the mother (Ruth Nelson) of a patient, Leonard Lowe. He is by far the youngest patient in the ward, and she visits him every day, providing a quiet conversation about daily life that forms a clear counterpoint to the harsh institutional background noise. Asked if he ever speaks to her, she responds, "Not in words." Sayer asks. "He speaks to you in other ways?" She responds, "You don't have children. If you did, you would know." Leonard's mother points to the importance of close observation in good medical practice, reminding Sayer to closely examine the evidence he has and use what he knows to produce more evidence.

He turns to the evidence he has on hand: case files. And they reveal an important shared characteristic beyond the clinical observations he made; every single patient that fits his symptom profile also had survived encephalitis lethargica. Encephalitis lethargic reached pandemic status in 1917, crossing Europe and then entering North America along with troops traveling around the globe for the World War I. The first cases likely occurred in Romania in 1915, and it reached epidemic status in Vienna in 1917 when it was also formally recognized as its own disease. "By 1919, the epidemic had overrun most of Europe, the USA, Canada, and India" (Hoffmann and Vilensky 2247). 1921 and 1924 saw the highest numbers of cases, and the disease has not reached epidemic status again since the 1930s. Despite this, sporadic cases occasionally appear, and patients originally affected by the disease can experience neurological deficits long after the acute phase of the disease dissipates. Sayer learns about the epidemic in the glow of the microfiche machine, where he also discovers the identity of its foremost expert, Peter Ingham (Man von Sydow). He arranges to meet with the chain-smoking, intellectually vibrant but clearly elderly physician. A filmstrip of a younger Ingham plays behind them as they talk about "children who fell asleep," showing him manipulating the inert legs of a sheet draped body on a gurney on a lecture hall stage. He reports that most patients recovered perfectly, but within a decade, they returned to his attention, increasingly incapacitated. The flickering screen shows a horror film of damaged bodies displaying the end stages of a progressive neurological disease: a standing child is held by the arms, then released. She falls. An elderly woman stands perfectly still until she grasps a pencil, when she begins to shake. He smokes his cigarette and says, eyes glued to the screen where a man stands inert, mouth open in a silent scream, before another gathering of seated physicians: "Families went mad. People who were normal were now...elsewhere." For any medical historian, this parade of neurologically defective bodies on display unerringly raises the specter of Charcot and his performing hysterics, an episode of patient subjugation in the name of psychiatric research we might prefer to forget. But it does so to demonstrate the difference between Sayer and Ingham. Sayer asks rhetorically what it was like to be them, what they were thinking. Ingham responds "They're not. The virus did not spare their higher faculties." Sayer asks whether he knows that and is told, "Yes. The alternative is unthinkable." But for someone embedded in the scientific method, there cannot be an "unthinkable" alternative, and it is clear that Sayer does not believe that there is sufficient evidence to allow this answer to stand. He leaves Ingham and returns to the ward and the heart of clinical practice: patient observation.

Lucy again brings Sayer a crucial piece of evidence. He observes her shuffling across the ward and repeatedly stopping at the edge of the black and white linoleum pattern, her eyes fixed on the wall about ten feet away. That wall contains a water fountain and a barred window. Sayer believes Lucy wants to use the fountain and even offers her water from it, but she does not respond. He continues to observe her slow walk and its repeated end, where the black and white pattern stops at an ocean of white. He and Evelyn, the nurse most closely associated with his work, spend the night painting the rest of the floor with black and white squares, and they are rewarded with Lucy walking across the entire ward – not to the water fountain, as he thought, but to look wistfully out the window while the breeze stirs her hair. Had she only wanted to satisfy thirst, he still would have been demonstrating an active mind. But the will to feel the sun on her face and watch the world passing outside, to take part – even from a distance – in the swirl of human activity flourishing outside the ward's walls, demonstrates a very active mind limited by its ability to control a neurologically disordered body.

The need to better understand how encephalitis lethargica progressed and was experienced by the patients and their families drives Sayer back to Mrs. Lowe, Leonard's mother. She is the only family member who regularly visits, and her quiet conversations with her son are the only non-medical human interactions in the ward. Sayer arranges to meet her at her home. His words on her doorstep speak volumes about the information he seeks: a voice to tell him who these people were before they got sick and to narrate their disease to him. He says, "Tell me about your son." She does: an 11-year-old whose hands shook too much for him to write, and then too much for him to stay in school. A boy who spent nine years in his childhood bedroom looking at the walls covered in ribbons and photographs from "before," the life he had before his body was hijacked by encephalitis lethargica. Nine years in which he read, proving that his mind stayed engaged and active even while his body froze. Mrs. Lowe's plaintive assertion, "He loved to read. Of course, it was all he could do," reflects the world he lost first – of children, baseball, and school – and then his final freedom – books that allowed his mind to range even while his body's cage tightened. He spoke his last word, "Mom," in 1939 at the age of 20. His mother checked him into Bainbridge hospital shortly thereafter, as she was still working, and he could not care for himself while she was out.

An EEG becomes the next voice to attest to Leonard's mental acuity. Sayer uses a strobe light for the first section of the test, and it produces absolutely no results. The response comes at the end, when Sayer says, "Leonard." If you choose to read this, as I do, as Leonard's mind finally finding some release, some means of contact, this is his first word, the first direct sign of his agency, in the film. The second comes when Sayer, having collected all the Bainbridge patients who appear catatonic until thrown a ball, is sitting in a circle with them as they pass a ball around. All the other patients throw the ball to the person directly opposite them. Leonard throws it to Sayer. And Sayer seizes the opportunity. He enlists the ward's nurses and orderlies in a campaign to find what engages these people, and in so doing, he slowly brings their personalities out. One woman is moved by opera, others find their groove in swing and – memorably – Hendrix. Several engage with each other over a game of cards, as long as a nurse plays the first one to get them going. Bert makes it clear that human contact can also reach these people, allowing them to become mobile. All of these findings reflect the medical staff's genuine desire to know more about these patients and their disease; they experimented with different stimuli – all from the realm of normal living. Many of the patients engaged. Uplifting! Amazing! Until you remember that, in the decades those people had been sitting in wheelchairs, no one on the staff had bothered to try to treat them like interactive equals. They had been fed, cleaned, put to bed, and woken up. But they had not been treated like humans. For a ward of people with no voices, it took a good physician and several excellent nurses to treat them first as people with histories, preferences, and desires.

Leonard's first words come from this attention and diligence. Sayer brings a Ouija board to his bedside, hoping he will spell his name. Instead, he hijacks the pointer and spells "Rilke's panther." This poem, about a wild panther stuck in a cage, mirrors Leonard's experience with encephalitis lethargica. Sayer reads about Leonard's imprisonment at the zoo, watching a panther pace in an excruciatingly small, concrete-floored cage. "His powerful strides are like a ritual dance/around a center where a great will stands paralyzed." Sayer reads the words while the camera closes tightly on the panther, and both the doctor and the cat stand in for Leonard's still missing voice, bringing his narrative ever more clearly into definition. Then the camera turns to Leonard sitting frozen in his wheelchair, mouth open, eyes turned elsewhere. "At times the curtains of the eye lift without a sound and a shape enters/slips through the tightened silence of the shoulders/reaches the heart and dies." Time in Leonard's cage has passed in a different way than it has for people still capable of making their will known, but it can be measured in the failed attempts to communicate with medical staff who did not notice, and the slow acceptance – heart death – that comes with knowing you are truly alone. Sayer is the first person to aggressively invade that quiet space, to navigate around Leonard's prison, listen at the walls for any sound coming from within. Unlike Leonard's mother, who quietly accepts her son's limited interaction as all that is left of him, Sayer hopes to break through the walls and bring Leonard out. To do so, however, he needs to figure out a treatment that might work. He turns to neurological research on another disease that causes increasing aphasia and dyskinesia, Parkinson's, and the use of a synthetically derived dopamine to control its symptoms. That research is new at the time, has limited clinical application, and is a dramatic reach given that the subjects who experienced positive results had only been suffering from mild symptoms. But Sayer has few other options to try, and through a combination of research, perseverance, and his assertion that – while he might not know how he knows – the patients are alive inside, he convinces his department chief to permit him to treat one patient, pending family consent.

Leonard, the only one of the patients who seems to have any involved family, is the obvious choice. His mother asks the questions that I hope will come to join, "What do we think, what do we know, and what can we prove" in the pantheon of medical epistemology. "What will the medicine do for him? What do you think it will do for him? What do you hope it will do for him?" Sayer uses all his medical training to truthfully answer the first two. The third brings out his own humanity and the intelligence and will that have driven him to the forefront of a difficult profession. "I hope it will bring him back from wherever he is." Seated at her beautifully polished dining table, china cups of tea in hand, these two people discuss the possibility of bringing a third – always seated with them, though silent – into the conversation. Mrs. Lowe asks what there is left for Leonard after three decades at Bainbridge, and Sayer says, "you." That gets her permission, reminding her that the son she talks to and cares for every day might actually be able to talk back. But Sayer has a bigger goal in mind: he wants to bring Leonard back "for the world": a world that has moved farther and farther from Leonard's grasp, drowning out the memory of his voice, his passions, his character as he receded beneath the weight of his damaged neurons. Sayer's hope is that he can regain the place he lost, find his feet, and move back into the stream of life. And, for a brief time, he does. Leonard's first words, spoken in the darkened ward while he sits drawing in the middle of the night after his fourth (very high) dose of L-dopa, are spoken very quietly and accompanied by an impish grin that breaks through his Parkinsonian mask. "I'm not asleep," he says. Sayer responds with wonder, "No, you're awake." His awakening continues with a wonderful reprise of his final words to his mother, "Mom, Mom, Mom," this time spoken while tottering across the room with wide open arms to hug her. And with the wonderful exchange he has at the office door with nurse, Eleanor. She offers him her hand and says, "My name is Eleanor. It is a pleasure to meet you." She has seen this man every day during her employment at Bainbridge, cared for him, fed him, and been in his life, but she is only meeting him now. Leonard is, to use his own words, back. But the body to which he has returned has aged in his absence, and his first heartbreak is to learn that he has been missing for a very long time. He is also consumed by fear that should he sleep, he will not wake up. His mother sits beside his bed in the dark ward stroking his hair, singing a lullaby whose refrain is, "don't forget to sail back to me."

The awakenings of the rest of the encephalitis lethargica patients introduce many new voices to the medical chorus contained in this film. These people, roused from their neurological fugue states through Sayer's experimental protocol, gain opinions, memories, relationships, and lives. They contribute a great deal of personal as well as clinical information about the disease, narrating their experiences with it to Sayer, Eleanor, and the other medical practitioner. One patient narrates as a nurse takes notes: "I was aware of things, but none of it meant anything to me. It was no connection to me." None of them are aware, at first, of how much time passed while they were missing. Dr. Sayer asks Lucy what year it is, and she responds with a grin and the expression of one a bit worried about her doctor's mental state, "What year is it? It's '26 silly." Later, she admits to Eleanor, "I know what year it is. I know it's not 1926. I just need it to be." And while there are some lovely reunions between patients and their families, not everyone gets one. Asked how he feels Frank (George Martin) responds, "My parents are dead, my wife is in an institution, my son has disappeared out West somewhere. I feel old and I feel swindled." Mrs. Lowe does not fully recognize the person who her son has become. His interest in women is certainly a shock to her, as is his new desire for independence and rebellion against authority. She gestures to the change that the years – and, as it turns out, psychosis brought about by the dopamine – have wrought. "I don't know who that is up there; I don't think he knows." She turns to Sayer and accuses, "You've turned Leonard into something he's not."

Even as they return to consciousness, however, these patients' humanity is not fully recognized. Leonard petitions the hospital's physicians for permission to freely leave and return without a chaperon. Asked what he would do, he indicates his need for freedom: "I would go for a walk; I would talk to people. I would turn left or turn right. You woke a person, not a thing." Despite his impassioned and articulate plea, the physicians turn him down. In a heartbreaking scene, he attempts to leave anyway, and, warned by Dr. Sayer, the guards will not allow it. He resists, and they wrestle him to the ground while Sayer stands by, objecting to the physical assault on the basis that he is not violent but not intervening. Leonard slowly falls back into a compromised neurological state, characterized by increasingly violent tics and paranoia. Sayer comes to appreciate how infuriating it would have been to be chemically brought back to the world only to have limited freedom and experience a slow descent back into neurological disease. He attributes Leonard's reactions, like his physical symptoms, to the medication's failure. But Leonard sees it as a larger failure, that of the medical profession to acknowledge that there are some things it cannot cure. In a rousing speech to the psychotics on ward 5, he declares, "We remind them that there's a problem that they don't have an answer to." Leonard's voice, raised in rage and fear to an audience of rapt mental patients, coming from a body racked by paroxysms and spasms, becomes a devastating part of this disease narrative.

The final reminder that Leonard is a highly observant man comes from his personal attack on Sayer, once again delivered through a body shaking barrage of involuntary movement: "I had a sickness that took me out of the world, and I fought to come back. I fought for thirty years and I'm still fighting. But you, you have no excuse. You're just a scared and lonely man with no life, nothing, nothing, you're the one who's asleep." Sayer's threat reminds the viewer – and Leonard – who possesses the control in this relationship: while Leonard might see them as equals, Sayer can deny Leonard access to the medication that keeps him awake. He later promises not to do this, but only when Leonard has fallen to the floor and beseeches him, "Help me." These human exchanges between two men reaching across the divide of experience, personality, education, and diagnosis are paired with the shot of Dr. Sayer helping a stricken Leonard stand and move across the floor, their two pairs of polished shoes moving across the institutional linoleum – one walking, one staggering. As his body continues to betray him and the efforts to fix his medication levels fail, Leonard engages as a partner in the clinical process. He insists Sayer get the video camera when he is gripped by a seizure. He insists, against Sayer's objections, that he "Watch and learn, learn from me." He narrates his experiences of intermittently going blank and feeling "nothing." He even makes a joke of the tics that turn his daily experience into a St. Vitus dance. But he is unflinching in his commitment that, having finally regained his voice, he remain an equal voice in the medical chorus describing and defining his existence. His mother intervenes when he is so consumed by tics that he can no longer read and pronounces, "This isn't me, I'm grotesque." She delivers the speech that continues to define my interest in scientific and medical epistemology. Once again, a small woman surrounded by medical men declares her voice as the central one in this story: "When my son was born healthy, I never asked why. Why was I so lucky? What did I do to deserve this perfect child, this perfect life. But when he got sick, you can bet I asked why? I demanded to know why. Why was this happening? There was nothing I could do about it; no one I could go to to say 'Please stop this, can't you see my son is in pain?'" Turning to face those doctors, she repeats, "Please stop this! Can't you see my son is in pain?" Sayer defends Leonard's agency, saying, "He's fighting, Mrs. Lowe." She responds, "He's losing." Having lost her son once, she would prefer to spare him the pain of total physical degradation than keep him with her any longer. This time, he gets to say goodbye to the world and the connections he has made, and Sayer stands as witness as he slips back into silence and catatonia. Sayer returns to his office to watch the first video he made of Leonard after he woke up, in which he narrates his return to the world. Narrative again defines his experience of illness and health. Asked when he knew that his awakening was not a dream, Leonard responds: "When I spoke and you understood me."

Conclusion

Not every doctor has the combination of genius and humanity that characterized Oliver Sacks and his film double, Dr. Sayer. But more reflect a desire to understand and engage with their patients than Foucault's narrative of medical professionalism and silent patients permits. While I understand that the evidence I provide here can be countered and should be critically evaluated, the promise of *Awakenings* extends hundreds of years before and decades after the miraculous summer of 1969. Physicians are people. They struggle to understand their patients' disease using the categories and language available to them. They labor under the assumptions that challenge all of us. Some are better than others at their jobs. But being a physician cannot be considered a wise way to dominate other human beings. I have argued here for the importance of multiple voices and multiple sources of narrative in medical encounters from the 17th century to the present. I hope you too can hear them.

Works cited

Ackerknecht, Erwin. 1955. *A Short History of Medicine*. Baltimore: Johns Hopkins University Press, 1982.

Didi-Huberman, Georges. *Invention of Hysteria: Charcot and the Photographic Iconography of the Salpatriere*. Translated by Alisa Hartz, Cambridge, MA: MIT Press, 2008.

Eamon, William. *Science and the Secrets of Nature: Books of Secrets in Medieval and Early Modern Culture*. Princeton, NJ: Princeton University Press, 1996.

Fissell, Mary E. *Patients, Power, and the Poor in Eighteenth-Century Cambridge*. Cambridge: Cambridge University Press, 1991.

Foucault, Michel. 1963 (French), 1973 (English). *The Birth of the Clinic an Archaeology of Medical Perception*. Translated by A. M. Sheridan Smith, New York: Vintage Books, a division of Random House, 1994.

Geun-Han Suk, Gyeong-Moon Kim, Kwang Ho Lee, Chin-Sang Chung, and Ki-Young Jung."Reflex Movements in Patients with Brain Death: A Prospective Study in a Tertiary Medical Center." *Journal of Korean Medical Science*, vol. 21, no. 3, June 2006, pp. 588–90.

Gramshaw, Lindsay Patricia and Roy Porter. *The Hospital in History*. New York and Abingdon: Routledge, 1989.

Hoffmann, Leslie A. and Joel A. Vilensky. "Encephalitis Lethargica: 100 Years after the Epidemic." *Brain*, vol. 140, no. 8, August 2017, pp. 2246–51.

Jewson, Nicholas. "The Disappearance of the Sick Man from Medical Cosmology, 1770–1870." *Sociology*, vol. 10, no. 2, 1976, pp. 225–44.

Jones, Colin and Michael Sonenscher. "The Social Functions of the Hospital in Eighteenth-Century France: The Case of the Hotel-Dieu of Nimes." *French Historical Studies*, vol. 13, no. 2, Autumn 1983, pp. 172–214.

Kassell, Lauren. "Casebooks in Early Modern England: Medicine, Astrology, and Written Records." *Bulletin of the History of Medicine*, vol. 88, no. 4, 2014, pp. 595–625.

Kavey, Allison B. *Books of Secrets: Natural Philosophy in England, 1550-1600*. Champaign-Urbana: University of Illinois Press, 2007.

Monette, Paul. *Borrowed Time: An AIDS Memoir*. San Diego: Harcourt Brace Jovanovich, 1988.

Montgomery, Kathryn. *Doctors' Stories: The Narrative Structure of Medical Knowledge*. Princeton, NJ: Princeton University Press, 1991.

Ojanuga, Durrenda. "The Medical Ethics of the 'Father of Gynecology,' Dr. J. Marion Sims." *Journal of Medical Ethics*, vol. 19, no. 1, 1993, pp. 28–31.

Park, Katharine. *Doctors and Medicine in Early Renaissance Florence*.Princeton, NJ: Princeton University Press, 1985.

Pomata, Gianna. *Contracting a Cure: Patients, Healers, and the Law in Early Modern Bologna*. Baltimore: Johns Hopkins University Press, 1998.

Sacks, M. D. Oliver. 1973. *Awakenings*. New York: Vintage Books, 1999.

Wall, L. L. "The Medical Ethics of Dr. J. Marion Sims: A Fresh Look at the Historical Record." *Journal of Medical Ethics*, vol. 32, no. 6, 2006, pp. 346–50.

11

BENEATH THE COVERS

The illness of sex as depicted in film

Julie M. Aultman

This chapter provides a critical analysis of three films that illustrate the disembodiment of persons as sexual beings because of dysfunction, disability, paraphilic deviancy, and disempowerment, thereby constructing illness narratives. Such disembodiment can produce devastating effects on a person's bodily integrity, mental and physical well-being, social status, and basic liberties. The complex illness narratives of sex speak to the multiple ways that "illness" is understood (albeit insufficiently or inaccurately) in the context of sex, such as: abnormal functioning, the imbalance of goals or abilities, immorality, or insufficient states of (well)being, i.e., suffering. While an abundance of literature on sex and sexual identity as related to health and illness proliferates, along with extensive reviews and analyses of relevant film genres and tropes (e.g., sexploitation films, rape revenge films), a lack of critical examination on the illness narrative of sex and its impact on the character either on or off the screen continues. Thus, this chapter addresses the limitations of such an illness narrative, particularly when "illness" is insufficiently or inaccurately understood, which is described within the film diegesis or as a result of the film narrative itself.

Little Children (Field 2007), *The Sessions* (Lewin 2012), and *The Nightingale* (Kent 2018) all compel audiences to see how an illness narrative of sex negatively impacts whole persons and their relationships with others even when there is no self-identifiable illness as suggested otherwise within medical, religious, and cultural-social communities. That is, the illness narratives presented in these films depict sexual behavior and activity (or the lack thereof despite having a sexual desire) as illness, and hence, suggest that persons need to be removed from society, fixed, or cured, or whose suffering should be ignored. The success of these films in representing sexual violence, deviancy, perversion, impairment, and the efforts characters take in healing their sexual selves rests on how directors depict the illness narrative: its mimicry of reality, the believability of the actors, the creative process of shaping raw material and film editing, and audience and critic reception. I selected these three films because their master narratives and complex stories force audiences to question the meaning and representation of sex as it intersects with concepts of illness. For film artists and viewers alike, some of these films have the power to re-traumatize victims of sexual abuse or violence, and thus, the films' illness narratives not only illustrate the disembodiment of persons as sexual beings but also directly contribute to the very illness that they describe.

The concept of illness, used here, is not merely the absence of health but rather involves "those perceived problems which are experienced, recognized, and communicated by persons,

DOI: 10.4324/9781003007661-15

and often to their caregivers or doctors 'via the illness language,' who, in turn, try to help and cure them, while looking to find causes" (Aultman 325; Nordenfelt "Understanding the Concept"). This is especially a concern when disability is conflated with the concept of "illness" to reinforce medical models that aim to "fix" that which is perceived to be "abnormal," and which consequentially devalue persons and the capabilities they possess. Alternative to other conceptual accounts of illness, such as Christopher Boorse's value-free concept of health and disease that rests on biological function and statistical normality (Boorse), Lennart Nordenfelt presents a holistic account of health and illness with two interconnected phenomena, including suffering (mental distress and/or physical pain) and disability (Nordenfelt, "Understanding the Concept," "The Concepts of Health"). When examining these illness narratives of sex, what is then presented is how sex is experienced, recognized, and communicated as something that needs attended to; it is how and why the story of the sexual behavior, desire, or encounter is viewed and interpreted by film artists, actors, critics, and general audience viewers as a "problem" that can include mental distress, physical pain, and/or a disability (e.g., the physical and/or mental inability to have sex with another person). The illness narrative as presented in film may present a character's emotional suffering, the physical damage done to his/her body, and the overall disabling effects to the individual unable to engage in future sexual acts that align with clinical and social norms. An illness narrative of sex may not be told without sociocultural, ethical, financial, or legal contextual features that contribute to the many featured sex-related tropes in film (e.g., rape tropes). In addition, the illness narrative of sex often prompts individuals to prevent and/or address their suffering and disability on their own rather than seek direct support or care from others, and such acts of "self-care" can lead to further harms or risks of damage to one's self or others (e.g., self-mutilation).

The three thematic sections in this chapter examine narrative threads within the selected films including: deviancy and perversion; dysfunction and disability; and disempowerment. Due to both the relational aspects of sex and the causes and effects of sexual harms, these themes, at times, intersect and thereby represent the *absence of* a holistic nature of illness (of sex) and the illness role or are simply inaccurate portrayals of sex as illness. They, instead, define the illness of sex based on insufficient definitions or classifications of illness (e.g., Boorse's functional and statistical normalcy) or sociocultural models, including moral assumptions, religious values, and mainstream standards that marginalize persons and groups. My final section explores how a holistic understanding of persons as sexual beings and the illnesses they might experience related to sex ought to be fostered to minimize harms, critique our social (and clinical) standards of what is or is not "normal" about sexual behavior, and promote social justice.

The chapter is organized in three sections, each beginning with a description of the film followed by a deeper examination of identified core themes and their historical, sociocultural, and ethical relevance to the illness of sex. The first selected film, *Little Children*, presents a spectrum of sex as illness, ranging from emotional suffering that serves as both a cause and effect of infidelity and the absence of "healthy" sex within monogamous relationships to sex addiction and pedophilia. Illness here is defined by social norms and morality, as well as the medical establishment; the film artists of *Little Children* aim to illustrate how society's perception of sex as illness negatively impacts sufferers and their relationships.

Little Children: sexual desires and deviancy in suburbia

> It's not the cheating. It's the hunger – the hunger for an alternative and the refusal to accept a life of unhappiness.
>
> Sarah Pierce (Kate Winslet) *Little Children*

In *Little Children* (2007), a film adaptation of the Tom Perrotta's 2004 novel, director Todd Field intermingles the infidelity of characters Sara Pierce (Kate Winslet) and Brad Adamson (Patrick Wilson), the addiction of Sarah's husband, Richard, (Gregg Edelman) for online pornography, and the local pedophile's insatiable desires (Jackie Earle Haley). The characters' stories fuel an examination of the intersections of deviancy, perversion, and mental illness, and the reparations to each other and to society that these characters attempt to make. *Little Children* requires audiences to address their biases and reflect on their sympathetic responses to the most unlikely characters, those deemed outside the bounds, and consequently the sympathetic consideration of conventional society because of their desires. Here, the impact of suburban society's response to taboo realms of sex and sexual desire emerges as a significant theme.

Set in a suburb in Boston, Massachusetts, the film begins with a child's voice set in a black background, followed by a flurry of houses and white picket fences as if being viewed by a passenger in a vehicle traveling at 25 miles per hour, immediately placing audiences into the setting of a middle-class, suburban neighborhood. The voices of children and images of suburbia are disrupted and audiences are visually and auditorily hit by a throng of animated cuckoo clocks and rows of Hummel porcelain figurines. The opening film credits end with a television news alert describes the recent release of Ronnie McGorvey, who was sentenced for two-years for exposing himself in the presence of children. Viewers are then transported back to a more serene suburban landscape – a lush green park on a summer's day. Here, three friends, Theresa (Trini Alvarado), Cheryl (Marsha Dietlein), and Mary Ann (Mary B. McCann), sit on a park bench talking about spas, motherhood, and scheduling sex with their husbands (so as to avoid falling asleep in the process) as their children play. The camera shifts to Sarah, sitting on a nearby park bench "smiling politely," as our omniscient narrator (William "Will" Lyman) describes what she is feeling and thinking. The "authoritative voice" of Will Lyman that we hear throughout the film sets a tone described as both "compassionate and severe" (Scott). It is in this park where Brad appears with his four-year-old son, Aaron (Ty Simpkins), referred to as the "Prom King" by Theresa, Cheryl, and Mary Ann. Brad, as a handsome stay-at-home father, challenges their sexist ideologies about parenting and fuels their fantasies. In making a bet with the three women to get Brad's phone number, Sarah walks over to the swing set where Aaron and her daughter Lucy are playing, supervised by Brad. Unintimidated by his good looks, Sarah converses with Brad as they swing their children in unison. Before Brad and Aaron leave the park, Sarah discloses the bet, and, in an effort to scandalize the women, she and Brad kiss. The kiss sparks something within them both, and the quest for passion, companionship, and a way to fill a void within each of them emerges as a primary plot within the film.

Ronnie's story, the second plot of the film, is initially overshadowed by the growing relationship between Brad and Sarah; however, at the film's mid-point, these two storylines intersect as Ronnie decides to enter the neighborhood pool "to cool off" on a hot, sunny day where children are playing, including Aaron and Lucy. From children's laughter to parents' panicked screaming, the neighborhood children are immediately called out of the pool and gathered for their safety. Brad, Sarah, along with the other parents and their children stand in silence staring down at Ronnie, who has emerged from the water with snorkel gear, highlighting his underwater voyeurism. The police intervene and haul Ronnie out of the pool area. At this point, a torrential rainstorm breaks through the clouds, and Brad and Sarah, with their kids in tow, run to Sarah's house. While the kids take a nap, Brad and Sarah have passionate, adulterous sex in the laundry room of the basement. Though a predictable end to a building sexual tension between the two characters, the intriguing story between Brad and Sarah continues as viewers begin to question the mores of monogamy and the causes and effects of infidelity on persons and their partners.

Throughout the film, Larry (Noah Emmerich), a former police officer and one of Brad's friends, is disgusted with a pedophile living in his midst and harasses Ronnie. Larry, like many of the families in the neighborhood, is concerned for the safety of the local children, despite his own equally horrific past of killing an unarmed child, forcing his retirement from the police force. Jackie Earle Haley feeds into viewers' biases about what a pedophile looks and acts like; he is a creepy, socially awkward, scrawny man with a balding head and pock marked face, who is dependent on – if not inappropriately attached to – his mother, May (Phyllis Somerville) with whom he lives[1]. May takes care of Ronnie as though he were a child (cooking, cleaning, advising, and seeking out women whom he could date); simple tasks such as washing dishes are not done by Ronnie until after May passes away, further revealing the co-dependency issues that might have contributed to Ronnie's deviancy.

Nevertheless, over the course of the film, viewers begin to sympathize with Ronnie. Particularly in the pool scene, viewers can imagine themselves in the parents' flip-flops, looking horrified at a convicted pedophile emerging from their children's aquatic playground after swimming beneath the surface and moving about the children. However, at the same time, viewers cannot help but feel pity for a sad, lonely individual who just wanted to cool off on a hot summer day. (Of note: Ronnie does not physically touch children but exposes himself or masturbates thinking about children.) As the film progresses, we learn that Ronnie's paraphilia prohibits him from having a successful date with a woman at the insistence of his mother, who desperately wants Ronnie to have a "normal" life and find a woman to settle down with and raise a family. While it is a challenge to feel sympathy in the moments in which he masturbates in front of a dimly lit playground as his date, with her own set of mental health crises, sits next to him in complete horror, audiences also witness the effects of Ronnie's untreated illness. We bear witness to his uncontrollable sexual desires and the deep suffering he experiences from his illness; he does not want to live this way. We also see the suffering of those closest to him – his mother – who, despite the aforementioned co-dependency issues, is concerned about Ronnie's ability to take care of himself and "be a good boy" (which are her final words to him). Her home is vandalized because of irate vigilantes, and eventually she dies from a heart attack after trying to defend her son from Larry's persistent harassment. The handwritten note with only the directive to be good sends Ronnie into a fit of rage as he smashes the carefully shelved Hummel figurines and cuckoo clocks that are now forever silenced.

Audiences begin to see Ronnie as a person and not simply a social deviant, who emotionally crumbles after his mother dies and genuinely wants to curb his sexual desires. Although our omniscient narrator does not permit viewers to get inside Ronnie's mind, we can imagine the magnitude of guilt that he is feeling; after all, if he did not have these sexual urges and criminal status, his mother would most likely still be living. Audiences feel sadness, guilt, and even disgust as set designers cleverly use dark color schemes and nighttime filming in many of Ronnie's scenes, especially when compared to the vibrant green lawns, stark white houses, clear blue pools and brightly colored bathing suits we see in Brad and Sarah's scenes. For example, May's house is dark and drab with various shades of browns and yellows with wall-to-wall wooden clocks; Ronnie's date night ends on a dark, barely lit street in front of a playground; Ronnie is harassed by Larry in the late evening hours where dark houses, broken sidewalks, and parked vehicles lining the streets make it seem as though Ronnie is living on the "other side of the tracks."

To end his suffering, he castrates himself with a kitchen knife, then heads to the local park and playground from which he is banned, nearly hidden from view by the night. Sitting, nearly bleeding to death, his bully, Larry, comes to his rescue after apologizing for contributing to his mother's death. By castrating himself, Ronnie commits the very act that many in society, such as Larry, demand when they learn of "a pedophile living among them." But here, Ronnie's story of illness shows us that he is a person suffering from Pedophiliac Disorder, that he is socially and cognitively disabled from leading a life that he desires without hurting others. Unfortunately, it takes a physical act of self-mutilation to drive the point that pedophilia is a complex "illness of sex" and not simply one man's erotic desire for children; he is someone's son and a member of a community who is not afforded the clinical, emotional, and social help that he needs.

Interestingly, the title, *Little Children*, is not just applicable to Ronnie's story and the subject of his paraphilia and how May treats him but also aptly applies to the suburban parents who, at times, lack emotional maturity and motivation. They are needy, self-absorbed, unable to commit, and divert any opportunity for open and honest communication. Brad, for example, has failed the bar exam twice, and instead of telling his wife, Kathy (Jennifer Connelly), that he simply does not want to study for this examination and commit to the law profession, he lies about studying at the library. In his deception, Brad watches local skateboarders or spends the evening playing on a local football team with Larry, while Kathy believes he is studying. Understandably, some viewers might sympathize with Brad as a demasculinized stay-at-home father who takes care of his son while Kathy is at work as a documentary film producer. Kathy and her mother financially support the family and control all aspects of Brad's life from having a cell phone to insisting on having their son in their bed at night, which prevents any intimacy between the couple. When tensions rise, neither Brad nor Kathy talk about their needs, desires, or concerns as adults. And here, viewers might further question the mores of monogamy, and whether such social expectations place further pressure on couples, even designating persons as "ill" if they are unable to have a "healthy" sex life with their partners or commit acts of infidelity. Instead of creating environments so that partners can feel comfortable discussing their needs and concerns or even recognizing that monogamy and marriage might not be valued by all persons, society creates an illness narrative, suggesting persons who divert from social norms are broken or abnormal and need fixed.

Similarly, we find that Sarah and her husband, Richard, are not communicative and appear to be in a loveless marriage. Sarah, who gave up her doctoral work in English to raise Lucy, appears lonely, disorganized, and not fully committed as a parent or a spouse. Viewers learn that Sarah is Richard's second wife and living in the first wife's decorated home, which has remained the same apart from a small study where Sarah has her books and remnants of her prior life. Only her study, along with nightly scheduled walks with a neighbor or the occasional book club, provide Sarah with the opportunities to form a personal identity that she longs for beyond mother or wife. While some viewers might sympathize with Sarah despite her absent-minded parenting skills and general lack of commitment or her privileged life living in the suburbs, it is difficult to condone Sarah's infidelity based on sociocultural influences (e.g., religion) that serve as barriers to how we value and define sex (and illness). We learn that Sarah's husband, Richard, has been addicted to his favorite online porn star, Slutty Kay, at work and at home. He even orders a pair of her dirty underwear to enhance his erotic experience with her digital images. Sarah witnesses Richard masturbating in his home office while watching Slutty Kay (with her panties on his face), and despite asking to have a talk later that evening, no mature conversation takes place between them. Audiences feel Sarah's frustration as she takes a brisk walk with a friend, who she does not confide in but who senses that Sarah is upset about something at home. This is yet another example illustrating the difficulty of talking about sex, of desires, interests, and needs. A society that makes sex and sex talk taboo impairs persons and relationships, perpetuates stigma, and contributes to the medicalization of sex and our inability to discern what is truly an illness or not.

While the acts of infidelity between Brad and Sarah and Richard's intense porn watching might be disturbing to viewers, such acts are not necessarily symptoms of an illness of sex. Brad and Sarah are two, unhappy people who reminisce about their lives prior to kids and their struggling marriages; their infidelity is a symptom of their emotional immaturity to address their own personal needs and concerns and a symptom of a rigid, morally arrogant society. Through an unsuccessful attempt to escape their unsatisfying lives and run away together, they each gain perspective of the importance of their lives and the need to "grow up" (regardless of their returning to monogamous relationships or not, which viewers are not privy to).

Richard's infatuation with online Slutty Kay may simply be a perversion, i.e., a digital object of desire and a pair of underwear for self-stimulation and arousal. However, if Richard's sexual activities interfere with his work, his marriage, and his emotional stability in that he develops a diagnosable sexual addiction, then with additional context to his character and insight into *his* story, we can begin to unravel the complexities of this perversion, exploring whether it ought to be defined as an illness. Rather than present a deeper narrative thread, our omniscient narrator details Richard's thoughts: *Lately Slutty Kay had become a problem. He thought about her far too often and spent hours studying the thousands of photographs available to him. Some of Kay's practices struck him as bizarre, even off-putting. She had a thing about kitchen utensils, spatulas, and dressing up like a little girl and playing with balloons. But who was Richard to judge?* Describing Richard's infatuation with Slutty Kay as a "problem," with obsessive or *addictive* behaviors that pull Richard away from work and family, we can begin to see the emergence of an illness – a sex addiction. However, we must be cautious in "diagnosing" or defining Richard given that perhaps the real problem is not his desire for online porn but his inability to share with Sarah his sexual fantasies, fearing her inability to understand and accept them. It is unclear from the film whether his obsessive-compulsive behaviors are, in fact, symptoms of an illness.

From Sarah's perspective, however, Richard has neglected her and their daughter, evidenced by his lack of interaction (if not deliberate hiding from his family in his upstairs office); her short-term trysts with Brad simply cannot change her loveless marriage and overall unhappiness, and audiences might have conflicted feelings about Sarah's and Richard's sexual behaviors and infidelity. From narrow attitudes of sex and marriage, such as what is traditionally viewed as morally and socially acceptable to the medicalization of sex such as sex addiction as illness, we begin to understand the complexity of sex from social, moral, and medical perspectives and its impact on persons and their relationships with others.

Social stigma and the medicalization of sexual deviancy and perversion

Sexual deviancy or perversion can be identified as a behavior or desire that departs from conventional standards or is considered abnormal. As suggested by the definition, society establishes models to guide what is or is not acceptable, while the identification of what is or is not deemed "normal" might be best described by medical professionals who are equipped to diagnose and treat abnormal behavior or desire such as Paraphilia Disorder. The most recent Diagnostic and Statistical Manual for Psychiatric Disorders (DSM-5) classifies Paraphilia, previously known as sexual deviation and perversion, under a family of Paraphilic Disorders including Voyeuristic Disorder, Exhibitionistic Disorder, Frotteuristic Disorder, Sexual Masochism Disorder, Sexual Sadism Disorder, Pedophilic Disorder, Fetishistic Disorder, Transvestic Disorder, Unspecified Paraphilic Disorder, and Other Specific Paraphilic Disorder. A paraphilia "denotes any intense and persistent sexual interest other than sexual interest in genital stimulation or preparatory fondling with phenotypically normal, physically mature, consenting human partners" (DSM-5 685). Sometimes the sexual interest focuses on the individual's erotic activities (spanking, whipping, cutting, binding, or strangulating another person) or on the target of the individual's sexual interest (children, corpses, or amputees [as a class], as well as intense or preferential interest in nonhuman animals) (685).

To be diagnosed with a paraphilic disorder, the paraphilia causes significant distress or impairment to the individual or involves personal harm or risk of harm to others. Having a paraphilia does not necessarily mean that the individual has a paraphilic disorder, illustrating how an individual might not have an "illness of sex" until suffering or harm to self or other is experienced and/or identified (e.g., Pedophilic Disorder). In other words, an individual spanking or whipping a consenting adult might simply focus on this erotic activity (rather than the sexual partner) for arousal, which would be deemed a paraphilia (i.e., sadism). But according to the psychiatric community, if the individual experiences distress or impairment in social, occupational settings or acts on their intense urges with a nonconsenting person, they have a Sexual Sadism Disorder. The individual might recognize the illness and seek clinical help or might be criminalized for the act with or without required clinical care. Despite the distinctions between paraphilia and paraphilic disorder according to the psychiatric community, however, an individual may still feel "ill" regarding any emotional distress in the experience of causing physical harm to another consenting individual who, in turn, desires this sexual interaction. Alternatively, some individuals might not feel ill but are regarded as such by medical, religious, and other social communities (e.g., homosexuality). Such emotional distress, for example, can stem from society's belief that sadism is a sexual perversion and that by failing to uphold social expectations, an individual contends with feeling that they are is abnormal or exhibit unnatural sexual behavior.

Philosopher Thomas Nagel writes that "if there are any sexual perversions, they will have to be sexual desires or practices that are in some sense unnatural, though the explanation of this natural/unnatural distinction is of course the main problem" (9). What is "unnatural" can vary from culture to culture, but "it is not a pure expression of disapproval or distaste" (10). Nagel purports a psychological perspective of perversion based on a theory of sexual desire and human sexual interactions. "The concept of perversion implies that a normal sexual development has been turned aside by distorting influences" (17). Consistent with contemporary views on paraphilic disorder, he further writes: "If the object is not alive, the experience is reduced entirely to an awareness of one's own sexual embodiment. Small children and animals permit awareness of the embodiment of the other, but present obstacles to reciprocity, to the recognition by the sexual object of the subject's desire as the source of his (the object's) sexual self-awareness. Voyeurism and exhibitionism are also incomplete relations..." (17).

However, Nagel philosophically struggles with cases of sadism, masochism, and homosexuality, questioning whether sadism and masochism ought to be deemed perversions simply because they fall short of interpersonal reciprocity. For example, "Sadism concentrates on the evocation of passive self-awareness in others, but the sadist's engagement is itself active and requires a retention of deliberate control which may impeded awareness of himself as a bodily subject of passion in the required sense" (18). However, consenting adults who agree to sadist/masochist eroticism, including the "rules" of the sexual encounter, are, in effect, participating in a sort of interpersonal reciprocity; arguably, in some cases of sadism and masochism, it is questionable if it is genuinely a paraphilia or a perversion in Nagel's sense of the word. Nagel, who initially wrote his essay on "Sexual Perversion" in 1969 (revised in 1979) at the time the DSM deemed homosexuality a pathological disorder, argues that while homosexuality is complex, he doubts that it is a perversion given the reciprocity of sexual desire and sexual interactions, "though like heterosexuality it has perverted forms" (18). Of note, it was not until 1973 that the American Psychiatric Association (APA) removed the diagnosis of homosexuality from the second edition of the Diagnostic and Statistical Manuel. Homosexuality, thought to deviate from "normal" heterosexual development and divert from moral, social behavior, was pathologized based on several biased perspectives based on theories of pathology, immaturity, and normal variation (Drescher).

Despite medical experts' denial of homosexuality as an illness, religious groups and social organizations still aim to "fix," "cure," or "treat" it; films such as *But I'm a Cheerleader* (Babbit 1999), *Save Me* (Cary 2007), *Boy Erased* (Edgarton 2018), and *The Miseducation of Cameron Post* (Akhavan 2018) depict characters facing prejudice, being ostracized from their families and communities and forced into therapy such as Conversion Therapy to rid them of their perceived sinful or unnatural homosexuality. The stories of these characters shed light on the emotional and physical harms inflicted upon the LGBTQ community and the continued belief that homosexuality is an illness, but what might it be like for a person who has a known and unmanageable diagnosable illness of sex – such as Ronnie's pedophilia?

Questions about sexual deviancy and perversion, along with the illness of sex in the context of paraphilic disorders, emerge throughout *Little Children* in a thought-provoking, non-authoritative manner. The film is an accessible and easy to watch Hollywood movie with intersecting narrative threads and often witty narration that challenges adult audiences to consider not just what constitutes sexual deviancy and perversion but also to understand the illness of sex through the film narrative. The film elicits a deeper understanding of and sympathy for a person who suffers from a morally abhorrent paraphilic disorder (i.e., Pedophiliac Disorder). The social suffering and mental anguish of an individual who is criminalized and generally ignored as a person is central to an examination of the film and might prompt viewers to envision a future where supportive care (e.g., mental health counseling) is offered, and blame, fear, and harm (including self-harm) is avoided.

Audiences are prompted to examine their own views of sex and how those views are shaped by social norms and expectations that perpetuate stigma, sexual repression, and feelings of being "ill" or "broken." *Little Children* pushes viewers to examine sex through multiple lenses and the need for a holistic understanding of the illness of sex beyond our social fears, bias, and uninformed opinions about the suffering of others. Such an understanding can contribute to empathic responses, while challenging audiences to look deeper within themselves and question their own sexual behaviors and desires, redefining what is (or is not) normal similarly to what audiences gain in our next film, *The Sessions*.

The Sessions: disabled desires

> I wanted to be loved. I wanted to be held, caressed, and valued. But my self-hatred and fear were too intense. I doubted I deserved to be loved. My frustrated sexual feelings seemed to be just another curse inflicted upon me by a cruel God.
>
> Mark O'Brien 1990, *The Sun Magazine*

The Sessions (2012), inspired by poet and journalist Mark O'Brien's autobiographical article, "On Seeing a Sex Surrogate" (O'Brien), explores the intersections of sex, disability, and religion when polio-paralyzed poet, Mark O'Brien (John Hawkes), hires a sex surrogate to lose his virginity before his "expiration date" is up. Complicating Mark's story is his Catholic guilt about having sex before marriage to which his friend and spiritual advisor, Father Brendan (William H. Macy), expresses: "I think God will give you a pass on this one." Directed and written by Ben Lewin, a polio survivor himself, the film addresses the social injustices among persons living with disabilities who are ignored as sexual beings and often are not afforded the opportunities to express their sexuality. The recognition of abled sexual bodies and the value of healing the sexual self through social support, advocacy, and disability rights awareness challenges the illness narrative and prompts a deeper understanding of the meaning and representations of sex.

Set in 1988 in Berkeley, California, Mark O'Brien, a 38-year-old virgin paralyzed from the neck down and dependent on an iron lung, feels unworthy as a man. He is able to get physically and emotionally aroused but has not been able to find a sexual partner. His love for his caretaker, Amanda (Annika Marks), gives Mark hope, but with an unsuccessful marriage proposal and her desire to leave the U.S. to study abroad, Mark seeks help from his therapist, Dr. Laura White (Blake Lindsley). Dr. White connects him to sex surrogate, Cheryl Cohen Greene (Helen Hunt), who has been trained in addressing issues of sex, intimacy, and clients' bodies, including addressing fear and anxiety surrounding sex.

Mark seeks out approval from his friend and priest, Father Brendan, and support from his close friend, Carmen (Jennifer Kumiyama), a woman born with arthrogryposis who advocates for the disabled community and expresses the importance of sex in the lives of persons with disabilities. Carmen opens her home to Mark, encouraging him to enjoy this sexual experience with Cheryl; though appreciative of Carmen's bold commentary on sex, Mark is guarded because of his Catholic guilt, his virginal status, and his upbringing closed to discussions about sex.

Mark's aid, Vera (Moon Bloodgood), takes him via gurney to Carmen's house for his first session. Sensing his trepidation, she exclaims, "Will you stop acting like you're going to your own execution!" To which Mark responds, "I'm not acting." Vera waits until Cheryl comes to the home, and during this scene, viewers can see the panic-stricken Mark, feeling almost as awkward as he appears. Explaining the nature of sex surrogacy and establishing a set of rules to maintain professional boundaries, Cheryl starts the first session by undressing in front of him and trying to get Mark to be comfortable with his own body and his emotions surrounding sex (fear, feelings of guilt, embarrassment). Mark is visibly and even physically uncomfortable as Cheryl awkwardly tries to remove his shirt as this is her first client with extensive paralysis. She remarks how she likes Mark's shirt; he replies that this is the second time she's made the remark, emphasizing her nervousness. He lets out a painful cry because of the mismanagement of his clothing removal, but Cheryl senses that his reaction is more emotional than physical and recognizes the need to slow down and learn from Mark as much as he wants to learn from her.

Cheryl is deeply sensitive to Mark's physical and emotional needs, his abilities, and his limitations; her therapeutic insights and ability to uncover Mark's fears of sex help him emerge as a fearless, sexual being fully capable of intercourse. Interesting to note, in researching her role of Cheryl, Helen Hunt met several times with the real Cheryl Cohen Greene who stayed friends with Mark O'Brien until his death. Hunt explained that she was not that comfortable being completely nude and pretending to engage in sexual acts. In a *Vanity Fair* interview, Hunt explained: "I was as comfortable as I could be, and then after that, I pretended. I think [my] character's desire to make [John Hawkes's character] comfortable and my desire to embody a sex-positive human being was what I hung on to" (Miller). In another interview with film critic and entertainment reporter, Stephen Schaefer (2012), Hunt stated: "I hope people take their 16 and 17-year-olds to see it [*The Sessions*]. His disability makes sex the way it is in real life for all of us…It isn't some perfectly orchestrated ballet that one knows exactly what the other one wants and it all is executed perfectly. It's clumsy, silly, scary and wonderful. His disability actually serves a real purpose in the story" (Schaefer).

In his article, "On Seeing a Sex Surrogate," Mark explains that seven years prior (1983), he wrote about sex and disabled people. However, as he interviewed sexually active men and women for his article, he "felt removed" and "envied these people ferociously." He learned that it was fear that separated him from those he interviewed, "fear of others, fear of my own sexuality, and a surpassing dread of my parents" (O'Brien). Mark tells his readers that sex was never talked about in his home growing up, and despite not living with them as a young man, he "continued to live with a sense of their unrelenting presence, and their disapproval of sexuality in general, mine in particular" (O'Brien). Ben Lewin not only captures the seriousness of sex, how it is viewed as a social taboo but also brings some humor into the film to reveal that regardless of a person's background and ability, there is always something to learn about sex. For example, at one point in the film, Mark is unable to use Carmen's home for the sessions, and so Vera takes Mark to a nearby hotel. The hotel clerk (Ming Lo) is curious about Mark, Cheryl, and the hourly rate that Vera works out with him. Though Vera is upfront and indicates that Cheryl is a type of sex therapist, the clerk does not believe her. "Now come on, what type of therapist is she?" "I told you, she is a sex therapist. Today they are working on simultaneous orgasm," Vera responds. "What's that?" questions the clerk. Comic relief opens the door for viewers to ask questions not just about sex and disability but also about their own knowledge (or lack thereof) and experiences.

Additionally, Mark's story pushes audiences to think deeply about the value of sex and sex surrogacy, as well as the professional boundaries crossed in the effort to promote care for another person. For example, a love is felt between Cheryl and Mark over the course of four sessions and interactions outside of the bedroom such as coffee at a local restaurant. Mark further challenges the professional boundaries that were initially established by sending Cheryl a love poem to her home address, which is found by Cheryl's husband, Josh (Adam Arkin). Despite having an open marriage, Josh throws the poem in the trash (later retrieved by Cheryl) and childishly pouts. Feeling the intensity of his love for Cheryl, Mark stops the sessions before finishing all six of them. Audiences are left to assume that Mark no longer needed the sessions nor wanted to be emotionally hurt, knowing he could not have a relationship with Cheryl. Both Cheryl and Father Brendan place their relationship with Mark above the expectations of their professions; Cheryl cherishes Mark's love poem, allowing herself to become emotionally close to him, and Father Brendan spends time with Mark as a friend, giving him advice counter to his priesthood and supporting sex outside of marriage. These crossing of boundaries established by social mores and religious attitudes challenge audiences to think more critically about their own views of sex and recognize that persons are not necessarily ill, disabled, immoral, sinful, or abnormal because they do not fit within society's parameters of what is or is not acceptable sex.

Sex and disabled bodies

While *The Sessions* does not explore the depths of Mark's "surpassing dread", his guilt for wanting sex as an unmarried man and the fear of his own sexuality are evident throughout the film. The complex illness narrative presented in this film shows audiences, on the surface, the importance of sex among disabled bodies. But as Mark O'Brian's story unfolds, we learn about his emotional illness – the barriers of fear, anxiety, and feelings of unworthiness that contribute to his suffering – rather than those physical disabilities of paraplegia, which are not, for him, barriers to a healthy sex life. Audiences are challenged to confront their biases surrounding both sex and disabled bodies and to look at the entirety of a person's life, including his sexual needs, and sexuality. Mark's illness of sex is not due to the direct physical effects of polio but to the disabling mental states, encouraging audiences to think more holistically about persons and to recognize that they might have multiple disabilities (and abilities), which may or may not require attention. Equally, when delving into Cheryl's character and her role of a sex surrogate, inquisitive audiences learn about the different roles among sex workers and sex surrogates; they are also exposed to what it might be like to be in an open marriage and having to establish good communication and boundaries just like any partnership.[2]

Alternatively, however, audiences seeing this film might easily assume a medical or functional model of disability where Mark's polio-caused paraplegia prevents him from having a "healthy" functional sexual relationship, unable to caress his lover or to engage in intercourse without assistance. Some may also interpret Mark's inability to have sex because of a "mental disability" such as anxiety and, therefore, can simply be "fixed" through therapeutic interventions including sex therapy and surrogacy. Both of these perspectives support conventional societal biases insufficiently addressed in the film despite the fact that audiences witness the fullness of Mark's life and an adaptable disability that neither defines him nor his sexual desires. For example, toward the end of the film, Mark starts a relationship with Susan Fernbach (Robin Weigert), whom he meets at the hospital following a near death experience: his iron lung stops functioning due to a power outage. However, before learning more about his newfound love, Lewin ends the film with Mark's death; Susan delivers the eulogy at his funeral, reading the love poem that Mark gave to Cheryl. Even in death Mark remains surrounded by friends and those he deeply loved. Despite our cultural assumptions, therefore, the film encourages audiences to understand that Mark lived a fulfilling, complete life as a journalist, poet, friend, and lover. As such, he generated economic stability, independence, spirituality, and several meaningful relationships, including (presumably) a sexual relationship with Susan.

Lewin implicitly but successfully shows a social model, if not holistic model, of disability understood more as a complex collection of conditions and not simply a "dysfunction" – some of which might be created by social environments. Audiences can readily recognize that we fail as a society in creating unnecessary barriers for our disabled community. First, often because of biases or short-sidedness, society fails to understand and accept the importance of sex and sexuality within disabled communities and, as a result, to provide support and opportunities. Further, religious communities too frequently create an environment in which persons feel as though their disabilities are punishments from God or that their differences cannot afford them with opportunities that able-bodied persons usually take for granted (e.g., sex). Due to such social environments, emotional distress becomes heightened, adding additional barriers that could have been prevented and often irrelevant to the physical disability itself. In Mark's disclosure to Father Brendan, he describes his disability in this way: God was punishing him, and to make matters worse, as a devout Catholic, he felt guilty thinking about sex outside of marriage, feelings of shame heightened by seeking it out and paying for it.

Alternatively, the environments that support Mark include friends' homes and a hotel that was physically accessible so that he could participate in the sessions (rather than at his residence that only contained the iron lung). Having access to a therapist and a sex surrogate who supported Mark's needs and focused on his abilities rather than his disabilities sends an important message to audiences to take a careful look at our environment to break down psychological biases and social barriers in the effort to be inclusive and promote better opportunities for our disabled community. While critics might be concerned with the casting of John Hawkes, not a disabled person himself, Lewin did meet with actors with disabilities to play the role of Mark O'Brien. In an interview with Lewin, Jada Yuan (2012) wrote that "some of them [disabled actors] he thought were terrific and he'd put in the movie, but none of them felt quite right for the character" (Yuan). Lewin as a polio survivor himself was able to relate to Mark, as well as work with the disabled community and Susan Fernbach to maintain the integrity of Mark's story. Mark's narrative of the illness of sex reveals how psychological barriers imposed by religion, society, and family can impair persons from fulfilling their capabilities, thus intensifying existing disabilities and leading to disembodiment of a sexual self. Seeking support to achieve his sexual goals, gaining confidence, and coming to know and appreciate his sexuality, the film demonstrates how Mark fosters future relationships, and no longer feel ill, but rather complete. By addressing the social stigma of sex, particularly surrounding disabled bodies, audiences are better equipped to understand and value those atypical sex needs and practices (e.g., sex surrogacy, pornography, open marriages) that can help persons flourish as sexual beings.

One of the most poignant scenes in *The Sessions* is when Cheryl, who was also raised Roman Catholic, decides to convert from Judaism and enters the *mikveh* with the support of the *mikveh* attendant (Rhea Pearlman). It is here where Cheryl undresses as part of the ritual and immerses herself in the spiritual waters. The *mikveh* attendant tells Cheryl, "This is your body. This is the body God crafted for you." This scene, which is juxtaposed with another scene where Cheryl affirms Mark's sexual identity by holding up a mirror for him to gaze upon his own nakedness is a reminder to viewers that humanness comes in all shapes, sizes, forms, and abilities and that we cannot deny, ignore, or silence ourselves as sexual beings nor be impaired by narrowly defined social mores.

In turning to our next and final film, *The Nightingale*, which details the devastating effects of colonization and acts of sexual violence, this particular historically situated rape narrative is essential for illustrating that such acts are neither sexually motivated nor a symptom of a sexual illness despite public perceptions to the contrary. By understanding that even though rape is, by definition, an act of "sex," the person committing the act is not expressing himself as a sexual being; instead, he is exerting power and control over others, traumatizing victims, who are likely to become physically and/or emotionally ill (e.g., post-traumatic stress disorder).

The Nightingale: an illness narrative of sexual violence and colonization

> I'm not your whore. I'm not your nightingale, your little bird, your dove. I'm not your anything. I belong to me and no one else!
>
> Clare Carroll (Aisling Franciosi), *The Nightingale*

The fight to feel whole – to achieve power when it has been taken away from you – is the theme of the final film, *The Nightingale* (2018). Set in 1825 in Australia's penal colony, Van Dieman's Land (Tasmania), the film is written, co-produced, and directed by Jennifer Kent. In this film, Irish convict Clare Carroll (Aisling Franciosi) seeks revenge after being held in servitude, brutally and repeatedly raped, and bearing witness to the murders of her husband, Aiden (Michael Sheasby) and her baby, Brigit (Addison and Maya Christie). Themes of racism, sexism, and post-traumatic stress arise from the brutishness of being violated within this illness narrative of sexual violence. The realities of rape and its repetitiveness throughout the film have sent some audiences fleeing from theaters and feeling discomfort and outrage. The illness of sex – of deviant perpetrators and disembodied victims – however, is at the forefront of this film where "rape is not sexualized nor the violence eroticized" (O'Malley) but, combined with murder, ignites Clare's revenge and quest-like illness narrative (Frank).

Known as the "Nightingale" for her beautiful voice among colonizing British soldiers, Clare is asked to sing to the unit. Following her vocal solo, Clare goes to Lieutenant Hawkins to ask him about a letter of recommendation to free her and her family from their years of servitude. Hawkins asks her sing to him to which she reluctantly complies. After making unwanted sexual advances toward Clare, to which she refuses, he hits her and rapes her. The initial rape scene is in Hawkins' dimly lit room where Clare's borrowed green dress (the color of Ireland) for her solo is the only bright color, drawing attention to her emotional and physical pain and suffering. The rape is not gratuitous and speaks loudly to the power differential between Hawkins and Clare. After she is raped, Clare is initially unable to tell her husband, despite his sensing that she has been harmed in some way. Aiden confronts Hawkins, and a brawl between them fuels Hawkins' further need for power and control.

A visiting officer who witnesses the brawl, meets with Hawkins and not only denies his upcoming promotion because of his treatment of Aiden but also questions Hawkins' abilities as a leader. The officer sends Hawkins through the dangerous bush to the town of Launceston where they meet to reconsider his status. Sergeant Ruse (Damon Herriman) and Jago (Harry Greenwood) are asked to accompany Hawkins. However, before leaving for their journey, Hawkins, Ruse and Jago go to the Carroll's rustic, dark home to confront Aiden, demanding an apology for the brawl and disclosing having sex with his wife. Naturally, Aiden becomes angry and lashes out as Hawkins grabs Clare, holds her down, and rapes her again as Aiden is held by Ruse and Jago. With Clare screaming and her baby girl crying, Hawkins stops penetrating Clare, turns, and shoots Aiden dead. Clare, screaming and crying over her husband's murder, is then gang raped by the men and forced to witness her baby's death. Jago shakes baby Brigit and forcefully slams her against the wall in a desperate need to follow Hawkins' orders to "stop the crying". Finally, they hit Clare and leave her for dead. It is at this point where disturbed, if not angered, audience members walked out of theaters worldwide after witnessing Clare's rape and the murdering of her family. The scene is filmed in a dimly lit room without close-ups, nudity, blood, or gore but the emotional and physical performance of the five adult actors and the sound effects of gun shots and physical violence feels "too real" (note: I cleared a room of viewers with my own screening of this film for purposes of this chapter).

Awaking the next morning to two lifeless, murdered bodies – her dearest loves – Clare angrily sets out to find Hawkins and his men. While the rape scene is, again, not gratuitous, and occurs in a darkly lit, thatched home, it *feels* disturbingly real and timeless as a violent act of power over a woman. After already losing her freedom, Clare is left with nothing but a physically damaged body (evidenced by slow, rigid body movements), stringy and lifeless hair, tattered clothes and the building rage within (evidenced by a rigid jaw, pursed lips, and grinding teeth). Her identity of mother and wife has been viciously taken away from her, but she finds the strength to fight and seek justice. To help guide her through the bush to find Hawkins, Clare offers two shillings to a black Aboriginal guide named "Billy" Mangana (Baykali Ganambarr). Interestingly, Mangana means "Blackbird." Clare as a "Nightingale" and Billy as "Blackbird" (both who sing in the film in their own languages) are "a rigid handling of potential metaphors" as critic Sheila O'Malley (2019) writes. However, as a widowed and childless woman traveling through the bush alone (and unable to trust men), she initially tells Billy that she is headed to Launceston to see her husband; he is unaware of the rapes and murders, seeing her as simply a White woman who has hired him. Early in their travels, they pass two Aboriginal figures hanging by their necks high in the tree line, a cruel reminder of the racial genocide leading up to and during the Black War and of the racial differences between Clare and Billy. Clare explains that she is Irish and not English and that her people are not involved with the mass killings. But viewers still see Clare's White privilege as she travels with Billy, such as calling him "boy" and treating him less than a person, sending the message to audiences that even those who are mistreated and oppressed disempower others seen as "lower" than themselves.

Through their journey, however, they come to understand each other – their loss of family and home and their vengeance against those who disempowered them. While Billy plays a pivotal role in the themes of racism and genocide because of blackness and the colonization by Whites and their racial cruelty toward Aboriginal people, this is Clare's story. Kent provides viewers with the female gaze to present sexual and physical violence that Clare endures as well as her vengeance, transformation, and empowerment. Unlike a typical rape revenge film, presented from a male gaze where unmarried women are presented as sex objects or presented as culpable targets of rape because of naivete, ignorance, or arrogance (e.g., walking alone, visiting male establishments) and seeking vengeance through violence ("an eye for an eye") without a transformative experience, Kent alternatively presents us with a married, feisty, prisoner of war whose only appeal to men is her singing voice. Clare carries the physical and emotional trauma she endures throughout her transformative journey; she does not ultimately seek vengeance, but the reclamation of self.

As the story progresses, Clare eventually trusts Billy, confronts her own racial biases and recognizes how to help him with the White privilege she possesses to keep him safe from the colonists. On their way to Launceston, Hawkins, Ruse, and Jago expand their traveling party with Charlie (Charlie Jampijinpa Brown), an Aboriginal guide, and a small band of hired convicts. Encountering an Aboriginal woman named Lowanna, Ruse kidnaps her in the effort to make her a sex slave. She is raped, and, to escape a group of Aboriginal men coming to her rescue, Hawkins kills her. Despite criticism by Larissa Behrendt (2019) for the "perfunctory and superficial interrogation of how that dynamic [colonial violence against women] plays out for Aboriginal women...a serious flaw that plays into a colonial cinematic tradition...[that] may well hit raw nerves with Indigenous women, who have long felt marginalized in Australian cinema," Lowanna's scene highlights what is going on in the periphery of Clare's quest. Kent's examinations of the violence and oppression of Aboriginal people are powerful and appropriately brief, signifying her own progress of learning and developed awareness without assuming what it is like to be a marginalized Aboriginal person in the 1800s or today.

Jago eventually is separated from his group and found by Clare, who brutally kills him; her anger and trauma are apparent as she repeatedly delivers blows to his face, crushing his skull. After murdering Jago, Clare finally discloses her true intentions for traveling to Launceston, which contributes to the growing trust between her and Billy. Billy, desperately wanting to see his family and describing the violent colonization of his land, then shares his story with Clare, giving context to her lack of understanding and privilege. Tragically, he later learns from a group of Aboriginal men held captive by colonists that he is the last remaining Letteremairrener man after his people, including his own family, are slaughtered by the colonists. Through shared suffering, a friendship emerges.

At one point in the journey, they are temporarily separated from one another, and Clare finds her way back to the main road toward Launceston after seeing a black bird and following it out of the wilderness. One of the few times she is alone, Billy is symbolically present and guiding her; she is transforming, becoming stronger, more aware, and perhaps recognizing her own biases. Eventually Clare finds Billy, and they travel together with their newly forged friendship to Launceston when they run into Hawkins. In front of Hawkins, who is surrounded by his superiors, she discloses what he has done and then abruptly leaves having said her piece. She and Billy (who hides from the men) leave town on horseback where they find a safe place in the bush to stay for the night. In the middle of the night, Billy ritualistically prepares himself (e.g., puts on body paint, arms himself) to go back to town to kill Hawkins. Awaking to his absence, Clare goes after Billy in the effort to stop him; and audiences see that she cares about his welfare. Upon her arrival, she witnesses Billy killing Hawkins in the town hostel, followed by Ruse shooting Billy in the abdomen. She flees the scene with her injured friend on horseback toward freedom; the film ends with Clare singing and Billy injured but dancing on a beach looking at the sun rise.

Neil Vickers (2012) states that identity is "almost always embedded in networks of relationships and its survival in both the subtle and the basic senses depends in part on what happens in those networks" (1070). Upon confronting Hawkins, Clare expresses that she is not the person who she was. Transformed by her suffering, her illness that has the "effect of making others forget your past self and its bearing on who you are now" (1070). And though initially seeking vengeance, she neither kills Hawkins nor seeks revenge, she transforms into a strong, empowered woman because of her illness journey, gaining knowledge of herself in relation to her environment and its people, and her friendship with Billy.

In one of the most powerful scenes, Clare, representing all that is loathed by Hawkins (prisoner, mother/female, and now ally – if not friend – of a black Aboriginal guide) confronts him in front of his superiors, and his fellow soldiers, all of whom are at a dimly lit, local all men's tavern, discussing politics over drinks. She stands above a seated Hawkins, looks him directly in the eye and states: "…That girl you raped, whose husband and baby you murdered, that girl died. But you cannot kill what's already dead." Hawkins tries to tell his superiors that she is a drunken whore who tried to steal his horse. The soldiers in the tavern are silent, looking and listening without a stir. Clare retaliates: "…Look at you all dressed up and shiny…what's the matter little soldier boy, didn't your mommy love ya." Hawkins strikes her hard, and after recoiling from his blow, she finds her voice again and sings. After she finishes, she briefly looks over to Hawkins' superiors and quietly leaves the tavern back through the darkened door frame from which she came through, which also frames the back of her body that stood tall, with her stringy, dirty hair, and filthy clothes. As she leaves, she is lit by the day's sun and in a daze, collapses to her feet on the outside street. Billy quickly comes to her aid, alerting her, and taking a horse (for which she was earlier accused of stealing). Clare's justice does not have to be as violent as the harm he has done to her and her family, or to the very persons he is colonizing. Confronting him, Clare reduces Hawkins to the very savage he really is, fulfilling her quest – not through a violent, vengeful act – but of taking back her power. The director captures this moment by having Clare stand above a seated Hawkins, symbolically and literally capturing the redistribution of power between the two. As Cara Buckley 2019 writes, "Revenge tales typically have a catharsis. *The Nightingale* looks at what happens after revenge is exacted, and the toll it takes when you try to rid yourself of pain by inflicting it on others. Kent latched onto these themes in response to a modern-day world filled with outrage and lashing out" (Buckley).

The harmful effects of a rape film trope with integrity

Rape and revenge films are typically structured with a female character raped and brutally harmed or left for dead, followed by her survival in the effort to seek vengeance and, in many films, kill the rapist. The rape trope is used in several horror films such as *I Spit on Your Grave* (Zarchi 1978), *Demented* (Jeffreys 1980), and *Teeth* (Lichtenstein 2007), and the rape is often gratuitous. Alexandra Heller-Nicholas (2011), however, writes that a film-specific approach to the rape-revenge genre reveals that this narrative structure is more complex; its complexity is understood by paying attention to how the rape or sexual assault is presented, the motivations of the characters in seeking justice, and the acts of revenge (e.g., killing of the rapist) and whether they are morally justified.

Wayne Wilson (1988) examined 26 films covering a span of nearly 60 years and draws upon three film categories, including classics, docudramas, and exploitation films. The classics are films of artistic merit that "use rape to make a significant statement about life, possessing integrity in characterization and story," showing how rape causes turmoil and anguish for the victim and their social and sexual relationships (e.g., *A Streetcar Named Desire* [Kazan 1951]) (608–9). For docudramas or melodramas, the focus is on the acts of sexual assault, presenting rape as real or with the appearance of reality. Within this category of rapist rehabilitation, there is the legal ambiguity of rape (e.g., marital rape), or confusion centering on consent. The final category, exploitation, are "overstated dramas" that range from sleazy, low-budget vehicles (e.g., *I Spit on Your Grave*) to "slick productions that deceptively use rape for gratuitous effect" (e.g., *Lipstick* [Johnson 1976]). Here we also see the genre of revenge films. Wayne Wilson (1980) writes, "Because *Lipstick* boasts higher production values and better performances, making the use of sexual assault appear more credible" (609). Wilson purports that when rape is used for entertainment purposes, there are at least four sexual myths about the victim including (1) an overemphasis on false reports of rape; (2) the futility of resisting the rapist; (3) the desirability of attempting personal revenge; and (4) the assumption that rape produces no prolonged aftereffects of suffering (610). It is this fourth myth that Kent debunks as she portrays the unrelenting physical and emotional suffering Clare carries with her throughout the film.

Wilson (1988) further explains that film and television distort aggravated rape, which involves sexual assault by a stranger(s) and includes "severe violence and threat with a weapon," and alternatively neglect simple rape that occurs by a known person or party that is not physically violent (607). He writes: "Movies opt for aggravated rape because of its greater dramatic value through violence. We know then that rape as entertainment services an illusion and that this illusion misses the mark of reality. But how damaging is this miss to the integrity of a real rape?" (608). For him, a rape story possesses integrity "when it conveys a natural and logical action, perfectly suitable and credible in the scheme of things… from the rapist's motivation to the victim's aftermath of suffering…Regrettably, movies that use rape for entertainment do not respond well to this standard of integrity" (608).

In the article "What Does It Mean for a Rape Scene to Be 'Done Well'?" Angelica Jade Bastién (2019) describes Jennifer Kent's perspective about the rape scenes in *The Nightingale*: "I don't see those scenes as rape scenes…it's a scene of someone's soul being destroyed." Kent, as a female director, did not want to present rape from the male gaze, i.e., gratuitous scenes with a woman's naked body and wanted to present rape from a woman's point of view. Bastién (2019) writes: "But I think the truth is more complicated…It's a reductive way to look at women's art to assume that they will eschew the very issues that make the male gaze such a problem… More broadly, we haven't created a sufficient theory to discuss this kind of cinematic violence…Is it merely the absence of nudity? Or more fully placing the audience in the perspective of the survivor? What does it mean when sexual violence is handled from a woman's perspective?" The rape story in *The Nightingale* arguably possesses integrity even if critics felt that the film lacked depth and character development with Luwanna's rape; the film presented an accurate portrayal of rape as an act of power and control of another and the pain felt – the *illness* experienced – and less about the act of sex.

This, of course, was not the first film that sparked controversy because of violence and rape scenes. In *Something Wild* (1961) directed by Jack Garfein and based on a 1958 novel, the emotional trauma of Mary Ann Robinson (Carroll Baker), who is raped in a New York Park, attempts suicide, and then is "rescued" by Mike (Ralph Meeker) who takes her back to his apartment and keeps her captive. *Something Wild* was one of the first films showing an on-screen rape. Audiences witnessing the rape and emotional trauma for the first time on film, endured these scenes hoping for positive resolution or justice, which was never accomplished. Critic J. C. Macek III (2017) describes the film as a "disturbing, uncomfortable, beautifully shot film that largely goes nowhere" and "ultimately comes off as incomplete, and perhaps even misogynistic and mean-spirited." Audiences critically described the inappropriate or "too real [a rape scene]," possibly re-traumatizing victims of sexual assault and rape, or even blaming them for "not being more careful." Wanda Hale (1961) began her review by stating "1961, the year that movie makers became infatuated with rape, will not pass without another on the subject slipping in for Christmas holiday presentation by the Plaza theater" and without giving further thought about the impact of rape on victims, and ignoring the broader social issues, writes "*Something Wild* carries a moral for the feminine sex: Don't walk in the city's parks alone after dark." Though the film makers of *Something Wild* did not intend to frighten women into changing their behaviors, sexist commentary from media critics and audiences, such as Wanda Hale's review, placed blame on those who are sexually assaulted. Rather than receiving empathy, rape victims who experience physical and emotional trauma are viewed as culpable; they are blamed for their actions and inadvertently any illness that results from sexual assault and violence such as PTSD, depression, physical trauma, sexually transmitted infections.

Depicting a realistic rape scene with integrity in film has its risks beyond economic ones because of negative audience and/or critic reception. Sexual violence in film can desensitize viewers, retraumatize viewers and actors playing the roles of victims and change perceptions about violence among youth and adults. Thus, the illness narrative of sex in film can impact the real lives of audiences, critics, and film artists and possibly extend their own illness narratives surrounding sex and sexual violence. In viewing *The Nightingale*, Bastién writes, "It isn't that such scenes of brutality have no place in cinema. But I often struggle to sit through scenes like this; they only bring back memories" (Bastién). For some audiences, they were drawn to see the film because of hearing reports of the "outraged walkouts" (Buckley).

Several studies have shown that exposure to violence, including sexual violence, in film and other media has both short-term and long-term negative effects such as desensitization and reduced empathy for others (Romer et al.), heightened aggression, and risky sexual behaviors (Anderson and Bushman; Anderson et al; Gentile *Media Violence*, Gentile "Are Motion Pictures Ratings"; Brown). As Bleakley et al. (2014) explain, "Through observational learning and the acquisition of scripts that inform adolescents' thoughts and associations, the behavioral context in which violence is presented in films may change the nature of adolescents' perceptions about violence, potentially teaching youth that violence is as acceptable as these behaviors…Because violence is prevalent in most top-grossing films, this conceptualization of potentially harmful content is critical in understanding the effects of violent media exposure and the portrayal of risk behaviors in general" (7X). To reduce such risks, film ratings are used to guide parents' decisions about whether the film content is suitable for their children or not (Gentile "Are Motion Picture Ratings").

Charles Mullin and Daniel Linz (1995) write: "Viewing violence may increase desensitization to violence, resulting in calloused attitudes toward violence directed at others and a decreased likelihood to take action on behalf of the victim when violence occurs" (449). The authors explain that eroticized or sexualized violence against women, such as rape, is particularly troubling but when such violence is reinforced in the environment or through messages, it is difficult for individuals to come back from a traumatic experience and be re-sensitized. Emotional desensitization occurs when viewing films of violence against women and their objectification; individuals become less empathic toward victims of sexual violence, and violence becomes more acceptable (Mullin and Linz).

In a study by Weidmann et al. (2009), reactions to distressing films were compared in the context of a stressful film paradigm (SFP). The authors specifically explored whether different responses in 100 five male and female study participants were produced when exposed to four different stressful films, including a film with a rape scene. Levels of distress, heart rate, and mood states were measured immediately after the film and during a diary phase of three days. The goals of the study included determining what type of film would "constitute an analogue traumatic situation," whether there would be gender differences in regard to intense reactions, and the experience of intrusive memories as a symptom of post-traumatic stress disorder (PTSD).

Weidmann et al. (2009) further found that, in contrast to other film clips, one "depicting rape elicited the most consistent reactions that were characterized by a higher heart rate, more distress and more intrusive memories, compared to the other three clips" (549), as well as a more intense emotional response regarding anger and disgust (564). The clip from the film *Irreversible* (2003) by Gaspar Noé, portrays the assault of a young woman on her way home from a party; she is brutally raped and beaten. Weidmann et al. (2009) in citing Kessler et al. (1995), purport experiencing sexual assault is commonly associated with the highest risk of PTSD. They write, "Our study suggests that also becoming a witness of sexual assault may have a greater impact on an individual than witnessing another type of traumatic event" (567).

For the actors and production crew in *The Nightingale*, the scenes were emotionally difficult and often with lasting effects. Cara Buckley explains, "Franciosi spent time with sexual assault victims to prepare for her role and worked closely with a psychologist ...Some of the scenes left the production crew in tears. Ganambarr said he would hear the screams and cower. After production wrapped, Franciosi canceled travel plans and instead stayed home for two months in Dublin, where she dreamed every night that she was still on set and sometimes woke up crying" (Buckley).

Filtering rape scenes or altering stories to reduce the traumatic impact they have on audiences and film artists, such as actors, might be done in ways that can preserve their integrity including viewers' exposure to the motivations and feelings prior to, during, and following an act of sexual violence. But one might argue that depending on the level of filtering, it can destroy the integrity of the scene by failing to reveal the truth of the sexual violent act between perpetrator to victim, leading to genuine feelings of empathy, compassion, etc. Trigger warnings for audience members is another alternative besides the rating system, which often does not provide explicit details regarding the level of violence, the nature of the rape, etc. Some audiences are even turning to streaming technologies such as VidAngel aimed at filtering certain scenes, e.g., sex and sexual images from films (despite not having permission to alter copyrighted material). Artistic freedom is important, but it should be balanced with monitoring the welfare of film artists and giving audiences the opportunities to make an informed decision about whether to view a film or not. Not only did *The Nightingale* have the required MPAA ratings: "Rated R for strong violent and disturbing content including rape, language throughout, and brief sexuality" but some sites such as IMDB.com have created parental guides that go into greater detail of the violence, gore, sex, and language.

Conclusion

This critical examination of the illness of sex in film and of those marginalized, victimized, and disembodied characters prompts advocacy and action toward a contemporary sexual revolution and a shift from the medicalization (and criminalization) of sex and illness to a more holistic understanding that challenges social norms and stigma and contextualizes sexual experiences and needs. The illness narrative of sex is broadly examined here, illustrating how it can be misunderstood within communities who victimize persons in need of care despite their sexual perversions and criminality, who create social barriers failing to see the capabilities and sexual needs of disabled persons, or who see sexual violence through a single lens or not at all due to filtering its reality.

The three chosen films, *Little Children*, *The Sessions*, and *The Nightingale* depict characters who are more than their clinical diagnoses, their disabilities, or their victimization; they are sufferers, and their emotional and physical suffering is further complicated with self-inflicted injury, emotional guilt, revenge, and anger. Some of the most unlikely relationships contribute to our characters' healing including a bully, a sex surrogate, and an Aboriginal guide. It is critical that we adopt a holistic understanding of persons as sexual beings without defining them by the illnesses (of sex) they experience, or the illness labels unjustly given to them by society and used for purposes of criminalization and marginalization. These films push audiences to see the characters as persons, to empathize with their plight, to recognize and critically evaluate society's standards of what is or is not "normal" about sexual behavior and desire, to break down structural and social barriers due to bias, ignorance, imbalance of power, or simply a lack of understanding and vision, and to promote justice. The concept of sex is complex, and how it is understood in clinical, legal, and social contexts as abnormal, unnatural, immoral, etc. ought not define the person who may or may not be ill.

Notes

1 Earle Haley played Freddy Krueger in the 2010 version of *A Nightmare on Elm Street* and has a talent for the macabre roles.

2 Interesting to note, Amy Kaufman (Los Angeles Times, 2012) writes about how the real Cheryl Cohen Greene ended her marriage with her first husband, Michael Cohen, who she had an open marriage with, and married her former client, Bob Greene. Cheryl had crossed professional boundaries with Bob, a Veteran who came to her for erectile issues, first by accepting an expensive gift (a camera) and then by starting a relationship.

Works cited

American Psychiatric Association. *Diagnostic and Statistical Manual of Mental Disorders*, 5th edition (DSM-5). Arlington, VA, American Psychiatric Association, 2013.

Anderson, Craig A. and Brad J. Bushman. "The Effects of Media Violence on Society." *Science*, vol. 295, no. 5564, 2002, pp. 2377–9.

Anderson Craig A., et al. "The Influence of Media Violence on Youth." *Psychol Sci Public Interest*, vol. 4, 2003, pp. 81–110.

Aultman, Julie. "The Diseased Embodied Mind: Constructing a Conception of Mental Disease in Relation to the Person." *Medicine, Health Care, and Philosophy*, vol. 13, 2010, pp. 321–32.

Bastién, Angelica Jade. "What Does It Mean for a Rape Scene to Be 'Done Well'?" *Vulture*, August 9, 2019, www.vulture.com/2019/08/rape-scenes-movies-nightingale-classic-hollywood.html. Accessed December 4, 2020.

Behrendt, Larissa. "The Nightingale Review – Ambitious, Urgent and Necessarily Brutal. But Who Is It For?" *The Guardian*, August 20, 2019, www.theguardian.com/film/2019/aug/20/the-nightingale-review-ambitious-urgent-and-necessarily-brutal-but-who-is-it-for. Accessed August 29, 2021.

Bleakley, Amy, Daniel Romer, and Patrick E. Jamieson. "Violent Film Characters' Portrayal of Alcohol, Sex, and Tobacco-Related Behaviors." *Pediatrics*, vol. 133, 2014, pp. 71–7.

Boorse, Christopher. "On the Distinction between Disease and Illness." *Philosophy and Public Affairs*, vol. 5, 1975, pp. 49–68.

Brown, Jane D. "Sexy Media Matter: Exposure to Sexual Content in Music, Movies, Television, and Magazines Predicts Black and White Adolescents' Sexual Behavior." *Pediatrics*, vol. 117, no. 4, 2006, pp. 1018–27.

Browne, Kevin D. and Catherine Hamilton-Giachritsis. "The Influence of Violent Media on Children and Adolescents: A Public-health Approach." *The Lancet*, vol. 365, no. 9460, 2005, pp. 702–10.

Buckley, Cara. "When Rape Onscreen is Directed by a Woman." *The New York Times*, August 2, 2019, www.nytimes.com/2019/08/02/movies/rape-film-nightingale.html. Accessed December 16, 2020.

Cline, Victor B, Roger G. Croft, and Steven Courrier. "Desensitization of Children to Television Violence." *Journal of Personality and Social Psychol*, vol. 27, no. 3, 1973, pp. 360–5.

Drescher, Jack. "Out of DSM: Depathologizing Homosexuality." *Behavioral Sciences*, vol. 5, no. 4, 2015, pp. 565–75.

Frank, Arthur W. *The Wounded Storyteller: Body, Illness, and Ethics*. Chicago, University of Chicago Press, 1995.

Gentile, Douglas A. *Media Violence and Children: A Complete Guide for Parents and Professionals*. Westport, CT: Praeger, 2003.

Gentile, Douglas A. "Are Motion Picture Ratings Reliable and Valid?" *Journal of Adolescent Health*, vol. 47, 2010, pp. 423–4.

Hale, Wanda. "Something Wild on Plaza Screen." *New York Daily News*, December 21, 1961, p. 171m, www.newspapers.com/clip/63831305/daily-news/. Accessed July 1, 2021.

Heller-Nicholas, Alexandra. *Rape-Revenge Films: A Critical Study*, North Carolina and London: McFarland, 2011.

Kaufman, Amy, "Sex, Love, Surrogacy and 'Sessions'." *Los Angeles Times*, November 6, 2012, https://web.archive.org/web/20140503060203/http://articles.latimes.com/2012/nov/26/entertainment/la-et-mn-sex-surrogates-sessions20121126/2.

Macek III, J. C. "Something Isn't Right with Criterion's Release of 'Something Wild'." *PopMatters*, 2, March 2017,www.popmatters.com/something-wild-jack-garfein-something-isnt-right-criterion-2495399164.html. Accessed July 1, 2021.

Miller, Julie. "Helen Hunt on Overcoming Inhibitions for The Sessions, the Difficulty of Playing a Real Person, and 'the Sexiest Quality There Is'." *Vanity Fair*, October 18, 2012, www.vanityfair.com/hollywood/2012/10/helen-hunt-the-sessions-interview. Accessed June 10, 2021.

Mullin, Charles R. and Daniel Linz. "Desensitization and Resensitization to Violence Against Women: Effects of Exposure to Sexually Violent Films on Judgments of Domestic Violence Victims." *Journal of Personality and Social Psychology*, vol. 69, no. 3, 1995, pp. 449–59.

Nagel, Thomas. 1969. "Sexual Perversion." *The Philosophy of Sex*, 4th edition, edited by Alan Soble. Lanham, MD, Rowman and Littlefield, 2002, pp. 9–20.

Nordenfelt, Lennart. *Health, Science and Ordinary Language*. Amsterdam, Rodopi, 2001.

Nordenfelt, Lennart. "Understanding the Concept of Health." 2007, www.fil.lu.se/HommageaWlodek/site/papper/NordenfeltLennart.pdf. Accessed January 3, 2019.

Nordenfelt, Lennart. "The Concepts of Health and Disease Revisited." *Medicine, Health Care and Philosophy*, Vol. 10, 2007, pp. 5–10.

O'Brien, Mark. "On Seeing a Sex Surrogate," *The Sun Magazine*, May 1990, www.thesunmagazine.org/issues/174/on-seeing-a-sex-surrogate. Accessed November 11, 2020.

O'Malley, Sheila. "*The Nightingale*, Roger Ebert Reviews." August 2, 2019, www.rogerebert.com/reviews/the-nightingale-2019. Accessed July 1, 2021.

Romer, Daniel, et al. "Parental Desensitization to Violence and Sex in Movies." *Pediatrics*, vol. 134, 2014, pp. 877–84.

Schaefer, Stephen. "Helen Hunt Was Mad about Sex Surrogate Role." *Boston Herald*, October 21, 2012. www.bostonherald.com/2012/10/21/helen-hunt-was-mad-about-sex-surrogate-role/. Accessed June 10, 2021.

Scott, A. O. "Playground Rules: No Hitting, No Sex." *New York Times*, September 29, 2006. www.nytimes.com/2006/09/29/movies/playground-rules-no-hitting-no-sex.html. Accessed August 29, 2021.

Thomas. Margaret H., et al. "Desensitization to Portrayals of Real-life Aggression as a Function of Exposure to Television Violence." *Journal of Personality and Social Psychol*, vol. 5, no. 6, 1977, pp. 450–8.

Thompson, Zoe Brigley and Sorcha Gunne. "Introduction – Feminism without Borders: The Potentials and Pitfalls of Re-theorizing Rape." *Feminism, Literature, and Rape Narratives: Violence and Violation*, edited by Sorcha Gunne and Zoe Brigley. Thompson. New York and Abingdon, Routledge, 2010, pp. 1–22.

Vickers, Neil. "Narrative Identity and Illness." *Journal of Evaluation in Clinical Practice*, vol. 18, no. 5, 2012, pp. 1070–1.

Weidmann, Anke, et al. "Using Stressful Films to Analyze Risk Factors for PTSD in Analogue Experimental Studies which Film Works Best?" *Anxiety, Stress and Coping*, vol. 22, no. 5, 2009, pp. 549–69.
Wilson, Wayne. "Rape as Entertainment." *Psychological Reports*, vol. 63, 1988, pp. 607–10.
Yuan, Jada. "John Hawkes on His Standing-Ovation-Worthy Sundance Film, *The Surrogate*." *New York Magazine*, 2012, www.vulture.com/2012/01/john-hawkes-on-his-standing-ovation-worthy-sundance-film-the-surrogate.html, Accessed December 12, 2020.

12

"STEREOTYPES," FOCALIZATION AND MODALITY

Mainstream cinematic images of disability

Nigel Morris

Context: the last liberation movement

The complex role film plays in the evolving development of disability politics remains controversial and increasingly contentious. Many scholars and activists assert that disability – treated as a single issue – is underrepresented in mainstream movies. While some statistical truth undergirds this claim, given that 20 percent of the population are disabled according to official definitions (longevity of previously non-disabled people in wealthy countries balancing lower life expectancy of people with impairments in poorer economies),[1] there is and has been no shortage of disability representations on screen, particularly when compared with other minority groups such as women in classical cinema, racial and ethnic communities, and LGBTQ+ characters. Countless movies have portrayed disabilities, grounded in impairments of different kinds and degrees experienced individually across the full range of other identities. Often when writing about these movies, activists strenuously object to what they term "stereotypes." But many of these critiques seem determined to homogenize that richness of experiences into simplistic categories approved or, more often, rejected as false to the genuine experience of disability, as if such a unified entity exists. This categorization, paradoxically based on a fundamental mistrust of categorization of people, is a self-fulfilling reduction. It arises out of well-intentioned desires to address widespread injustices as if they are common to all people with impairments – rather than to celebrate the richness and diversity they wish to honor. I believe, as I illustrate below, that the most effective way to counter these reductive tendencies is to scrutinize films which generally do not represent disabilities in such standardized ways and to demonstrate that these examples are not exceptional.

Disability politics – "The last liberation movement," according to sociologist and bioethicist Tom Shakespeare (*Disability: The Basics* 144) – in many ways echoes earlier (and ongoing) equal rights campaigns concerning race, gender, and sexuality. What the Creative Industries Policy and Evidence Centre (2021) calls "presence, prominence and portrayal" (https://pec.ac.uk) are complexly interconnected yet methodologically separate

DOI: 10.4324/9781003007661-16

issues too often simplistically and impressionistically linked in struggles that involve screen representations. Certainly historian Paul Longmore (1985), among others, has correlated disabled people's emergent "socio-political consciousness" with increasingly favorable screen characterizations (133). Yet respect for diversity, both onscreen and beyond, contrasts with medical commitments to rectifying anomalies. This contradiction, which people affected by disabilities negotiate daily, rigidifies when condemnations of objectification confront scientific rationality. Separate sociological and medical understandings of disability cause methods and discourses of film theory and cultural criticism, popular reviewing, and audiences' actual or imputed responses to clash with each other. Real-life dilemmas and paradoxes inform cinematic representations and criticism alike, but competing priorities and strategies can stoke disagreement, while irreconcilable experiences and interdisciplinary agendas exacerbate confusion.

Let me quickly acknowledge that direct effects of single films are rarely demonstrable: production schedules lag behind social attitudes, as media scholar Martin F. Norden highlights (107). Yet their combined recirculation of dominant ideas is clearly a factor in our perception of both people and the circumstances they inhabit. Films that radically challenge common worldviews often elicit displeasure and result in commercial failure, while familiar characters and situations endorse widespread beliefs. Nevertheless, claims that movies' "powerful influence" *perpetuates* negativity (Norden 7, 8) may be exaggerated, even if some individual examples are objectionable. That "historical tendencies … led to numerous socio-cultural influences" today (11) is inconclusive – "led to" means "preceded" or "prefigured" beside "continued into" or "caused." Shakespeare tempers such generalizations appropriately: "high status disabled people were sometimes very successful," while "venerated people in myth and legend" had impairments (*Disability: The Basics* 26). That said, however, inadequate postulations about attitude construction reproduce misunderstandings of communication and inadvertently perpetuate prejudice. This chapter contextualizes such assumptions, proposes moving beyond them, and considers a contemporary illustration.

Definitions, scope, and focus

Multitudinous impairments underlie disability: physical, mental; perceptual, motor; visible, invisible; congenital, acquired; permanent, temporary; debilitating, differently manageable; degenerative, stable; variously distressing; at different or all life stages. Important, as well, are institutional factors and roles within popular culture. Thus, fundamental to representation is visibility through inclusion. Theater access and facilities for people with limited mobility; discounts for carers; signing for Deaf people; captions and induction loops for hearing impaired moviegoers; verbal description for those visually impaired; and autism-friendly screenings: all foster community. Cultural identification potentially encourages more disabled people into a notoriously closed production industry, arguably to influence worldviews projected. Nevertheless, personality, background, beliefs, relationships, aspirations, and opportunities complicate outwardly similar situations.

Representation of differences embraces different definitions. One is that individuals "stand for" groups – a character might illustrate an entire minority. So, for example, *Whose Life Is It Anyway?* (Badham 1981), released against a backdrop of concerns around escalating costs of providing care, allegedly implies suicide's preferability to quadriplegia, as does the popular, lauded *Million Dollar Baby* (Eastwood 2004). *The Sea Inside* (Amenábar 2004), about the first Spaniard assisted legally to die, examines effects on close acquaintances, setting religion against human rights. Another biopic, *The Diving-Bell and the Butterfly* (Schnabel 2007), portrays French writer Jean-Dominique Bauby's life-affirming experience despite suffering through locked-in syndrome. *The Theory of Everything* (Marsh 2014) celebrates Stephen Hawking's achievements notwithstanding his degenerative illness.

Representations can metaphorize, appear neutral (unmarked aspects of characterization or performer), or advocate for all people with disabilities or those with specific conditions. Generalization, however, requires caution. No definitive representation encapsulates any condition. Considerations involving films include a sense of accordance with reality. Aside from common subjection to discrimination – crucial for movies to tackle – diversity multiplies dramatic possibilities. Conversely, minority filmmakers, held accountable for perceptions of their social category, implicitly bear a burden of representation – restricting them to pertinent topics. Yet a mainstream entertainment, *Silver Bullet* (Attias 1985), tacitly fails for not explaining why its hero uses a wheelchair (Norden 296): disability apparently requires justification. In the statistical sense, merely including more disabled characters in secondary roles or as extras, without necessarily dramatizing their experience every time, would normalize their social presence and overcome tendencies for them to be – as 1980s feminists argued women on screen generally were – muted, sidelined, or omitted. That said, the striking prevalence of disabled protagonists and popularity of movies featuring them question the efficacy of transcribing principles and assumptions between different minority activisms. Statistical usage sometimes overlaps the Media Theory concept "representation": how signs make meanings. Mediating technology does not automatically capture truth but communicates interpretations: within economic, cultural, and political determinants; for defined audiences; amid medium-specific constraints; serving ideological functions.

Disagreements complicate, yet can often enrich, understanding: within scholarship, Marxist-influenced "materialist" investigations; "critical realism," embracing qualitative autoethnography to acknowledge researchers' individual experiences, unlike traditional academic claims to objectivity; and Humanities-based "critical disability studies" (Shakespeare, *Disability: The Basics* 158–9), with which this chapter broadly aligns. Many activists and advocates question non-disabled actors playing disabled characters, likened to blackface or to inauthentic drag falsifying communication between stigmatized "insiders" (Siebers 115). Nevertheless, actors almost always play people different from themselves: Lionel Barrymore, Herbert Marshall, Ronald Reagan, Esmond Knight, Hugo Weaving, and Bill Nighy perform roles that ignore their impairments, of which audiences may be unaware – respectively: hip fracture and arthritis, permanently necessitating wheelchair mobility; leg amputation; hearing loss; severe visual impairment; epilepsy; and Dupuytren's Contracture, a progressive deformity of the fingers. Casting entails finding the best available performers for any given production, but disagreement concerns who that is. In *Stalag 17* (Wilder 1953), a non-professional employed for his missing leg (essential narratively although his character served little other function) spoke no lines. However, a real-life World War II veteran (Harold Russell) with artificial hands took an Oscar-winning role in *The Best Years of Our Lives* (Wyler 1946). Acquired impairment narratives often compare "before and after," one actor portraying both. Commercial imperatives demanded that *Born on the Fourth of July* (Stone 1989) needed Tom Cruise as paraplegic Vietnam War veteran, Ron Kovic. Granted Shakespeare's acknowledgement that certain occupations are incompatible with some impairments (*Disability: The Basics* 6, 20, 30), could anyone with severe cerebral palsy sustain the ability and possess the sheer physical stamina necessary to play painter Christy Brown as Daniel Day-Lewis managed in *My Left Foot* (Sheridan 1989)? Could someone with learning difficulties, autism, and attention deficit perform as Sean Penn did in *I Am Sam* (Nelson 2001), having learned from people with impairments, acting alongside two (playing characters, not themselves)? Could any disabled soldier perform as Marlon Brando did, living with paraplegic veterans before appearing with 45 of them in *The Men* (Zinnemann 1950)? All these performances garnered critical accolades that compounded discomfort for some commentators on disability.

However, criticism that "Academy Award winners ... are received (and hailed) as representing 'true' disability experience" (Chivers and Markotic 5) oversimplifies this complex situation: "[W]hat constitutes misrepresentation or correct representation is fraught with the impossible determination of reality" (Kim 150). Conscious illusion recognizes Day-Lewis, Cruise – or Jane Wyman depicting a mute character unable to speak in *Johnny Belinda* (Negulesco 1948), the physically and mentally vulnerable Laura in *The Glass Menagerie* (Rapper 1950), or a woman blinded by the protagonist's carelessness in *Magnificent Obsession* (Sirk 1954). Some criticism compounds social disability – the disabled "community's" experience (although many refuse definition by impairment) – with implied interchangeability. Thus Nicholas Ray's monocular vision supposedly helped utilize his "experiences" to represent blindness in *On Dangerous Ground* (1951) (Norden 208); actually, impaired depth perception and distance judgment are incomparable with congenital blindness lacking visual memory. Conversely, nobody without achondroplasia could, discounting unnecessary CGI, play characters with restricted growth as Peter Dinklage does; yet increased respect for difference means he undertakes roles where disability is marginal, even irrelevant – or should be, as his characters remark (Figure 12.1).

Shakespeare laments that critical disability studies reduces experience to discourse (*Disability Rights* 52–3). Nonetheless discourse – including cinematic codes – establishes mindsets. Consider sociologist Robert Bogdan's once appropriate title: "The Exhibition of People We Now Call Mentally Retarded" (119). Codes defining disability assume deviance: "de-formed, dis-eased, dis-abled, dis-ordered, ab-normal, and most telling ... in-valid" (qtd. Norden 12). Nowadays, "person with disabilities" stresses individuality, yet "*people-first* language" arguably trivializes disability as "contingent add-on" (Shildrick 42). Shakespeare qualifies the slogan "disability is no tragedy": "it's not just an irrelevant difference" and can cause more "misery and suffering than the average human should have to endure" (*Disability: The Basics* 22, 49).

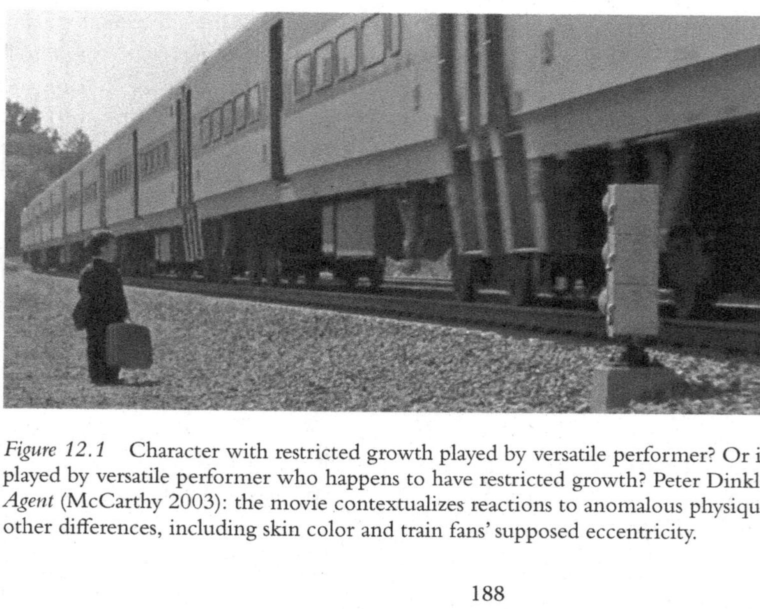

Figure 12.1 Character with restricted growth played by versatile performer? Or intriguing character played by versatile performer who happens to have restricted growth? Peter Dinklage in *The Station Agent* (McCarthy 2003): the movie contextualizes reactions to anomalous physique among attitudes to other differences, including skin color and train fans' supposed eccentricity.

"Disabled person" embraces "disabled by society": preconceptions and inadequate adjustments exacerbate impairment.

An infamous example concretizes such concerns. Benshoff and Griffin survey pre-cinematic othering of "people with congenital impairments and/or other physical anomalies." Freak shows "*sometimes* exhibited" these for audiences "to laugh, jeer, pity, or otherwise be entertained"; early cinema "*sometimes*" analogously "frighten[ed] or titillate[d]" (363, emphases added). Assumed responses to spectacles where context, address, and possibly unease, were crucial suggest diverse perceptions. "Freak" described a purveyed image, not the person. (Bogdan recounts a showman asking a tall student, "How would you like to be a giant?" [3].) Bogdan's research and reactions to *Freaks* (Browning 1932), demonstrate historical contingency. Cruelty often exacerbated impairment, as *The Elephant Man* (Lynch 1980) with John Hurt as the highly disfigured but gentle and artistic John Merrick recalls. Yet many exhibits were affluent entrepreneurs, controlling their careers, and scarcity of "people with anomalies strange enough to make them a premier attraction" (38) commanded favorable terms. Promotional strategies made some "upstanding, high-status," with "achievements, talents, family, and physiology" variously "fabricated, elevated or exaggerated" (Bogdan 108). For example, fame and patronage made Charles Stratton ("Tom Thumb") an international celebrity and socialite; his wife Lavinia Warren, reputedly the world's most photographed woman, hosted Civil War generals, the Astors and the Vanderbilts. Acceptance into showmen's values and argot othered such people more than physiology. *Freaks*, initiated by the "short-statured actor" portraying Hans (Norden 115), punishes not "normals" indiscriminately – only disrespectful co-performers.

Spuriously scientific or educational presentations pre-echoed film. Socially disabling objectification and staring, reinforcing inequalities, underlie anxieties around exploitative entertainment. The "pit show" – where *Freaks'* villainess ends – literally abjects. So, too, in other films, when adventitiously impaired characters flounder on the ground, do temporary metaphorical abasements, particularly following loss of legs or their use: in *Fourth of July*; by WW2 heroes Ted Lawson (Van Johnson) in *Thirty Seconds Over Tokyo* (LeRoy 1944), Monty Stratton (James Stewart) in *The Stratton Story* (Wood 1949), John Hoskins (Sterling Hayden) in *The Eternal Sea* (Auer 1955) and Douglas Bader (Kenneth More) in *Reach for the Sky* (Gilbert 1956); as well as fictional Long John Silver (Robert Newton) in *Treasure Island* (Haskin 1950), psychologically traumatized Tommy (Roger Daltrey) in *Tommy* (Russell 1975), paralyzed sculptor Ken (Richard Dreyfuss) in *Whose Life...?*, wounded veteran Captain Dan (Gary Synise) in *Forrest Gump* (Zemeckis 1994), and sea life park trainer Stéphanie (Marion Cotillard) in *Rust and Bone* (Audiard 2012), who loses her legs to a killer whale. As Bogdan concludes of attitudes to freaks, discomfort, exacerbated by terminology, expresses how "social institutions managed these people's identities" (x).

Hostility to freakshows, Bogdan insists, stemmed not from exhibition of anomalous people but from "deception and stealing" that showmen encouraged (81). Twentieth-century medicalization then discredited even "fashionable and most legitimate" shows (62). Simultaneously, welfare programs countered fraud with quantifiable clinical definitions, and eugenics drove "counselling, sterilization, and incarceration," despite the fact that many with congenital abnormalities produce healthy offspring. Formerly "benign and interesting," freaks were now considered inferior, pitiable, threatening, needing prevention and cure (62–4). Neutral terminology (designating freak occurrences) became derogatory. Institutional scrutiny supplanted public gaze, and individuals, reduced to diagnoses, lost agency in their presentation. Simultaneously, cinema's increasing respectability meant movies featuring "oddities" failed. Fifty years on, *The Elephant Man* changed that. Valorizing benign medicalization, it re-explores familiar territory through Joseph Merrick's transition from abasement to aggrandizement, challenging audiences to question their fascination and its makers'.

Freaks begins: "Never again will such a story be filmed, as modern science and teratology is rapidly eliminating such blunders of nature." This *The Greatest Showman* (Gracey 2017) belies. Its disabled characters are vocal among minorities previously marginalized, underrepresented, objectified, patronized, or vilified. They queer disability, sex, class, race, gender, sexuality, and nationality against puritanism and intolerance, singing "This is Me" – not *Us*, as *Freaks* insisted. Yet they require permission from a white, socially mobile, patriarchal, American Dreamer, P. T. Barnum (Hugh Jackman) whose perspective renders them massed others, albeit internally differentiated. Whether journeying from abjection to pride is progressive (mainstream acceptance) or regressive (visibility conditional on confidence trickery, crusading, patronage, and supporting player status) remains moot. American belief in "positive mental outlook … therapies, psychologies, and sects" continues, whereby " 'successful' handicapped people" exemplify "personal adjustment, striving, and achievement," while "individualistic claptrap" coopts disability (Longmore 139; 257).

Problems with "stereotyping"

A "stereotype" is "a group concept," often irrational, held by a social group about a social group; imposing "simple structure," it "frequently conceals complexity" (Perkins 80). A dubious metaphor, its claims usually evaporate once uttered. The term can be omitted without loss. "Stereotypes" supposedly are objective, thoughtlessly applied, inherently false, and harmful. Unexamined dogmas – that "stereotypes" are fully-formed, immediate, consistent – preempt comprehension of image functioning. Ideas Perkins challenged persist: that "stereotypes" necessarily denigrate, categorize other (usually minority/oppressed) groups, are unchanging and influence attitudes. Kneejerk indignation inculcates superiority and immunity, compounding inequalities that struggles over representation express. Martin Barker, although affirming arguments "stereotyping" claims support, terms it "useless," even "dangerous," for understanding media texts (89). Consider O'Sullivan and Jewkes' reference to "use of stereotypes to put across information" in "shorthand and easily decoded form" (Qualter Introduction 154). "Use of" implies selection from available templates. Yet every representation is constructed. "Stereotypes" are concepts, not relayed signs. Emphasis on form sidelines response, context, and medium specificity. "Decoded" implies ideas "encoded": wrapped up. Receivers unwrap them. Absent is the framework integral to process models, usually incorporating feedback. Representations, rather than imposed, *circulate*. Despite being editors of a Media Studies book, acknowledging that "assumptions" about "stereotypes" are "questionable," O'Sullivan and Jewkes refer to "the recipient group" (Perkins Introduction 75). Accordingly, common sense assumes influence, while psychology, measuring behavior, reinforces assertions that films "convey" "messages" (Norden 4).

Audiences may not recognize particular "stereotypes." Cataloging subjective, indefinable beliefs supposedly widely shared, paradoxically not by oneself, consolidates them. Labeling, useful heuristically to make distinctions and identify tendencies, constructs or perpetuates the representation and mindset purportedly explained. *Synecdoche* (part for whole; one image representing a classification) conflates with *metonymy* (attributed qualities). Synecdoche highlights a character's disability; metonymy imposes expectations. Confirmation bias encourages selection bias, impeding evaluation of discrete representations and their components. Among humanly diverse disabled characters, *some* are "angry and obnoxious, wallowing in self-pity and unwilling to take responsibility"; noticing three implies a pattern – thereafter visible if sought. Subsequent writers amplify Longmore's generalization, questionable originally, untrue now: "disabled people are inevitably shown" thus (123). Identifying disability "stereotypes," as Benshoff and Griffin (after Norden) do with "fake cripple," "Sweet Innocent," "Saintly Sage," "Noble Warrior," and "Tragic Victim," implicitly renders retrospective classifications current and objective. Application to contemporary output is disingenuous – as with the "particular (and particularly nasty) … Obsessive Avenger" "stereotype" that, "although attitudes … have changed," shapes "every *Phantom of the Opera* remake" (365). Obsessive avengers are *not* exclusively disabled.

Representations also associate villainy with physical disability: impairment entails "loss of self-control" (Longmore 135). If selfhood holistically embraces the body, disability's definition includes this. Everyone dreads losing control. "Triumph over tragedy" narratives are no more concerned with challenges associated with disability than with intensifying human stories that reinforce ideological imperatives to be determined, proactive, and self-reliant. Meanwhile villains, imposing *their* control, elicit fear. Moreover the small incidence of congenital impairments (Shakespeare, *Disability: The Basics* 50) contributes to mystery, associated with widespread mistrust of difference. As Bogdan reports a child observing, you know villains are bad because they appear different (vii). They do not represent actual people any more than James Bond is real.

Snyder and Mitchell contend "disabled bodies" threaten "integrity of the able body. … Bodies are subjugated to [audience's] worst fears of vulnerability, and/or the already disabled body is scripted out of control" (186). Yet they stress *Forrest Gump*'s Captain Dan climbing into his wheelchair, deftly, in control. Insistence that this allows "opportunity to stare at the dynamics of a physical transition we rarely witness" and "marvel at the special effects" (179) overlooks an editing illusion beyond momentary levitation with legs digitally erased; cutting to Gump elides the transition – implausible like the entire film. The example triply marginalizes disability: a non-disabled actor performs impossibility, offscreen. Snyder and Mitchell describe not "stereotypes" but "scripted social formulas" and "visual shorthand," nevertheless unquantifiable (189). As with genre, no research embraces all examples. Recognizing tendencies, though, educated hunches, permits exploration. Yet suspicion of misrepresentation does not need "stereotyping" to explain what is wrong or how to rectify it.

Naming "stereotypes" rather than explicating processes or trends that representations uphold demands logical contortions. Qualities of the "impoverished, orthopedically impaired" Porgy (Sidney Poitier) in *Porgy and Bess* (Preminger 1959) distinguish that hero's "more resonant character" from "the standard Sweet Innocent"; "he's an adult black male who conspicuously avoids the passivity so long associated with the stereotype" (Norden 212). Evading what constitutes this "stereotype" means that a construct implicating simplified mental association simultaneously evokes rich connotations. So flexible is "stereotyping" that Norden identifies "new" ones (307), references three "modernized if widely varying versions of the Sweet Innocent" (229) and observes in *Cutter's Way* (Passer 1981) the protagonist's "embodiment of two stereotypes" (275). Longmore spots in a TV show another "stereotype" – "mitigated and complicated" because she champions disability rights (143). Concerning *Whose Life…?*," Darke explains that medicalization assumes normality to which bodies should conform; problems result from "corporeal deviance, not … social perception of deformity and disease." Darke continues: "despite social change, the archetypal and stereotypical persist" (97) – without explicating "change," "archetypes," "stereotypes," or persistence. He claims the quadriplegic protagonist is effeminized. Yet flirting and sexual banter to an extent nowadays considered abusive as well as an erotic fantasy flashback characterize Ken against emotional, sexualized women. Darke contrasts a "stereotypical WASP" doctor with her male adversary whose darker skin evidences an "additional stereotype ... that constructs certain ethnicities as evil" – confirming how "stereotypes ... are often interdependent and/or work interdependently" (98, 99). This might persuade without the African-Caribbean orderly Ken befriends. While "disability oppression includes gender, race, sexuality and class" (Kim 147), inconceivably multi-faceted "stereotyping" muddies how "The film problematically uses disability ... to examine medicalization" (Darke 99).

"Sweet Innocents" are "constructed as undeserving" their "disease or genetic condition" (Benshoff and Griffin 368). Who then *is* deserving? Why? *How* are they "constructed"? That "moviemakers found" this characterization "most serviceable ... for perpetuating beliefs about physically disabled people" (Norden 35) confuses intention, effect, and function. That "Sweet Innocents" – alongside "Saintly Sages" (370) – are "almost saint-like" (Benshoff and Griffin 369) betrays hesitancy. *Are* they "saint-like"? When a character suffers "ableist and homophobic slurs (offered unfortunately by another disabled person)" the parenthesis assumes disabled persons should be (Norden 237). Shakespeare's claim that "Negative images and attitudes about disability derive from a range of stereotypes" (*Disability: The Basics* 77) – provides occasion for pause. Narratology categorizes around eight character types. Disabled characters, among whom Norden identifies five further categories, thus appear comparatively diverse, yet they match non-disabled characters: in *The Birth of a Nation* (Griffith 1915), "Obsessive Avenger" describes Colonel Cameron (Henry Walthall) *and* Silas Lynch (George Seigmann); "Sweet Innocent," Little Sister (Flora Cameron); "Saintly Sage," Abraham Lincoln (Jos. Hanebery), with Elsie Stoneman (Lillian Gish) saintly if less sagacious. Both sides' officers are "Noble Warriors"; almost everyone, "Tragic Victim."

Benshoff and Griffin unwittingly affirm diversity: disabled characters evoke "sympathy and/or victimization" *and* "violence, sagacity, and/or tragedy" (363). That increasingly these represent "living and breathing" humans, sharing "joys and sorrows of so-called 'normal' or able-bodied people" (363), does not require "stereotyping." Shakespeare overloads disquiet about "bitter" villains who "associate disability with negativity," generating "fear and hostility from non-disabled viewers" (*Disability: The Basics* 77). This implies that disabled viewers, notwithstanding diverse impairments, respond uniformly. Non-disabled viewers, accordingly, would not despise non-disabled villains. Unwarranted assumption that spectators identify with their like, however loosely determined, denies textual positioning. *Psycho* (Hitchcock 1960), portraying a criminal woman and a man with dissociative identity disorder, would fail for males and anyone without psychosis. Feminist male gaze theory would be untenable.

Rejecting caricature does not necessitate shortcutting how and why representations offend. When "Saintly Sage" "bleeds into the social perception that blind people are gifted 'seers'" (Benshoff and Griffin 369), imprecise "stereotypes" *solidify* representations, and "stereotypes" become "social perceptions." Shakespeare reports suspected "sham cripples" among American Civil War veterans (*Disability: The Basics* 34). These concerns addressed begging, not disability. That films rendered "such character types" (Benshoff and Griffin 364) comedic did not "stereotype": their *non*-disability was the point – invalidating claims they perpetuated a "generations-old" "suspicion or fear" of disabled people (364). Mendicancy laws exempted disabled ex-servicemen (Norden 7). Disability in the 1890s was widely visible; other reasons underlay taking false representation seriously. While "stereotypes" often imply intellectual inferiority (Perkins 83), here dupes – including unpopular police – not perpetrators were ridiculed; narratives exploited anxieties concerning deception. "Stereotype" terminology reifies, without elucidating, conflation and confusion.

"Things hav[ing] changed" since freak shows, "stereotypical images," Benshoff and Griffin reiterate, "linger"; "anomalies" are "staples of mystery and horror films, while acquired disability" is "foundational" in "war movies" (363). Genre noted, they examine differences, but "elements," inseparable from mood, tone, and purpose, including offensive aspects, do not require homogenization. Genres evolve *and* repeat. Historical representations do not necessarily influence contemporary injustices.

One "stereotype" maintains that "poverty somehow causes disability" (Benshoff and Griffin 363). Correlation is undeniable: employers' prejudices, lower productivity, workplace inaccessibility, unequal or interrupted education, inadequate medicine, punitive welfare regulations, workers quitting to become carers, and class (dangerous employment in factories, mines, construction, and armed forces) compound disadvantage. "Somehow" misleads: inverting "effect into cause" resolves "contradiction" in oppressed groups' socialization, as Perkins argued (83). The World Health Organization reports poorer people's increased impairments and disabled people's greater risk of poverty (Shakespeare, *Disability: The Basics* 8, 91). Variously disabled characters in immediately recollected movies nevertheless overwhelmingly counter any such "stereotype": a wealthy doctor's widow, blinded by the irresponsible playboy (Rock Hudson) who killed her husband, regains sight after he self-funds surgical training to cure her himself in *Magnificent Obsession*; wheelchair users such as press baron *Citizen Kane* (Orson Welles) (Welles 1941), oil mogul General Sternwood (Charles Waldron) in *The Big Sleep* (Hawks 1946), financier Potter (Lionel Barrymore) in *It's a Wonderful Life* (Capra 1946), Presidential advisor *Doctor Strangelove* (Kubrick 1964), automotive tycoon "Number One" (Laurence Olivier) in *The Betsy* (Petrie 1978), and the Dude's (Jeff Bridges) millionaire namesake, *The Big Lebowski* (Coen 1998); Henry Fonda's railroad-building boss-turned-adversary (Gabriele Ferzetti) whose coach is adapted to help him walk in *Once Upon a Time in the West* (Leone 1968); a blind tourist seer (Hilary Mason) in *Don't Look Now* (Roeg 1973); an autistic gambling wizard and inheritor of millions (Dustin Hoffman) in *Rain Man* (Levinson 1988); *Hook*'s amputee pirate captain (Dustin Hoffman) (Spielberg 1991); bipolar or stuttering monarchs (Nigel Hawthorne and Colin Firth respectively) in *The Madness of King George* (Hytner 1994) and *The King's Speech* (Hooper 2010); numerous Bond villains physically stigmatized; orthopedically impaired Bella (Gina McKee) among *Notting Hill*'s bright young things (Michell 1999); blind music star *Ray* (Jamie Foxx) (Hackford 2004); physically- and intellectually-impaired Howard Hughes (Leonardo di Caprio) in *The Aviator* (Scorsese 2004); a magazine director capable of moving only one eyelid after a massive stroke (Mathieu Amalric) in *The Diving-Bell...*; *Iron Man*, a millionaire inventor (Robert Downey Jr.) who overcomes massive injury (Favreau 2008); *Avatar*'s protagonist (Sam Worthington), who – "vet benefits" rendering spinal surgery unaffordable – serves an advanced military-industrial complex (Cameron 2009); the world's most famous academic played by Eddie Redmayne in *The Theory of Everything*, surrounded by "personal assistants" and research "technology" (Shakespeare, *Disability: The Basics* 48) while becoming progressively paralyzed; *Untouchable*'s millionaire quadriplegic (François Cluzet) (Nakache and Toledano 2011); and a former linguistics professor – *Still Alice* (Julianne Moore) despite early onset Alzheimer's (Glatzer and Westmoreland 2014).

Exaggerated make up means *The Da Vinci Code*'s (Howard 2006) assassin (Paul Bettany), gunmen (Neil and Adrian Rayment) in *The Matrix Reloaded* (Wachowski 2003) and Voldemort (Ralph Fiennes) from *Harry Potter* (Columbus 2001) share pallidity. Rather than signifying disability – these characters lack other symptoms of albinism, notably visual impairment – aberration enhances their difference from society: paleness alongside villainy reverberates with, yet reverses, Nazi notions of Aryan superiority. "Stereotyping," which explains correlations of appearance with villainy, presupposes stock characters, automatically discounting other roles that might tackle challenges interestingly. Yet "fair" connotes both justice and beauty. In *Blade Runner* (Scott 1982), complexion exemplifies complexity and contradiction. Pale, white-haired replicant Roy Batty (Rutger Hauer) is hardly one-dimensional. Villainous from the protagonist's perspective, this super-powerful visionary achieves martyrdom, replete with religious symbolism, by fulfilling fate and redeeming his intended assassin. While his outward appearance signals impairment, he, railing against his minority's life-expectancy, is neither disabled nor real. Tom Hanks's AIDS sufferer in *Philadelphia* (Demme 1993), appearing similarly, signifies direct association with death, embodying real fears the movie challenges.

The Usual Suspects' (Singer 1995) "fake cripple" narrator, Verbal Kint (Kevin Spacey), pretending he is not prime mover, villain, and protagonist, proffers no claims about actual disabilities. Generosity, bravery, and wise utterances make Forrest Gump (Tom Hanks) "Sweet Innocent" *and* "Saintly Sage," but "stereotypes" cannot explicate rewritten history or Gump's unremitting success despite low IQ, even shedding orthotic calipers through willpower. *Reach for the Sky*, once Britain's most popular film – its epigraph calling real-life "Noble Warrior" double amputee Bader inspirational – is "an albatross round the neck of every [British] person ... conditioned to believe that it would take unadulterated heroism to cope with their disability" (qtd. Karpf 120). "Inspiring" – which victim-blames those who cannot "cheerfully 'overcom[e]'" impairments – downplays social disablement, Longmore explains (129–30). Inspirational examples disavow that most lives involving disability are "not filled with dramatic accomplishments" (qtd. Norden 222), but that describes non-disabled people too. "Stereotyping" – invoking an assumed category, not exceptions – stifles debate.

Objections to "Tragic Victim" forget that victimhood rationalizes misfortune. "Victim" is acceptable terminology when someone else's incompetence or neglect – especially governmental or corporate – causes impairment. It describes a *role*, not an individual or a generalized image, and, in certain circumstances, how some disabled persons consider themselves or advocates present them. Bauby calls his life-changing "suffering" (78) "monstrous, iniquitous, revolting, horrible" (79). Depression, sometimes suicidal, frequently follows impairment. Yet "quality of life returns" (Shakespeare, *Disability: The Basics* 47, 136); the "so-called 'disability paradox'" (46) renders life "as good as, or sometimes better than, that of non-disabled people" (122).

Mentally, sometimes physically, traumatized "Obsessive Avengers" abound. Common traits, which "stereotype" requires, hardly exist. Some are heroes; others villainous; many ambiguous. All lack the ability to function socially, but also most lack explicitly acknowledged medical impairments. Examples include John Wayne's battle-scarred Confederate veteran in *The Searchers* (Ford 1956); a childhood abuse survivor turned serial murderer (Carl Boehm) in *Peeping Tom* (Powell 1960); a conscientious objector driven to vigilantism (Charles Bronson) in *Death Wish* (Winner 1974); Travis Bickle (Robert De Niro) in *Taxi Driver* (Scorsese 1976) and John Rambo (Sylvester Stallone) in *First Blood* (Kotcheff 1982), unappreciated Vietnam veterans whose psychological troubles undermine values of the culture that trained them; Darth Vader (David Prowse), kept alive with cyborg prosthetics after light-saber injuries in *Star Wars* (Lucas 1977); Fred Kreuger (Robert Englund) in *A Nightmare on Elm Street* (Craven 1984), whose badly burned reincarnation explicitly embodies other characters' collective fantasy; "The Bride" (Uma Thurman) in *Kill Bill* (Tarantino 2003), already an assassin before eliminating former accomplices; anti-fascist freedom fighter "V" (Hugo Weaving) in *V for Vendetta* (McTeigue 2005), whose mask obscures facial burning; any Batman film, in which the hero, fighting for justice, is motivated similarly to his adversaries; and Amy (Rosamund Pike) in *Gone Girl* (Fincher 2014) whose ruthless manipulation of others stems from insecurities induced by her upbringing.

Unease rests upon assumption that categorizing humans is inherently wrong, while attributing "*individual physical or personality traits*" to groups (Barker 89) self-perpetuates an academic industry around unsustainable theory. Misguidedly, " 'Stereotyping' dissolves all sense of social organization. In protesting against category-inclusions, it dissolves all categories" (89), thereby obscuring structural inequalities. Assertions that "media etc should 'reflect' society" compound problems. Accusers complain when inequalities are represented other than as desired, even if truthfully. This Barker considers reasonable, but then " 'stereotype' has disappeared as a criterion" (86). Slipperiness makes empirical studies unreliable. Visual metaphors – "images," "representations," mental "pictures," distorted "perceptions" – posit thinking as mediation of reality, accordingly falsified, and equate mental with audio-visual representations. "Positive group-images" bolster "collective self-defense," Barker stresses. This contradicts condemnation of "stereotyping" because of categorization itself rather than objection to "content of a certain category" (87). As with *Reach for the Sky*, positivity can also exacerbate inappropriate expectations and role modeling, as when denying welfare to people arbitrarily deemed work-capable. Concerning "triumph over tragedy," recall that movies, including *The Diving-Bell…*, *Greatest Showman*, *I Am Sam*, *The King's Speech*, *Theory of Everything*, and *Sex and Drugs and Rock and Roll* (Whitecross 2010) – about punk star Ian Dury (Andy Serkis), bullied in childhood after contracting polio and who released a song protesting what he considered patronizing motivation behind 1981's International Year of Disabled Persons – generally prioritize exceptionality. Furthermore, superheroes embrace impairments, as in *Iron Man* and *X-Men* (Singer 2000) franchises. *Reach for the Sky* does not consider disability "a problem of emotional coping, of personal acceptance" – Bader handles this – but rather recognizes how "social stigma and discrimination" (Longmore 139) delayed heroic opportunities. Such narratives temper Chivers and Markotic's generalizations that onscreen disabilities metaphorize "emotional and spiritual deficiency" or characters "unable to [advance the plot]" (2). Disabilities often kindle, at least do not suppress, protagonists' talents, mostly in congenial or privileged environments. A possible result is to stigmatize disabled people who, like most individuals, lack similar determination, competitiveness, creativity, or enterprise, beside opportunity. Unclear is what "stereotyping" accusations add, even while some activists' "super crip" label (Shakespeare, *Disability: The Basics* 77–8) expresses unease.

Quantifying categories assumes frequency of encountering them magnifies their effects. Subtlety, complexity, and constructive contradiction are preempted. Checking boxes confirms expectations, consolidating inequalities that discussion could expose. Recurrent representations are facets of storytelling, subject to conventions best explored and challenged individually. Chivers and Markotic condemn *I Am Sam* as predictable "triumph over tragedy" whose hero " 'overcomes' disability to end up 'just like' everyone else": Sam manages to "draw on aspects of his cognitive disability to parent 'just like' other parents" (7). Yet his daughter's behavior convinces her foster mother she cannot substitute for him (which he never doubted). However, Sam believes Lucy needs a mother. Once Sam accepts he cannot parent alone, they share custody. He further integrates socially, not because of his neurodiversity but after it is accepted and accommodated. In *It's a Wonderful Life*, Potter's immobility, greed, isolation, and dependence counterpoint George's (James Stewart) frustrated wanderlust, generosity, community spirit and independence. Potter's villainy no more generalizes disability than does George's partial deafness.

Qualter deems "stereotypes" as "active and powerful guides to behavior"; "learned responses," albeit changeable, supplant "contact with, and relevance to, the world" (160). That, however, describes all ideology. Signs reinforce assumptions. The expression "little people," although labeling individuals whose differences encompass 400 conditions, designates distinct shared personhood. Derogatory references to "dwarfs" and "midgets" – interchangeably misused medical and showbusiness categories – help explain why Billy Barty, a movie actor with restricted growth, so named the Little People of America. Yet that organization's nomenclature, perhaps knowingly, infantilizes or denigrates in terms of importance or power. Contemplate this accidental patronizing of an Oscar-nominated little person: "despite his acting talents, Michael Dunn also played villains and sidekicks" (Bernshoff and Griffin 368) – absurd if applied to Anthony Hopkins or other Supporting Actor nominees.

Representation and focalization

Questions of representation center on who has agency within the narrative and externally in shaping it; to simplify an early communication studies formula: who represents whom, in what ways, and with what effect and purpose (Braddock). Films are not primarily "about" disabled people when responses toward disability inform non-disabled characterization – *Truly Madly Deeply* (Minghella 1990); *The Sweet Hereafter* (Egoyan 1997); *The Wolf of Wall Street* (Scorsese 2013); *A Man Called Ove* (Holm 2015) (which presents strikingly differentiated wheelchair users); *The Forty-Year-Old Version* (Blank 2020) – or signify fantasized alternate realities: *The Wizard of Oz* (Fleming 1939); *Twin Peaks: Fire Walk With Me* (Lynch 1992); *Big Fish* (Burton 2003). Typical filmmaking "reflect[s]" non-disabled "point of view" (Norden 1). More enlighteningly, *focalization* distinguishes a narrator, "who speaks" – in film, where narration can seem invisible, "enunciates" – from a character, "who sees" (Genette 186). Who speaks for whom separates "insider" from "outsider" (Longmore 231). Focalization's lens metaphor implies angle, distance, focus, filtering, clarity, distortion, inclusion or marginalization. Accordingly, rejecting "contemptible trends" – "disability as a source of humor" (Norden 15), as in Farrelly Brothers' productions (whose disabled actors in supporting roles arguably normalize disability) – unhelpfully could exclude people with impairments. Spectatorship, positioned without "stereotyping's" dismissiveness, distinguishes experience from attitude, inferred overall meaning from dramatized opinions.

Narrators, temporally detached, recount, not live, stories from outside. They do not look or learn *with* characters. Viewers follow alongside characters, informed of more or less; knowledge is identical, separate, or shifting. Some experiences – pain or fear – viewers infer. Focalization privileges one or more characters, switches, or stays aloof. An aspect of narration, it establishes attitude or tone. In *Fourth of July* – adapted autobiography – retrospective regret, cynicism, or anger unite author, filmmaker, and audience against blind patriotism. Distance, offering contradictory perspectives more than sole identification, encourages judgment, as when young Kovic's attitudes counter a former classmate's.

A center of consciousness "sees." Narration "shows." In *Still Alice*, the film and its audience understand better Alice's video memos to her older self than the latter does. Soft focus conveys her detachment; delayed or startling cuts her disorientation. But audiences judge from her former perspective rather than her advancing dementia, inaccessible hence uncommunicable. *The Diving-Bell...*'s perceptions, memories and internal monologue exemplify restricted focalization. *I Am Sam* commences with optical close-ups: Sam's experience leads. Objective camerawork can focalize internally: *Johnny Got His Gun* (Trumbo 1971) presents a limbless battle casualty, Joe (Timothy Bottoms), lacking all senses beyond feeling, whose thoughts and attempted communication feature aurally against his shrouded body and flashbacks.

Facets of focalization interact (Rimmon-Kenan). The *perceptual* defines sensory range. *I Am Sam* approximates cafe customers' viewpoints, confirming Sam's self-aware competence, friendliness and popularity. The *psychological* narrates knowledge or emotion. Embracing Sam's subjectivity, eccentric music and Beatles' songs indicate his tastes, establish commonality with culture, heighten childlike sensibility, yet acknowledge awareness of difference. In the hospital, handheld flash-pans, zooms, jumpy editing and a cold blue cast disorientate; calmer cinematography verifies his acceptance of his newborn daughter. Successive reflections fracture his existence as her mother departs. The *ideological* facet reinforces values: Sam's individualism, determination, empathy, honesty and trust; or Joe's and Kovic's anti-war sentiments. *Untouchable* defamiliarizes prejudice, celebrating commonality through opposed protagonists' mutually evolving perceptions. *Philadelphia* contrasts Andy's experience with others' reactions, encouraging viewers to question their own.

External focalization narrates outward behavior. Spectatorial empathy and projection nevertheless render characters without inferred thoughts, motivations, emotions and attitude unimaginable. *Still Alice* presents coping strategies such as Alice's tracking a script with a highlighter during a speech; her professionalism simultaneously stresses the psychological facet, focalized internally when she loses her place. *The Peanut Butter Falcon* (Nilson and Shwartz 2019), social drama rendered feel-good comedy by its Down syndrome hero's optimism, focalizes through Zak (Zack Gottsagen), and others whose humanity gains by encountering him, yet externally as well as from the implied audience perspective that recognizes his fantasies' limitations alongside dramatized debate around social disability. Outlaws on a raft evoke the classic American novel *Huckleberry Finn*'s themes and constructive duplicity, while visually Zak's initial escape from institutionalization suggests rebirth – unstated narratorial commentary outside his knowledge (Figure 12.2). *Greatest Showman* – primarily Barnum's focalization – implies

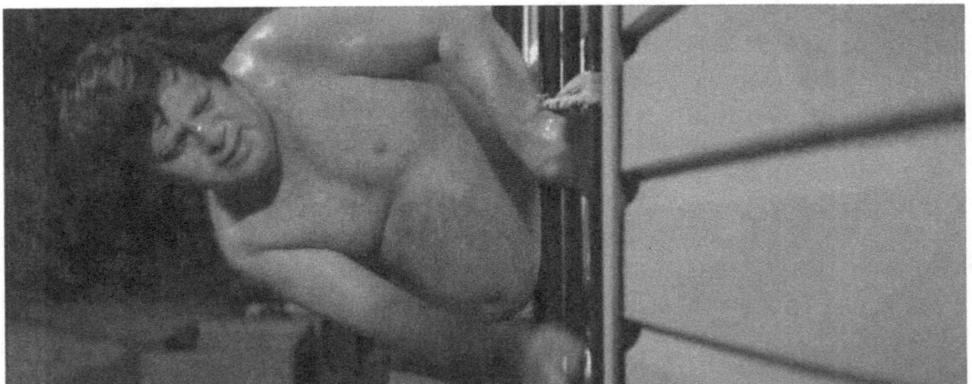

Figure 12.2 Zak in *The Peanut Butter Falcon*, played by an actor with Down Syndrome (Zack Gottsagen), escapes from an unsuitable care home. External focalization narrates, through composition and camera position, a metaphor of rebirth separate from his immediate awareness – yet, as internal focalization, expressive of his unfolding experience.

psychological meaning through an external view when Tom Thumb appears. Little beyond his stature being known, he challenges: "What are *you* looking at?"

Representation and modality

Longmore, citing his severe impairment, corrects reviews in which, he contends, movies were "completely misunderstood." *Whose Life…?* he rejects for neoliberalist arguments that, supporting assisted suicide, ignore possibilities of rehabilitation, "adaptive methods and special equipment" that helped Longmore beat institutionalized prejudice (120, 230–59). Predating critical realist disability studies' autoethnographic turn, he reads the film as a morality play, evidencing its shortcomings against his own positive medical encounters. Ascribing essayistic tone and intention, Longmore emphasizes what has become known as *modality*: attitude toward, investment or belief in a representation's "ontological status, or … value as truth or fact" (Hodge and Kress 124). Imputing effects is problematic. In contrast, Longmore praised *My Left Foot*, a social realist biopic. Day-Lewis's Method approach – living as if paralyzed – constructed a hero "fierce" in rejecting condescension (126). While promotional materials stressed working-class upbringing, artistic expression, and recognition (because disability might appear "depressing or saccharine"), modality and focalization, "down to the camera angles," were "utterly true" to disabled people's "point of view" (125, 126). Nevertheless, "capturing" Brown's "emotional directness and strength and vulnerability," alongside his future wife's initial ambivalence, lauded by Longmore as "fidelity" to disabled people's experience (127), indicates successful filmmaking, not anything easily generalizable. Countering "stereotypical" *critical responses*, Longmore differentiates this film from any " 'triumph-over-adversity' tale"; rather it chronicles a "life-long struggle against prejudice" (129). Such matters need greater consideration when seriously discussing representations. Filmgoers presumably recognize fantastic, artificial elements of cinematic pleasure, as ubiquitous instinctive yet logically evasive assertions about "escapism" suggest.

As modality strengthens, it increasingly affects responses "emotionally and cognitively as though it were reality" (Hodge and Tripp 116); weaker modality less. Multimodality better describes texts – different discourses often dramatically conflicting. Modality, "individually constructed" (106), is not exclusively textual. Deeming any film "realistic" encompasses its construction and critical- or marketing-led expectations, beyond relationship to actuality. "Signs of realism," Kress argues, "are semiotic navigational devices … . They allow us to ask …, 'Is this … to be taken seriously?', 'Should I get outraged that this has been said?'" (106). Modality implicates genre and indicated or inferred intentions. Filmmakers', viewers', or analysts' circumstances shape anticipation. Meanings, none automatically primary, differ.

Analyzing modality acknowledges social and functional requirements: questioning, not assuming, the recognition of rhetoric in audiovisual conventions, including promotional materials and paratextual features such as title typography. For example, whether Bond villains' differences impair their fictional lives congruently to real-world definitions of disability is unapparent. Abnormalities signifying "moral corruption" (Benshoff and Griffin 375), including lachrymal bleeding in *Casino Royale* (Campbell 2006), are hardly "stereotypes" in most recognized senses. Anomalous embodiment enhances opposition to 007's state-sanctioned, elite-nation, liberal-democratic, patriarchal norms. Whether anyone takes seriously (high modality) Bond's idealized, if flawed, characterization – lighthearted exaggerations (low modality) of outdated masculinity – remains moot. World domination desires are insane, yet villainous "assorted lethal oddities that pass[…] for humans" (Norden 220) are rarely considered intellectually impaired. Fantasy-adventure modality foregrounds wickedness over psychological problems. Social realist dramatization of delusional disorder would tell another story, focalized and presented differently. Nevertheless, baddies, adept at asserting power, are judged demeaning "stereotypes." Jaws' (Richard Kiel) metal teeth in *The Spy Who Loved Me* (Gilbert 1977) and *Moonraker* (Gilbert 1979) are alarming weapons, much as Captain Hook's prosthesis threatens Oedipal castration. (Anathema to psychiatry but familiar from film theory, this explains "psychosexual significance" of linking "badness, amputation, and artificial arms" [Longmore 134] – something Freud addressed [1919], and Norden pursues illuminatingly.)

Mask (Bogdanovich 1985), a "welcome departure," operates different modalities. Its visually anomalous protagonist, Rocky Dennis (Eric Stoltz), refuses social disablement. The true story, deemed commercially risky, was marketed as family melodrama, coming-of-age high school romance, biker movie (with puppies), star vehicle and auteur offering. Popular success raised consciousness, highlighting disability activism's "growing militancy" (Longmore 125).Modality is concerned with assumed status, not truth. *Rain Man*, *Sea Inside*, *The Diving-Bell...*, *Still Alice*, *Untouchable*, *Theory of Everything*: all have input or endorsement from clinicians, advocacy organizations, or individuals portrayed. As with *The Elephant Man* and *My Left Foot*, their awards enhance credibility – or justify cynicism. Films elicit existing but not universal associations. Interpretation, always contestable, requires analysis – *as films*: textually – identifying specific discourses.

Bringing it together: *Joker*

Joker (Philips 2019) unreliably focalizes multi-discursive complexity through its protagonist. Modality compounds comic-book expectations with psychological thriller. Articulated socio-economic concerns explain, without justifying, Arthur's (Joaquin Phoenix) victimhood – not outright villainy – as titular lead rather than disruptive force. Hardly important is whether Arthur's laughter accurately portrays a genuine condition. Familiar assertions, deeming weighty matters high modality, reckon *Joker* "dangerously misinformed." Psychiatrists Annabel Driscoll and Mina Husain consider "toxic" *Joker*'s "hackneyed association between serious mental illness and extreme violence": "Portrayals of mental illness in film can perpetuate unfounded stereotypes." Yet, discounting Original Sin, what explains violence? Legally, insanity mitigates criminality.

"[T]hat ... mental deterioration necessarily leads to violence against others – implied by the juxtaposition of ... Arthur stopping his medication with his increasingly frequent acts of violence – ... further amplifies stigma and fear," so Driscoll and Husain, assuming transparent linear causality, contend. Actually, *Joker*'s chronology reorders and fragments. Heartbeats and applause accompany flashbacks or hallucinations. Many believe the ending – Arthur receding, leaving red footprints – suggests he murders his therapist. This ignores absence of bloody clothing and the footprints' continuation. Transitory external focalization here invokes theories that neurological disease manifests physically: Tourette (who identified a syndrome Arthur's laughter resembles) tested these, powdering patients' feet red to imprint their gait on paper (McCance 90).

Considering pharmaceutically suppressed violence inherently Arthur's, detaching it from broader causes, reasserts medicalization. Kids assault him, accordant with real concerns: Driscoll and Husain insist association between psychological problems and violence "is exaggerated [because] people with severe mental illness are more vulnerable to violence from others." Yet, inconsistently, the result "is to – disappointingly – remove Arthur's agency and divert attention from a potentially more stimulating conversation about wealth inequality and its responsibility for societal collapse"; recognition, after all, of the social model that insists unjust and uncaring society disables persons with impairments. That is for audiences to debate, not a blockbuster entertainment (which nevertheless, untypically, prompts such interpretation) to decide. Viewers judge whether Arthur is the *Batman* Joker, which the movie evades, or a delusional patient obsessed with comics and De Niro. The first train scene, featuring murderous retribution, is morally objectionable, if logically justified according to vigilante movies from the represented period, and includes realistically motivated blackouts. Electricity interruptions cannot explain these in the second, daylight, train scene. Such punctuation, foreshadowing a fade to black between the movie's climax and coda, reaffirms fractured fantasizing.

Arthur writes: "The worst part about having a mental illness is that other people expect you to behave as if you don't." Ironically, this describes critics assuming his imaginings are consistent. Arthur's punctured hand suggests intravenous medication. Medical incarceration is revealed before he headbutts a door – not conclusively flashback – repeated after he steals hospital records and again after killing a co-worker. Frequently observing through screens and bars, metaphorical or actual imprisonment, he traverses signed exits. As in *Still Alice*, soft focus emphasizes detachment (Figure 12.3). Arthur inhabits harshly-lit tiled or whitewashed spaces recalling prisons or hospitals. Even his wallpaper resembles tiles. Shouting "I love you Murray!" in the studio, bookended by TV watching, is clearly fantasy. Why shouldn't passively receiving a gun be delusion, especially as his boss insists: "Randall told me you tried to buy a .38 off of him"? Arthur projects problems and solutions onto others, even proclaiming, "I love Doctor Sally!" He asserts, "Everyone's telling me my standup's ready for the big clubs," although encouragements are not shown. "Smile, though your heart is aching" quickly supplants his performance. (The tune comes from *Modern Times* [Chaplin 1936] – social commentary as entertainment – a gala screening of which Arthur gatecrashes effortlessly.) When Sophie finds him funny, his words are obscured. A pitiful standup, his nonverbal clowning and magic are lithe. Bemoaning universal craziness, Sophie's gunshot suicide gesture (or his – mirroring it, resembling Travis Bickle) means *Joker* starts where *Taxi Driver* ends: ambiguously.

Allegory and fantasy entangle with social realism – strikes, moral panics concerning media effects, cutbacks. However, unlikelihood undermines period detail. Do audiences seriously

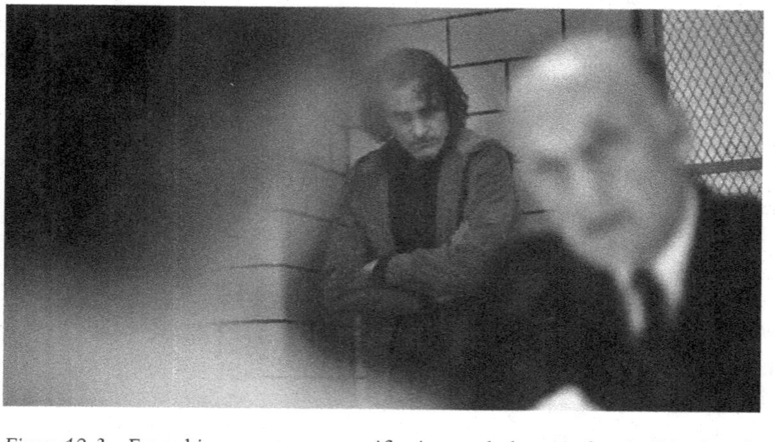

Figure 12.3 From his current non-specific time and place, Arthur in *Joker* imaginatively projects himself into a scene (during his early childhood) that he was not present at. The context, and the wall tiles, indicate the same secure prison where he is incarcerated at film's end—and likely throughout. The highly blurred interlocutors in the foreground and differential lighting suggest his dissociation and confusion concerning the traumatic yet misunderstood event

accept Arthur is uninjured when vehicles hit him or is sprung from a patrol car by deliberate collision? Unchallenged he enters a secure hospital and Sophie's improbably unlocked apartment. Sophie, despite accusing him of stalking, accompanies him to his show immediately after he has watched a comedian describing role play fantasy. Later she implausibly exclaims: "What are *you* doing here? You're in the wrong apartment!" Arthur, visiting the Wayne mansion, informs Alfred, through bars, that his act is "not real; it's magic," before learning his mother "was delusional." Alfred's surname is Pennyworth; Arthur's mother is Penny Flack; Stephen King's dancing clown in *It* is Pennywise: logic spins uncontrollably.

When a cop questions whether Arthur's laughing compulsion is genuine, he asks, "What do you think?" before walking into a glass door: classic mime clowning – except the door exists. A white-uniformed nurse or orderly comes out. Arthur, having departed the clown agency through a signed exit – pre-echoing departure from the screening – enters through the exit (as does Chaplin's waiter, prompting slapstick chaos), ahead of an elaborately planned television entrance prefacing his fantasized onscreen slaying. In his mother's tiled hospital room, Sophie miraculously materializes, then disappears as Arthur relives his broadcast humiliation, the TV recalling the comedy club monitor. The screen is behind a plastic curtain, evoking the studio stage entrance used by Murray (De Niro, significantly) and *Psycho*'s shower in this tale of a loner who seemingly without consequence murders his mother, before final hospitalization. After meeting Wayne – "I need a doctor," Arthur exclaims – a graphic match cut positions him identically at home. Other represented disabilities include a workmate's restricted growth and his mother's "delusional psychosis and narcissistic personality disorder," an actual or projected condition matching his. Unmentioned, but supporting initially empathetic characterization, Arthur's anorexia – that Phoenix lost 52 pounds suggests its centrality – and the actor's shoulder deformity and microform cleft lip resist supposed expectations of Hollywood stars' appearance.

Joker begins with tears of a clown, initially anonymous, amid vast inequality, casual employment, business failures, degrading work, welfare cuts, helpless professional cynicism, urban sprawl, crime, bullying, predatory misogyny, cruel television hosts, weak politicians, advertised movies about anti-heroes exploiting misfortune or violently tackling corruption – *Blow Out*'s (DePalma 1981) rating would actually prevent young Bruce's attendance – and discontented hordes craving a cause, symbol, uniform and leader. Arthur later, among crowds reflecting his persona, pushes his face into a *V for Vendetta* grimace – another DC Comics-Warner Bros franchise by the writer of an earlier Joker origin story.

To claim *Joker* unequivocally medicalizes mental health misses the point. Such reviews resemble "diagnostic overshadowing": prioritizing someone's "primary condition" over "general health problems" (Shakespeare, *Disability: The Basics* 94). Driscoll and Husain's assertion – Arthur's psychopathology "is foggy at best: his apparent lack of disordered thinking means the attempt to illustrate psychosis is half formed" – ignores textual specificity. In *Joker* social disablement symptomizes cultural malaise. Arthur writes: "What do you get when you cross a mentally ill loner with a society that abandons him and treats him like trash? You get what you fucking deserve!"

Conclusion

Movies considered here, although predominantly one type – mainstream features, ultimately profit-oriented – originate from different national cinemas within a global market, address various audiences diversely (distracting entertainment, expressive art, dramatic advocacy, or whatever), and command accordant budgets and production values. Some play around the edges of received wisdom, generating publicity by stoking controversy or incorporating progressive elements. In latter instances, given that long production cycles mean they lag behind the culture that they purportedly "reflect," films more likely endorse ongoing attitudinal changes. Notwithstanding tendencies, including cultural prejudices, they may embody, it is as reductive and stultifying to homogenize and judge films "stereotypically" as it is with disabilities represented. Reinforcement of any unfair stigmatization requires constant challenge, for which semiotic understandings are necessary and adequate. Recourse to "stereotypes" – a wall of mystification – never helps.

Note

1 Statistics compiled in different ways that include or exclude certain groups, support various agendas, even often embrace people who most of the time would not consider themselves disabled, are undoubtedly contestable. It is beyond the scope of this chapter to comment, other than to note broad consensus among four reputable sources:

www.cdc.gov/ncbddd/disabilityandhealth/infographic-disability-impacts-all.html
www.st-andrews.ac.uk/hr/edi/disability/facts/
https://bit.ly/37lUrIL
https://fullfact.org/health/how-many-people-have-disability/

Works cited

Barker, Martin. 1989. "The Lost World of Stereotypes." *The Media Studies Reader*, edited by Tim O'Sullivan and Yvonne Jewkes. London: Arnold, 1997, pp. 86–90.

Bauby, Jean-Dominique. *The Diving-Bell and the Butterfly*, translated by Jeremy Leggatt. New York: Harper, 2008.

Benshoff, Harry M. and Sean Griffin. *America on Film: Representing Race, Class, Gender and Sexuality at the Movies*, 2nd ed. Hoboken, NJ: Wiley-Blackwell, 2009.

Bogdan, Robert. *Freak Show: Presenting Human Oddities for Amusement and Profit*. Chicago: U of Chicago Press, 2007.

Braddock, Richard. "An Extension of the 'Lasswell Formula'." *Journal of Communication*, vol. 8, 1958, pp. 88–93.

Chivers, Sally and Nicole Markotic. "Introduction." *The Problem Body: Projecting Disability on Film*, edited by Sally Chivers and Nicole Markotic. Columbus, OH: Ohio State University Press, 2010, pp. 1–21.

Darke, Paul. "No Life Anyway: Pathologizing Disability on Film." *The Problem Body: Projecting Disability on Film*, edited by Sally Chivers and Nicole Markotic. Columbus, OH: Ohio State University Press, 2010, pp. 97–108.

Driscoll, Annabel and Mina Husain. "Why *Joker's* Depiction of Mental Illness is Dangerously Misinformed." *The Guardian,* October 21, 2019, www.theguardian.com/film/2019/oct/21/joker-mental-illness-joaquin-phoenix-dangerous-misinformed. Accessed May 7, 2020.

Freud, Sigmund. "The 'Uncanny'." *The Standard Edition of the Complete Psychological Works of Sigmund Freud,* Vol. XVII (1917–1919): *An Infantile Neurosis and Other Works*. London: Hogarth, 1955, pp. 217–56.

Genette, Gérard. *Narrative Discourse: An Essay in Method*, translated by Jane E. Lewin. Ithaca, N.Y.: Cornell University Press, 1980.

Goodwin, Andrew. "Understanding Media Stereotypes." *Media Studies for Adults*, edited by Jim Cook and Nicky North, BFI, 1988, pp. 29–32.

Hodge, Robert and Gunther Kress. *Language as Ideology*. London: Routledge and Kegan Paul, 1979.

Hodge, Robert and David Tripp. *Children and Television*. Oxford: Polity Press, 1986.

Karpf, Anne. 1988. "Crippling Images." *The Media Studies Reader*, edited by Tim O'Sullivan and Yvonne Jewkes. London: Arnold, 1997, pp. 114–24.

Kim, Eunjung. "'A Man, with the Same Feelings': Disability, Humanity, and Heterosexual Apparatus in *Breaking the Waves, Born on the Fourth of July, Breathing Lessons*, and *Oasis*." *The Problem Body: Projecting Disability on Film*, edited by Sally Chivers and Nicole Markotic. Columbus, OH: Ohio State University Press, 2010, pp. 131–58.

Kress, Gunther R. *Multimodality: A Social Semiotic Approach to Contemporary Communication.* New York and Abingdon: Routledge, 2010.
Longmore, Paul K. 1985. *Why I Burned My Book and Other Essays on Disability*. Temple University Press, 2003.
McCance, Dawn. "The Wild Child." *The Problem Body: Projecting Disability on Film*, edited by Sally Chivers and Nicole Markotic. Columbus, OH: Ohio State University Press, 2010, pp. 83–96.
Norden, Martin F. *The Cinema of Isolation: A History of Physical Disability in the Movies*. New Brunswick, NJ: Rutgers University Press, 1994.
Perkins, Tessa. 1979. "Rethinking Stereotypes." *The Media Studies Reader*, edited by Tim O'Sullivan and Yvonne Jewkes. London: Arnold, 1997, pp. 75–85.
Qualter, T. H. "The Social Role of Advertising." *The Media Studies Reader*, edited by Tim O'Sullivan and Yvonne Jewkes. London: Arnold, 1997, pp. 154–64.
Rimmon-Kenan, Shlomith. *Narrative Fiction: Contemporary Poetics*. New York and Abingdon: Routledge, 1983.
Shakespeare, Tom. *Disability Rights and Wrongs Revisited*. New York and Abingdon: Routledge, 2013.
Shakespeare, Tom. *Disability: the Basics*. New York and Abingdon: Routledge, 2018.
Shildrick, Margrit. "Critical Disability Studies: Rethinking the Conventions for the Age of Postmodernity." *Routledge Handbook of Disability Studies*, 2nd ed., edited by Nick Watson and Simo Vehmas. New York and Abingdon: Routledge, 2019, pp. 32–44.
Siebers, Tobin. *Disability Theory*. Ann Arbor, MI: U of Michigan P, 2008.
Snyder, Sharon L. and David T. Mitchell. "Body Genres: An Anatomy of Disability in Film." *The Problem Body: Projecting Disability on Film*, edited by Sally Chivers and Nicole Markotic. Columbus, OH: Ohio State University Press, 2010, pp. 179–204.

PART IV

Documentary film

The order of chapters in this section roughly corresponds to the life span of a human person: from pubescence to senescence, from fighting to live to struggling to die.

In the first chapter, **"From corporate discourse to menstrual equality? A history of menstruation films,"** Christie Milliken writes how, after World War II, North American educators began to rely on films to teach adolescent girls about menstruation. Such films were either sponsored by makers of feminine hygiene products or by companies in the business of making sex education films for widespread classroom use. Beginning with the first of these films, the 1946 distribution of *The Story of Menstruation*, financed by the Kimberly-Clark Corporation and produced by Walt Disney Studios, and concluding with the 2018 Oscar-winning documentary short, *Period: End of Sentence,* which touches upon the taboos and prohibitions around menstruation for women in India, Milliken interrogates the ways in which menstrual health and coming of age have been visualized and narrativized across this sub-genre.

In the second chapter, "**Crip wisdom in the time of insulin crisis: performing #insulin4all in short documentary film,"** Bianca Frazer begins with a snapshot of protesters delivering "blood money" to the entrance of the pharmaceutical company, Eli Lilly, in response to a 300 percent increase in the price of insulin. What is now known as the "insulin crisis" in the United States prompted people with diabetes to experiment with different approaches for mobilizing the public and pressuring lawmakers to change legislation. This includes documentary film, and Frazer introduces readers to three shorts published by established news organizations that lend authority and validity to a group of people determined to change public understanding about diabetes and to circumvent oppressive healthcare systems' practices.

Over the past decade, the emergence of digital storytelling has become another medium for sharing individual experiences of health and illness – one that is both powerful and accessible. As Andrea Charise writes in **"Aging, remixed: intergenerational storytelling in the digital realm,"** the typical format of sharing personal and collective memories of lived experience from one generation to another is itself an adjacent form of health-related storytelling. In this chapter, she offers a critical assessment of digital storytelling practices with a focus on their application in the aging and intergenerational context including an overview of recent scholarship; a discussion of the intersection of digital media with age studies; and an introduction to *The Resemblage Project,* a Toronto-based initiative.

DOI: 10.4324/9781003007661-17

In contrast to the imitated death usually depicted in fiction films, documentary images, however they might be manipulated, can and do show real death, and when it appears, it is sobering in a way that even the most naturalistic death in a fiction film can never be. In the final chapter of this section, **"Documenting the American way of dying: the *Near Death* experience,"** Barry Keith Grant argues that the most penetrating documentary on death and dying is Frederick Wiseman's monumental film, *Near Death,* which takes place in the Medical Intensive Care Unit at Beth Israel Hospital in Boston, Massachusetts. Although made in 1989, the film remains powerfully relevant today, especially given biomedical science's ever advancing ability to maintain life or life functions and the ethical questions that process raises for health professionals, patients, and their families.

13

FROM CORPORATE DISCOURSE TO MENSTRUAL EQUITY?

A history of menstruation films

Christie Milliken

Since the emergence of early classroom sex education productions, which proliferated in the post-World War II period, educators in both Canada and the United States have relied on films to teach adolescent girls about menstruation. As a subgenre, menstruation films were part of a cluster of hygiene films made specifically for premenarchal and adolescent girls. These films were frequently sponsored by makers of feminine hygiene products with titles including: *The Story of Menstruation* (Walt Disney Company and Kimberly-Clark 1946), *Growing Girls* (Film Producers Guild and Southalls Sanitary Wear 1949),[1] *Molly Grows Up* (Personal Products Corporation 1953), *It's Wonderful Being a Girl* (Johnson & Johnson 1968), *Naturally...A Girl* (Johnson & Johnson 1973), *Growing Up on Broadway* (Personal Products Company 1984), *Who Am I Now?* (Tambrands 1987), *Kids to Kids: Talking about Puberty* (Tambrands 1991), and *Always Changing, Always Growing* (Proctor & Gamble 1995), all of which were widely distributed as classroom films. While not sponsored by feminine care companies, multiple contemporaneous titles including *Girl to Woman* (Churchill Films 1961, 1965, 1976, 1984, 1993 and Churchill Media 2005), *Personal Health for Girls* (Coronet 1952, 1972), and *Girl Stuff* (Churchill Films 1982) were all made by companies in the business of producing educational films for widespread classroom use.

Two somewhat unique texts not sponsored by business or educational film enterprises emerge later: *Linda's Film on Menstruation* (Linda Feferman 1974) and *Dear Diary* (Boston Family Planning Project and Copperfield Films 1981).[2] These two films prefigure the emergence of more independently produced menstrual equity and advocacy documentaries produced in the last few decades. Many later films tend to be directed to a wider audience and reflect the rise of second wave feminism, departing from the previous preoccupation with menstruation as fundamentally a hygienic crisis and striving – variously – to recast and de-stigmatize the cultural meanings of menstruation, consider problems with access to and regulation of menstrual products, and visualize activist lobbies against their taxation. Others tackle newer issues around menstrual suppression and the pharmaceutical industry, as well as the environmental impact of menstrual products. Some of these titles include *Period Piece* (Jennifer Frame and Jay Rosenblatt 1995), *Under Wraps* (Teresa MacInnes, National Film Board of Canada 1998),[3] and *Period: The End of Menstruation?* (Giovanna Chesler 2006), as well as advocacy films targeting specific geopolitical menstrual issues, including the India-focused, Oscar-winning documentary short,

DOI: 10.4324/9781003007661-18

Period: End of Sentence (Rayka Zehtabchi 2018). This chapter interrogates the ways in which the menstrual health and coming of age have been visualized and narrativized across this subgenre, highlighting competing discourses – corporate, patriarchal, biological, medical, feminist, social justice – that have framed the meanings of menarche and menstruation across seventy years of educational film production devoted explicitly to the topic.[4]

Hygienic bodies

In 1946, the Kimberly-Clark Corporation hired the Walt Disney Company to make the first of these educational films, *The Story of Menstruation,* which remained in active distribution for over 25 years. With versions made in several languages and shown around the world, Kimberly-Clark estimates that *The Story of Menstruation* was viewed by more than 100 million young women in the United States alone, veritable blockbuster status for a ten-minute classroom film (Kennard 1990, 67).[5] While unique as one of the few fully animated menstruation films, *The Story of Menstruation* becomes a prototype, reflecting the post-World War II shift in menstrual marketing and promotion from mothers directly to young girls as a strategy for cultivating brand loyalty (see Bobel 34). Although it is only one of several significant physical changes experienced by adolescent girls, menstruation is accorded greater cultural significance than budding breasts or the appearance of body hair. Paradoxically, despite the significance of this maturational event, hygiene remains the focus of instruction in these films. When issues of reproduction and egg fertilization come up in discussion of the whys and the mechanics of menstruation, the uterus is typically described as the place "where fertilization takes place" with no specificity about how and where sperm arrives. In her analysis of the social and cultural history of menstrual discourse as a culturally constructed script, Joan Jacobs Brumberg argues that instead of seeing menarche as a marker of an important internal change for girls – specifically in their new capacity for reproduction, the tendency has been instead to stress the importance of outside appearances, "keeping clean, avoiding soiled clothes, and purchasing the 'right equipment.'" In *The Body Project: An Intimate History of American Girls*, Brumberg contends:

> The script that we follow in late-20th-century America involves mothers, doctors, and the producers of new technologies, all of whom have collaborated over the past hundred years to produce a distinctly American menstrual experience that stresses personal hygiene over information about adult womanhood or female sexuality. In the 1990s, the sanitary products industry is a more-than-$2 billion-a-year business, built on scientific and popular beliefs about personal cleanliness as well as changes in contemporary women's lives: earlier menarche, fewer pregnancies, and later menopause – all of which foster more periods and more sales. The way we menstruate in America today not only affects the economy, it also contributes to the way in which adolescent girls make the body into an intense project requiring careful scrutiny and constant personal control.
>
> *(30)*

Along precisely these lines, *The Story of Menstruation* offers a seemingly transhistorical narrative about the "natural" and "normal" cycle of life for females which ultimately and essentially suggests that reproduction in the context of white middle-class heterosexual conjugality is the desired, inevitable consequence of maturity, part of nature's so-called "eternal plan." Fertility is limited to instruction that focuses primarily on hygiene as if it were part of the natural order of maintaining female health, indeed of femininity itself, with childbearing as a preordained destination. This animated film begins with credits to Walt Disney and Kotex as white flowers float across the screen and into the bedroom of a baby girl. A female voice-over intones:

> Why is nature always called Mother Nature? Perhaps it's because like any mother she quietly manages so much of our living without our ever realizing there's a woman at work. Why, right from the beginning, we breathe and sleep and wake up with no more conscious planning than we use in sprouting teeth. Mother nature controls many of our routine bodily processes though automatic control centers called glands. The story of menstruation really begins with one particular gland....the pituitary gland.

The invocation of nature, of "*Mother* Nature," from the beginning of the film narrativizes menstruation within a model which reflects an ideological position of femininity as one of passive/objecthood rather than of active subjectivity. Far from being a subject in her own right, this biological model maintains that "As a girl grows up from blocks to dolls to books, that means her body is obeying the orders issued by the pituitary gland." From a series of animated sketches giving general views of the pituitary gland and the reproductive organs, the film goes on to emphasize the sociocultural aspects of menstruation, such as the importance of body cleanliness, good posture, regular exercise, and a healthy, balanced diet, all of which are displayed through the obedient performance of a female figure who resembles a cross between Snow White and Cinderella. Although product placement is not significant in *The Story of Menstruation*, the pamphlet created to accompany the film (and featured in it), entitled *Very Personally Yours*, is certainly a more obvious hard sell for Kotex products, free samples of which would have been distributed to contemporaneous classes seeing the film.[6] In fact, many of these films mention accompanying pamphlets and products intended to be distributed by teachers, school nurses, or public health workers who presided over the screenings. It is interesting to note that the anatomical information provided in these pamphlets, complete editions of which can be found on the Museum of Menstruation web site, does not show the clitoris until 1981, when it is named in the glossary of terms, but not shown in any of the anatomical diagrams. Similarly, the companion pamphlet by Modess accompanying *Naturally a Girl* appears to omit the clitoris from all iterations available up until 1991.[7]

In a review of *The Story of Menstruation* published in *Educational Screen* (a trade publication for educational professionals and film librarians), the film's use of animation is lauded as "a happy solution to most of the problems posed by the subject matter." The review states:

> With this medium of expression, "glass-figure" technique could be employed to show the internal organs. A half-real and half-diagramatic rendering of these was developed in order to avoid any unpleasantness. Thus the technical clarity of straight diagrams was maintained, and the ghastly effect of a realistic rendering was avoided. No nude figures were shown. Medical language was simplified, and unnecessary terms eliminated without the loss of essential accuracy. A gynecologist of the highest reputation checked the story in detail at every stage of its development: words, pictorial representation, animations, and implications.
>
> *("New Biology Film" 215)*

This paternalistic review reflects the misogynistic attitude toward the "ghastliness" of menstruation which frames this corporeal event within the rhetoric of naturalized, essentialized experience legitimated by the patriarchal invocation of medical science. Similarly, a review of the film in the *Journal of the American Medical Association* praises *The Story of Menstruation* for presenting "material related to the reproductive processes without creating an atmosphere of tension, not to say fear and disgust" (1033). Interestingly, although a mother is shown in the film as she tends to her baby in a brief image, no mother is shown imparting information here.[8] Moreover, in anatomical sketches which explain the mechanics of the cycle itself, only internal organs are shown, a common trope at this time which avoids any specific naming and description of female genitalia.[9]

To be sure, menstruation films are generally targeted to a specific and "age appropriate" audience, but their tendency to veer into euphemism and indirection is a characteristic of these early texts. *Molly Grows Up*, released seven years after *The Story of Menstruation*, offers a live-action, character-driven portrait of a white middle-class adolescent, Molly, chronicling her experience of menarche, which includes the supportive acceptance of her school nurse, proud parents and older sister. The film provides background on Molly (as a typical adolescent) via direct address and voice-over conveniently narrated by her school nurse who also gives Molly's all-girl class instruction about menstruation, including demonstration of sanitary products. While an earlier scene shows Molly handling her sister's sanitary pads (where the Modess branding is clearly visible), no branding promotion is included in the nurse's demonstration which shows the use of pads, belts and tampons. It is worth noting that when tampons first entered the market in 1936, they were viewed as a problematic product for adolescent girls because they were controversially linked to hymen disruption and thus a threat to virginity, so their appearance in this and subsequent films from the 1950s onward would be viewed as progressive to some degree.[10]

In a 1989 unpublished dissertation, *The Corporation in the Classroom: The Struggles over Meanings of Menstrual Education in Sponsored Films*, Margot Kennard points out that sponsoring corporations enjoyed little competition from noncommercial producers of menstrual films during this era. Among the number of companies created in the postwar period to enter the business of sex education, very few made films dealing exclusively with menstrual education which, when handled explicitly, was more typically framed within the broader context of female urogenital education and coming-of-age. To some degree, this must necessarily reflect the uneasy place of menstruation in the public and private spheres. In addition, problematically tied to sponsorship is the question of what role the sponsor might play in the deployment (or concealment) of information. In Kennard's view, the significant and often central role such films play in the history of menstrual education practices begs the question of what and whose meanings are privileged in these texts. Her cultural studies framework addresses issues concerning the construction and circulation of meanings within various menstrual education films with the goal of unearthing contradictory moments in these texts, sites where corporate authority is contested (however briefly) in the struggle for meanings within the films themselves.

While her study is an important one, Kennard downplays the degree to which virtually all menstruation films from the late 1940s well into the 1990s deploy upbeat, positive messaging. Hygiene discourse pervades virtually all postwar sex education, *including* menstruation education. To be sure, a corporate discourse on menstrual education wants its image and products to be associated with primarily "positive" images of menstruation which results in a "sugar coating" or white washing of the process whereby menstrual "problems" (pains, irregularities, fears and phobias, product risks, and failures) are barely touched upon. In other words, these films are designed to promote a positive viewing experience. That said, even a film made without femcare industry sponsorship, such as *Dear Diary* (Boston Family Planning Project 1981) – which deals more complexly with the ups and downs of coming-of-age with both poignancy and humor (and notably features a white adolescent girl with a racially diverse group of friends), the complete avoidance of any discussion of hygiene products and how to use them is a glaring omission. Even the offbeat and humorous engagement with menstruation proffered by the independently-produced, *Linda's Film on Menstruation*, explicitly addresses the use of sanitary products, including animations of tampon insertion and best practices for how to use them.

Linda's Film also – neutrally – shows a range of consumer brands and types, staging a discussion about product choice between protagonist Judy and a store owner whom she consults. This educational moment is interrupted by the coincidental (and comical) arrival of Judy's boyfriend who has been sent to pick up femcare products for his mum. When the package of pads he purchases is far too big for the shopping bag, Johnny is compelled to leave the store with visible evidence of this purchase in a scenario mocking male anxiety over menstruation as well as the practices of anxious concealment with respect to both consumption of menstrual products and menstruation itself that pervade our culture. *Linda's Film* is interesting for the ways in which it involves Johnny's growth and maturity in dealing with the subject of menstruation alongside Judy, who is portrayed as thrilled and relieved to menstruate finally for the first time at age 15, considerably later than all of her friends. That said, it's hard to determine the target audience for this film: for one thing, the talking heads of people on the street (women and men) who are interviewed at various points in the film about meanings of menstruation discuss more adult behaviors. One woman, for example, talks about growing to accept her body and its processes gradually over time, eventually becoming comfortable having intercourse while menstruating. Presented by the Los Angeles Public Library with AFI funding, *Linda's Film* is an anomalous text in the history of menstrual education films that predate it and was perhaps made as a more adult sendup and a counterpoint to so many of the prosaic, hygiene-focused films preceding it.

The titles of these films are suggestive: *Molly Grows Up*, *It's Wonderful Being a Girl*, *Naturally...A Girl*, and *Growing Up on Broadway* were all produced by Personal Products, a subsidiary of Johnson & Johnson and promote an ancillary pamphlet, *Growing Up and Liking It*, produced by the company and distributed with the films. A consistent trope within these films related to a corporate agenda more broadly would seem to be the tension between the sponsor's need to privilege "accurate" medical/scientific knowledge with the need to win approval from schools which have often been pressured on many sides to regard the explicit processes of fertilization and detailed genitalia as too controversial for the elementary classroom. These films and those made by educational film companies like Coronet, Churchill and Crawley Films are remarkably similar for the ways in which they seek to avoid controversy and advocate hygienic messaging. Even a film such as *Growing Up on Broadway*, which addresses toxic shock syndrome – something that would have been impossible (and irresponsible) to avoid in a menstruation film released in the 1980s. That said, the film merely states that it is rare but serious see below. that it is rare but serious and that girls should seek medical information about it outside of the film itself, which is woefully inadequate. Although perhaps less known to a younger generation today, toxic shock syndrome is a rare bacterial infection linked to high absorbency tampons introduced in 1978 which contained synthetic fibres. This product led to serious illnesses in over 2,000 women, including at least 38 deaths in the United States and recurred again in the late 1990s following the introduction of new high absorbency tampon products. Toxic shock syndrome had a mobilizing effect on menstrual activism as women increasingly began to question the FemCare industry's lack of commitment to menstruator safety. Finally, racial diversity also begins to show up in some of the films made from the 1960s onward (*Dear Diary*, *Growing Up on Broadway*, and *Naturally...A Girl*), although minority characters are frequently given supporting roles in service of a white lead and prototype. Gradually, as menstruation films feature a broader range of voices, no one single experience continues to dominate. Films like *Kid to Kids* (1991) and even *Always Changing, Always Growing* (1995) – while blatant in its product placement for Proctor and Gamble – at least show a multiracial mix of girls (and also boys) in their menstruation messaging.

Another marker of change across these films is the portrayal of young women's prospects for maturity in a gendered world. Rather than assuming that female maturity automatically leads to marriage and family as is the case with *The Story of Menstruation*, *Growing Girls*, and *Molly Grows Up*, *Naturally*... .*A Girl* concludes with a the onscreen appearance of the woman who has voiced-over the film. As she directly addresses the camera from a film set, reflecting on her past and her dreams, she observes how "being is so much better than dreaming" now that she has matured into the woman and actress she had fantasized about becoming. The film then shows a montage of women performing career options – nurse, teacher, flight attendant, traffic officer, utility worker, office assistant and mother, concluding with a plucky young girl who says of her gender: "It's better than being a boy!" While it otherwise trafficks in the tropes of hygiene, appearance, menstrual concealment, and good health/exercise practices as well as upbeat messaging, *Naturally...a Girl* reflects, to a limited degree, the influence of second wave feminism and female empowerment. It also offers, via a broad range of young racially mixed voices who talk about menstruation throughout the film (including boys), the visual analogue of a consciousness-raising frame by privileging the experiences of a diverse group of young girls rather than one specific character, thereby gesturing toward a communitarian, inclusive approach to understanding adolescence reflective of its historical context.

From hygiene to critical menstrual discourse

The expanse between the unrealistic (and poorly acted) menstrual practices in some of the older films is thrown into sharp relief by the inclusion of this footage in more recent independently produced films. For example, footage from *Molly Grows Up* and *Social Sex Attitudes in Adolescence* (both from 1953), *It's Wonderful Being a Girl* (1968) and *World of a Girl* (unknown) is woven throughout Jennifer Frame and Jay Rosenblatt's film, *Period Piece* (1996), in ways which add structure to the various topics that the interviewees discuss, underscoring dated menstrual advice and myths (such as prohibitions against riding horseback or swimming while menstruating). The juxtaposition of old footage and titles thematically structures the film which includes testimony from a diverse range of women (young, old, as well as racially and ethnically mixed) who share their varied experience with menarche and menstruation. This includes a young girl of eight who knows very little about it and hasn't yet started her period, as well as women well into menopause who reflect back on their experiences. The use of archival footage to frame the film has the effect of revealing what one critic calls "the brutality of a culture which on the one hand professes rational enlightenment in the guise of biological knowledge and on the other, categorically ignores the complexities of embodied experience" (Goslinga-Roy 68). Through candid testimony that is in parts funny and profoundly sad, *Period Piece* gives voice to a more polyvocal portrait of the meanings of menarche from a diverse range of Euro and Asian-American women and girls, signifying a move away from exclusive preoccupation with menstruation as primarily and merely a hygienic crisis in need of "buck up camper"[11] management to one often rife with pain, shame, concealment, and ambivalence. *Period Piece* ends on an upbeat note as a series of women envision how they would teach their own daughters about menstruation and its meanings; how to change the script and embrace this transition into young female sexuality without shame and embarrassment.

Unlike the other films mentioned thus far which conform to the classroom film length of 30 minutes or less, *Under Wraps* (1998) is a feature length documentary sponsored by the National

Film Board of Canada that covers a range of issues related to menstruation, interviewing journalists, scholars, activists, doctors, patients, small business makers of reusable, organic femcare products and artists to address the emotional, cultural, medical, and environmental impact of menstruation and the femcare industry. The film begins with the pioneering work of Judy Chicago whose iconic 1970 photo litho, "Fed Flag," and 1972 Womanhouse exhibit entitled, "Menstruation Bathroom," represented controversial, pathbreaking public displays of this culturally private female experience. The double valence of the film's title alludes to products always discreetly marketed to promote their concealment and the myriad injunctions women are indoctrinated to accept by keeping their menstrual cycles private, preferably silent, under wraps. The film interviews Judy Blume, author of *Are You There God? It's Me Margaret* (1970), a canonical young adult novel about menarche, the impact of which continues to resonate with generations of young women and fans who often contact Blume, seeking advice and expressing their gratitude to her for writing the book. Blume talks about visiting elementary schools well into the 1990s who celebrate her long career as a YA author yet refuse to stock that particular book in their school libraries (Figure 13.1).

Moving around North America, *Under Wraps* is very much a talking heads documentary. The filmmakers interview gynecologists who discuss Toxic Shock Syndrome (TSS) and who sound the alarm about the continued lack of sufficient regulation of synthetic and toxic ingredients used by the femcare industry. They interview survivors of TSS and pay homage to several young women who died from the illness and lawyers who continue to doggedly battle powerful corporations to make them accountable. One scene features Harry Finley, founder of the Museum of Menstruation (1994–98) as he tours a small group through the installations in his suburban Washington D.C. home (his huge collection is now archived and online). They profile makers of organic reusable pads and environmental activists and artists who use tampons, pads and disposable applicators in their work and who visit a water treatment facility to draw attention to the huge problem with nonrecyclable applicators that clog treatment plants across the continent. As they visit a plant in Toronto, the authors of *Whitewash* – Liz Armstrong and Adrienne Scott – discuss the unnecessary and continued use of chlorine in wood pulping and in femcare products, stating that 12 billion tampons and pads are sent to landfill or incinerated each year in North America alone and that most Western menstruating women will use about 10,000 products over the course of their menstruating lives. They also show the workshops of advocates at the Menstrual Health Foundation in Baltimore who coach parents about how to address coming of age for their adolescent girls in ways that are celebratory rather than strictly about hygienic management and product consumption.

Another important feature length documentary to emerge in recent decades is *Period: The End of Menstruation* (2006) by Giovanna Chesler which tackles, among other things, the issue of menstrual suppression enabled by the FDA approval of Seasonale in Fall 2003, a drug that reduces the number of menstrual cycles to four per year (Figure 13.2). As with *Under Wraps*, *The End of Menstruation* involves travel across multiple cities in Canada and the United States where Chesler interviews racially diverse women about their attitudes toward menstruation, gynecologists who advocate for the benefits and convenience of using Seasonale, and others who argue against its use and the need for more expansive study. They talk to a woman who deliberately and happily suppressed her menstruation with DepoProvera due to the debilitating severity and pain of her periods. Chesler catches up with her a year later to discover that she has stopped using the drug after experiencing severe bone loss in her lower spine because of its hormonal suppressing side effects. The film shows groups who participate in Women's Wisdom Weekends in Northern California, a form of feminist activism striving to reclaim menstruation as healthy, spiritual, and empowering. Chesler also interviews scholar/activist/health educator

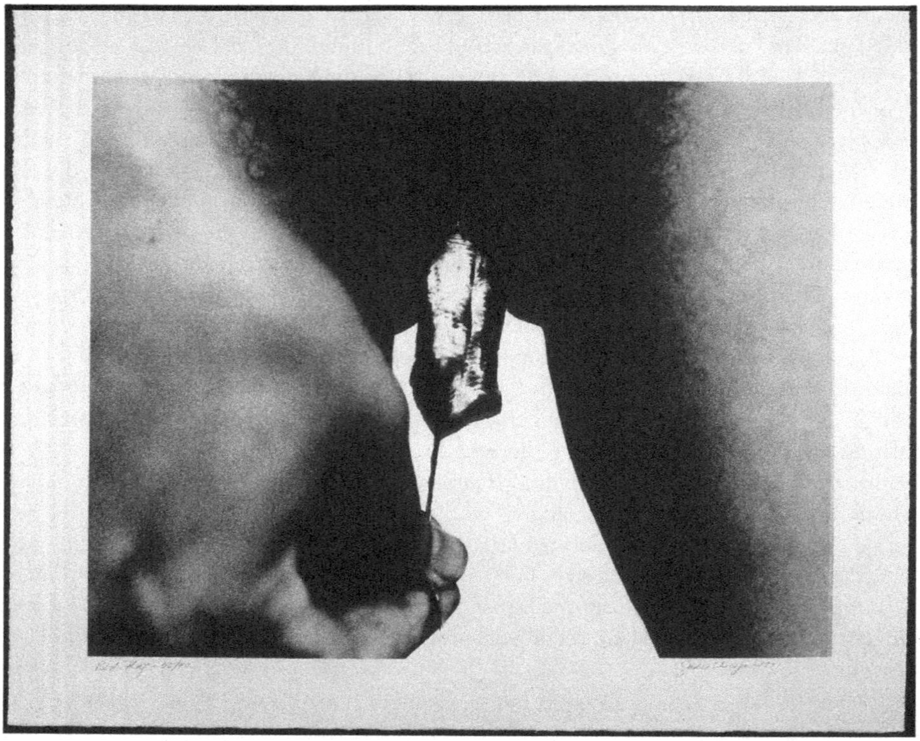

Figure 13.1 Judy Chicago's "Red Flag" is one of the iconic, provocative and path-breaking examples of second wave menstrual visibility and advocacy

Terri Kapsalis and artist Vanessa Tiegs who uses her own menstrual blood in her canvases. Their interview with transman, Morty Diamond, and his continued investment in menstruation (he deliberately modulates his testosterone intake to be able to menstruate), demonstrates a more inclusive gender queer view of menstruators. These and other films strive to find ways of visualizing and thinking about corporeal practices that are powerfully reflective of interrelated social change movements – feminism and women's health, consumer rights, LGBTQ and race, as well as environmental – that have led to the emergence of what Chris Bobel calls a "critical menstrual consciousness" (46). This involves moving beyond thinking about menstruation hygienically as a consumer and taking critical self-directed action that allows menstruators to proactively experience their bodies in ways that are healthy, sustainable, and enjoyable. Like *Under Wraps*, *The End of Menstruation* is probably not an age-appropriate elementary classroom film. Nevertheless, the film is a noteworthy text for healthcare educators, practitioners, high school and college students alike and represents an important contribution to the menstruation film subgenre.

The last film I want to address in this brief history is a short Netflix documentary about menstruation in India which won a 2018 Academy Award entitled *Period: End of Sentence* (hereafter referred to as *End of Sentence*). Directed by Iranian-American Rayka Zehtabchi, *End of Sentence* begins in a classroom at a rural school in Hapur, a small town in the northern state of Uttar Pradesh 60 miles from Delhi when a teacher asks her adolescent students what periods are. A montage of awkward silences and embarrassed efforts at a response ensues.

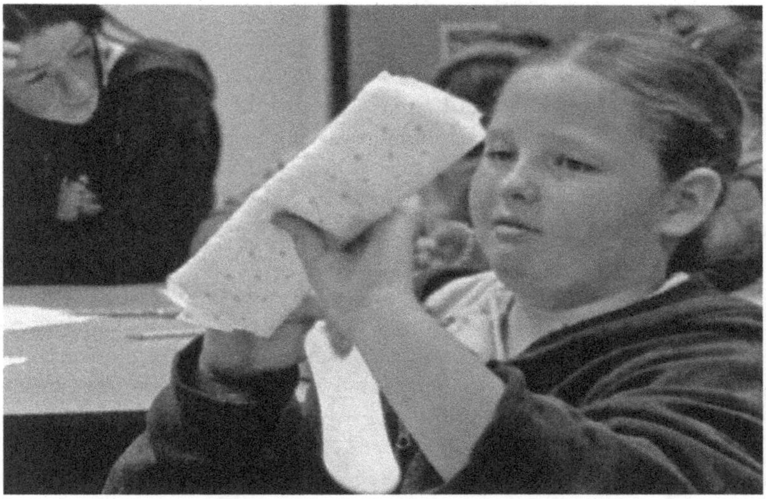

Figure 13.2 A student at Cesar Chavez Elementary School in San Diego participates in a hands-on approach to menstrual education in *Period: The End of Menstruation*

The film cuts to a group of young men sitting outside on a bench who feign ignorance about the word "period" until one of them speaks up: "It's an illness that affects ladies." A young woman recounts how she had to miss school so frequently after she began to menstruate that she eventually dropped out. While the film makes clear that sanitary protection has been a fraught domain in India for both economic and cultural reasons, it does not offer illuminating statistics. For example, an estimated 23 percent of girls in India drop out of school after reaching puberty both because they are humiliated by their peers and unable to afford or access proper products and private toilets. About 70 percent of women in India cannot afford sanitary products, and 300,000,000 use unhygienic alternatives like newspapers, rags and dry leaves to cope with their flow, which often leads to serious infection and illness (*The Economist Online*).

Despite advances that have been made for women in recent decades, the taboo against menstruating women in India persists. The film touches upon these taboos and prohibitions and shows a broad range of women – young and old – who discuss menstrual prejudices and inequities. For example, one scene shows women leaving a temple as voice-over describes being barred from entering such spaces when they menstruate because their bodies are deemed dirty and contaminating. One of them, amusingly, argues that they should be especially welcomed in temples honoring goddesses, since goddesses are females! Another woman – Sneha – talks about her desire to join the police so that she can avoid marriage and its constrictions. Later in the film, we see her doing physical training for the academy in ways that invoke older menstruation films depicting girls engaged in strenuous physical activity while menstruating. This is about the liberatory potential of using sanitary products. The film introduces us to Arunachalam Muruganantham, an enterprising school dropout who has famously succeeded in inventing a pad machine that can manufacture sanitary biodegradable pads in India for a fraction of the cost of the branded ones made by multinational corporations.[12] Muruganantham demonstrates how to work the device to a group of women and girls in the village and from here, the film focusses on the liberatory effect this machine has on the women who acquire the device and begin to manufacture and sell the pads on their own.[13]

End of Sentence is ultimately an upbeat and powerful message film about menstrual hygiene and microenterprise, using interviews across a wide generational swathe of Indian women in this rural locale to advocate for the transformative effect of the pad machine as a low-cost sanitary option for dealing with menstruation. It also, comically, shows several men being asked about the device and what it is used for who feign varying degrees of ignorance and discomfort. One insists that they are making diapers for babies. This is less a film exploring the social, cultural and religious taboos that persist in denigrating menstruators and more one that conveys an upbeat message not unlike menstrual hygiene films of old which represent the process as a hygienic crisis to be solved with little attention to the gender inequalities that persist around the fact of menstruation itself. One of the women involved in the pad machine enterprise says: "The thing is, when there's patriarchy, it takes time to talk about something that's related to women. It's taking time even amongst us women, but we'll get there." As a short film, *End of Sentence* cannot engage in a complex way the cultural taboos and misogynistic beliefs that persist in Indian culture, and it appears designed primarily for a North American audience. Nevertheless, it is a positive film that aims to re-write the story of menstruation as it gets told in India today by highlighting a hugely successful microenterprise and the socioeconomic empowerment it offers to the community of women who work within it. The degree to which it can meaningfully remove the stigma of menstruation is beyond the scope of the film's agenda or focus.

Conclusion

This general overview of menstruation films shows the ways in which competing discourses have participated in the construction of menarche, menstruation, and female sexual health over the past 70 years. While the connection between menstruation and hygiene (or menstruation as hygienic crisis as Brumberg notes) persists, recent decades have shown an expansion of discussion – particularly in independently produced films – of the taboos of secrecy, embarrassment, and indirection as well as engagement with the myriad issues that menstruators face (beyond a world of consumer choices) as women address body shaming and naming, pharmaceutical technologies and malpractices, economic realities of product use and consumer advocacy, environmentalism, and so on. From more dated conceptions of good grooming and menstrual disguise in the postwar period, it is clear that North American culture is slowing moving into Bobel's "critical menstrual discourse" framework where the menstrual script has expanded, however small those steps might be.

Notes

1 A British film directed and narrated by Winifred Holmes included because it appears to have been widely distributed in both Canada and the United States and remains part of many educational film collections/archives.

2 *Physical Aspects of Puberty* and *Social Sex Attitudes in Adolescence* (1953 Crawley Films) are frequently mentioned in discussion of menstruation films but geared to both sexes and produced in conjunction with a McGraw-Hill Family Life Education textbook, *Adolescent Development* by Elizabeth Hurlock. Clearly this list is by no means complete and this short paper can hardly offer a detailed analysis of so many titles. Many of these films are now available on DVD, through streaming services, archives.org, and on YouTube.

3 Distributed in the US under the title *Menstruation: Breaking the Silence* by Films Media Group.

4 This list is not an exhaustive one. Several recent papers constitute part of a growing field of useful research on this subject. See Martin "Postmodern Periods" and Vostral "Advice to Adolescents."

5 This essay is an extract from Kennard's doctoral dissertation, *The Corporation in the Classroom: The Struggles over Meanings of Menstrual Education in Sponsored Films, 1947-1983*. *The Story of Menstruation* has achieved almost a cult-like status and can be viewed on archives.org and even YouTube.
6 Complete versions of the 1948, 1961, and 1981 manuals can be found of the Museum of Menstruation website (mum.org).
7 The editions available on the MUM site include 1944, 1964, 1970, 1972, 1976, and 1991.
8 For a more expanded analysis of medical discourse in the film see, McFarland, "And that's the story": Themes of Medicalization within Disney and Kotex's *The Story of Menstruation*.
9 This includes the clitoris which, of course, would complicate the narrative that menstruation films stage (paradoxically privileging biological sex while diminishing sexuality). The clitoris is virtually absent from all menstruation and sex education films directed to youth until the early 1960s when, for example, in *Girl to Women* it is described succinctly "a small, highly sensitive organ" with no further elaboration. The same language is used in the 1982 menstruation film *Dear Diary*.
10 Tampons were also reviled by some as "nothing more than a dildo," thus as a form of sexual stimulant. See Brumberg, 160–3 and Vostral 55–7. It is noteworthy that comedian Amy Schumer's series of smart, humorous advertisements for Tampax in 2020 includes a mythbreaking sequence where she asks young teens if they think using a tampon affects their virginity.
11 I borrow this phrase from Sharra Vostra.
12 Muruganantham has been the subject of several films, including a mainstream Hindi film released in 2018 entitled *Padman* (R. Balki). *Padman* was one of the top grossing films in India in 2018, and sparked a much-needed national conversation about menstruation in that country.
13 The film credits tell us that the money for the Pad Machine was raised by the students at the Oakwood School in California via bake sales, Kickstarter and yogathons. In other words, it's a "developed" world film in English for a Western audience about "developing" world menstrual issues.

Works cited

"A New Documentary Addresses the Stigma of Menstruation in India," *The Economist Online*, January 22, 2019, www.economist.com/prospero/2019/01/22/a-new-documentary-addresses-the-stigma-of-menstruation-in-india.

Armstrong, Liz and Adrienne Scott. *Whitewash: Exposing the Health and Environmental Dangers of Women's Sanitary Products and Disposable Diapers – What You Can Do About It*. New York: Harper Perennial, 1992.

Bhadare, Namita. "Breaking New Ground: Films on Menstruation Shatter an Old Silence," *Indian Journal of Gender Studies*, vol. 26, no. 1&2, 2019, pp. 196–206.

Bobel, Chris. *New Blood: Third-Wave Feminism and the Politics of Menstruation*. New Brunswick, NJ: Rutgers University Press, 2010.

Brumberg, Joan Jacobs. *The Body Project: An Intimate History of American Girls*. New York: Vintage Books, 1997.

Delaney, Janice et al. *The Curse: A Cultural History of Menstruation*. Urbana, IL: University of Illinois Press, 1988.

Goslinga-Roy, Gillian. "Menarche in the Euro-American Traditions (Makes Us Bleed), a Review of Period Piece." *Visual Anthropology Review*, vol. 13, no. 1, 1997, pp. 68–9.

Kennard, Margot. "The Corporation in the Classroom: The Struggles over Meaning of Menstrual Education in Sponsored Films, 1947–1983," unpublished PhD dissertation, Madison, WI: University of Wisconsin, 1989.

Kennard, Margot. "Producing Sponsored Films on Menstruation: The Struggle over Meaning." In *The Ideology of Images in Educational Media: Hidden Curriculums in the Classroom*, edited by Elizabeth Ellsworth and Marianne Whatley. New York: Teachers College Press, 1990, pp. 57–73.

Martin, Michelle H. "Postmodern Periods: Menstruation Media in the 1990s." *The Lion and the Unicorn*, vol. 23, no. 3, September 1999, pp. 395–414.

McFarland, Christina Shipma. "'And That's the Story': Themes of Medicalization within Disney and Kotex's The Story of Menstruation." Unpublished thesis, Auburn University, 4 April2019.

"New Biology Film Helps Girls," *Educational Screen*, vol. 26, no. 4, April 1947, p. 215.

"Review of The Story of Menstruation," *JAMA*, vol. 133, no. 5, April 1947, p. 1033.

Vostral, Sharra L. "Advice to Adolescents: Menstrual Health and Menstrual Education Films, 1946–1982." In *Gender, Health and Popular Culture: Historical Perspectives*, edited by Cheryl Krasnic Warsh. Waterloo, Ontario: Wilfrid Laurier University Press, 2011, pp. 47–64.

Filmography

The Story of Menstruation (1947 Walt Disney Productions with Kimberly-Clark Corporation)
Growing Girls (1949 Film Producers Guild)
Molly Grows Up (1953 Personal Products Corporation)
It's Wonderful Being a Girl (1960 Johnson & Johnson)
Personal Health for Girls (1972 Coronet Instructional Films)
Naturally…A Girl (1973 Johnson & Johnson)
Dear Diary (1981 Boston Family Planning Project)
Girl Stuff (1982 Churchill Films)
Growing Up on Broadway (1984 Personal Products Corporation)
Linda's Film on Menstruation (1974 Linda Feferman)
Period Piece (1999 Jennifer Frame and Jay Rosenblatt)
Under Wraps (2004 National Film Board of Canada) Distributed in the US under the title *Menstruation: Breaking the Silence* by Films for Humanities and Sciences)
Period: End of Menstruation? (2006 Giovanna Chesler)
Period: End of Sentence (2018 Rayka Zehtabchi)
The Price of Getting Your Period in America (2019 CBSN Originals)

14

CRIP WISDOM IN THE TIME OF INSULIN CRISIS

Performing #insulin4all in short documentary film

Bianca C. Frazer

Introduction

On November 16, 2019, a group of protesters delivered blood money to the doorstep of the pharmaceutical company, Eli Lilly (Alliance, "Doctors, Family of Dead"). Lilly is one of three companies in the United States with the patent to produce and sell the drug insulin, a hormone that people with diabetes take to regulate their blood glucose levels. For people with Type 1 diabetes, the body does not produce any insulin, so they must take the hormone externally to survive. In the image from the protest, an older, white male stands on the steps and extends his right arm to pour out a pale of red paint, meant to symbolize blood, on a white poster on the concrete steps in front of him. The red paint lands on a white banner laid out on the steps with Lilly's name on the front. On the ground on either side of the man are large canvas bags with black dollar signs on the front and red paint across the bottom. Behind him, the man is surrounded by other people in winter clothing who hold various signs, some of which say, "Drugs don't work if you can't afford them," "Stop insulin price gouging," and "Health care for people not for profits."

These people are protesting conditions in the U.S. known as the insulin crisis (Figure 14.1). Insulin was discovered in 1921 by Canadian scientists who sold their patents to the University of Toronto for $1 each (Fralick and Kesselheim). One of those scientists, Frederick Banting, famously said, "Insulin does not belong to me, it belongs to the world." However, in the 21st century, the list price of insulin in the U.S. increased over 300 percent. Three factors have contributed to the cost increases: first, U.S. law allows pharmaceutical manufacturers to price their products at whatever level they believe the market will bear. Second, U.S. law allows companies to raise prices over time without limit. Third, because of patent evergreening, companies will make changes to keep patent protections although the product isn't substantially different; in the case of insulin, there is no direct market competition from a generic (Fralick and Kesselheim 1793–4).

DOI: 10.4324/9781003007661-19

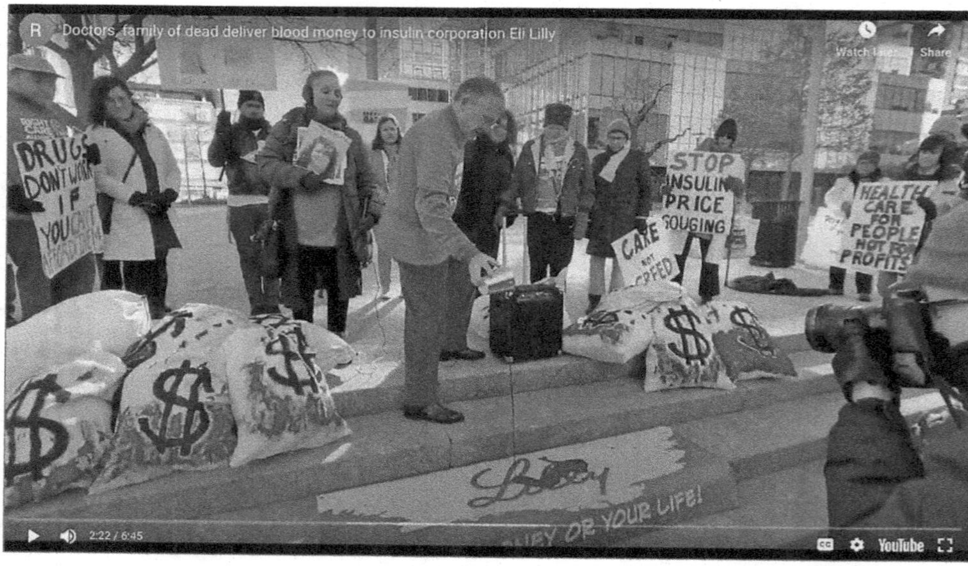

Figure 14.1 A protestor stands on the steps of Eli Lilly Innovation Center in Cambridge, MA. He pours out a small bucket of red paint, a symbol of blood, onto a white banner with Lilly's name on it. From the video "Doctors, family of dead deliver blood money to insulin corporation Eli Lilly" by Right Care Alliance, YouTube, 2019.

Source: Author's screenshot.

The cost-increases of this life-sustaining drug have led young people, both insured and uninsured, to ration insulin and in some cases, to die. Recent reports show that due to cost, one in four people with diabetes rations insulin (Herkert et al.). In 2019 alone, at least four young people including Jesimya David Scherer, age 21; Jada Renee Louis, age 24; and Josh Wilkerson, age 27 died from insulin rationing, delayed insurance coverage of insulin, an older, less effective versions of insulin available at Wal-Mart (Alliance "High Insulin Costs"). While having insurance might seem like the solution to affordable insulin, there are still variable co-pays. Even those with insurance are limited by which types of insulin their insurance covers. The brand or kind of insulin that one desires to take may not be the kind covered by insurance. As the situation grows more desperate, people with diabetes are experimenting with different approaches, including documentaries, to mobilize the general public's collective power to pressure lawmakers to change legislation.

In this chapter, I offer a performance analysis of three documentaries to demonstrate how people with diabetes use *crip wisdom* to change public opinion about diabetes and circumvent oppressive healthcare systems. After describing the concept of crip wisdom, I trace how activists perform it in documentary shorts. These shorts are each less than 20 minutes and released by established news organizations that lend authority and validity for the general public: "We Buy Insulin or We Die," released by *The New York Times* as an Opinion-Video in June 2019; "The Lethal Price of Insulin," by *NowThisNews* in June 2019; and "Insulin Quest: When Lifesaving Drugs Are Out of Reach," by the *Wall Street Journal* in December 2018. In these videos, subjects with diabetes show the camera the complex and creative behaviors they are performing to access affordable insulin. Short documentary film captures these acts and shares them with a broad audience, thereby building empathy and prompting action toward a shared goal of insulin for all.

A note on terminology: Disability Studies scholar Carrie Sandahl reclaims and incorporates the term "crip," from the derogatory epithet, "cripple," to signify disability identity, politics, and culture (25). "Crip wisdom" is a concept from disability justice advocates who say people with lived experience of disability are not objects to be fixed but whole human beings with skills, ingenuity, and brilliance. Patricia Berne, the executive director of the performance collective, Sins Invalid, explains crip wisdom as the difference between knowledge, which "is when we take information, facts, and create a system of understanding," and wisdom, which is "when we know something because it's in our bones. It's our experience" (Leibowitz). Crip wisdom, therefore, is an affirmation of the resourcefulness and authority held by individuals and communities with disability experience, not only the traditional information and facts held by healthcare providers. The crip framework of health critiques the U.S. healthcare system, exemplified by disability justice warrior Stacey Milbern's question: "Is medicine about quality of life or is it about social control and perpetuating this idea of a good body?" (Spade and Dector).

Performing disability, performing diabetes

Some readers may be surprised to consider diabetes within a disability framework. While the Americans with Disabilities Act considers it a disability, most members of the diabetes community themselves do not identity with diabetes as a disability. Still, I find several "points of affinity" between people with diabetes and the broader disability community (Kafer 11). For example, diabetic and disabled communities and activists foreground a non-able-bodied identity, challenge dehumanizing stereotypes, and value access in various forms. Another point of affinity with disability culture is the presence and value of crip wisdom. For those with a non-apparent disability, assessing when, and what, and how to reveal behavior dictated by an impairment is crip wisdom. Disability scholar Tobin Siebers remarks that "disabled people who pass for able-bodied are neither cowards, cheats, nor con artists but skillful interprets of the world from whom we all might learn" (324). Frequently, discourses of diabetes in medical institutions focuses on an individual who causes diabetes through a poor lifestyle, lack of exercise, unhealthy eating rather than naming systemic issues like the insulin crisis. Insofar as the project of medicine and health is about quality of life, then, the insulin crisis reveals the failures of U.S. health care. The subjects of these documentaries explain that the source of failure remains with profit driven pharmaceutical companies, not with diabetic individuals and their behaviors. The goal is for broader audiences to comprehend this reality with the hopes that understanding and empathizing will build a broader coalition of political pressure groups to demand legislative change

All of the following documentary shorts were released between 2018 and 2019. On December 3, 2018, the *Wall Street Journal* video platform, *WSJ | Video,* published the piece, "Insulin Quest: When Lifesaving Drugs Are Out of Reach," Episode 8 in Season 2 of *Moving Upstream*, a documentary video series focused on "trends, technologies, ideas and challenges that are headed our way" (Macnaughton and Jones). In this 09:58 minute-long episode, *WSJ* correspondent and senior producer "Jason Bellini takes a look at some of the unconventional steps Americans are taking to access the lifesaving drug."

Next, on June 13, 2019, the *New York Times* published the Op-Ed video titled, "We Either Buy Insulin or We Die." A note under the video describes it as piece that "reveals the lengths to which [people with diabetes] go to get a nearly century-old drug" (Cressman et al.). The film features recognizable activists and advocates from the diabetes community: Robin Cressman is a Type 1 diabetes advocate and creator of the group Liberate Insulin, and Laura Pavlakovich is a Type 1 diabetic who created a photojournalism account on Instagram of people with diabetes called "You're Just My Type." The video also includes Nicole Smith-Holt, a Charity Ambassador for T1 International. The video is 04:23 minutes long and was written and edited by the featured diabetics in the film.

Lastly, on June 17, 2019, *NowThisNews* published a 13:45 minute video to YouTube titled, "The Lethal Price of Insulin." *NowThisNews* describes itself as a "premier news outlet providing you with all the videos you need to stay up to date" and specializes in news, politics, and pop culture in documentary short format. In the video description, the filmmakers write that they "followed 29-year-old Paloma Kemak as she traveled across the U.S.-Mexico border to get the medication she needs to survive" (*NowThisNews*). Viewers have downloaded this video over 90,000 times. The following analysis is organized into themes that emerge across the three videos.

Performing the burden: crossing borders to access insulin

In the United States, the broad public believes individuals cause their diabetes through poor lifestyle choices and lack of self-control (Bock). The public perception maintains that such individuals need only follow three simple rules: eat better, exercise more, and lose weight (Walker and Frazer). As videos reveal the immense barriers and complex labor that individuals must perform to access their medication, they illuminate that living with diabetes is not as simple as the public believes. The activists reveal great effort, not laziness, and illuminate great complexity, not simplicity, as they navigate living with diabetes. These videos provide essential insights for healthcare providers who may hold a similar view of diabetes: it is relatively simple to manage with easy rules to follow and all within an individual's control. The notion of individual control is so central to health professionals' understanding of diabetes that they are taught to code for an individual's quality of diabetes management in terms of control (Dugan and Shubrook). However, these video stories evidence several factors outside of an individual's control, greatly impacting diabetes management. Health professionals would do well to attend to this complexity as they work with patients' fears, behaviors, and efforts to access the tools they need to live.

One example of significant labor revealed in two of the documentary shorts are people compelled to cross the U.S.–Mexico border to access less expensive insulin. In these segments, interviewees emphasize their desperation and frame the travel as an injustice. For example, to circumvent the high price structure established by big pharma companies and insurance markets, diabetes sufferers must travel long distances to obtain their insulin. Berne explains that "every time you spend money you shouldn't have to spend for healthcare" is an ableist encounter (Leibowitz). The broader public is not usually witness to such ableist encounters, but the footage that shows people traveling to another country to evade the U.S. market reveals how desperate costly health care has become for so many people. As the documentary reveals the distances people go to buy insulin, it also demands a public response to ameliorate this crisis. Such media and documentaries can influence public opinion, which in turn, can impact legislation around health care.

At the start of "We Either Buy Insulin or We Die," each speaker in the film describes his or her actions as absurd but necessary. The video begins with a series of camera shots: first, the film provides an establishing shot of the U.S.–Mexico border port of entry followed by a medium shot of a thin, white person named Robin Cressman. Cressman stands at a pharmacy counter in Mexico purchasing insulin. Cressman's voice speaks over the footage: "I should not have to cross a border to buy my insulin." Next, a low angle shot captures Paulius Podziunas' back as seen through the passenger seat of his car as he approaches the passenger side of another vehicle. His voice plays over the footage: "I should not have to buy my insulin off a stranger in a parking lot as if it were a drug deal." The footage then cuts to a medium shot of Laura Pavlakovich, a petite, white woman with long, dark hair and several tattoos, sitting indoors in front of her camera and speaking directly to the viewer: "None of us should fear death from a perfectly manageable disease, but we do because American drug makers can arbitrarily raise prices to line their pockets and Congress hasn't done anything to stop them." As they stress that the physical lengths they must go to are outrageous, these diabetics also condemn the greed of American drug makers and the inaction of Congress. As audiences witness this connection, the documentary reveals a crisis in need of a public response.

Description: Robin Cressman sits on a bench with her lap full of name-brand insulin. From the video "We Either Buy Insulin or We Die" by Laura Juncadella, *New York Times* Opinion, 2019

In one trip to Mexico, Cressman focuses on the arbitrarily high cost of insulin in the U.S. as she and Pavlakovich take the viewer on a journey with a group of other diabetics to "patronize[e] the good pharmacies of Tijuana, Mexico." An establishing shot captures the sunlit street in Tijuana. The camera technique then changes to show a long shot of three people walking down a concrete hallway. The long shot continues as Cressman and another person enter a pharmacy. The footage cuts to Cressman, surrounded by four other people, sitting on a park bench with her lap full of insulin boxes (Figure 14.2). An off-camera voice says, "Dang that's a lot of medicine," while Cressman, smiling and nodding, says: "So we have about $8,000–$10,000 dollars' worth of insulin sitting here in my lap and we got it for between 5–10% of U.S. retail price." As Cressman displays her haul of name-brand insulin at a fraction of the U.S. cost, she demonstrates for the viewer that high insulin prices in the U.S. are simply high because they can be. Other people surround Cressman, both to advocate for a larger diabetes community as well as to demonstrate that she has community support for

Figure 14.2 Robin Cressman sits on a bench with her lap full of name-brand insulin. From the video "We Either Buy Insulin or We Die" by Laura Juncadella, New York Times Opinion, 2019

Source: Author's screenshot.

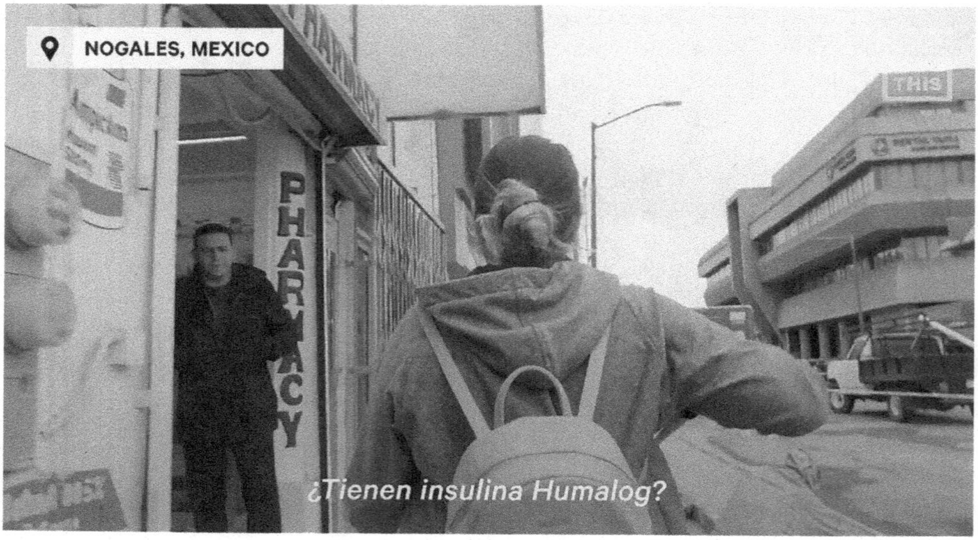

Figure 14.3 Paloma Kemak looks for insulin in pharmacies in Nogales, Mexico. From the video "The Lethal Price of Insulin" by NowThis Reports, NowThis News, 2019
Source: Author's screenshot.

her actions. This undertaking does not constitute an illegal sneaking off to another country to avoid paying a few more dollars but rather, a principal act of disability justice led by those most affected by commercial avarice, public apathy, and political inertia. In this video, Cressman leads a band of desperate diabetics to get what they urgently need. By bypassing the corrupt system, Cressman and her fellow diabetics prove that it does not have to be this way in the U.S.

In contrast to the *NYT Op-Ed* emphasis on community, the *NowThis* video features an individual traveling on her own to Mexico to obtain affordable insulin. The video footage of Paloma Kemak, a 29-year-old woman with long brown hair tracks her as she travels across the border and around the streets of Nogales, Mexico (Figure 14.3). Kemak, wearing a grey hoodie and tan backpack, enters a metal turnstile with the words, "To Mexico," above it. Kemak's voice plays over footage of her walking: "Going to Mexico to buy insulin is kind of a last resort to be able to live another month or two, that's my only option at this point." The viewer can see a long shot of Kemak as she approaches the doorway of a pharmacy and asks a man standing in the entrance, "Tienen insulina Humalog?" He replies, "no," and Kemak keeps walking down the street. At the conclusion of the short, the *NowThis* correspondent, CC Allen, stands on a pedestrian street with Kemak and asks, "Is it what you expected?" Kemak replies, "I expected it to be a tiny bit easier. There was plenty of insulin, just not the specific kind that I prefer to use. I did get one box. This was $45." This exchange emphasizes that people crossing the border to access insulin is not a total fix: in many ways, diabetic people are still relatively powerless when seeking affordable insulin in Mexico. Kemak explains that there is a brand of insulin that she prefers to use, but not every pharmacy carries the insulin brand of her choice. The film shows Kemak approaching several strangers to ask about pharmacies and then entering pharmacies to ask if they sell Humalog. In several shots, pharmacists tell Kemak repeatedly, "no." By sharing this harrowing journey with the camera, Kemak engenders empathy from the viewer, a key aspect for transforming public opinion. The burden of U.S. drug costs is so extreme that people have no choice but to go to another country to get insulin. This is crip wisdom, the resourcefulness and brilliance that enable people to find easier ways to survive and to be empowered.

Documenting the cost: emotional vulnerability as activism

Filmmakers like Laura Juncadella capture people sharing emotional confessional-style stories about the stress of the insulin crisis, providing audiences with insider knowledge. The documentary format also focuses on intimate spaces such as Kemak's empty fridge with her dwindling insulin supply; an anonymous mother's stockpile of supplies in her kitchen cabinets; and Podziunas in a parking lot buying supplies from a stranger. The documentary footage captures authentic, intimate moments while also offering contextualizing information to give audiences previously unknown information and new knowledge. Such portrayals convey the crisis with contextual, intimate settings rather than with testimonials filmed in settings like doctor's offices or congressional hearings. This technique generates the empathy that is essential for changing public opinion of diabetes. The public pressure effects public health decisions around access to health care.

Each of the documentaries expounds on the emotional weight of the insulin crisis. By centering emotion, subjects challenge the ableist notion that one should strive to minimize disability and "try to be as able-bodied as possible all the time" (Siebers 316). For many complex reasons, a person with diabetes may hide its emotional toll. However, if the broader public does not know the painful stories, then they might maintain the belief that the problem of disability is "best solved through strength of character and resolve" (Kafer 4). However, these stories of pain and loss help convince the public that unaffordable insulin is not an issue of individuals overcoming but of an injustice that requires broad attention and legislative change. By communicating the human cost of the insulin crisis, the subjects aim to galvanize a broad audience who holds the power to pressure lawmakers.

Nicole Holt-Smith appears in both the *NYT* and *NowThis* videos to share the story of the death of her son, Alec Smith. As Berne notes, "Some things you just have to live through to really f***ing get it," and Smith-Holt brings the moral authority of a mother whose son died because of unaffordable insulin (Leibowitz). In the *NYT* video, we first hear Holt-Smith's voice over photos of her son as a young adult, remembering him as, "energic, fun-loving. He was just so full of life." Holt-Smith's voice continues to tell Alec's story: after he was kicked off his mother's insurance, he went to purchase insulin at a cost of $1,300. Unable to afford that amount, he left the pharmacy, tried to eat low carb, but was unable to ration his insulin until his next paycheck. Three days before payday, Smith's body was found in his apartment with all of his insulin used. Nicole Smith-Holt appears in the *NowThis* video to share her son's story again. The pain of this story is undeniable. Smith-Holt demonstrates that her son's death was preventable if he could have afforded insulin, and she enacts crip wisdom by sharing her son's story with a broad audience, who upon learning how his death was preventable, is encouraged to shift the blame narrative from individuals with diabetes to the U.S. healthcare system.

Contrasting Smith-Holt's loss, the *WSJ* episode focuses on Karyn Wofford, a Type 1 diabetic who again generates affect and authority grounded in her lived experience. In the video, Wofford, a 29-year-old white woman with long brunette hair, describes the impact of unaffordable insulin to correspondent and senior producer, Jason Bellini. Wofford tells Bellini that she and her husband have moved back in with her parents so that they can afford her insulin. The two-shot footage shows Wofford and Bellini sitting at a kitchen table, and Bellini asks if Wofford thinks this disease will shorten her life. She tears up and answers, "I think it probably already has, I go to sleep you know wondering, sorry, I'm not really a crier that much, sorry.

I think about, you know, like if my sugar is high, like what kind of damage is being done, like you know, is it going to damage my heart." Wofford shares a metaphor to convey the gravity of her need for insulin: "This is our oxygen, it's our water, it's as essential as those things." As a formulation of crip wisdom, Wofford foregrounds rather than hides her thoughts and emotions around diabetes to transform public conceptions of diabetes, vital to the activism projects of regulating drug prices. These documentaries in which subjects share their emotional vulnerability born of struggle and loss can increase pressure on public opinion and lawmakers.

Creative strategies: the underground network

Crip wisdom also emphasizes community and working together to fight unjust systems. Each documentary not only focuses on one person's story but also brings together multiple stories from different people. The documentaries present a broader picture of the effect in the U.S. For example, Bellini talks to Wofford in Georgia but connects her experience with Di Franco's actions in California. As activists seek federal reform of drug pricing policy, it matters how people are affected by the crisis in different settings across the country. The power of documentary puts individual stories in the context of communities and reveals the underground networks of supply sharing and survival strategies that are necessary to circumvent the price gouging, which often characterizes the U.S. healthcare system.

Each of the documentaries shows people with diabetes creating modes outside of traditional systems to access insulin. Some of these measures, such as persons sharing or selling extra insulin from prescriptions are, in fact, illegal. However, such illegal measures are represented as preferable to what U.S. healthcare offers, demonstrating the need to regulate if not completely dismantle these systems. As Sins Invalid performer Leah Lakshimi Piepzna-Samarasinha puts it: "Crips are geniuses" (Leibowitz) and have authority from their lived experience with their bodies. People with disabilities "are often smarter and more skilled at navigating both our bodyminds and ableism than most medical professionals." The *NowThis* short provides a telling illustration of Piepzna-Samarasinha's point when correspondent CC Allen asks Dr. Joshua Miller, who is also a Type 1 diabetic, "It's almost, like, can you afford to be diabetic?" Dr. Miller looks at Allen and says, "I have patients come and see me, and I don't know what to tell them." This interaction highlights that even experts in the medical establishment are powerless in the face of pharmaceutical companies and insurance systems. Piepzna-Samarasinha's concept only highlights the skills and the risks many crips have to "game" systemic barriers.

Another example of people who reveal going outside of traditional systems is through the underground exchange of diabetes supplies. This exchange occurs when a person shares or sells extra medication or supplies leftover from a prescription. While illegal, these acts have become increasingly common. A 2019 study confirms that over 50 percent of participants had donated supplies, while only 34.6 percent had received donations (Litchman et al.). While social sciences researcher can quantify the phenomenon of prescription sharing, documentary film can communicate the humanity and crip wisdom of community more affectively and viscerally than the data as well as what is at stake without community efforts.

Another example of community knowledge that emerges from these underground networks is a sense of humor and generosity about the exchange. Humor lets the audience in on a joke and creates community as what preceeds in the video enables the viewer to get it. In the *NYT* Opinion video, Type 1 diabetic Paulius Podziunas uses humor to talk about the person he buys illegal insulin from as his drug dealer. Speaking as a talking head to the camera, he explains how he began buying insulin in an "underground world" through a website called OfferUp. Podziunas describes the person he buys from: "He constantly has insulin on deck." Then the shot switches to close up images of the site OfferUp: a disembodied user scrolls down the page displaying post after post of diabetes supplies for sale at lower prices. The footage cuts to a long shot of Podziunas stepping out of the driver's seat of a vehicle to approach a stranger in a car parked next to him. Podziunas calls this stranger his "number one drug dealer."

The scale of the underground network expands as each video includes multiple examples of people taking part in an underground exchange. Another example in the *NYT* Op-Ed piece occurs when Pavlakovich talks about her Instagram account, "You're Just My Type," evolving into "a platform for people to donate and trade diabetes supplies." In the *NowThis* video, correspondent CC Allen goes inside the suburban home of an anonymous mother who does not want her face filmed but who agrees to take Allen around her kitchen where she sells and donates extra supplies leftover from her young son's prescriptions. In the *WSJ* film, the narrator, Jason Bellini, accompanies Wofford to a local café where they meet another person wishing to remain anonymous who sells Wofford his extra insulin over coffee. Sitting in the café, the seller explains the situation to Bellini, "I don't take all my insulin all the time. If I can help someone else out, I just want to do it." This attitude expresses the willingness of the broader diabetic community to do whatever they can to help others in need. This sharing is a form of getting outside the capitalist pharma structures, but it is worth noting that these subjects are taking illegal actions to work around the system as is.

In the *WSJ* episode, Bellini captures another fascinating, albeit rarer, formulation of crip wisdom meant to get around the medical establishment's stranglehold on the insulin market. Bellini travels to California and tours the lab of Anthony Di Franco, the Founder of the Open Insulin Project. The Open Insulin Project is "doing the research and development necessary to put insulin production under the control of the people who need it to survive and restore access to this crucial drug" (Di Franco). Again, these stories challenge the assumption of authority held by pharma and supply companies. The "do-it-yourself" element of crip wisdom shows that people are not always and only beholden to the official medical establishment. Stories, captured and shared in documentary format, help others imagine new ways of getting what they need, supporting other community-led efforts, and showing crips working together.

Conclusions and future work

While these documentaries provide urgent and compelling portrayals of the insulin crisis, they also present several thorny considerations. The makers of these documentaries focus on white, predominantly thin people with Type 1 and their activist strategies. Of course, the breadth of the insulin crisis impacts people outside these identities. For example, *ProPublica* and *The New York Times* published a 2018 article that details how unaffordable insulin causes harm to people with Type 2 diabetes forced to choose between medications they need based on what they can afford (Thomas and Ornstein). Traditionally, the public has viewed Type 1 diabetes as a more sympathetic disease (Bock 156–7), and even within the diabetic community, people with Type 1 have resisted solidarity with people with Type 2. The erasure of people with Type 2 diabetes from the documentaries maintains the public perception of them as lazy and undeserving of public sympathy or resources.

When these filmmakers focus exclusively on white and mostly thin bodies, they do not address the complications of medical racism or weight bias as a part of the insulin crisis. Given that a smaller number of Black and Latanx people in the U.S. are insured, the increasing cost of insulin has a more devastating impact in these communities (Chalabi). Future diabetic activism may consider a more intersectional exploration of the many examples of crip wisdom within communities of color who are navigating this crisis. Additionally, these films do not comment on the privilege that allows white subjects to perform illegal acts in public, believing that the behavior can be interpreted as a justified response to unjust systems rather than criminalized and punished. Another area where privilege shapes the premise of activism is the idea that insulin in Mexico is much more affordable than the U.S. This proposition does not address insulin affordability as a global issue, as many people with diabetes in Mexico do not consider those prices affordable relative to their income.

Still, the efforts of advocates and activists are beginning to yield results. In 2018, the Senate Special Committee on Aging included a hearing on "Insulin Access and Affordability: The Rising Cost of Treatment." In February 2019, the U.S. Senate Committee on Finance announced a bipartisan investigation into insulin prices. In May 2019, Colorado enacted a law that limited monthly insurance copayments for insulin to $100. On March 4, 2019, Eli Lilly announced it would begin to sell, "a generic version of its most commonly prescribed insulin – Humalog® – for half the name-brand's cost" (Young). This drug, called Insulin Lispro, will have a list price of $137.25. Rather than being met with gladness, many activists criticized this action as evidence of the arbitrariness of high costs; they noted how easily pharmaceutical companies lowered prices under public pressure and described this amount for a life-sustaining drug as completely unacceptable.

Activists point to the larger issue that despite the modifications to the crisis of insulin affordability, none of these changes completely addresses the barriers to insulin for anyone who needs it. As of this writing, Congress has not passed compressive federal legislation that makes insulin accessible. In the meantime, people with diabetes go on navigating this complexity in order to stay alive. These short films document the crip wisdom of diabetics at this time of crisis as they find ways to get what they need, to care for community, and to perform themselves for a public audience in order to achieve social change.

Works cited

Alliance, Right Care. "Doctors, Family of Dead Deliver Blood Money to Insulin Corporation Eli Lilly." November 17, 2019, www.youtube.com/watch?v=-TsGzleU3XE.

Alliance, Right Care. "High Insulin Costs Are Killing Americans." Rightcarealliance.org, https://rightcarealliance.org/actions/insulin/. Accessed July 15, 2020.

Bock, Sheila. "Contextualization, Reflexivity, and the Study of Diabetes-Related Stigma." *Journal of Folklore Research*, vol. 49, no. 2, 2012, pp. 153–78,

Chalabi, Mona. "Insulin Costs Are Rising – and Diabetic Americans of Color Are Hit Hardest | Mona Chalabi." *The Guardian*, July 14, 2019, www.theguardian.com/us-news/datablog/2019/jul/14/diabetes-insulin-mona-chalabi-data-blog.

Cressman, Robin et al. " 'We Either Buy Insulin or We Die'." *The New York Times*, June 13, 2019, www.nytimes.com/2019/06/13/opinion/insulin-price-costs.html.

Di Franco, Anthony. "About the Project." *Openinsulin.org*. https://openinsulin.org/about-the-project/. Accessed July 22, 2020.

Dugan, Joy and Jay Shubrook. "International Classification of Diseases, 10th Revision, Coding for Diabetes." *Clinical Diabetes: A Publication of theAmerican Diabetes Association*, vol. 35, no. 4, 2017, pp. 232–8.

Fralick, Michael and Aaron. S. Kesselheim. "The U.S. Insulin Crisis – Rationing a Lifesaving Medication Discovered in the 1920s." *The New England Journal of Medicine*, vol. 381, no. 19, 2019, pp. 1793–5.

Herkert, D. et al. "Cost-Related Insulin Underuse among Patients with Diabetes." *JAMA Intern Med*, vol. 179, no. 1, 2019, pp. 112–14.

Kafer, Alison. *Feminist, Queer, Crip*. Bloomington, IN: Indiana University Press, 2013.

Leibowitz, Tovah. "Sins Invalid's 'Birthing, Dying, Becoming Crip Wisdom' Features Crip Art, Activism, Love & Liberation | Autostraddle." *Autostraddle*, October 13, 2016, www.autostraddle.com/sins-invalids-birthing-dying-becoming-crip-wisdom-features-crip-art-activism-love-and-liberation-354749/.

Litchman, M. L. et al. "The Underground Exchange of Diabetes Medications and Supplies: Donating, Trading, and Borrowing, Oh My!" *Journal of Diabetes Science and Technology*, 2019, pp. 1–10.

Macnaughton, Spencer and Conall Jones. "Insulin Quest: When Lifesaving Drugs Are Out of Reach." *Moving Upstream*, edited by Jason Bellini, *The Wall Street Journal*, 2018. www.wsj.com/video/series/moving-upstream/high-insulin-prices-drive-diabetics-to-take-extreme-measures/1AB7653D-D0F8-4441-9218-5668D1BC62A7.

NowThisNews. "The Lethal Cost of Insulin." 2019. www.youtube.com/watch?v=Ow8lCYPPzNY.

Sandahl, Carrie. "Queering the Crip or Cripping the Queer?: Intersections of Queer and Crip Identities in Solo Autobiographical Performance." *GLQ: A Journal of Lesbian and Gay Studies*, vol. 9, no. 1–2, 2003, pp. 25–56, https://muse.jhu.edu/article/40804.

Siebers, Tobin. "Disability and the Theory of Complex Embodiment – for Identity Politics in a New Register." *The Disability Studies Reader*, edited by Lennard J. Davis, 5th edition. New York and Abingdon: Routledge, 2017, pp. 313–32.

Spade, Dean and Hope Dector. "Ableism Is the Bane of My Motherfuckin' Existance." *BCRW Videos*, Vimeo, 2017. https://vimeo.com/216562627.

Thomas, Katie and Charles Ornstein. "The Price They Pay." *ProPublica and The New York Times*, March 5, 2018, https://features.propublica.org/drug-prices/high-cost-drugs-the-price-they-pay/.

Walker, Heather and Bianca Frazer. "The Metanarrative of Diabetes: Should You Be Eating That?" *Metanarratives of Disability: Culture, Assumed Authority, and the Normative Social Order*, edited by David Bolt. New York and Abingdon: Routledge, 2021, pp. 156–68.

Young, Ayana. "Eli Lilly Announces Lower-Cost Generic Insulin." *JDRF*, March 4, 2019, www.jdrf.org/blog/2019/03/04/eli-lilly-announces-new-lower-cost-generic-insulin/.

15

AGING, REMIXED

Intergenerational storytelling in the digital realm

Andrea Charise

"Storytelling" is a vital element of humanities-based health research, education, and practice that involves the sharing of individual experiences of health and illness. Over the past decade, the emergence of *digital storytelling* has provided another medium for opening important windows into health-related experiences, vastly enhancing the "spreadable" qualities of such stories (to use media scholar Henry Jenkins' evocative term). While aging and older age must not be collapsed with ideas of illness or decline, intergenerational storytelling may be considered an adjacent form of health-related storytelling, given its typical format of personal and/or collective memories of lived experience as told by one distinct generation to another. Intergenerational storytelling is well positioned to benefit from the affordances of the digital realm, as reflected by the emergence of "born digital" intergenerational storytelling initiatives across North America and Europe – and this is particularly true in the context of Covid-19, which has introduced significant obstacles to in-person research and knowledge creation.

Yet, if the medium remains the message (as per Marshall McLuhan's enduring maxim), what critical issues – for digital storytelling, age studies, and health humanities alike – might the digitization of intergenerational practices solicit, address, or elide? This chapter offers a critical assessment of the emergence of digital storytelling practices, with a particular focus on their applications as they relate to aging and the intergenerational context. It provides an overview of current scholarship in health-related digital storytelling, explores the intersection of digital media and age studies, and discusses one recent award-winning exemplar, the Toronto-based Canadian initiative *The Resemblage Project* (www.resemblageproject.ca), to provide a critical analysis of digital intergenerational storytelling – and crucially, the conceptual, ethical, and social justice concerns related to its current and future practice.

Aging, remixed: intergenerational storytelling in the digital realm

"Storytelling" is now a widespread feature of arts- and humanities-based approaches to health research, education, practice, and knowledge translation. Personal narratives that highlight the profoundly individual human experience of health, illness, and their sociocultural contexts are increasingly recognized as a vital creative resource for making sense of how ill health disrupts what might be considered "life-as-normal" (Frank 195). As established by canonical works like Rita Charon's *Narrative Medicine: Honouring the Story of Illness* (2006), Arthur Kleinman's

DOI: 10.4324/9781003007661-20

The Illness Narratives: Suffering, Healing, and the Human Condition (1988), and Arthur Frank's *The Wounded Storyteller: Body, Illness, and Ethics* ([1995] 2013), health-related storytelling has conventionally taken the form of narrative textual accounts. More recently, the pull of visual media has further expanded the creative modalities available for such work, as evinced by the popularity of comics, graphic medicine, TV programs, and, of course, documentary and fictional film.

Over the past decade, ***digital storytelling*** has emerged as yet another medium for generating evocative openings into health-related experience. In its most basic form, digital storytelling refers to the creation of a short (usually two- to five-minute) audiovisual clip combining photographs and/or video, a (typically first-person) narrative voiceover, and other audio like ambient or outdoor sounds and music. It is an amalgam of several media types, engaging elements of documentary film, visual diaries, collage, autotheory, and oral history. Its origin is attributed to the collaborative efforts of Joe Lambert, Dana Atchley, and Nina Mullen who founded the San Francisco "Center for Digital Media" in the mid-1990s, which was renamed the "Center for Digital Storytelling" in 1998 and then StoryCenter in 2015. Scholars have offered multiple histories and accounts of digital storytelling (see Lambert; de Jager et al.; Moreau et al.; and Gubrium et al.), but StoryCenter's core mandate, reflected in their online mission statement, is worth underscoring here: "When we listen deeply, and tell stories, we build a just and healthy world" (www.storycenter.org).

Digital storytelling engages a broad range of topics including education, social justice, civic engagement, and human rights. While it is not exclusively dedicated to matters of health and illness, a significant genre within digital storytelling involves detailing an individual health experience in its embodied ***actuality*** (significantly, a term originally used to describe what we now call "documentary" films). In line with Douglas Crimp's assertion of documentary video as fundamental to affirming processes of self-representation in AIDS-related activism, digital storytelling has emerged as a creative, and potentially therapeutic, mode of self-expression. It is often used within the context of ***participatory research***, defined by Diane Conrad and Anita Sinner as knowledge-making work conducted and designed "with" rather than "on" participants. Because of their intimate insights into human vulnerability and marginalization, digital stories have also been employed in the service of knowledge translation and for the purposes of health education, training, and professional development although its impact in these domains remains somewhat undefined (Moreau et al.).

In the following discussion, I explore the emergence of health-related digital storytelling, with a special focus on its critical applications to aging, older age, and intergenerational interaction. While aging and older age must not be collapsed with ideas of illness and decline, ***intergenerational storytelling*** (digital or otherwise) can be considered an adjacent practice that involves the oral sharing of personal and/or collective memories of lived experience, often as told by one distinct generation to another. In place of more conventional oral sharing techniques such as "life review" (Butler, 529) or "reminiscence therapy," defined by the American Psychological Assocation (APA) as older people's "use of life histories – written, oral, or both – to improve psychological well-being," digital storytelling offers a more contemporary iteration of such practices – as the emergence of "born digital" intergenerational storytelling initiatives (i.e., originally produced in and for the digital realm rather than converted from print or other media) across North America and Europe suggest.

Even before the Covid-19 pandemic introduced significant obstacles to in-person research methodologies (Chivers), intergenerational storytelling was especially well-positioned to benefit from the affordances of the digital realm. It has the potential to destabilize dominant ideologies of ageism and the default white, often cis-female, subject of aging research (Charise 191). But if the medium remains the message, what critical issues – related to digital storytelling, health humanities, and age studies – might such digital mediations solicit, address, or elide in the case of intergenerational storytelling? This chapter blends critical insights drawn from current scholarship in health-related digital storytelling, the intersection of digital media and age studies, and one recent exemplar, *The Resemblage Project*. It offers a comprehensive analysis of digital intergenerational storytelling – and, crucially, conceptual, ethical, and social justice concerns related to its current and future practice.

Digital storytelling: situating ethical media practice

In her classic essay, "What is Documentation" (1951), Suzanne Briet defined a document as "any concrete or symbolic indication, preserved or recorded, for reconstructing or for proving a phenomenon, whether physical or mental" (Briet 10). While documentation may appear a principally academic activity, Briet notes that it in certain cases it can "end in genuine creation, through the juxtaposition, selection, and the comparison of documents, and the production of auxiliary documents. The content of documentation is, thus, inter-documentary" (16). In multiple ways, digital storytelling is both a product and process of ***documentation***: a memorialized representation of thought but also, considering its etymological roots in the Latin *documentum*, a "teaching" or "lesson" (from *doceō,* "to teach").

Due to its inventive assembly and deliberate arrangement of multiple media forms, digital storytelling is clearly a genuinely creative process of documentation. However, its contemporary context and application invites more rigorous framing and theorization. For example, 21st-century research in the arts, humanities, and social sciences has undergone what has been called a ***visual and sensory turn***, which is associated with the potential for "de-colonizing knowledge" by shifting "away from linguistic and discursive ways of knowing the world, to engaging with the visual, the sensorial, and the embodied ways of 'seeing' the other, and allowing them to see and know themselves" (Rajan-Rankin, 37). Digital storytelling initiatives such as Project Re•Vision (https://revisioncentre.ca/) are consistent with this kind of framework in their foregrounding of the body as a source of knowledge production: particularly in the service of challenging dominant narratives of ableism (in the case of persons with disability), colonialism (Indigenous peoples), healthism (bodies that are read as "unwell"), and ageism (where age, especially older age, is understood in terms of illness and decline). By evoking the affordances of visual and sensory materials, practices of digital story creation help interrupt the marginalization of individuals and communities who are in some way "regarded as failing to qualify as 'fully human,' as lacking vitality, productivity, and the capacity to contribute to culture and society" (Rice 342).

Stemming from the visual and sensory knowledge-making impulse of digital storytelling, we might further sense its realization of ***multimedia storytelling in the lyric mode***. While "narrative" remains a key word in arts- and humanities-based approaches to health (e.g., *narrative medicine, patient narratives, narrative competency*), the poetic latency of digital storytelling – its brevity, lift, musicality, and conventions of a single speaker with an indeterminate audience – incorporates a vital lyricism into this multimedia form. This lyrical quality differentiates digital storytelling from the dominant *narrative* paradigm of much medical- and health-humanities work, as well as from more instrumentalized applications of short film, documentary, and digital media more overtly intended for the purposes of health education, promotion, or knowledge translation.

In light of these distinctive qualities, how might digital storytelling be leveraged for health-related research? In a recent systematic review, de Jager and colleagues assessed the use of this "sensory visual research method" in a range of peer-reviewed research settings (2573). Typical features include the association of digital stories with counter-narratives; participatory research; therapeutic aims (or potential); knowledge translation; preservation of cultural heritage; education, training, or professional development; and community development. *Counternarrative* is a familiar term within qualitative health research, describing stories "that splinter widely accepted truths about people, cultures, and institutions as well as the value of those institutions" (Mutua 132). Counternarratives within health-related digital storytelling often reflect what might be called social determinants of health and sources of health inequity more generally (including sexism, racism, ableism, physical and mental health status, lower socio-economic and/or refugee status, and sexual orientation). Other scholars have provided further insights into the counternarrative potential of digital storytelling, including its alignment with what Linda Tuhiwai Smith and others have described as decolonizing research practices, which challenge "Eurocentric research methods that undermine the local knowledge and experiences" of Indigenous peoples especially (Keikelame and Swartz, 1).

However, in light of such claims to digital storytelling's decolonizing potential, it is crucial to recall Eve Tuck and K. Wayne Yang's 2012 essay, "Decolonization is Not a Metaphor." "When metaphor invades decolonization," they write, "it kills the very possibility of decolonization; it recenters whiteness, it resettles theory, it extends innocence to the settler, it *entertains a settler future*" (3). (I will return to this issue of settler futurity as it relates to aging and intergenerational work later.) While digital storytelling methods may contribute to ***decolonizing health research methods***, there is nothing intrinsically liberatory in its deployment as a research method – nor should "decolonizing" be used interchangeably with social justice or human rights-based imperatives, as Tuck and Wang argue (36). Instead, the capacity of digital storytelling to generate counternarratives to longstanding realities such as colonization and ageism is entirely dependent upon a facilitator and storyteller's intentional – and temporally intensive – commitment to (1) de-metaphorizing decolonization, (2) deliberately unsettling form and content, and (3) attending carefully to the space, place, and land(s) on which such stories are generated, rather than only the method itself.

Certain ethical considerations arise within this context. For example, what constitutes "ethical conduct" in a formal academic setting (i.e., as defined by an institutional review board) may not align well with the objectives of participatory research or the advocacy goals common to arts-based methods (as Susan M. Cox and Katherine M. Boydell have argued), or the expectations of the digital storytelling process, which involves extensive rapport-building between facilitators and storymakers. In a 2014 study, Aline Gubrium and colleagues identified six ethical concerns relevant to digital storytelling for health: fuzzy boundaries, recruitment and consent to participate, representation and harm, power of shaping, confidentiality, and release of materials. Regarding ***fuzzy boundaries*** (of research, practice, and advocacy), ethical practice standards for digital storytelling relate to relationships between participants, facilitators, community members, field-site and partner organizations, funders, and researchers and their supporting institutions. Specifically, it is important "to (1) address the impact of power differentials on methods, knowledge production, and outcomes; (2) build rapport, reciprocity, and trust; (3) ensure transparency about potential risks and benefits of digital storytelling; and (4) acknowledge the complex politics of representation surrounding visual media" (Gubrium et al. 1608–9). Regarding ***recruitment and consent to participate***, facilitators of digital storytelling initiatives may need to determine participants' appropriate stage of engagement, particularly in cases where participants might still be in the midst of "experiencing their stories" as in the case of traumatic experience (1609).

This is relevant to the issue of ***representation and harm*** – the potential for both emancipatory and oppressive outcomes – which requires facilitators to acknowledge "the seamier side of visual and digital technology" (1609). A critical assessment of digital storytelling must also recognise that "it can be used to spread 'uncivil' stories [and] create . . . its own forms of exclusion and risk' (Gready 180). Related to this, during the storymaking process facilitators must be acutely aware of the ***power of shaping***: namely, how the collaborative environment of digital storytelling might influence a participant's decisions "about whether to create a story, when to speak up, what to say, what story topics or visual images are viewed as appropriate, and how they feel their stories should or should not be shared" (Gubrium et al. 1610).

At the other end of the making process, institutional health research conventions regarding ***confidentiality*** may not permit for digital stories to be published or screened, even in the workshop where they are produced. In contrast to typical requirements of confidentiality in health-related research, workshop participants may find that "digital storytelling offers a utile arena for exploring the terrain between the right to personal privacy and the right to lay claim to knowledge production" (1611). Similarly, ***release of materials*** must remain "a dynamic concept" (1611) rather than a prescribed plan of action (as is typical to institutional ethics board requirements). For example, the public sharing of stories and personal information might be raised during recruitment, at the commencement of storymaking, throughout the making process (e.g., when participants are selecting images and personal footage), when stories are shared within the storymaking circle, and prior to further publication (e.g., in academic journals or on a public-facing website). Integrating all these ethical considerations significantly adds to the time-intensiveness of the digital storytelling process, which may be problematic within the "publish or perish" discourse of academic productivity. Moreover, scholarly publication venues tend to be unwelcoming to creative, participatory, arts-based methodologies. Together, these features present considerable obstacles to generating a robust evidence basis for supporting the goals and intentions of digital storytelling, particularly in health-related contexts.

A partial solution to these issues may be to frame digital storytelling as an arts-based media practice with relevance to health-related issues, rather than as a health-research method. By combining visual, sonic, and musical elements to produce a lyrical narrative of personal experience, digital stories hold rich potential as a ***research assemblage***: a multimedia document capable of (re)animating the dynamic convergences of "things, people, ideas, social collectivities and institutions" (Fox and Alldred 1). In combination with what Lawrence Lessig called *remix culture,* which refers to combining existing creative materials to produce new and often original work, the goals of digital storytelling are well aligned with the creative process and product of assemblage. These include disrupting the conventional flow of intellectual authority, information, and creative ownership of health-related experiences – from centralized, institutional, or ideological practices to the highly individualized personal context. The next section builds on these issues related to form, content, and ethical practice in the specific application of digital storytelling to aging, older age, and intergenerational relationships.

Digital mediations: spreadable age studies

Scholars working in the field of ***age studies*** focus on the critical interlinkages of *age* (the chronological number of years a person has lived); *aging* (the ongoing temporality of the body, including mental and physiological changes often associated with post-midlife); and *older age* (a vague, context-dependent designation generally starting at 65 years of age) (Charise 188). Age studies differs from cognate fields such as gerontology by emphasizing forms of knowledge that are not primarily quantitative or clinical. Within aging research, arts- and humanities-based interventions are increasingly deployed as health- and wellness-supportive practices such as cultural arts initiatives, social prescribing, expressive and creative writing workshops, and participatory reading programs (Charise and Eginton 81).

However, digital practices are rarely integrated into creative interventions involving older people. Older people's relationships with digital life are largely framed in terms of social isolation, vulnerability to online fraud, or personal data extraction (Rosales and Fernández-Ardèvol 1074). The aesthetic potential of human aging is still an undeveloped aspect of digital humanities, and digital storytelling has the potential to introduce aging as a critical concept within media studies. For example, storytelling around issues of age may serve as a compelling, accessible advocacy opportunity to address ***ageism*** (defined by Robert Butler as prejudicial behavior against people based on age, and particularly older age). Consider Stuart Campbell's 2015 Eisner Award-nominated digital webcomic, "These Memories Won't Last" (http://memories.sutueatsflies.com). While not a "digital story" in the sense described by Lambert, this multilayered intergenerational account relates Campbell's grandfather's experiences with dementia. In a remarkable interweaving of form and content, the narrative and accompanying images disappear as the reader scrolls vertically through the story. Furthermore, the digital comic itself was deliberately created to become unreadable by future web browser software technologies, thus weaving together human aging and technological obsolescence in the digital realm.

Such original counternarratives to ageism are forms of what Henry Jenkins, Sam Ford, and Joshua Green have called ***spreadable media***, referring to "the potential – both technical and cultural – for audiences to share content for their own purposes, sometimes with the permission of rights holders, sometimes against their wishes" (3). The intergenerational elements of digital storytelling – in terms of both process and product – have the potential to address one of the profound deficits of an ageist society: the blockage of intergenerational communion involving meaningful relationships between people from different generational cohorts. As Tamara Baker and Aimi Hamraie each note, however, the fundamental arguments and default subject of age studies are predominantly attuned to white, Western, and often cis-female experiences; technology scholars including Ruha Benjamin, Nehal El-Hadi, and Jennifer Wemigwans have further shown that digital spaces because of their ostensibly neutral construction and their ubiquitous presence consistently amplify the ideological architectures of colonial hierarchies and racial segregation. Together, these factors can aid with the proliferation of racist and colonial violence – and their detrimental health effects – across global networks.

Intergenerational storytelling is a shared opportunity both in terms of digital practices and age studies. It can lead to forms of analysis that "reanimate" older bodies of color (Rajan-Rankin 32). One evocative example of such work is Lan A. Li's short film, "Liao Jialun" (http://lan-a-li.com/on-aging), which portrays a lyric meditation by the film's protagonist on the nature of aging, creativity, and later life as an example of "medical poetics." "As scholars of the humanities," Li writes, "we use lots of conceptual tools to assess human data. My tools include microphones, cameras, battery packs, miscellaneous adapters, and editing software that shape how I move in the world and how I understand the ethical implications of my work" (170). This intersection of health (and health-adjacent) practices with media production and theory demonstrates the necessity of ensuring the fields of age studies and health humanities – and the digital work performed in these fields – are thoroughly invested in intersectional analyses and commitments. Li continues, "As an editor, I see my value in collaborative projects to refashion narratives of 'global' health humanities . . . I join the digital and medical humanities as an exercise in ethics and aesthetics" (170). As "Liao Jialun" makes clear, age is more than "a different difference" (Gullette 111): it is an intersectional axis of personal and collective identity amplified by race and geography.

The intergenerational resituation of aging as a *life course issue* – that is, as an issue of concern and relevance to all persons across age identities – invites further consideration of digital forms of storytelling related to age. Age-related digital storytelling may also be an ideal research-creation method given Covid-19 and the consequent restrictions to on-site research (especially in the long-term care context) as well as the increased emphasis on online pedagogy and curriculum delivery at all levels of education. Across the Western world, digital media are increasingly being used for touchless yet socially intimate purposes: isolation and social distancing may increase the appeal of creating and disseminating digital stories of aging across generations. It may also underscore the capacity for such work to further the aims of anti-ageist knowledge creation.

However, when applying digital storytelling as a promising, pandemic-compatible research-creation method, it is essential to remain alert to potential issues regarding its deployment for the purposes of enhancing age consciousness. For example, younger participants may be characterized as *de facto* technologically competent "teachers" of older participants, thus affirming, rather than undermining, longstanding generational stereotypes associated with ***digital ageism*** (whereby younger people are regarded as "digital natives" in opposition to "technologically incompetent" older people (Sawchuk and Crow 157)). Overall, it is insufficient to engage in intergenerational storytelling in the digital realm without considering how it might contribute to oppressive practices of racism, colonization, and ageism.

Two Canadian aging-related initiatives have responded to the suite of affordances and concerns presented by digital storytelling methodologies. The first, *Aging Activisms*, (www.agingactivisms.org/) based at Trent University, "explores the diverse ways that activists of different ages, abilities, genders, and backgrounds resist injustices and create change across different movements and throughout their lives" (Chazan and MacNab). Specifically, it applies the concept of the ***feminist intergenerational mic***, meaning "the norm-challenging possibilities of our methodology . . . not, in other words, solely a matter of offering up 'the mic,'" but fostering "reciprocal, multi-directional connections across age and circumscribed possibilities for such connections" (Chazen and MacNab). The second project, *Aging Vitalities,* is part of the broader *Bodies in Translation* initiative (https://bodiesintranslation.ca/) and is committed to illuminating diverse representations of aging with difference by older adults and persons who identify as aging, settler, Indigenous, disabled, racialized, and/or queer in the city of Peterborough/Nogojiwanong (Anishinaabe). As project lead Nadine Changfoot noted, "We are socialized and shaped to think of a human life in singular terms, as linear, proceeding forward in time in an able-bodied and minded way, and also in an acquiring way . . . In contrast, the stories of *Aging Vitalities* tell viewers that a person need not fight aging. Instead, of fear and anxiety and 'fixes,' aging offers experiences to be welcomed, savoured, and shared" ("Aging Vitalities").

In addition to exploring the boundaries of aging and generational consciousness as embodied identities, these initiatives highlight a productive tension between the principles of "spreadable" media and the deeply situated contexts that give rise to digital storytelling about the life course. While digital storytelling is by no means immune or intrinsically opposed to the shadow-side of spreadable media, its ability to integrate embodied, sensory, visual, and lyrical methods holds promise for exploring how "the contours of how race, ethnicity and old age can be visualized and experienced" (Rajan-Rankin 37).

Case study: *The Resemblage Project*

resemblage (rɪˈzɛmbleɪʤ), n. A portmanteau that mingles *resemblance*, *assemblage*, and *age*.

How might creative responses to aging be shared across space, time, and generations? Drawing from Black feminist theorizations of difference (including Combahee River Collective and

Kimberlé Crenshaw), *The Resemblage Project* is an intergenerational digital storytelling initiative based in eastern Toronto, Canada. The resource (www.resemblageproject.ca) involves students, scholars, artists, activists, and community members from across the city – and the life course – who are imaginatively exploring what it means to grow older in Scarborough, particularly in terms of intersectionality and assemblage. Since launching in 2019, it has received the 2020 Digital Humanities (DH) Award for "Best Public Engagement," and the AVA 2021 Award (High Commendation), for "Best Visual Ethnographic Material Addressing Ageing and the Life Course" (jointly awarded by the Association for Anthropology, Gerontology and the Life Course (AAGE) and the European Association of Social Anthropologists (EASA)).

Why "resemblage?" The portmanteau reflects a creative mingling of *resemblance*, *assemblage*, and *age*, each key words for this intergenerational digital storytelling project. To resemble means to liken or sense similarity. Resemblance does not imply sameness or the flattening of difference, variation, and the dissimilar, instead: resemblance emerges when we assemble what is found or what can be shared for a moment in time, amid the abundance of bodies and things. Gender, race, ethnicity, class, ability, geography, citizenship, and migration all generate assemblages of selfhood that alter and reorganize our identity over the life course. *The Resemblage Project* thus responds to the need for stories of aging that reflect profound difference; yet, for all the particularities of personal experience, aging is also a kind of universalizing process. In this collection of digital stories, grandchildren and grandparents, educators and students, arts and sciences, activism and academia intermingle to yield new ways of seeing the world, while sensing how distinct aging experiences can involve the possibility of shared collective action.

Drawing from the postcolonial and decolonial work of G. K. Bhambra, Sweta Rajan-Rankin writes that in aging research, "epistemic decolonization of knowledge needs us to consider both the damaging effects of modernity and coloniality, but also of viewing modernity/coloniality *as* modernity" (36). This is particularly relevant to experiences of aging drawn from the global South and diasporic communities. Two cases created for *The Resemblage Project* illustrate the possibilities of intergenerational storytelling in the digital realm, and specifically integrate experiences of first and second-generation migration in the Canadian context: the grandfather-grandson dyad of Gulamhussein and Kaamil Khalfan (creators of "My Happy Days" and "The Contours of Generation," respectively), and Angelus Baliwas's "Departure."[1]

Gulamhussein Khalfan's "My Happy Days" recounts the story of his own migration from Mombasa, Kenya, to Toronto, Canada, at the age of 43. Gulamhussein describes the challenges and rewards that he has experienced since that time: the loss and gain of a homeland, the continuity of his ancestral roots, the intergenerational transmission of culture, music, and the intricate meanings of living through time. Finally, he frames his retirement as a concretization of his own aging: "I try to lead as normal and as active a life as possible. I have taken it in my stride that such health problems are part and parcel of growing old . . . My daily life routine consists of very basic rituals." One involves dropping off his granddaughter Asiya at school every morning: "Those twenty minutes with her make my day. We talk on different subjects and listen to our favorite Indian music . . . This is my very simple but satisfying retired life" (Figure 15.1). Gulamhussein's resonant, sonorous voice grounds his recounting of the past 30 years and the forward-looking trajectory of his grandchildren's lives, which is contextualized and situated in turn by the broader ancestral net woven by time, migration, and geography. His conclusion that his life, while possibly not "happy," is undoubtedly "satisfying," recalls the framework of what health sociologist Arthur Frank calls a "quest narrative" (115). While Gulamhussein's story does not equate aging and illness, the shape of his digital story, which interweaves his own aging with the occasion of his migration to Canada, aligns with Frank's description of "meet[ing] suffering head on . . . the occasion of a journey that becomes a quest" (115).

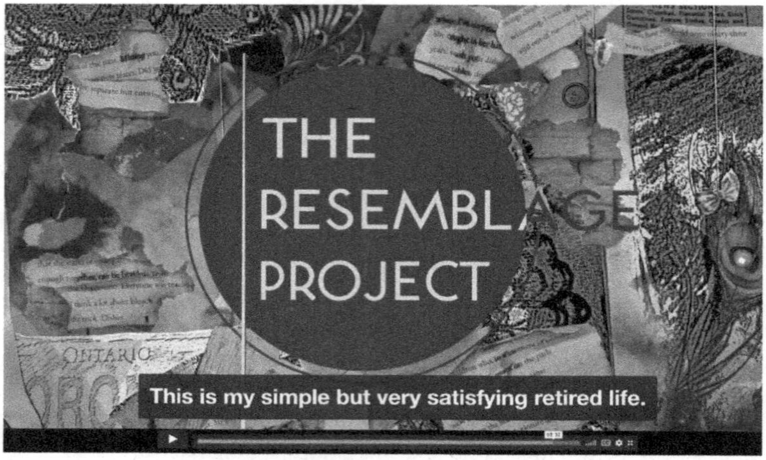

Figure 15.1 The Resemblage Project (1)

Gulamhussein's grandson, Kaamil Khalfan, created his own candid, deeply sensitive, reflection on the meaning of aging in "The Contours of Generation." Kaamil's reflections at the age of 21 serve as an evocative intergenerational pendant to his grandfather's story. From the standpoint of a younger generation, Kaamil notes that, "Overcoming a physical migration like [my grandfather's] is not my obstacle. Overcoming an imaginative migration is mine." The quest-like narrative structure of his grandfather's story – which began with the hardships of weather, economic precarity, and racial prejudice in Canada and resolved with Gulamhussein's affirmation of his decision to migrate – becomes an anxious inheritance, a story whose "contours" (to use Kaamil's word) seem unlikely to be reflected in his grandson's life course.

Kaamil was born in Canada, with no first-hand experience of his ancestral homeland. He sees his grandfather as an instantiation of both ancestry and cultural ties, a connection evidenced by the numerous photos of his grandfather Kaamil interlaces into his digital story. To Kaamil, the personal and cultural intergenerational legacy articulated in his grandfather's story seems tenuous and threatened – and perhaps impossible for Kaamil to continue:

> I fear that my Dada's outlook on aging will not resonate with me in my own older age. What if I am unable to achieve, what he calls, his *simple but very satisfying retired life*? What if I lack the ability to sustain and maintain a family as he has?
>
> I have always wanted to be a carbon copy of my Dada.
>
> I am afraid I might fail.
>
> *("The Contours of Generation" 1.25–1.32)*

Kaamil presents a photograph of his younger self and grandfather embracing (Figure 15.2), but his happy expression in the photograph is in stark contrast with his voiceover, which reflects his fear of failure. This is a moving example of the resonant layering of affect made possible by this multimedia storytelling method. The younger generation's fear of failure is manifold – encompassing economic, personal, and even imaginative connotations – and motivated by the sense that intergenerational communion may not suffice to bridge, meet, or otherwise sustain ancestral continuity.

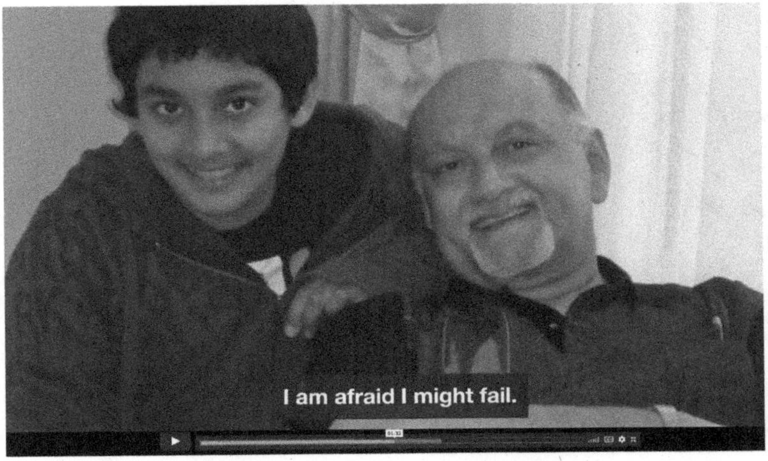

Figure 15.2 The Resemblage Project (2)

Box 15.1

Excerpt of voiceover from the digital story "Departure," by Angelus Baliwas (full digital story at https://resemblageproject.ca/our-stories/).

This is the part
Where I'm supposed to show you
A picture of my grandparents
But I don't have any
I left them back in my homeland
The same way I left the last grandparent that I have

We left reluctantly
But the desire for a better life
For this young family
Had to be prioritized by mom and dad
Migration took away my final chance
At a generational relationship
One generation's pursuit of a better life
Meant abandoning another
[...]

What does it mean to age in a world where globalization can interrupt the very possibility of intergenerational kinship? Angelus Baliwas's "Departure" explores how migration shapes – or erases – narratives of life course, aging, and conventional assumptions about

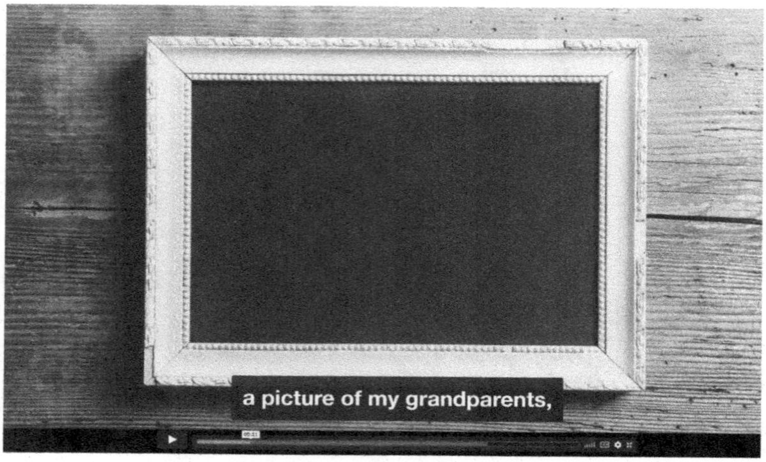

Figure 15.3 The Resemblage Project (3)

generational connection. In contrast to idealized portraits of multi-generational households and cultures where intergenerational interaction is normalized, in this moving, lyrical exploration of pain, loss, and self-reflection, Angelus realizes that "One generation's pursuit of a better life / Meant abandoning another" (see Box 15.1). Speaking over an image of an empty picture frame (Figure 15.3), Angelus acknowledges that her story diverges – departs – from the implied expectations of intergenerational storytelling itself ("This is the part / Where I'm supposed to show you / A picture of my grandparents"). As we learn, the digital story's motif of "departure" therefore points to the formal conventions of digital storytelling as much as content. Angelus's story of broken generational ties itself breaks with the implied, or at least emergent, conventions of intergenerational storytelling that would assume familial memories involving kin of another generation. The tension opened by this reality, and the digital story's refusal to suture such loss within the conventions of a conclusion, speak to the lyrical engine of digital storytelling as a disruptive, non-prescriptive space of storytelling.

In addition to hosting completed digital stories in a "Storybank" (https://resemblageproject.ca/our-stories/storybank/), what further differentiates *The Resemblage Project* from more conventional curations of digital film is the foregrounding and documentation of process. The "Documents" page (https://resemblageproject.ca/documents/) includes a comprehensive list of scholarly references and creative resources, as well as a description of the creative decisions that influenced the design of the project logo. For example, the logo shown in Figure 15.1 reflects the project's core concerns: the final three letters, "AGE," are placed on the threshold of the logo's inner and outer boundaries, just as older age and ageing are situated on the fringes of society. *The Resemblage Project* is intended to bring age back into the common fold of thought. Even the choice of font, called "Toronto Subway," deliberately evokes Toronto's city transit infrastructure, thereby situating this particular intergenerational storytelling work within a particular national and civic context – and the decades-long controversy regarding inequitable access to public transit that has long been part of Scarborough's deeply racialized and socio-economic marginalization within the "Greater Toronto Area."

By foregrounding the documentation process alongside creative outputs, *The Resemblage Project* deliberately iterates multiple layers of remixing. In this case, this includes the material form of the online "scrapbook" style of the project's documentation and resources, in addition to the aesthetic and multimedia remixing involved in the creative process of the digital stories themselves.[2] The centrality of counternarratives to the purpose and aesthetic of digital storytelling extends beyond the decisions of storymakers about the content of their health-related experience. Digital storytelling uses form, method, and ethos to explore alternatives to the dominant genres of health-related storytelling (i.e., narrative), and challenges conventional wisdom regarding whom stories of aging are typically created by – or for. By involving undergraduate students, most of whom were in their early twenties, *The Resemblage Project* explores how generationally defined cohorts might "other" matters of aging, and provides space for the possibility of shared, or at least speculative, collectivities of past, present, and future.

Beyond the specifics of media practices, additional transformative potential exists in digital storytelling's ability to expand the idea of *who has the right to make things*, particularly compelling stories of selfhood over time: for example, makers who might identify as younger or older; as members of racialized communities with aging experiences not typically represented within white, Western, and/or settler and medicalized portraits of aging and intergenerational experience; or as members of disciplinary traditions (STEM and otherwise) that do not conventionally involve creative storytelling practices. By attending to the convergence of health and media practices, digitally spreadable stories of aging can encourage viewers to confront whether conventional modes of health training, research, and practice can engender practices of storytelling, making, and creativity across the life course – in the service of assembling diverse, vital, communities of aging across race and ethnicity.

Conclusion: acknowledging endurance

In her 1985 essay, "Poetry is not a Luxury," Audre Lorde notes that "The quality of light by which we scrutinize our lives has direct bearing upon the product which we live, and upon the changes we hope to bring about through those lives" (371). *The Resemblage Project* signals an ongoing commitment to changing the quality of light by which we view aging, and each other, across generational selves. Drawing from the insights of postcolonial, Black, and feminist theorizations of difference, *The Resemblage Project* and similarly informed digital storytelling initiatives generate "spreadable" media related to aging and intergenerational experience, while simultaneously holding the very notion of spreadable media up for critique. As Angelus Baliwas's story illustrates, the conventions within intergenerational digital storytelling itself risk ossification by colonizing the imagination of aging: whether in the form of visual iconographies (i.e., photos of grandparents) or the assumption that intergenerational relationships are necessarily proximal, accessible, and familial (as opposed to, for example, chosen kin). In light of theoretical frameworks that address racism, colonization, and ageism (either as separate or interacting axes of identity), we might further consider just how "spreadable" media forms, like digital storytelling, demand more precise and nuanced terminologies for addressing the entangled facts of migration of people, stories, aging, and individual and community-centered experiences in the embodied realm.

The spreadable qualities of intergenerational digital storytelling invite further consideration of what a decolonial approach to age studies (and health research more generally) might entail. For example, it is important to challenge assumptions about access to the internet, which is clearly affected by class, socio-economic status and, indeed, age. It is also important to better understand what media messaging is being spread, how, for whom, and by means of what kinds of material and digital communications infrastructure. To this end, I must acknowledge that much of this research, including the creative work and collaborations that contributed to *The Resemblage Project*, was conducted on the traditional territory of the Huron-Wendat and

Petun First Nations, the Seneca, and the Mississaugas of the Credit River. This chapter was written while I was an uninvited visitor on the traditional lands of the St. Lawrence Iroquoians, Anishinabewaki ᐊᓂᔑᓈᐯᐧᐊ, Mohawk, and Omàmìwininìwag (Algonquin). As a white settler scholar and educator, I assume responsibility for acknowledging my relationship to the land on which I conduct my research and for recognizing the ways this work has been directly enabled by Canada's colonial history of land removal, including the University of Toronto's ongoing institutional occupation of Treaty 13 territory. While this chapter has focused on digital modalities of intergenerational storytelling, it remains imperative to reckon with the material realities of land, land rights, and land theft involved in making and dissemination of digital work: from the destructive practices of resource extraction that enable the manufacture of digital tools; to the significant consumption of unrenewable energy necessitated by data centers, search engines, and online activity; to the construction of internet and communication infrastructure on Indigenous territory.[3]

Ultimately it is insufficient to merely "acknowledge" the digital translation of systemic oppressions. Without a more capacious attention to temporal endurance and longevity, such acknowledgements are little more than an admission of withdrawal – they are, in effect, a refusal to age alongside the lengthy timeline of settler accountability. This idea resonates with key language and concerns of health humanities more generally: consider how the limiting imperatives of "remedy" and "cure" can impose premature closure on an individual's experiences of illness, often promising far more than can be delivered. In a similar way, settler scholars might understand "acknowledgements" as risking too-hasty remedies and one-sided drives to "reconciliation" that erase complex, enduring, transformative possibilities for more reciprocal and ongoing community relations within colonization's long durée.

The question thus becomes: how to live in best relationship with the digital realm and similar forms of new media across the life course? How might we live, and age, in an ongoing state of reciprocity that recognizes the nourishing, even liberating, potential of digital engagement, on one hand – and, on the other hand, acknowledge the potential this medium has to maintain the same extractive, exploitative, inequitable practices associated with conventional spaces of health-related practice? The materialities of media, documentation, health, and aging converge in this nexus, as do the systemic effects of colonialism and ageism: both of which have been enabled, in the Western context, by centuries of extractive capitalism and its fantasy of perpetual, everlasting planetary resources. A critical analysis of intergenerational digital storytelling must therefore be prepared to reckon with its entanglement in past, present, and future global networks of colonization. In turn, realizing the transformative possibilities of digital storytelling for health – indeed, of health-engaged media in all its forms – depends upon recognizing its deep, enduring, and vital engagements with aging: from aging bodies to aging methods, aging social practices, and aging worlds to come.

Acknowledgments

This chapter is the outcome of an ongoing collaborative research project made possible by the creative efforts and intellectual generosity of many key contributors. Special thanks to Angelus Baliwas, Kaamil A. Khalfan, and Gulamhussein Khalfan, who granted me permission to discuss their extraordinary digital stories in this venue. Enduring appreciation extends to Celeste N. Pang, Mia Sanders, and each of the storytellers who have shared their insights with *The Resemblage Project*; and to illustrators April Brust and Iqra Mahmood for designing *The Resemblage Project*'s evocative banner image and inspired logo, respectively. I am grateful to Nehal El-Hadi for early discussions of the potentials and pitfalls of media practices old and new; and to Jeff Gagnon, whose postdoctoral research on decolonization and digital sovereignty has fundamentally informed my understanding of digital storytelling. Early financial support for this work was received from the Jackman Humanities Institute and, more recently, the University of Toronto Scarborough's Clusters of Scholarly Prominence program.

Notes

1 Digital stories from *The Resemblage Project* cited in this chapter can be accessed via the "Storybank": https://resemblageproject.ca/our-stories/storybank/

2 I encourage readers to consult "Critically Unpacking The Resemblage Project: A Conversation" (https://resemblageproject.ca/critically-unpacking-the-resemblage-project/) is a transcription of a roundtable (2019) involving a number of storymakers and researchers, with introductory remarks by Celeste Pang.

3 I am motivated here by the insights shared in "Praxis Sessions for Virtual Collaboration: Land Acknowledgements" (featuring Claudia Alick, Roo George-Warren, Jessica Schacht, Tara Moses, Andrea Kovich, Carmen Papalia, and mia susan amir), posted online in March 2020. For more on Indigenous knowledge, community resurgence, and its relationship to fields including health, law, and social wellbeing in the virtual context, see Wemigwans.

Works cited

"Aging Vitalities." April 17, 2019, https://bodiesintranslation.ca/aging-vitalities-an-interview-with-nadine-changfoot/. Accessed May 29, 2021.

Alick, Claudia, Roo George-Warren, Jessica Schacht, Tara Moses, Andrea Kovich, Carmen Papalia, and mia susan amir. *Praxis Sessions for Virtual Collaboration: Land Acknowledgements*. March 31, 2020, https://howlround.com/happenings/praxis-sessions-virtual-collaboration-land-acknowledgements. Accessed May 29, 2021.

Baker, Tamara A. "The Importance of Aging Studies: Understanding the Influence of Diversity and Culture." January 2014, https://ageculturehumanities.org/WP/the-importance-of-aging-studies-understanding-the-influence-of-diversity-and-culture/. Accessed May 29, 2021.

Benjamin, Ruha. *Race after Technology: Abolitionist Tools for the New Jim Code*. Polity, 2020.

Briet, Suzanne. *What Is Documentation? English Translation of the Classic French Text*. Translated by Ronald E. Day, Laurent Martinet, and Hermina G. B. Anghelescu, Lanham, Md: Scarecrow Press, 2006.

Butler, Robert N. "Successful Aging and the Role of the Life Review." *Journal of the American Geriatrics Society*, vol. 22, no.12, 1974, pp. 529–35.

Charise, Andrea. "Resemblance, Diversity, and Making Age Studies Matter." *Teaching Health Humanities*, edited by Olivia Banner, Nathan Carlin, and Thomas Cole, Oxford University Press, 2019, pp. 188–206.

Charise, Andrea and Margaret L. Eginton. "Arts and the Aging Mind." *The Wiley Handbook on the Aging Mind and Brain*, edited by Matthew Rizzo and Steven W. Anderson, Hoboken: Wiley, 2018, pp. 78–99.

Combahee River Collective. *The Combahee River Collective Statement*. 1977, www.blackpast.org/african-american-history/combahee-river-collective-statement-1977/. Accessed May 29, 2021.

Charon, Rita. *Narrative Medicine: Honoring the Stories of Illness*. Oxford: Oxford University Press, 2006.

Chazan, May and Maddy Macnab. "Doing the Feminist Intergenerational Mic: Methodological Reflections on Digital Storytelling as Process and Praxis." *Forum Qualitative Sozialforschung / Forum: Qualitative Social Research*, vol. 19, no. 2, Art. 8, 2018. www.qualitative-research.net/index.php/fqs/article/view/2949/4209. Accessed May 29, 2021.

Chivers, Sally. "Aging Together and Apart: From the Pivot to the Pirouette." *Synapsis*, July 29, 2020, https://medicalhealthhumanities.com/2020/07/29/aging-together-and-apart-from-the-pivot-to-the-pirouette/. Accessed May 29, 2021.

Crimp, Douglas. "Introduction." *October*, vol. 43, Winter, 1987, pp. 3–16.

Conrad, Diane, and Anita Sinner. *Creating Together: Participatory, Community-Based, and Collaborative Arts Practices and Scholarship across Canada*. Wilfrid Laurier University Press, 2015.

Cox, S. M., and K. M. Boydell. "Ethical Issues in Arts-based Health Research." *Creative Arts in Public Health: International Perspectives*, edited by Stephen Clift and Paul Camic, Oxford: Oxford University Press, 2015, pp. 83–91.

de Jager, Adele et al. "Digital Storytelling in Research: A Systematic Review." *The Qualitative Report*, vol. 22, no. 10, 2017, pp. 2548–82.

El-Hadi, Nehal. "Death Undone." *The New Inquiry*, May 2, 2017, https://thenewinquiry.com/death-undone/. Accessed May 29, 2021.

Frank, Arthur W. *The Wounded Storyteller: Body, Illness, and Ethics*, 2nd edition. Chicago: U of Chicago P, 2013.

Fox, Nick J., and Pam Alldred. "Inside the Research-Assemblage: New Materialism and the Micropolitics of Social Inquiry." *Sociological Research Online*, vol. 20, no. 2, 2015, pp. 122–40.

Gubrium, Aline et al. "A Situated Practice of Ethics for Participatory Visual and Digital Methods in Public Health Research and Practice: A Focus on Digital Storytelling." *American Journal of Public Health*, vol. 104, no. 9, 2014, pp. 1606–14.

Gullette, M. M. *Aged by Culture*. Chicago: University of Chicago Press, 2004.

Gready, P. "Introduction: Responsibility to the Story." *Journal of Human Rights Practice*, vol. 2, no. 2, 2010, pp. 177–90.

Hamraie, Aimi. "Inclusive Design: Cultivating Accountability toward the Intersections of Race, Aging, and Disability." *Age, Culture, Humanities*, vol. 2, 2015, https://ageculturehumanities.org/WP/inclusive-design-cultivating-accountability-toward-the-intersections-of-race-aging-and-disability/.

Jenkins, Henry, Sam Ford, and Joshua Green. *Spreadable Media: Creating Value and Meaning in a Networked Culture: with a New Afterword*. New York: New York University Press, 2018.

Keikelame, Mpoe Johannah, and Leslie Swartz. "Decolonising Research Methodologies: Lessons from a Qualitative Research Project, Cape Town, South Africa." *Global Health Action*, vol. 12, no. 1, 2019, pp. 1–7.

Kleinman, Arthur. *The Illness Narratives: Suffering, Healing, and the Human Condition*. New York: Basic Books, 1988.

Lambert, J. "Where It All Started: The Centre for Digital Sorytelling in California." *Story Circle: Digital Storytelling Around the World*, edited by John Hartley and Kelly McWilliam, Malden: Wiley-Blackwell, 2009, pp. 79–90.

Lessig, Lawrence. *Remix: Making Art and Commerce Thrive in the Hybrid Economy*. New York: Penguin Press, 2008.

Li, Lan A. "Medical Poetics: Representing Global Health Humanities and the Case of 心." *The Routledge Companion to Health Humanities*, edited by Paul Crawford, Brian Brown, and Andrea Charise. New York and Abingdon: Routledge, 2020, pp. 163–72.

Lorde, Audre. "Poetry Is Not a Luxury." *Women's Voices, Feminist Visions: Classic and Contemporary Readings*, edited by Susan M. Haw and Janet Lee, New York: McGraw-Hill Education, 2015, pp. 371–3.

Moreau, K. A., K. Eady, L. Sikora, et al. "Digital Storytelling in Health Professions Education: A Systematic Review." *BMC Medical Education*, vol. 18, no. 1, 2018, p. 208.

Mutua, Kagendo. "counternarrative." *The SAGE Encyclopedia of Qualitative Research Methods*, edited by Lisa Given, Thousand Oaks, CA: SAGE Publications, Inc., 2008, p. 132.

Rajan-Rankin, Sweta. "Race, Embodiment and Later Life: Re-Animating Aging Bodies of Color." *Journal of Aging Studies*, vol. 45, 2018, pp. 32–8.

"reminiscence therapy." APA Dictionary of Psychology. https://dictionary.apa.org/reminiscence-therapy. Accessed May 29, 2021.

Rice, Carla. "Digital Storytelling." *The Routledge Companion to Health Humanities*, edited by Paul Crawford, Brian Brown, and Andrea Charise. New York and Abingdon: Routledge, 2020, pp. 341–5.

Rosales, Andrea, and Mireia Fernández-Ardèvol. "Ageism in the Era of Digital Platforms." *Convergence*, vol. 26, no. 5–6, 2020, pp. 1074–87.

Sawchuk, Kim, and Barbara Crow. "Tactical Restriction: Seniors and Cell Phones." In *Technologies of Mobility in the Americas*, edited by Phillip Vannini, Lucy Bud, Ole Jensen, Paola Jirón, and Christian Fisker, New York: Peter Lang, 2012, pp. 157–74.

Smith, Linda Tuhiwai. *Decolonizing Methodologies: Research and Indigenous Peoples*. London: Zed Books, 1999.

Tuck, Eve and K. Wayne Yang. "Decolonization Is Not a Metaphor." *Decolonization: Indigeneity, Education & Society*, vol. 1, no. 1, 2012, pp. 1–40.

Wemigwans, Jennifer. *A Digital Bundle: Protecting and Promoting Indigenous Knowledge Online*. U of Regina Press, 2018.

16

DOCUMENTING THE AMERICAN WAY OF DYING

The *Near Death* experience

Barry Keith Grant

Introduction

As preeminent documentary film theorist Bill Nichols observes, in fiction films "death is imitated; it is presented as fact but not in fact" (Nichols, *Representing Reality* 81). Fiction films cannot show actual death and dying, but documentary images, however they might be manipulated subsequently, can and do show real death because of their "indexical bond," their origin in our world (28). Thus, the sight of actual death or dying, when it appears in the documentary film, is always sobering and in a way that fiction films, however naturalistic, can never be.[1] Some documentaries are notable in their focus on the process of dying and its medical management, such as *Dying at Grace* (2003) and *On the Bridge* (1992), in which fiction filmmaker Frank Perry documented his own unsuccessful battle with cancer, as well as the many films about dying with AIDS such as *Silverlake Life: The View from Here* (1993), but certainly the most penetrating is Frederick Wiseman's monumental 1989 film, *Near Death*. Its subject is the Medical Intensive Care Unit (MICU) at Beth Israel Hospital in Boston, one of the most technically sophisticated in the United States, known for its emphasis on the process of family consultation and a consensual approach regarding life-support treatment (Kleinman). Although made in 1989, it remains as relevant today, if indeed not more so given medical science's ever advancing ability to maintain life, or life functions, as a teaching tool in medical ethics and end-of-life care, and more generally for the ethical questions it examines for physicians, staff, patients, and families alike.[2]

Recognized as a major figure in American documentary filmmaking, Frederick Wiseman has been making films consistently since 1967. His work has garnered numerous awards, and appreciative critics have praised him as "the most sophisticated intelligence in documentary" and even "the most interesting of American directors" (Kael 204; Bromwich 508). Impressively, Wiseman has made more than 40 feature-length documentaries in approximately as many years, developing a distinctive style and approach to the form. In his films, there is no narrator, either as voiceover or within the events being filmed, nor is there any clear indication of temporal

DOI: 10.4324/9781003007661-21

relations between sequences (wipes, dissolves, titles), unless it happens to arise in the dialogue. Editing, though, is crucial for Wiseman. He edits his films himself, spending from four to six weeks shooting each film on location and as many months or more in the editing room sifting through and giving shape to the footage. Wiseman claims that he enters an institution with inevitable preconceptions, but the experience of being there reveals a greater complexity about it. In the editing, he works out a "theory" about the events, which is then reflected in the film's structure. He sees the process as a "voyage of discovery," and the end result as "a report on what I've found" (Graham and Garrett 31; Halberstadt 22). Wiseman readily admits the creative manipulation in his films in his own frequent description of them as "reality dreams" or "reality fictions" (Robb 28; Berg 26). In this editing process, elements of profilmic reality are compressed, reordered; in all his films, while it is true that these profilmic events (that which happens before the camera) are always real, never staged, recreated or rehearsed for the camera, the footage remains for Wiseman only a record of the events, textually meaningless until he structures it at the editing table.[3]

Each of Wiseman's films focuses on a different American institution – as he says, in his work the institution is the star (qtd. Rosenthal 69) – ranging from those concentrated within individual buildings (*High School* 1968) to those international in scope (*Sinai Field Mission* 1978), from institutions set up and maintained by government (*Juvenile Court* 1973; *City Hall* 2020) to those less tangible ones organized by principles of ideology and culture (*Canal Zone* 1977; *Model* 1980). Wiseman has broadly defined an institution as "a place that has certain kinds of geographical limitations and where at least some of the people have well-established roles" (Janis and MacNeil 67). Together, Wiseman's films offer the most comprehensive account of American institutional life to be found in any medium. The filmmaker regards his films as a series of works that present "a natural history of the way we live" (Eames 97), and one might view Wiseman's documentaries as individual sections of one magnum opus in process.[4] These films demonstrate the shaping force of institutions themselves, which dictate to as much as they serve both clients and administrators. Wiseman's sense of what defines an institution is perfectly realized in *Near Death* by the dynamics of Beth Israel's MICU, a place where the process of institutional processing operates with particular intensity: the ICU context encourages, even requires, the kind of depersonalization Wiseman has found in so many other institutions, for the medical staff must distance themselves from their patients and become detached to some extent in order to function efficiently in their jobs. "It's all the way you look at death," says one nurse in the film, "whether you look at it legally or emotionally."

Wiseman had focused on issues of health and the American healthcare system earlier in his career in his controversial first film, *Titicut Follies* (1967), shot at the Bridgewater, Massachusetts Hospital for the Criminally Insane, and in *Hospital* (1970), filmed in the emergency room of New York City's publicly-funded Metropolitan Hospital. While the two earlier films largely view public health care as impeded, even subverted, by the nature of bureaucracy itself, *Near Death* is more attentive to the complex interrelationships among patients, families, doctors, and nurses as they confront the personal, ethical, medical, psychological, religious, and legal issues involved in making decisions about whether or not to give or withdraw life-sustaining treatment to dying patients. Dr. Weiss explains in the film, "Everything here is sort of built on the Quaker concept of consensus." But, he adds significantly, difficulty arises when, in the context of "what is easily one of the most agonizing questions in medicine" (Broodman), "one of those elements is out of sync." And *Near Death*, like all of Wiseman's films, seeks out and examines that lack of "sync," the gaps between institutional theory and practice. Yet in its emphasis on the human dimension, "although *Near Death* is a movie in which death is omnipresent and hope rarely rewarded; as such, it is an antidote to the two other Wiseman films set in hospitals" (Neugeboren 127). The film's balance of perspectives makes it especially relevant today when more people (encouraged in part by the availability of medical information on the internet) are becoming proactive about their medical treatment, and as the medical technology for maintaining life continues to evolve.

The *Near Death* experience

If Wiseman's previous films have documented "a natural history of the way we live," in *Near Death,* he examines aspects of what Jessica Mitford calls "the American Way of Death." Epic in scope, *Near Death*'s six hours running time plunges the viewer into real life-and-death dramas. Like Wiseman's own *Deaf and Blind* (four feature length films released in 1986 about training at the Alabama Institute for the Deaf and Blind),[5] *Near Death* is "less a viewing experience than a total immersion." (Maslin 11) Crucial to this immersive experience is the film's ability to elicit complex and ambivalent responses from spectators who are shunted back and forth between the differing views of staff and patients. The film focuses on four specific patients whose cases provide applied variations of the ethical issues involved in decisions concerning life-support treatment. The four cases are presented sequentially, each taking about an hour of screen time. Preceding them is an "overture" sequence of approximately the same length that establishes the routine activities of the MICU and introduces the inevitably knotty ethical issues subsequently explored in more detail. Within each of the four case studies, Wiseman alternates between sequences featuring the patient (either with medical staff or family members) and sequences featuring the medical staff discussing the patient among themselves. Twice sections are divided by brief sequences showing parts of regular nurses' ethics meetings in which discussions of theoretical moral questions highlight or contradict what the medical staff actually do in the case studies.

Hospital concludes with a particularly powerful image: Wiseman cuts from patients praying in the hospital chapel to an exterior shot of the building from across a nearby highway. The hospital seems to recede with the slow reverse zoom of the camera while cars traveling on the highway fill the frame, moving across the frame in front of the hospital. The voices of the patients singing a hymn in the chapel can still be heard, but they gradually diminish in volume and are replaced by the "whooshing" of the automobiles going by in the foreground. The busy traffic expresses the peripatetic rush of contemporary life and how the immediate concerns of the material world cause us to forget spiritual values. *Near Death,* like *Hospital,* wants us to get past the clutter of this traffic to consider fundamental questions of health care. According to Wiseman, "Ordinary people don't have enough information to deal with the choices that high-tech medicine presents. . . . Yet more than half of us will die in a hospital. So, in a sense, *Near Death* could be regarded as a rehearsal" (Waters 52).

As in many of Wiseman's best films, such as *High School* and *Titicut Follies, Near Death* can be analyzed as a rhetorical example of what linguist Gregory Bateson calls the double bind – a situation wherein "the victim is sent inconsistent messages by those in authority. . . where the victim must make some response to the messages but is prohibited from drawing attention to the contradictory nature of the messages and from withdrawing from the situation" (Benson 238). As Bateson's concept suggests, Wiseman's films often force viewers to negotiate between apparently contradictory scenes. In *Titicut Follies,* for example, patients remain trapped in catch-22s regarding official opinion of their sanity, while in *High School* (set in Northeast High School in Philadelphia), students are caught within a number of double bind structures. In the case of *Near Death,* Dr. Weiss explicitly identifies the staff's double bind at the very beginning of the film: a split between an intellectual and an emotional response. This double bind, Dr. Weiss suggests, makes their job more difficult but is also necessary for coping in a context of constant death. The question before them, which ultimately is the same for all four of the patients documented in detail, involves whether and when to wean patients off the ventilator, and what to do if the process is unsuccessful. Dr. Weiss addresses the distinction between reason and emotion when facing death: referring to the family of the first patient, Mr. Gavin, he says they "knew intellectually that he wasn't going to make it, but emotionally. . .they were just not prepared to accept that." Like the mother and daughter we hear about who respond differently over each other's shoulder, this split informs the medical staff's situation and our experience of the film.

The film thematizes this split as a tension between technology and human contact. Throughout the film, the cold comfort of medical technology is contrasted with the simple and direct human contact that serves as the physical emblem of what Elisabeth Kübler-Ross calls empathy (Kübler-Ross 33). Numerous images in the film show hospital bed handrails visually separating patients from staff and family, but at the same time Wiseman incorporates many shots of hands touching those of other people. Doctors, nurses, and family members frequently touch patients and their relatives when they talk. Most of these touches are gestures of comfort, concern, and sympathy. Mrs. Factor, the film's second patient, is so weak that she can communicate only through feeble hand gestures. When a nurse discusses the condition of Mr. Sperazza, the fourth patient, with his wife, she touches the distraught woman's leg, while her friend, seated on her other side, also touches her. Sperazza himself is asked at different times by a nurse, his wife, and his son to respond with a squeeze of the hand. And there is the extraordinarily moving scene of Mr. Factor gently stroking and kissing his ill wife's hand. Wiseman underscores the importance of these gestures of contact in several ways. Sometimes images are carefully composed so that they are positioned in the middle of the frame, clearly the center of visual attention. He also emphasizes these gestures through editing, as when he cuts to a close-up of Mrs. Sperazza holding her husband's hand ("Here I am, honey") when she tries to soothe him and again when Dr. Taylor does the same with her. Elsewhere, Wiseman uses camera movement, as when Dr. Kurland's hand rests upon the chest of the supine Mrs. Factor, which is framed in a full shot before the camera moves in to a close up of her face.

A short montage early in the film inside patients' rooms in the MICU features a series of close-ups showing details of the various machines used in the unit – the ventilators, computers, and IVs that provide continual monitoring and life support for the critically and terminally ill patients there (Figure 16.1). On the soundtrack, bits of easy-listening instrumental versions of Stevie Wonder's "My Cherie Amour" and the theme from *The Way We Were* (1973) accompany the first of many images of monitoring machines, computer screens, tubes and IVs, presumably carried over the unit's sound system. The counterpoint between hearing the soft arrangements of these romantic tunes and seeing the cold, clean technological devices creates a disjunction between the sound and image tracks that expresses the confluence of love and death, the sad irony that life carries on even in the face of death. As well, the pleasant, unobtrusive quality of the music suggests the extent to which the MICU staff go to make patients "comfortable" (the importance of this word is discussed in more detail below). From one point of view, as explained in one of the ethics meetings, this technology is used to maintain life support largely in order to give families time to accept the likely possibility of death rather than as a phase in the treatment of illness. But this sophisticated technology creates ethical problems by, in effect, confusing the boundary between life and death. The alternatives of, as one doctor puts it, "Life in an institution with a tube in your throat on a machine, or you can die tomorrow," inevitably raises the question posed by Kübler-Ross and others as to whether health care should be

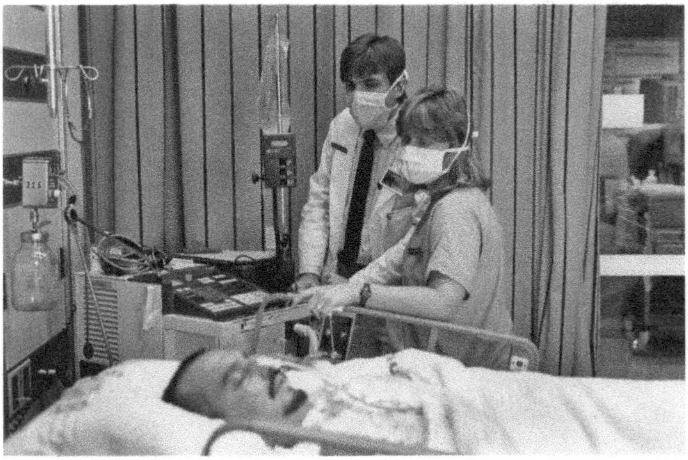

Figure 16.1 Medical technology extends life even as it physically isolates patients (*Near Death*). Copyright © 1989 by Zipporah Films. Used with permission

conceived as a humanitarian profession that reduces suffering or as an impersonal science for prolonging life (10).

Wiseman's films are always attentive to the specialized uses (and abuses) of language within institutions, and *Near Death* is a vivid example of, as Wiseman has observed, "the demeaning way in which words, which are essentially cliches, are used to categorize a person, so that as a result he will be treated as a member of a category, not a person" (qtd. Feldman 69). Dr. Weiss emphasizes the importance of their professional language in his comment that "There are a few situations, though, in life where the critical meaning of what you say and how you say it has [sic] as much ramifications as it does around this issue." (Hence, we inevitably wince when Dr. Taylor, trying to soothe a very upset Mrs. Sperazza, twice describes her husband's situation as "grave.") The staff's language is peppered with the peculiar euphemisms and phrasings of palliative health care that seem designed to downplay the real pain and fear of patients. Heart seizures, for example, are referred to as "episodes of pain," and the consideration of withdrawing life-support is described to patients as "reassessing goals." When Mr. Gavin explains his understanding of the treatment he is getting to Dr. Taylor as "experimenting" with different medications, the physician replies, "We shy away from the word 'experiment' 'cause it sounds like we're treating you like a guinea pig." The most frequently uttered euphemism in the film, though, particularly in the opening section, is the word "comfortable." Wiseman's editing gives the word a deliberate, almost rhythmic emphasis. Doctors and nurses alike constantly speak of "making people comfortable" and of "maximizing comfort" (Figure 16.2). Even the physicians themselves must "feel comfortable" with their decisions. We hear the word so frequently that we cannot help but become aware of it as a mantra of avoidance for the word that is never spoken. Like the title, their language only comes near death.

"Episodes of pain"

John Gavin, the first case shown in detail, is suffering from terminal heart disease with end-stage cardiomyopathy (an enlarged heart) and other complications. Dr. Weiss's bleak prognosis is that at best "we will probably be able to drag it on for a couple of weeks probably." Gavin's

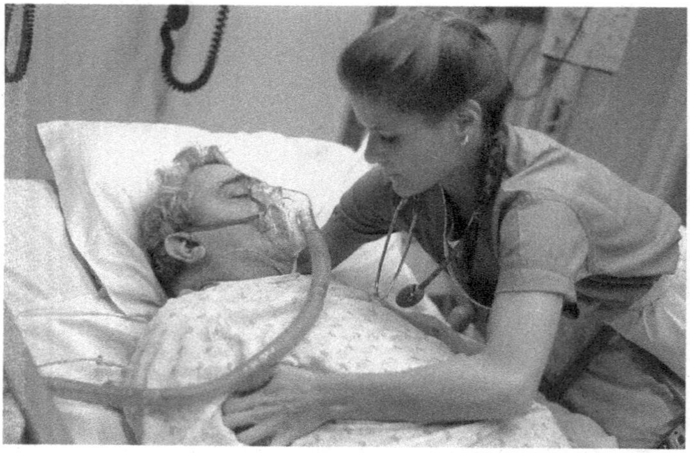

Figure 16.2 Human contact is crucial in palliative care despite the barriers of medical technology (*Near Death*). Copyright © 1989 by Zipporah Films. Used with permission

case foregrounds the ethical dilemma of maintaining life support when meaningful recovery is questionable, and the problem of defining what meaningful recovery is. As we learn, his case is "ironic" because some of the drugs he is receiving have the effect of counteracting others. Dr. Weiss agrees that the man's condition would be the same without any of the treatment he has had, and his preference would be to stop further therapy and give him morphine to make him "comfortable." The issue of informed consent is also raised by the question of Gavin's mental competence. Dr. Weiss questions whether Gavin should be involved in decisions regarding his treatment, since the high dosage of his medications may be clouding his judgment. To the surprise of all the medical staff, however, Gavin rallies and is able to be moved out of the ICU to a regular ward, trundled away in a wheelchair with his belongings stacked on his lap.

Bernice Factor has suffered a stroke with complications of pneumonia, and her prognosis is clearly poor. She has been intubated five times in the last six months, and this time she has already been on the ventilator for two weeks. Now, though, she seems to be asked so many times that she likely feels pressure to agree. In one discussion, she tries to speak and almost inaudibly whispers that she does not know. Ironically, a nurse reassures her that it is alright because "you've got as much time as you want." From what we see, her response is ambiguous, and the two attending doctors finally have to admit that she is giving different messages depending upon how she feels at any given moment. For Dr. Weiss, the goal of her treatment is the inevitable "comfort," and he reaches the conclusion that he will have to confront Dr. Kurland, who disagrees, on the matter. Both doctors later discuss Mrs. Factor, but they interpret her responses differently, according to their own opinions: Dr. Weiss thinks she has agreed not to be reintubated, while Dr. Kurland is not convinced. As Dr. Weiss says when discussing the meaning of informed choice, "the problem is that, you know, it's always 'informed' in quotes." But by the time we are near the conclusion of this section of the film, Mrs. Factor seems to have decided to be given a tracheostomy (the implantation of a permanent tube in the throat) if necessary, even if "it would mean an institutional existence in a nursing home or a hospital" for the rest of her life. Like John Gavin, Mrs. Factor eventually comes to agree with the decision of the medical staff. At the end of *Near Death*, we discover from the final insert titles that "At the time of the completion of the film, Mrs. Factor was living at home with her husband" – the only surviving patient of the four chronicled by the film.

The situation with her husband, himself a doctor, reveals the extent to which institutional perspective shapes perception. Whereas in the next section Mrs. Cabra, whose husband is dying, is described as "great" because "she was really cooperative," Dr. Factor is perceived negatively because he refuses to acknowledge his wife's likely death or agree with the staff's opinion. The staff decide that they may have to keep Dr. Factor out of his wife's room if he is going to continue to behave in an uncooperative manner and "decide how things are going to be handled in terms of care." The disposition to view him ungenerously is revealed by Dr. Kurland's petulant comment to Dr. Weiss that Dr. Factor has been so upset he came to his office the day before "and he didn't have an appointment." Dr. Factor's devotion to his wife is constant. We are told he comes every day, like clockwork, bearing cookies. As he appears one day clutching his cookie bag, a slightly begrudging nurse gives him permission to see his wife; in one of the most moving scenes in the entire film, he shuffles across the frame, silently and stoically bearing the weight of his grief, hardly the intemperate man the nurses describe.

Manuel Cabra's case receives the shortest screen time of the four cases chronicled, but it is powerful nevertheless. In one scene where Cabra is being examined, Wiseman holds on his face for several seconds in silence, allowing time for spectatorial empathy to engage. But with each scene, Cabra seems to deteriorate further. The man is dying of lung and heart failure and has been on the ventilator for three weeks (a relatively lengthy time) when the section begins. He is the youngest of the patients shown in the film – only 33 ("he's a young man and he's otherwise quite healthy," as Dr. Taylor says), with a wife and three children, whose "heart-breaking" letters to "Dear Daddy" adorn the hospital room. Cabra was first seen for a genital infection which became cancerous; although it was a "highly curable" form of cancer, he developed pulmonary fibrosis as a rare reaction to his chemotherapy and antibiotics. Dr. Weiss refers to his illness as "the Andromeda Strain" and muses "what a horrible way to die."

Because Cabra's outlook seems so "hopeless," his chances of survival "maybe one in a million," the question is not whether but when to terminate life support and of how to broach it with his wife. The doctors agree that Mrs. Cabra understands what is happening; but, it is not at all clear that she understand what Dr. Schulman means when he says that there is not much they can do other than to keep him "comfortable." To Dr. Taylor, she confesses that she could not bring herself to make the decision to withdraw life support although subsequently she consents that there should be no CPR or shock therapy if he experiences cardiac arrest. Only a week and a half (but within a few minutes of screen time) later, Mrs. Cabra, initially opposed to withdrawing further measures, has come to grant permission to provide "comfort measures only." Two nurses discuss this decision, one explaining to the other that Dr. Weiss has "just been kind of gradually bringing her around."

The moment of Mr. Cabra's death is not shown; we merely hear about it, as if in passing, during one of the rounds discussions when a doctor says, "By the way, Mr. Cabra died yesterday about 5 P.M." The seemingly casual, understated manner in which he reports the news of a death that earlier was said to be of "tragic" proportions is likely to shock us. Yet a greater shock follows, as we next witness some of the mundane considerations that necessarily follow death. Orderlies wheel Cabra's body down the freight elevator and along a hallway to the morgue, his few personal effects stacked on his chest. In the morgue, prosaic instructions are posted on signs: "Place body feet first" and "Use middle compartment when available." The body – shown as physically, palpably present – requires the effort of four people – one of the two nurses wipes her brow from the strain – to put it in a morgue drawer. Then the drawer is tagged. The corridors of institutional pressures seem to extend even into the afterlife. Thankfully, we do not see the autopsy itself, but the post-autopsy examination forcefully exacerbates our inevitably conflicted reaction – a reaction that mirrors the double bind of the staff. Some of Cabra's internal organs are arranged neatly on a metal tray, like an artful collage. (The reference to images in Wiseman's earlier *Meat* [1976], an uncomfortably graphic look at animal slaughterhouses, is unavoidable.) Of course, the physicians have to examine the fibrotic condition of the patient's lungs in the hope of being able to find the cause and prevent it from happening to others, but the moment has an unavoidably ghoulish quality as hands reach in from all sides of the frame to touch the strangely hardened organs like one of the grislier scenes from *Night of the Living Dead* (1968). The discrepancy between this simple sum of bodily parts and the person to whom they once belonged cannot help but strike viewers unaccustomed to seeing such a sight.

The first image of Charles Sperazza, the fourth and final case Wiseman presents, shows him supine in readiness for emergency treatment, inevitably recalling the opening of *Hospital*. No fewer than 14 caregivers mill around the patient, working frantically to revive him. The man's heart and lungs have failed, and while his heart function has been resuscitated, he has not been weaned off the ventilator. He still has a blocked heart valve and aortic stenosis (hardening of the aorta), and his kidneys are also in the process of failing. Further, since he had been without oxygen for a while, Dr. Weiss seems certain that Sperazza has lost some brain function ("I don't think he's got everything there") although later Dr. Taylor says the brain scan showed no abnormalities. Then Sperazza surprises everyone when he is able to breathe without the ventilator although Dr. Weiss still does not give him more than six months to live.

Dr. Taylor's talks with Mrs. Sperazza are likely to seem ambiguous given the discussions about the nature of informed consent earlier in the film. The immediate question concerns whether to do a valvuloplasty for a blocked heart valve when the patient is already in serious difficulty and there may be no hope for meaningful recovery anyway. Surprisingly, though, Mr. Sperazza seems to be recovering. Now awake, he is informed that on this day he will finally be taken off the ventilator. After extubation, his wife at his bedside, we hear his raspy but regular breathing, and he seems to be doing better than anyone had expected. From this point on, Sperazza's condition seems, happily, to progressively improve. Having survived one close shave, he sits up and is shaved and combed by a nurse. His eyes, taped shut earlier, now flare wide open for the first time as he glares ferociously at the nurse because of her obviously rough manner of shaving. The scene recalls the rough shaving of one of the patients in *Titicut Follies*, of animals in *Meat* and *Primate* (1974), and of the recruits in *Basic Training* (1971) – all images of forceful institutional processing in Wiseman's work. After the shaving scene, we never see Mr. Sperazza again, except briefly in the coda, when he is being taken out of the MICU, but in the final credits we learn that he died a week later.

Near Death concludes with a brief montage that includes several quick shots of more rounds discussions, more patients. A corpse is wrapped in a body bag, and the identity of the deceased patient is checked (apparently mistakes have been made before). There are shots of people entering the hospital, but this is the only one of somebody leaving. The hearse pulls away, like the truck loaded with processed meats that once were live animals leaving the packing plant at the end of *Meat* or the funeral at the end of *Titicut Follies*. Dr. Factor is shown at his wife's side, still. With a formal symmetry of which art is capable but which life – and death – clearly lacks, the film concludes as it begins, with exterior shots of the hospital and the Boston skyline. The light of the sun glints reassuringly off the facade of the office buildings in the distance, and on the River Charles sailboats dot the water, life flowing on.

Conclusion

During several rounds and ethics discussions, members of the staff voice the opinion that it is better to give families the news of a patient's impending death directly, but the film does not show this happening in practice. As a result, the staff may seem, at least initially, to be somewhat dishonest, if not devious, in their indirect strategy of coaxing patients and families into agreeing that sustained dependence on life-support equipment is less preferable than a relatively comfortable death. While it is, of course, commendable that the doctors continually seek this consultation, it sometimes appears as if they are badgering people into submission. In a sense, the choice these patients and families are offered seems merely "the guise of real choice" (Kleinman 29). As *Near Death* proceeds, however, this response is inevitably modified, as various members of the hospital staff are seen genuinely to wrestle with the various ethical questions inevitably raised by the existence of life-support technology (Figure 16.3). Perhaps these lengthy discussions can themselves be understood as a method of avoidance or coping (Kübler-Ross 7). In short, viewers of *Near Death* are presented with the same emotional and intellectual split as the people in the film. Our shifting view of the medical staff gives us a direct sense of what those who must make such momentous decisions regarding their loved ones feel. In fact, the more we see, the more likely we are to think, as Avery Weisman asserts, that to insist upon full disclosure is "as dogmatic and inexcusable" as avoiding discussion (Kübler-Ross 7).

The constant talk by doctors in the film, their refusal to express hopelessness to families even when they admit it privately, is explicitly said by Kübler-Ross to be of great support at a time when people feel particularly helpless (26). And doctors, too, we learn, suffer from a sickness unto death. Several times the camera holds on Dr. Taylor, after a discussion with relatives about the poor prospects of a patient, walking alone away from the camera down one of the hospital corridors. An authority "endowed with magic and mystery" (Weisman 200), one to whom

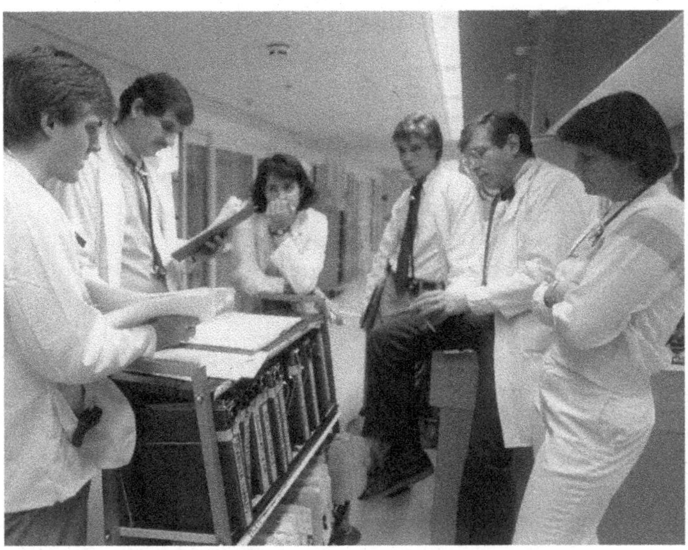

Figure 16.3 One of the many staff discussions shown in *Near Death*. Copyright © 1989 by Zipporah Films. Used with permission

family members look for solace and answers in a stressful time, he literally dwindles before our eyes as he walks into the background of the image, also bearing the emotional burden of death. In the last line of dialogue in the film, Dr. Weiss refers to the "psychological toll" exacted from working in the MICU. All four cases show a doctor as embodying the paradox of being both "a healer and someone equally baffled by inexorable death." (Kübler-Ross 200–1).

Wiseman never treats an institution in isolation but always suggests its connections to other institutions and aspects of American social life. Mr. Gavin is concerned about the financial implications of extended treatment: "I'm fortunate enough now as it is to have the Blue Cross and Blue Shield. . . otherwise I'd be cleaned out," he observes. As well, Dr. Weiss's discussion of the hospital's budget and the fact that it has been cut 5 percent as a result of state legislation contextualizes the ethical debate of life-support treatment within more pragmatic considerations – a factor that seems even more pressing today given the strains on the health system during the Covid-19 pandemic. Dr. Weiss observes that "Two thirds of all your health care costs are incurred during the final twenty-one days of life. . . . And the problem is we can't tell who's going to make it and who's not." His comment explicitly frames Beth Israel's MICU within the larger network of taxation, government policy, the various institutions of the social safety net, and questions of the welfare state and entitlement programs (and further connecting *Near Death* with *Titicut Follies* and *Hospital*). Certainly, the high cost of dying is a central part of American life, thus begging for such scrutiny.

Reviewers and critics generally agreed that *Near Death* is a documentary of great importance. Most commented that the film is an extremely intense experience and that it is lofty in principle. Wiseman was praised for his ability to empathize with his subjects and for making viewers aware of how many of us will spend the last part of our lives. Arthur Kleinman in *The New Republic*, for example, praised the film for the numerous ethical issues it forces viewers to consider. A bit of controversy developed in the *New England Journal of Medicine* when a flurry of letters to the editor followed in response to an article by Dr. Susan Wolf in which, responding to the film, she questions the ethics of the decision-making process and argues that the responsibility belongs to the families of dying patients. One of the letters, signed by two doctors from Beth Israel Hospital and Wiseman, asserted that the film is about "the process of coming to grips with making decisions and not the final decisions or their justification," and that Wolf misrepresents clinicians in the film by describing them as trying "to create substantial pressure to conform to the group view" ("Correspondence").

Near Death attempts to represent death in a way that is distinctly different from its treatment in fiction film, where death tends to be shown as graphic and violent or euphemistically sentimental. Susan Sontag has written that "All photographs are memento mori. To take a photograph is to participate in another person's (or thing's) mortality, vulnerability, mutability. Precisely by slicing out this moment and freezing it, all the photographs testify to time's relentless melt" (15). This is as true of *Near Death* as it is of any other film, but one might argue that in Wiseman's documentary life inevitably shines through the paraphernalia of death, like the nurse who loudly sneezes in a supposedly antiseptic environment. Indeed, the film challenges cinema's inevitable chronicling of mortality: because it is the patients and their families who command our attention more than the technology that always surrounds them, Wiseman's emotionally powerful footage testifies to the fact of their lives and will remain long after they have shuffled off their mortal coils. There is an unforgettable sequence in *Titicut Follies* in which Wiseman alternates between shots of an inmate being force-fed and shots of him, after his death from malnutrition, being embalmed and prepared for burial. Wiseman here makes a powerful point about institutional indifference, but we have little sense of the man himself. By contrast,

Near Death documents human behavior concerning death yet never sacrifices the dignity of its social actors, the real people who allowed their personal dramas to be made available for our inspection.

Toward the end of *Hospital* (1970) there is a scene in which a doctor tries to get the medical history of a woman who has suffered a severe heart attack from her daughter who responds with confusion and suspicion and so delays necessary emergency treatment. Perhaps she is simply in shock at the possible loss of her mother, but because she does not cope well with her mother's imminent death, she hinders rather than helps the medical staff in their efforts. Similarly, in *Near Death*, Mrs. Gavin wants to avoid discussing the likely possibility of her husband's death because, as she says, "It's a touchy subject." As one of the doctors remarks at the beginning of *Near Death*, presumably to a patient's spouse but of course to the film's audience as well, "I know this is a very difficult topic for you." Several writers on death and dying have noted that the subject is a difficult one to address because of its taboo nature.[6] According to Nichols, Wiseman's cinema is characterized by a "tactlessness," by which he means a disregard for "the ideological constraints of politeness, respect for privacy, queasiness in the face of the grotesque or taboo" (Nichols, *Idealogy* 209). *Near Death*, then, may be Wiseman's most "tactless" work.

Ultimately, *Near Death* raises several crucial questions that remain so in contemporary times as well, none of which it makes a pretense of resolving. What is an appropriate death in the era of life-support technology? When should technological intervention cease? Is euthanasia morally justifiable? With whom does responsibility for such decisions rest? What constitutes informed consent and how is it obtained? Having experienced *Near Death*, we have become more aware of these knotty questions and our own responses to them. Such questions grow more pressing when, as Kleinman puts it, "Death is no longer regarded as a natural event" (28). All of these issues involving the quality of death in *Near Death* really concern the quality of life, what Avery Weisman calls "the practical significance of mortality." As he declares, "If we can discover more significant and more acceptable ways of facing death, then perhaps we will also find a method of accentuating the values and goals of life" (4).[7] The life-affirming implications of thanatology are asserted by the film's opening shots of the bright cityscape on the horizon, connoting vibrant and teeming life. Dr. Weiss, too, is fully aware of the limits of his work: "If you wanted to give people quality of life," he remarks, "you could like be a furniture salesman or something; it's easy to fix things that are fixable."

Notes

1 My choice of the word "sobering" is deliberate in that it invokes Nichols' assertion that the documentary is a "discourse of sobriety," along with religion, education, politics, science, and others (Nichols, *Representing Reality* 3).

2 Wiseman shot the film over a six-week period, between September and November 1988, and then edited the film for approximately ten months. It was first broadcast on PBS in January 1990. Thirty years later, neurologist Dr. Eelco F.M. Wijdicks observed that it "might be suitable for a masterclass on medical ethics in urgent care and end-of-life decisions in the intensive care unit" and suggests several topics for class discussions. "Teaching Medicine through Film: Wiseman's Medical Trilogy Revisited," (p. 3). *BMC Medical Education*, https://dol.org/10.1186/s12909-019-1819-0.

3 For detailed readings of Wiseman's films, see: Thomas Benson and Carolyn Anderson, *Reality Fictions: The Films of Frederick Wiseman*, 2nd ed. (Carbondale: Southern Illinois University Press, 2002) and my *Voyages of Discovery: The Cinema of Frederick Wiseman* (Urbana: University of Illinois Press, 1992; 2nd edition forthcoming from Columbia University Press, 2023). Transcripts of five of Wiseman's films are available in *Five Films by Frederick Wiseman*, ed. Grant (Berkeley: University of California Press, 2006).

4 As Wiseman observes, they "are always the same film, by and large"; they "are all one film . . . ." Quoted in Anon., "Viewpoints: Shooting the Institution," *Time* (December 9, 1974), p. 95. See also Ira Halberstadt, p. 24.

5 The four films of the series are: *Blind* (132 min.), *Deaf* (164 min.), *Adjustment and Work* (120 min.), and *Multi-Handicapped* (126). The first two films emphasize viewer identification and involvement, while the latter two are more focused on occupational therapies.

6 See, for example, Weisman, *On Dying and Denying* and Elisabeth Kübler-Ross, *On Death and Dying*.

7 See also Weisman's *The Realization of Death: A Guide to the Psychological Autopsy* (New York: Jason Aronson, 1974), pp. 4, 16.

Works cited

Benson, Thomas W. "The Rhetorical Structure of Frederick Wiseman's *High School*." *Communications Monographs*, vol. 47, 1980, pp. 233–61.

Benson, Thomas and Carolyn Anderson. *Reality Fictions: The Films of Frederick Wiseman*. 2nd ed. Carbondale: Southern Illinois University Press, 2002.

Berg, Beatrice. "I Was Fed Up with Hollywood Fantasies." *New York Times*, February 1, 1970, sec. 2, pp. 25–6.

Bromwich, David. "Documentary Now." *Dissent*, October 1971, pp. 507–12.

Broodman, Sandra D. "A Look at the End of Life: Frederick Wiseman's Gripping New Documentary." *Washington Post*. January 16, 1990.

"Correspondence." *New England Journal of Medicine*, vol. 322, no. 22, 1990, pp. 1604–6.

Eames, David. "Watching Wiseman Watch." *New York Times Magazine*, October 2, 1977, pp. 96–102, 104, 108.

Feldman, Sylvia. "The Wiseman Documentary." *Human Behavior*, vol. 5, 1976, pp. 64–9.

Graham, John, and George Garrett. "How Far Can You Go: A Conversation with Fred Wiseman." *Contempora*, vol. 1, no. 4, 1970, pp. 30–3.

Grant, Barry K. *Voyages of Discovery: The Cinema of Frederick Wiseman*. Urbana: University of Illinois Press, 1992.

Halberstadt, Ira. "An Interview with Fred Wiseman." *Filmmakers Newsletter*, vol. 7, no. 4, 1974, pp. 19–25.

Janis, Eugenia, and Wendy MacNeil, eds. *Photography within the Humanities*. Danbury, NH: Addison House, 1977.

Kael, Pauline. "The Current Cinema." *New Yorker*, October 18, 1969, pp. 199–204.

Kleinman, Arthur. "The American Way of Medical Death: Do Not Go Gentle." *New Republic*, February 5, 1998, pp. 28–9.

Kübler-Ross, Elizabeth. *On Death and Dying: What the Dying Have to Teach Doctors, Nurses, Clergy, and Their Own Families*. New York: Scribner's, 1969.

Maslin, Janet. "Frederick Wiseman's *Near Death*." *New York Times*, October 7, 1989, p. 11.

Mitford, Jessica. *The American Way of Death*. New York: Simon and Schuster, 1963.

Neugeboren, Jay. "Near Death/Near Life." *Frederick Wiseman*, edited by Joshua Siegel and Marie-Christine de Navacelle, New York: Museum of Modern Art, 2010, pp. 122–30.

Nichols, Bill. *Ideology and the Image*. Bloomington: Indiana University Press, 1981.

Nichols, Bill. *Representing Reality: Issues and Concepts in Documentary*. Bloomington and Indianapolis: Indiana University Press, 1991.

Robb, Christina. "Focus on Life." *Boston Globe Magazine*, January 23, 1983, pp. 15–17, 26–34.

Rosenthal, Alan. *The New Documentary in Action: A Casebook in Film Making*. Berkeley, CA: University of California Press, 1971.

Sontag, Susan. *On Photography*. New York: Delta, 1978.

"Viewpoints: Shooting the Institution." *Time*, December 9, 1974, p. 95.

Waters, Harry F. "A Stiff Dose of Intensive Care." *Newsweek*, January 22, 1990, p. 52.

Weisman, Avery. *On Death and Denying: A Psychiatric Study of Terminality*. New York: Behavioral Publications, 1972.

Weisman, Avery. *The Realization of Death: A Guide for the Psychological Autopsy*. New York: Jason Aronson, 1974.

Wijdicks, Eelco F. M. "Teaching Medicine through Film: Wiseman's Medical Trilogy Revisited." *BMC Medical Education,* p. 3, https://doi.org/10.1186/s12909-019-1819-0.

Wiseman, Frederick. *Five Films by Frederick Wiseman.* Transcribed and edited by Barry Keth Grant, Berkeley, CA: University of California Press, 2006.

Wolf, Susan. "Near Death – In the Moment of Decision." *New England Journal of Medicine*, vol. 322, no. 3, 1990, pp. 208–9.

PART V

Television

Unlike most other forms of media, TV screens are part of our home setting, common pieces of furniture that, nonetheless, dispense hours of medical information via dramatic programs, seemingly endless commercials, and non-fictional broadcasting. The four contributors to this section examine several elements of television programming including advertising, reality TV, seasonal drama, and limited series.

In the first chapter, **"Early pharmaceutical TV ads and medicalized consumers,"** Rebecca Burditt and Leah Shafer scrutinize the 1996 commercial for the allergy drug, Claritin. While we've all been encouraged, countless times, to ask our doctor about certain pharmaceuticals, most of us are unaware of how that commercial created a precedent for the onslaught of Direct-to-Consumer (DTC) advertising that now characterizes 21st-century medical care. Burditt and Shafer represent the ad as a nodal point in the crucial transformation of media and culture in the late 1990s, arguing that it relies on both hegemonic discursive structures and consumerist internet aesthetics, which reflect the neoliberal turn of health care in the United States.

In the second chapter, **"Medical horror story: realism, reality, and the real on television,"** Catherine Belling begins with a truism: that most of us fear being sick and being subject to medicine's attentions and interventions. Our anxieties about and hopes for the future rise and fall as we try to predict it, extrapolating from a repertoire of plots from the best- and worst-case scenarios that we know or imagine have happened to others. Television is an extremely potent source of such scenarios, regardless of their accuracy or probability, and Belling explores the representation of health care in three television genres, focusing particularly on those aspects that make us most anxious and afraid.

In the contemporary pantheon of cinematic and televisual monsters, zombies hold a prominent place, metaphorically reflecting our fears about being ill and impaired. In his chapter, **"Unhealthy horrors: the biopolitical zombie in 21st century film and television,"** Erik Larsen writes that zombies have essentially infected mainstream culture, reflected in the immense volume of works produced since 2001. Increasingly, he argues, the figure serves to express our panic about endemic health crises, genetic susceptibilities, chronic disabling conditions, outbreaks of infectious diseases, aging populations, and neurological conditions such as Alzheimer's Disease.

DOI: 10.4324/9781003007661-22

Like Burditt and Shafer, JV Fuqua also begins her chapter with an historical account: the death of LGBTQ and trans rights activist, Marsha P. Johnson, in July 1992. Johnson's death and the public recognition of her contributions to civil rights and the political struggle of LGBTQ and trans people of color frame Fuqua's discussion titled, **" 'The category is *LIVE!*': transing care and the persistence of queer survival in F/X's *Pose*."** The series, *Pose*, is remarkable for many reasons: the critical acclaim it has received; its representation of two public health crises in the 1980s including AIDS and transphobic violence; and its industrial/ productive context that supports and celebrates queer, creative labors of care.

17

EARLY PHARMACEUTICAL TV ADS AND MEDICALIZED CONSUMERS

Rebecca Burditt and Leah Shafer

In 1996, Schering-Plough produced a television commercial for its prescription allergy drug Claritin that followed the letter but not the intention of the Federal Drug Administration's (FDA) regulations for Direct-to-Consumer (DTC) advertising. Following the first television commercial for a pharmaceutical product in 1983 (for Rufen, a branded ibuprofen) the FDA ruled that advertising for pharmaceuticals had to divide time equally between promotion and potential side effects. The Claritin ad evaded this regulation, focusing on the brand name and inviting viewers to conduct further research "on the internet," rather than explain what the drug was or what it did.[1] The Claritin ad forced the FDA to relax its regulations the following year, and the multi-billion-dollar DTC pharmaceutical advertising industry was born.

This chapter reads the Claritin advertisement as a nodal point in the crucial transformations of media and culture in the mid- to late 90s. The ad's surreal foregrounding of branding, scale, digital materiality, and interactivity anticipates the visual aesthetics that arose in the era when American television shifted toward digital distribution and American consumers began using the World Wide Web. The Claritin commercial (and Schering-Plough's profits off the drug after it was advertised) set precedents for the onslaught of televised DTC advertising of pharmaceutical drugs that characterizes 21st-century medical care. The ad's invitation for viewers to research and recommend treatments to their doctors reflects a significant shift in consumer orientation to pharmaceutical drugs. When it invites consumers to seek out the drug, it espouses a neoliberal, "Do It Yourself" (DIY) attitude toward medicine, which reflects what YooJin Chelsea Jang describes as the "consumer driven" healthcare system of the United States, "an assemblage of socio-political-economic principles and practices" rather than a system that treats the health of the populace (Jang 9). Supported by consumers' ability to search the newly available trove of medical information online on sites such as *WebMD* (which launched in 1996 as Healthscape), this emerging neoliberal system would eventually transform American medicine into an enterprise that reduces diverse consumer needs and behaviors into points of data. Debuting in an era when "good health" became an individualized and consumerist endeavor, the Claritin ad also demonstrates the long-held racial bias of television and the American medical system. As such, an analysis of the ad is uniquely suited to provide insight on the cultural shifts around medical consumerism in the 1990s. The following is a close reading of the Claritin ad and the ways in which its reliance on both hegemonic discursive structures and consumerist internet

DOI: 10.4324/9781003007661-23

aesthetics reflect a neoliberal turn in U.S. healthcare. Such a turn draws consumers into distorted relationships with medicine and with their bodies through a process of mediatized abstraction.

Pharmaceutical advertising and U.S. culture

The history of U.S. television advertising is as long and varied as that of television itself. This brief history of pharmaceutical advertising will demonstrate that mass marketing of drugs has been a part of American culture for well over a century; that the U.S. government has been reluctant to regulate marketing claims around drug sales; and, that shifts in advertising exhibition and distribution drove the FDA to embrace DTC pharmaceutical advertising. In television's earliest days, when programming was presented live, the boundaries between news or entertainment content and commercial content were blurry. The role of the sponsor in framing early televised programming was repeatedly performed for viewers. Not only were sponsors' logos and products frequently the most visible element of early television studio sets, audiences were directly addressed by television personalities, and programs themselves were identified by their sponsors' jingles and names: for example, NBC's news program, *Camel Newsreel Theatre* (1949–1956); ABC's variety show, *Texaco Star Theatre* (1948–1953); or, the opening sequence to CBS's *The Goldbergs (*1949–1951), which featured Gertrude Berg, as her character Molly Goldberg, encouraging viewers at home to take Rybutol, a multi-vitamin, as she leaned through the window of her tenement apartment.

In commercial moments like this, the homey, familiar voice of Berg's character, Molly Golberg, is abstracted from the image. Berg's finger, pointing both to the Rybutol and to the viewer, is literally an indexical endorsement of Rybutol. As we will see in the Claritin commercial, the abstraction of bodies and sound from images disorients viewers in order to orient their attention on the drug being advertised.

Americans, and by extension their health, are profoundly affected by television and television advertising. The national perception of television's commercial nature has long been significantly contradictory, especially regarding the boundaries between television's commercial content and its place in the home. As Pamela Pennock notes, "With the advent of commercialized … television, it became more difficult – some would argue impossible – to maintain the boundary between the home and the marketplace" (Pennock 620). As we will see, the Claritin commercial's visual aesthetics evoke a home and a marketplace without boundaries, an impossibly open space that invites consumers to transform their bodies into sites for self-directed consumption of medicine and health information.

Some of the earliest mass-market advertising campaigns were for drugs. Historically, pharmaceutical advertising has blurred the boundaries between medically useful information and marketing claims while exploiting the affordances of the media forms available during each era. For example, Lydia Pinkham's Vegetable Compound, a menstrual pain medication, was first marketed in 1875. Mrs. Lydia Pinkham's Medicine Company placed advertisements in magazines and newspapers, sent representatives to fairs, and produced trading cards, songs, and pamphlets. One memorable trading card pictured a sign for the Compound stretched across the Brooklyn Bridge and claimed that the compound could "dissolve and expel tumors from the uterus" ("Lydia E. Pinkham's"). The sign did not exist in real life: just on the advertisement, and, the Compound could not "expel tumors from the uterus." It wasn't until 1906 that the US government began to regulate such marketing claims. As Scott A. Mogull notes: "In the first major case regarding marketing claims (United States v Johnson [1911]), the Supreme Court ruled that the 1906 Food and Drugs Act required manufacturers and salespeople to accurately divulge the ingredients or identity of a drug" (107). This case did not, however, require that manufacturers or marketers make truthful claims about the therapeutic benefits of their products. The FDA did not gain authority over the regulation of prescription drug advertising until 1962 (Mogull 108). DTC advertising for pharmaceutical goods began with print advertisements for a Merck pneumonia vaccine in 1981 (Scott). That same year, then-FDA Commissioner Arthur Hull Hayes Jr. spoke to the Pharmaceutical Advertising Council at the American Advertising Federation Conference, saying "[drug advertising] may be on the brink of the exponential-growth phase of direct-to-consumer promotion of prescription products" (Thomaselli).

The era of exponential growth of the DTC market, the era when pharmaceutical commercials first aired on television, was an era of significant change in the television industry and U.S. media industries in general. This era also saw a significant shift in the economics of medical insurance from non-profit organizations to corporate entities: in the early 1980s, Ronald Reagan ended federal support for HMOs, which gave rise to "a system to promote HMOs as investment opportunities" (Gaffney 44). The rise of cable television is followed by the rise of internet culture in the 1990s. By 1996, the year when Schering-Plough aired its Claritin commercial, cable television modems were first being installed in U.S. homes ("Cable's Story"). A correlative shift in medical insurance "with deep roots in the neoliberal revolution" began, at this time, to focus on "consumer driven" healthcare (Gaffney 45). As might be expected for a commercial medium, the shift in exhibition platforms and modes saw a parallel shift in advertising modes, including advertising for pharmaceutical goods which targeted the market for American consumers who had no choice but to participate in a "consumer driven" health care system. The DTC phenomenon reflects the larger philosophical aims of the neoliberal, "consumer driven" health care system adopted by the United States, a system that is inextricable from marketing and advertising culture.

The DTC mode evokes discourses of medicalization, algorithmic advertising, and interactivity typical of the digital era. The rise of for-profit websites like *WebMD*, which was founded the same year as the Claritin commercial, reflects this move toward consumer-directed, interactive, for-profit commercial interfaces through which Americans can directly access health services and information. On sites like *WebMD*, DTC pharmaceutical advertising is delivered to consumers via quizzes, discussion threads, message boards and other tools that rely on an architecture of participation. *WebMD*'s editorial policy frames this participation as a kind of empowerment, saying

> We are committed to providing information on a wide variety of health topics, and rather than filtering certain types of information that may or may not be applicable to any one individual's personal health, we rely on you, our reader, to choose the information that is most appropriate for you.

The language of empowerment, choice and individual responsibility is predicated on what YooJin Chelsea Jang calls a neoliberal "market rationality," a structure in which "the population as a collective is obliged to become responsible for their own health" (Jang 57). *WebMD*'s rhetoric of individual responsibility extends to its framing of advertisements on the site, of which they note, "the Advertiser is responsible for the accuracy and objectivity of their Advertising" ("Advertising Policy"). *WebMD's* participatory, for-profit structure disaggregates the consumer's autonomous identity while reinforcing the neoliberal emphasis on individual responsibility; it "subjectivates users to become self-responsible in healthcare by equating health knowledge with empowerment" (Jang 37). The Claritin commercial models this in the technique it uses to evade FDA regulations on pharmaceutical advertising. By offering viewers the "empowering" ability to seek information about Claritin from their doctor and from the internet, they are able to promote their product as a site of knowledge rather than as a material object. The immateriality of the promises made by the commercial are evident in both its form and its aesthetics, which mirror the visual signatures of early internet style.

Claritin commercial and early internet aesthetics

DTC TV advertisements today follow a well-known pattern: actors move through clichés of happiness and fulfillment – dining out, walking the dog, laughing with grandchildren – while a disembodied voice discloses the ailment, the drug, and an uncomfortably long list of side effects. For those familiar with this formula, Claritin's first DTC advertisement is puzzling at best. At the start of the ad, a white tablet etched with the words CLARITIN 10 emerges in a star burst from a blue sky dotted with clouds, transforms into a clock with rapidly spinning hands, then becomes a White woman's face while a man's voice intones, "Claritin," and a woman's voice says, "It's time! It's time!" The ad then cuts to a part-digitally generated, part-live action doctor's office, where a bank of television sets playing the Claritin ad are featured in the corner. The final shot of the ad returns to the woman's face superimposed on a digitally produced green lawn and the same sky, while on-screen text exhorts the viewer to "call your doctor" and visit Claritin "on the internet." At thirty seconds, viewers encounter an ensemble of vague imagery and frustratingly nonspecific dialogue (Call our doctor about what? What is it time for? What is Claritin?). In spite of its ambiguity, the spot initiated one of the most successful drug marketing efforts in history. By 1997, annual sales climbed to $1.4 billion and by 2000, it was responsible for nearly one third of Schering-Plough's yearly profit (Li 85).

Understanding mid-90s television aesthetics can provide useful insight into the commercial's enigmatic visual style and its resonance with a contemporary audience. As media scholars Jay Bolter and Richard Grusin argue, television is often "hypermediated" – that is, it actively calls attention to its role in mediating information rather than pretending to be a completely transparent window onto reality (185–6). Compared to the relative realism of film, some televisual conventions – such as the stylization of sitcoms and elaborate graphics of news broadcasts and commercials – openly highlight television's hypermediated state (187). Such texts foreground the technological and cultural conditions under which they were produced and therefore become especially valuable objects of analysis. This Claritin advertisement provides vivid evidence of two mid-90s conditions: first, the convergence between internet and television aesthetics and second, national reckonings with racial disparity in health care and beyond.

Conditioned by the aesthetics of the newly available World Wide Web, audiences in 1996 likely recognized the ad's strange poetry. With its unabashed citation of digital form, style, and modes of address, the commercial is a key example of what Bolter and Grusin have famously termed "remediation," or the process by which older and newer mediums "honor, rival, and revise" each other's conventions as they evolve (15; Cooke 26). Newer mediums, like websites, mirror some of the design characteristics of television and newspapers (Cooke 37), while older mediums, like television, adopt the visual qualities of the internet in order to remain relevant (Bolter and Grusin 185, 189). This commercial is a key example of television's remediation of early digital culture. The waiting room is an architectural shell without walls or a ceiling, which overlays a scrolling cloud pattern reminiscent of the animated wallpaper that graced the early web. This layering of imagery reflects the modularity and interchangeability of each component – a key feature of digital culture that became more widely known through programs such as Photoshop (Manovich, *Language of New Media* 30–1, 229). Moreover, the ad's obsessive display of perspective through its checkered floor tiles, arches, and columns is a clear reference to early web-based realms, which compensated for their lack of spatial continuity by boldly highlighting each receding plane. As media theorist Lev Manovich notes, early online virtual worlds (which were limited by '90s bandwidth capacity) could not yet achieve seamless movement through three-dimensional space; instead, avatars were often placed over pre-fabricated backgrounds displaying Renaissance perspective (256–7). The awkward movement of objects within the commercial recalls this spatial quirk of early internet realms: like the clipboard that is pulled from thin air and the sculpture that hovers above the table on the right, human figures inexplicably materialize and vanish at different points on the screen rather than move continuously through a three-dimensional milieu.

Another telling parallel with '90s web culture is the ad's almost surreal experimentation with form and scale. As design scholar Ida Engholm argues, "The great avant-garde of the mid-1990s" (203) marked a period in which some leading web artists were inspired by "Dadaist collage-like nonsense paste-ups" (206). The Claritin ad mirrors this collage philosophy with its inexplicable repetitions and shifts in scale. At about the 15 second mark, the woman from the first few frames appears again but this time in massive profile, as if her close-up had been pasted onto the waiting room scene. Soon after, a female nurse suddenly appears as a frame-filling medium close up that floats horizontally across the screen, while her appropriately scaled doppelgänger appears in the waiting room with the male patients.

These moments are striking for their graphic juxtapositions and their very lack of spatial rationale. As the advertisement contains essentially no content, we may read this collapse of perspective and realism as an invocation of the body of the viewer, affixed to the surface of the screen, seeking information about a body that is becoming increasingly abstracted from the previously established medical system.

Throughout the mid to late 90s, television's remediation of the internet yielded a distinctly busy, layered aesthetic. Viewers' experience with surfing the web acclimated them to navigating many streams of information simultaneously. The Claritin commercial serves as an example of television's new mode of engagement. Quickly paced and featuring many points of interest on screen at once (or in rapid succession), it emulates the computer desktop that is crowded with open windows, moving banners, and scrolling text (Bolter and Grusin 189). Web influence is also evident in the many smaller screens in the waiting room, which act as different windows of information within the larger window of the frame. For 30 seconds, viewers have a choice of where to focus their attention: on the figures in the waiting room? The large faces that appear? The phone number? The brand name? The website URL? The dizzying pace of information serves as a reminder of television's need to capture viewers' ever-fleeting attention and figures the dense layers of information that characterize the consumer's experience of searching for medical information on the internet.

The commercial's suitability for a distracted, web savvy audience extends to the level of interactivity it requires from viewers, who must chart a path through its rush of information and interpret its intentional ambiguities. One would be hard pressed to find a narrative arc to anchor a particular reading, and because the commercial cannot convey crucial information to viewers – namely what the drug is and what purpose it serves – much of the iconography remains mysterious as well. For Manovich, this lack of narrative definition is foundational to the internet's operation. Using the database as a model for theorizing our engagement with the web, he argues that users' experience is much less linear, rational, or predictable than in narrative driven forms of media. Instead, he claims, the internet is where "the world appears to us as an endless and unstructured collection of images, texts, and other data records..." ("Database as a Symbolic Form" 2). The Claritin commercial embodies this unstructured, non-hierarchical model, in which "every item has the same significance of every other" (1). Without knowing anything about the product, we see a puzzling array of objects: pill, clock, clouds, floating room, smiling woman, door, phone number; sudden changes in scale elevate certain objects over others with no rationale. Rather than a story about a potential patient's struggle and then relief, viewers face a seemingly random set of images. It is as if the imagery, pulled from a digital database and now the subject of a pharmaceutical DTC commercial, encourages viewers to experience their bodies through this database logic.

Race and the Whiteness of health

While in large part the commercial's aesthetic strategies reflect the structure and design of the nascent internet era, the commercial's visual style evokes a long-established historical signature. Beginning with the snowy white Claritin tablet that emerges from a radiant sunburst, it is clear who the imagined "consumer" is in this direct-to-consumer advertisement. Throughout the spot, we encounter khaki clad White men in the waiting room, mammoth close-ups of a White nurse (dressed in a crisp white uniform), and the face of a smiling White woman – perhaps a satisfied customer. From the first few seconds of the commercial, the entire scene is awash with signifiers of Whiteness, making very obvious the cultural associations between race, health, and agency.

It is impossible to deny the longstanding health disparities between White and Black Americans. A 2021 study found that between the years of 2016 and 2018, the mortality rate for Black Americans was 24 percent higher than that of White Americans, amounting to 74,402 more Black deaths per year (Benjamins et al. 1; Robeznieks), and statistics reveal higher risk for diabetes, heart disease, AIDS, asthma, and cancer (U.S. Department of Health; Satcher 6–7).[2] These numbers reflect the country's race-based, structural inequities. While part of this imbalance stems from lack of insurance and inadequate access to resources (Satcher 1–2), another problem lies in the interactions between patients and doctors (who are overwhelmingly White; as of 2018, only 5 percent of doctors identify as Black) ("Diversity in Medicine 2019"). Black patients are routinely under-diagnosed and are less likely to receive appropriate medical care: research indicates disparities in cancer treatments, pain management, testing, the prescription of psychotropic medications, and access to transplants (Rouse 4; Penner and Dovidio 278).[3] African Americans also tend to have markedly different interactions with physicians, who in one study were less likely to suggest preventative care, testing, or ongoing care to Black patients[4] (Rouse 14) and tend to be more "verbally dominant" with Black patients than with White (Johnson et al. 2087).[5] Implicit assumptions about African Americans – beliefs that they are less intelligent, less capable of learning about good health, less trustworthy, or are drug seeking "malingerers" (Rouse 2) – continue to shape patient-doctor interactions (6–7; Penner and Dovidio 281; Moskowitz et al. 849–50). Patients' experiences of racial discrimination have resulted in early termination of treatment (Mays et al. 178–9), increased patient dissatisfaction, (Benjamins and Whitman, 409), and lower adherence to treatment plans (Cuffee et al. e58; Cuevas et al. 991).

As legal scholar Vernellia R. Randall argues, a central barrier to resolving these biases is the assumption that they no longer exist in a modern, post-civil rights America. Current civil rights law, established in the 1960s to ban overt and intentional acts of discrimination, does not account for the unconscious biases and often unintentional acts (such as those listed above) that drive health disparities in the U.S. (74). And, as studies have shown, even when White physicians attest to their own colorblindness and efforts toward equity, implicit biases can still lead to sub-optimal patient experiences (Penner and Dovidio 281–7).

Racial disparities in health were not new in the 1990s, but they were gradually becoming a larger part of collective consciousness due to increased media coverage surrounding the Tuskegee Syphilis Experiment. Major newspapers such as the *Los Angeles Times* and *The Washington Post,* as well as popular programs like *Nightline,* began to call attention to its grave injustices (Gamble 1773, 1777); similarly, in 1993, James H. Jones published an update to *Bad Blood,* his landmark 1981 book that helped expose the details of Tuskegee to a national audience. Readers were re-introduced to the horrors of the secretive study, which in the 1930s gathered 399 Black men with syphilis from Macon, Georgia, to examine how the disease, when left untreated, affected the human body. Under the guise of providing care, White researchers allowed the disease to run rampant in the unknowing subjects and continued the study for decades (Warren et al. 643; Jones 5–6). As Jones chronicles, a number of doctors had been protesting the study on moral grounds since 1965, and yet authorities from the U.S. Public Health Service allowed it to continue until the press exposed the story in 1972 (190–204).

In the years leading up to the Claritin commercial, awareness grew about Tuskegee[6] and became even more pronounced in 1996, given the highly publicized push for public recognition and reparations to the study's victims. Icons such as Bill Jenkins – a Black CDC epidemiologist who was one of the first to call attention to the study in the 1960s – joined other advocacy groups in the effort, and in 1997, President Bill Clinton issued a nationally broadcast formal apology (Warren et al.; Smith; Gamble 1773). While confronting this history exposed the need to dissolve structural barriers in medicine, it also brought to light long held ideological associations of Whiteness with care, agency, and good health – a belief that clearly influenced Claritin's casting decisions and imagery.

Noticeably, the Whiteness of the people in the commercial is matched by the whiteness of the rest of the color palette: the nimbus of light around the pill, the clouds, the nurse's uniform. All of these details play a role in conveying the message of good health and its associations with hygiene, wellness, and purity. So deeply ingrained are these ideas in our national ideology that few viewers, then and now, register how much this symbolism is culturally determined. In a society in which White people remain dominant, whiteness is often privileged as the positive half of a racial binary: white symbolizes purity and health, of course, but also rationality, goodness, progress, intelligence, order, and civilization. Blackness, on the other hand, has been constructed to represent the opposite: dirt, sickness, childishness, villainy, weakness, and savagery. Constructions of the racialized Other therefore protect the authority of Whiteness through stark contrast (Morrison 52).

Like many racial ideologies, however, the web of associations reaches deeper still, with dominant society mobilizing the cultural links between race, health, and cleanliness in order to deny the very humanity of non-White bodies. Ann McClintock's famous study of Pears soap advertisements, for instance, illustrates this conceptual leap by tracing how advertisements in the Victorian Era depicted soap as a savior of colonized peoples all over the world. To bolster British imperialism, these ads positioned soap as the key to not only clean, healthy bodies but also to British bathing rituals and therefore to civilization (McClintock 145). The presumed physical dirt of Black, colonized bodies became conflated with savagery, savagery with moral impurity, and moral impurity with being something less than human (Berthold 10). As Richard Dyer argues, while racial Others are "particular, marked, raced…the white man has attained the position of being without properties, unmarked, universal, just human" (27). Such ideas presume fundamental differences between races (human and not human) and thus draw disturbing parallels with 19th-century pseudo sciences such as craniology and physiognomy, which claimed that physical differences correlated to biologically rooted differences in intelligence and morality (Cartwright and Sturken 358–9).

For viewers of the Claritin commercial in 1996, such racist assertions would likely have seemed like relics from a shameful past. Yet the mid-1990s witnessed the resurfacing of similar ideas, even if called by another name. Just as Claritin was beginning to gain traction in the market (and the year after the debut of the commercial), a heart medication called BiDil failed to gain FDA approval (Kahn, *Race in a Bottle* 56). In the years before it came up for approval again, it was rebranded as a heart medication designed especially for African Americans and suited to what was believed to be their distinct biological difference: their extra susceptibility to congestive heart failure (Kahn, *Race in a Bottle* 50–1). Although the scientific community had long dismissed biological bases for racial difference, medical discourse around the time of the Claritin commercial's release began to reintroduce these assumptions, albeit amid great resistance from some in the field.[7] BiDil was eventually granted full FDA approval in 2005 and was the first medication approved for the treatment of a specific racial group (Kahn, *Race in a Bottle* 2). As such, it echoed the same racist beliefs that had for centuries associated Black bodies with disease and biological inferiority. As lawyer and medical researcher Jonathan Kahn concludes:

> [The assumption is that] a drug tested on white people was good enough for everybody. In approving BiDil as a drug only for African Americans, the FDA also implicitly adopted an assumption that drugs tested on black people are only good for black people. This sends the clearly unintended but nonetheless powerful message that black people are somehow less fully representative of humanity than are white people.
>
> *(Race in a Bottle 49)*

In language that strongly recalls Dyer's discussion of Whiteness as a universal, transcendent standard, Kahn stresses the dangerous slippage between scientific discussions in the mid-1990s and early 2000s, and racist notions about the biological specificity of non-White peoples.

A close reading of the Claritin ad demonstrates that late-90s televisual aesthetics continue a decades' long American obsession with Whiteness and efficiency. The history of American television advertising has long linked sponsorship to televisual aesthetics and an analysis of early DTC pharmaceutical advertising locates that style in service to a nascent neoliberalism in the medical field. Neoliberal principles of disaggregation and remediation permeate the commercial's style and, when read decades later, visibly figure the disturbing rise of a new, more insidious form of racism and disempowerment. The Claritin ad's savvy evasions result in an ad without audible side effects. Its collapse of perspective and realism is an invocation of the viewer's hand on the remote control, positioned on the surface of the screen, seeking information about a body that is becoming increasingly abstracted from healthy outcomes.

Ultimately, the Claritin ad is symptomatic of a fundamental neoliberal paradox in which the bodily agency of consumers is transformed into points of data beyond their control. This unimaginably vast system's algorithmic logic reconstructs cultural bias "in ways that disproportionately disadvantage women, people of color, and other marginalized groups" (Kenworthy et al. np.). Ruha Benjamin has described this web of new technologies as a "subtle but no less hostile form of systemic bias," and one that often is disguised by common perceptions of technology as objective, open, and non-biased" (Kenworthy et al. np.). The Claritin ad's waiting room without walls and infinite sky reflect the distortions of a reality in which consumers are offered control over their health while being pushed to participate in a system that forecloses the very agency it promises.

Notes

1 The only extant copies of this commercial are low resolution and therefore are not included as images in this article. Please visit https://www.youtube.com/watch?v=5ZWQp0Q6m8o to screen the commercial.
2 According to the U.S. Department of Health and Human Services Office of Minority Health, African Americans were twice as likely as Whites to die of diabetes in 2018 ("Diabetes and African Americans") and 30% more likely to die from heart disease ("Heart Disease and African Americans"); in 2019, African Americans accounted for 42% of HIV cases, even though they made up only 13% of the total U.S. population ("HIV/AIDS and African Americans"); in 2018, African Americans were 40% more likely to have asthma than Whites ("Asthma and African Americans"); and "African Americans have the highest mortality rate for all cancers combined" ("Cancer and African Americans").
3 For further information on disparities in access to cardiovascular disease care, transplants, pain management, antipsychotic medication, dialysis, and lumbar spine radiographs, see Rouse p. 4, and her references on p. 269; for articles on disparities in providing antibiotics to children, treatment for peripheral arterial disease, and cancer treatment, see references in Penner and Dovidio, p. 278.
4 Anthropologist Carolyn Moxley Rouse notes that lack of insurance coverage is responsible for many disparities in health care. Her observations of these physician behaviors, however, support her argument that lack of initial access to treatment is not the only potential barrier to quality care for African American patients (14).
5 Note that Johnson et al.'s study does not measure how racial discordance or concordance (whether the patient and physician identify as the same race) affects verbal dominance in patient-physician interactions. In this particular study, out of 61 total physicians, 30 identified as White, 21 African American, nine Asian, and one other. For more information on how racial discordance/concordance affects African Americans patients' health and communication with their doctors, see Cuevas et al. and their citation of other studies on p. 988 and 992.
6 In spite of this increased media coverage, studies have shown that White awareness of Tuskegee remains much lower than that of people of color (Katz et al. 1137).
7 As Jonathan Kahn notes, scholars criticized the re-emergence of philosophies supporting genetic distinction between races, noting uncomfortable resonances with a racist past, a lack of sound scientific support, and a neglect of the socioeconomic and structural inequities that could equally contribute to health disparities between Black and White patients (Kahn, "How a Drug Becomes 'Ethnic'" 34; *Race in a Bottle* 85–6). Kahn's study reveals that a confluence of legal and marketing conditions – rather than science – led to the designation of the drug as solely for African Americans ("How a Drug Becomes 'Ethnic'" 1–46; *Race in a Bottle* 48–70).

Works cited

"Advertising Policy." *WebMD*. www.webmd.com/about-webmd-policies/about-advertising-policy.

Benjamins, Maureen R., Abigail Silva, Nazia S. Saiyed, and Fernando G. De Maio. "Comparison of All-Cause Mortality Rates and Inequities between Black and White Populations Across the 30 Most Populous US Cities." *JAMA Network Open*, vol. 4, no. 1, 2021, e2032086, pp. 1–14.

Benjamins, Maureen R. and Steven Whitman. "Relationships between Discrimination in Health Care and Health Care Outcomes Among Four Race/Ethnic Groups." *Journal of Behavioral Medicine*, vol. 37, no. 3, June 2014, pp. 402–13.

Berthold, Diana. "Tidy Whiteness: A Genealogy of Race, Purity, and Hygiene." *Ethics and the Environment*, vol. 15, no. 1, Spring 2010, pp. 1–26. *ProjectMUSE,* muse.jhu.edu/article/381832.

Bolter, Jay and Richard Grusin. *Remediation: Understanding New Media*. MIT Press, 1998.

"Cable's Story." *NCTA*.www.ncta.com/cables-story. Accessed March 9, 2021.

Cartwright, Lisa and MaritaSturken. *Practices of Looking: An Introduction to Visual Culture*. 2nd ed. Oxford: Oxford University Press, 2009.

Cooke, Lynne. "A Visual Convergence of Print, Television, and the Internet: Charting 40 Years of Design Change in News Presentation." *New Media and Society*, vol. 7, no. 1, 2005, pp. 22–46.

Cuevas, Adolfo, Kerth O'Brien, and Somnath Saha. "African American Experiences in Healthcare: 'I Always Feel Like I'm Getting Skipped Over.'" *Health Psychology,* vol. 35, no. 9, September 2016, pp. 987–95.

Cuffee, Yandelela, J. Lee Hargraves, Milagros Rosal, Becky A. Briesacher, Antoinette Schoenthaler, Sharina Person, Sandral Hullett, and Jeroan Allison. "Reported Racial Discrimination, Trust in Physicians, and Medication Adherence among Inner-City African Americans with Hypertension." *American Journal of Public Health,* vol. 103, no. 11, November 2013, pp. e55–e62.

Dyer, Richard. *White*. New York and Abingdon: Routledge, 1997.

"Diversity in Medicine: Facts and Figures 2019." Figure 18. Percentage of All Active Physicians by Race/Ethnicity, 2018, www.aamc.org/data-reports/workforce/interactive-data/figure-18-percentage-all-active-physicians-race/ethnicity-2018. Accessed July 31, 2021.

Engholm, Ida. "Digital Style History: The Development of Graphic Design on the Internet." *Digital Creativity*, vol. 13, no. 4, December 2002, pp. 193–211.

Gaffney, Adam. "The Neoliberal Turn in American Health Care." *Jacobin*, April 15, 2014, www.jacobinmag.com/2014/04/the-neoliberal-turn-in-american-health-care/.

Gamble, Vanessa Northington. "Under the Shadow of Tuskegee: African Americans and Health Care." *American Journal of Public Health*, vol. 87, no. 11, November 1997, pp. 1773–8. *Proquest*, www-proquest-com.ezproxy.hws.edu/docview/215096365/abstract/110B9A98B058406EPQ/1?accountid=27680.

Jang, Yoo Jin Chelsea. "Health 2.0: A Symptom of the Neoliberal Healthcare." Amsterdam: University of Amsterdam, Master's Thesis, 2014, https://scripties.uba.uva.nl/download?fid=544317.

Jones, James H. *Bad Blood: the Tuskegee Syphilis Experiment*. New and expanded edition, New York: The Free Press, 1993.

Johnson, Rachel L., Debra Roter, Neil R. Powe, and Lisa A. Cooper. "Patient Race/Ethnicity and Quality of Patient-Physician Communication during Medical Visits." *American Journal of Public Health*, vol. 94, no. 12, December 2004, pp. 2084–90.

Kahn, Jonathan. "How a Drug becomes 'Ethnic': Law, Commerce, and the Production of Racial Categories in Medicine." *Yale Journal of Health Policy, Law, and Ethics* vol. 4, no. 1, February 2004, pp. 1–46. https://digitalcommons.law.yale.edu/yjhple/vol4/iss1/1/.

Kahn, Jonathan. *Race in a Bottle: The Story of BiDil and Racialized Medicine in the Post-Genomic Age*. New York: Columbia University Press, 2012.

Katz, Ralph, S. Stephen Kegeles, Nancy R. Kressin, B. LeeGreen, Sherman A. James, Min Qi Wang, Stefanie L. Russell, and Cristina Claudio. "Awareness of the Tuskegee Syphilis Study and the U.S. Presidential Apology and their Influence on Minority Participation in Biomedical Research." *American Journal of Public Health*, vol. 98, no. 6, June 2008, 1137–42.

Kenworthy, Nora et al. "A Cross-sectional Study of Social Inequities in Medical Crowdfunding Campaigns in the United States." *PLoS ONE*, vol. 15, no. 3, 2020. https://journals.plos.org/plosone/article?id=10.1371/journal.pone.0229760.

Li, Jie Jack. *Blockbuster Drugs: The Rise and Decline of the Pharmaceutical Industry*. Oxford: Oxford University Press, 2014.

"Lydia E. Pinkham's Vegetable Compound: The Great East River Suspension Bridge." WH183F. William H. Helfland Collection of Pharmaceutical Trade Cards, The New York Academy of Medicine, https://digitalcollections.nyam.org/islandora/object/digital%3A764.

Manovich, Lev. "Database as a Symbolic Form," http://manovich.net/content/04-projects/022-database-as-a-symbolic-form/19_article_1998.pdf. Accessed July 30, 2021.

Manovich, Lev. *The Language of New Media*. Cambridge, MA: MIT Press, 2001.

Mays, Vickie M., Audrey Jones, Ayesha Delany-Brumsey, Courtney Coles, Susan D. Cochran. "Perceived Discrimination in Healthcare and Mental Health/Substance Abuse Treatment among Blacks, Latinos, and Whites." *Medical Care*, vol. 55, no. 2, February 2017, pp. 173–81.

McClintock, Ann. "Soft-Soaping Empire." *Consumer and Society Reader*, edited by Juliet Schor and Douglas B. Holt. New York: The New Press, 2000, pp. 129–52.

Mogull, Scott A. "Chronology of Direct-to-Consumer Advertising Regulation in the United States." *AMWA Journal*, vol. 22, no. 3, 2008, pp. 106–9.

Morrison, Toni. *Playing in the Dark: Whiteness and the Literary Imagination*. New York: Vintage Books, 1992.

Moskowitz, David, David H. Thom, David Guzman, Joanne Penko, Christine Miaskowski, and Margot Kushel. "Is Primary Care Providers' Trust in Socially Marginalized Patients Affected by Race?" *Journal of General Internal Medicine*, vol. 26, no. 8, August 2011, pp. 846–51.

Penner, Louis A. and John F. Dovidio. "Racial Color Blindness and Black-White Health Care Disparities." *The Myth of Racial Color Blindness: Manifestations, Dynamics, and Impact*, edited by Helen A. Neville, Miguel E. Gallardo, and Derald Wing Sue. Wshington, D.C.: American Psychological Association, 2016, pp. 275–93.

Pennock, Pamela. "Televising Sin: Efforts to Restrict the Televised Advertisement of Cigarettes and Alcohol in the United States, 1950s to 1980s." *Historical Journal of Film, Radio and Television*, vol. 25, no. 4, 2005, pp. 619–36.

Randall, Vernellia R. "Dying While Black in America: Maslow's Hierarchy of Need and Racial Policy Making." *Reconsidering Law and Policy Debates: A Public Health Perspective*, edited by John G. Culhane. E-book, Cambridge: Cambridge University Press, 2010, pp. 69–88.

Robeznieks, Andis. "Inequity's Toll for Black Americans: 74,000 More Deaths a Year." *AMA,* February 22, 2021. www.ama-assn.org/delivering-care/health-equity/inequity-s-toll-black-americans-74000-more-deaths-year. Accessed July 30, 2021.

Rouse, Carolyn. *Uncertain Suffering: Racial Healthcare Disparities and Sickle Cell Disease.* 1st ed., Oakland, CA: University of California Press, 2009.

Satcher, David M. "Securing the Right to Health Care and Well-Being." *The Covenant with Black America: Ten Years Later*, compiled and edited by Tavis Smiley. Carlsbad, CA: Hay House, 2016, pp 1–17.

Scott, Dylan. "The Untold Story of TV's First Prescription Drug Ad." *STAT*, December 11, 2015, www.statnews.com/2015/12/11/untold-story-tvs-first-prescription-drug-ad/.

Smith, Harrison. "Bill Jenkins, Epidemiologist Who Tried to End Tuskegee Syphilis Study, Dies at 73." *Washington Post,* February 27, 2019. www.washingtonpost.com/local/obituaries/bill-jenkins-epidemiologist-who-tried-to-end-tuskegee-syphilis-study-dies-at-73/2019/02/27/2319e142-3aa2-11e9-a06c-3ec8ed509d15_story.html. Accessed August 5, 2021.

Thomaselli, Rich. "Ten Years Later: Direct to Consumer Drug Advertising." *Ad Age*, October 1, 2006, https://adage.com/article/news/ten-years-direct-consumer-drug-advertising/112215.

United States, U.S. Energy Information Administration, "Average Number of Televisions in U.S. Homes Declining." *Today in Energy*, December 22, 2017, www.eia.gov/todayinenergy/detail.php?id=34252.

U.S. Department of Health and Human Services Office of Minority Health. "Asthma and African Americans." https://minorityhealth.hhs.gov/omh/browse.aspx?lvl=4&lvlid=15. Accessed May 23, 2021.

U.S. Department of Health and Human Services Office of Minority Health. "Cancer and African Americans." https://minorityhealth.hhs.gov/omh/browse.aspx?lvl=4&lvlid=16. Accessed May 23, 2021.

U.S. Department of Health and Human Services Office of Minority Health. "Diabetes and African Americans."https://minorityhealth.hhs.gov/omh/browse.aspx?lvl=4&lvlid=18. Accessed May 23, 2021.

U.S. Department of Health and Human Services Office of Minority Health. "Heart Disease and African Americans." https://minorityhealth.hhs.gov/omh/browse.aspx?lvl=4&lvlid=19. Accessed May 23, 2021.

U.S. Department of Health and Human Services Office of Minority Health. "HIV/AIDS and African Americans." https://minorityhealth.hhs.gov/omh/browse.aspx?lvl=4&lvlid=21. Accessed May 23, 2021.

Warren, Reuben, David Hodge, and Ann Gallagher. "Reparation, Bill Jenkins, and a Legacy of Courage." *Nursing Ethics,* vol. 26, no. 3, 7 May 2019, pp. 643–5. *Proquest.*

"WebMD Editorial Policy." *WebMD*. www.webmd.com/about-webmd-policies/about-editorial-policy.

18

MEDICAL HORROR STORY

Realism, reality, and the real on television

Catherine Belling

Max, a small boy, has a fever, a rash, and a sore throat. The pediatrician, Dr. Alex Lowe (Chloe Sevigny), makes a diagnosis: "Your son has the measles" ("Chutes and Ladders" 00:09:00). Max's mother is relieved: "Oh, the measles! Thank God. I thought it was something serious." Dr. Lowe corrects her: "The measles *are* serious, Mrs. Ellison. And completely unnecessary. If you had followed my advice and had Max vaccinated, then we wouldn't be–."Now the mother interrupts: "We did what we thought was right… all that stuff out there about how vaccines can lead to autism, how they can actually kill people– "Dr. Lowe corrects her again: "*Measles* kills people."

A television show engages a contemporary public health controversy in one of its plot lines, establishing both the well-intentioned parent's misinformed fears and the pediatrician's exasperation. "All that stuff out there" – the media in its various forms – has overridden Mrs. Ellison's trust in direct medical advice. But this looks like an allopathic cautionary tale, a counternarrative to anti-vaxxers, because soon Max is hospitalized with measles complications. Again, the pediatrician admonishes the mother – "I don't understand why you didn't call me the second his fever went over 103" – but she in turn blames the doctor for thwarting effective communication: "I guess I just felt ashamed after our last conversation. You made me feel pretty terrible" ("Mommy" 00:05:50). An interesting clinical–ethical tension is illustrated here, regarding a pediatrician's responsibility for acknowledging parents' concerns and not alienating their trust while helping them reach a medically appropriate decision.

But Max gets sicker. He is dying, and things take a turn: Dr. Lowe draws some of her own blood and transfuses it into Max. He quickly recovers. His mother hugs Dr. Lowe, calling it a miracle ("Room Service" 00:08:00). Then, when Max goes back to school, he infects his classmates with something presenting like rapid onset measles. By the end of the day, the sick children have attacked a teacher. We see them clustered around her body, drinking her blood. It makes them feel better.

How should we read this? Is this a sensible public health story that's gone off the rails? In the television series of which it is a part, the clinical realism is the surprise, not the preternatural violence that follows, for Dr. Lowe is a character in *American Horror Story*, an anthology series that systematically plays out the tropes and conventions of horror fiction in increasingly extreme, and archly camp, plot lines. In season 5, Dr. Lowe is the wife of a noirish detective tangled up with the inhabitants of a haunted Los Angeles hotel, a group

 DOI: 10.4324/9781003007661-24

including vampires whose condition is caused by a virus giving them both a "super-charged immune system" and an addiction to fresh blood. Dr. Lowe is infected, and the transfusion of her blood to Max is a kind of super-inoculation, wiping out his measles and turning him into a vampire. The medical scenes stand in stark contrast to the majority of the show, probably alerting the regular viewer that their stable setting of science-based authority is being established as vulnerable to the disruptions of a different, gothic, kind of medicine, both biological and supernatural.

The implausibilities in this narrative, and the tonal shift from decorous to extreme, mean that this representation of health care is likely to be dismissed by medical educators, for instance, as silly and irrelevant. *American Horror Story* is clearly not realistic: it does not try to resemble the actual world or to persuade us that its plot events are probable. It does, however, establish vivid touchstones for the imaginings that underpin illnesses and treatments. It makes explicit the terrors that lurk just beneath the surface of many television accounts of health care, approaching some medical truths more effectively than realist representations can.

Max's mother's fear and his doctor's assertions find a triangulation point in the body – the sick child's but also bodies in general – as a mysterious site of unpredictable power. What else lurks beneath tense conversations between parents and pediatricians but the potential for horror, specifically here the all-too-imaginable realization that things have gone wrong, that, say, a child has been harmed: *what have I done?* What, worries the mother, if the doctor's syringe contains something that will change my child into my worst nightmare? What, worries the doctor, if my power is inadequate in the face of a virus? (Dr. Lowe has herself, after all, been infected in an effort to retrieve her own lost son: she is a mother as well as a doctor, and the two roles are, for her, in traumatizing conflict.) What if the decisions we (clinicians, parents, patients) make (to consent, to decline, to wait), being dependent on our efforts to convert statistical probabilities into predictions of an as-yet unknown future, lead us to horror? The monstrous outcome of Max's measles may come closer to the phenomenological experience of vaccine anxiety (both for and against) than any more "realistic" anecdote or case history.

Most of us fear being sick. We also tend to fear being subject to medicine's attentions: trust and hope usually pull against an undertow of terror. Both optimism and anxiety arise because we predict the future by extrapolating from an existing repertoire of plots: fear is predicated on imagining worst-case scenarios constructed from what we know, or imagine, has already happened to others. Television, both fiction and non-fiction, is a potent source of such scenarios, the effects of which, regardless of their accuracy or probability, can, in influencing patients' (and professionals') healthcare decision-making, have emphatically real effects.

So how does television mediate our fears? Here are three scenarios: We see a man's eyeball fill with blood and extrude from its socket. We listen as plans are made to bisect a child's brain. And, while a child is dying of complications from measles, the pediatrician chides the child's mother for failing to have him vaccinated. All three are from television representations of medicine but from distinctly different genres. The first scene is from a realist drama, *House, M.D.* (2004–2012). The second is from a medical reality show, *Diagnosis* (2019). The third, as we have seen, is from *American Horror Story* (2011–present). Each representation both illustrates and complicates the relationship between actual health care and the stories television can tell about it.

We must note that "television" is of course a medium in transition. Many quite recent accounts view television as a mainstream medium, assuming that "prime time" network shows have a large and predictable viewership. With first cable and then online and social media viewing communities, the production and consumption of "television" have changed immensely. Here I consider "television" to refer to a "show" screened serially (even if "dropped" all at once on a streaming service), with multiple episodes connected by a shared genre, title, theme, structure, and/or cast of characters and actors. I will also refer to television shows in the present tense, even if they are no longer "on the air" in broadcast terms. This is because all the episodes I refer to remain available to view on streaming services as of late 2020. My intent here is to question assumptions about realism in the representation of health care in three television genres, focusing particularly on the aspects of medicine that make us afraid.

Because most viewers have at least some experience as healthcare consumers, many feel capable of evaluating some aspects of what they see and may therefore be inclined to trust other aspects about which they have less direct knowledge. In the same way, healthcare providers will quickly and critically notice discrepancies in representations of conditions and procedures with which they are professionally familiar.

Medicine on TV is thus a useful place for thinking about tensions between the false ideal that media representations should or can transparently and faithfully replicate the actual world (close to impossible) and its opposite, the frankly stylized and fictionalized representation of truths about health and medicine that exist beneath the surfaces of that actual world, far less rare but generally dismissed as "unrealistic." Medicine itself, in its reliance on the positivist epistemologies of bioscience, tends to overlook, or be suspicious of, the constructivist implications – the textuality – of all representation and can be quick to dismiss the unrealistic as irrelevant or obviously misleading. This can leave its practitioners vulnerable to the assumption that the "realistic" is a reliable index reality and that the fantastical cannot possibly refer to what is true. In the clinic and in public health, though, very real healthcare decisions are made based on expectations, aspirations, and, perhaps most significantly, fears that emerge from how we imagine health, suffering, and death as they are manifest in bodies over which medicine has only a tenuous and temporary control.

Realism

A patient presents with a swollen tongue. Dr. House, medical detective (Hugh Laurie), and his team attempt to identify the cause. While House is observing the patient undergo a lumbar puncture, we see that the patient's face has become distorted not only by his swollen tongue but by an increasingly bloodshot eye which, as we watch, bulges and then extrudes with an audible pop from its socket ("No Reason" 00:13:20). The scene has been mentioned in online discussions as the most gruesome and disturbing episode of *House*. It is presented as shocking but also as something that *might* happen to a hospital patient as the result of some as-yet unexplained pathophysiological crisis.

A typical realist medical drama, *House* gives us longitudinal accounts of the health providers' experiences, both professional and personal, while focusing each episode on a particular patient plot, in *House* the story of a mysterious illness embodied by a specific patient whose case is almost always solved and concluded in that episode. This format – the clinical detective case – keeps audience identification with providers rather than patients (even though most viewers are likely to take the latter role in real world interactions with health care) and, in presenting the bodily disruptions caused by disease in the narrative structure of the case, makes extreme physical events a primarily intellectual problem. With its layered analogies to Sherlock Holmes detective stories, *House* makes the link between medical and other investigative case studies even more pervasive, part of the show's attraction lying in the tension between the unruly chaos of sick bodies and medicine's efforts – within the show almost always successful – to control them. But how much of *House* applies outside the parameters of the show, and should this question matter?

Representations of the *content* of health care – disease, disfigurement, death, and the scary gross stuff we all have inside us – tend to generate horror as a powerful emotional, visceral, and affective response. Yet such representations, when situated in a realist clinical diegesis, temper that response with credulity: this is happening in a hospital not a horror movie. (No vampires here.) Our visceral response to the sudden shift of the patient's eye, from a reassuring, albeit bloodshot, part of his already-threatened facial identity (his lips cannot close around his swollen tongue) to a small round ball lying on his cheek attached to a thick bloody string, is thus both tempered and exacerbated by the clinical setting. A thought like *He's in a hospital, so this is under control* is set against *This is happening to a normal hospital patient even though it looks like something from a horror movie. Must I believe this? Could it to happen to my eye?* A question of plausibility disturbs the viewer here more than in, say, an overtly gruesome horror movie that makes no claims that this shocking sight could be integrated into the routine work depicted in the show. It's harder to say, "it's only a movie," about a movie we think of as realistic rather than fantastical.

We do not identify with or care much about the patient, who, like most "cases" in realist medical television dramas, is the transient object of the clinicians' attention. Instead we watch the patient's eye from the detached perspective of Dr. House and his team. This reversed identification may explain why questions about such shows' correspondence with the real medical world seem to preoccupy both media critics and medical professionals. Viewers – both the general public and healthcare insiders – tend to fixate on how much these representations correspond with actual biotechnical facts and actual patient or provider experience. Popular television criticism turns frequently to evaluating the accuracy of medical shows, inevitably judged by health professionals. For instance, in a 2020 *Insider* magazine article, "Doctors and Nurses Rate 10 Popular Medical Shows Based on Accuracy" (Mitrokostas), the magazine's "expert panel" gave *House* the top score, rating it 9.5 out of 10.

Accuracy suggests an absence of errors, as if the show should precisely transfer the actual world into its representation. A more complex criterion (though the *Insider* article uses the terms interchangeably) is *realism. House* is a realist text in the literary sense: its characters function in a world that largely abides by the same laws as ours, reinforced through the accretion of seemingly random minor detail – what Roland Barthes describes as the "reality effect" – that make the fictive *feel* like real life. Literary realism therefore concerns not the reality of the subject matter or the referentiality of the text but the opposite: its verisimilitude or capacity to create the illusion of reality. This illusion should not be mistaken as claiming non-fiction status, but the overlap between *House* cases and actual clinical cases – those paradoxical non-fiction constructs – can be misleading.

In a *New York Times* op-ed titled, "Magical Medicine on TV," cardiologist Sandeep Jauhar complains that *House* is "unrealistic." His criteria are based on the assumption that TV fiction ought to work the way many published clinical cases do. Composite or anonymized accounts of patients, identifying details changed in the interest of confidentiality, are treated as if they are essentially real-world events. The fact that the patient in a clinical case never actually existed as described is not seen as diminishing the real-world applicability of a case in which certain facts are invented. Such cases are seen as scientific, and doctors trust that the "medical facts" of a case are, as presented, wholly trustworthy, that the case is not a construct but simply a transparent container for reality. It is unsurprising, then, that a case-based show like *House* might be subjected to the same criteria, despite its frank fictionality and its entirely different rhetorical purpose.

Jauhar's observations reveal the difference between clinical experience and the satisfying control that narrative, both as case-writing and as realist fiction, can impose on it. He notes, wistfully, that the show "portrays a world where doctors have time to solve problems."

Television, that is, manipulates the reality of the clinic – lots of different cases all going on at once – to the demands of the production – fewer plots per episode. The objection, then, is to what differentiates representation from experience, and, as he concludes, he *prefers* the representation, sad that his real world is different from this "unrealistic" drama, not because the medical facts are inaccurate but because the storytelling is better done.

The case format of realist medical drama has led healthcare professions educators to treat such television plots *as if* they were clinical cases, as especially appealing conduits for vicarious experience of real medical practice. Medical educators periodically publish accounts of such teaching, praising the way such shows "contextualize illness and disease within narrative arcs … and story-line intrigue, and for this reason many students appreciate them as entertaining ways to learn – as enjoyable accompaniments to their clearly more substantive and supervised formal education" (Goodman 182). Teachers are then disgruntled when such shows seem to betray their trust. The author of one guide to using TV drama to teach primary care notes "some serious limitations": such representations are "rife with egregious deviations from the norm," so there is "potential for unexpected learning outcomes and insights due to social and cultural backgrounds distracting from the desired learning" (Williams 48). The one account I found that recognized TV medical dramas as "cultural texts," in particular as developing fantasies that reinforce students' emerging professional identities, still focuses primarily on the use of such shows for conveying medical information and criticizes them for failing to deliver content reliably (Goodman 183).

The expectation that realist television can be trusted as showing us what the real world is like is not, of course, limited to medically-trained viewers. In the 1970s, social scientists began to study "cultivation effects," the role of television in enculturating audiences into a mainstream view of what the media, specifically realist drama, presents as social reality (Chung 333). Especially concerned with television's effect on public acceptance of violence, they viewed realist drama as a dangerous source of indoctrination: "However contrived television plots are, viewers assume that they take place against a backdrop of the real world. … The premise of realism is a Trojan horse which carries within it a highly selective, synthetic, and purposeful image of the facts of life" (Gerbner and Gross 178). Similar concerns about misleading the public continue to be of interest to researchers working on medical TV drama now: "individuals who watch medical melodramas tend to perceive the representations of both the healthcare industry and doctors specifically as realistic," by which the authors mean actual or authentic, rather than presenting an illusion of reality (Meyer and Yermal 6). This "realism" is questioned by attempting to quantify correspondences, asking, for example, "at what rate do the fictional medical diagnoses on [*Grey's Anatomy*] align with contemporary trends in U.S. hospital diagnoses and how might these representations narratively frame our understanding of health and medicine?" (2). These authors object that "only 6% of the diagnoses/patient experiences represented on *Grey's* [*Anatomy*] are at all representative of an average individual's reasons for seeking health care" (6) – and that, therefore, the show is not realistic. But, of course, no individual narrative – no single dramatic "case" – can ever have a comparable sample size, and such shows never make any claim to being referential to or representative of external population-based health care reality.

Nonetheless, cultivation theory continues to influence studies of how television might affect popular assumptions about public health and expectations of medical care. There have been studies measuring the effects of television on patients' hopes and fears. Perhaps best known was the one showing how much more successful – or "miraculous" – CPR was on television than in the real world (Diem, Lantos, and Tulsky 1578). A more recent study names the "Gray's Anatomy Effect" as leading patients and their families to expect faster and easier recovery after major physical trauma or surgery (Serrone et al.). Stories about health care can also of course frighten potential patients, possibly discouraging them from seeking care and increasing a patient's preoperative fear (Witzel et al.).

Of course, frequent viewers of fictional medical dramas *do* tend to perceive what they're watching as correlating to some extent with actuality. Studies have found that trust in the accuracy of the dramas tends to correlate with these viewers' trust in their own physicians and in medicine in general, but this trust is modified by a viewer's "health literacy," with more "literate" viewers less likely to view television representations uncritically (Tian and Yoo 46). Like medical educators, such studies want to capitalize on the trust TV viewers seem to have in order to develop public health campaigns manipulating viewers' health perceptions and behaviors. Such authors turn only infrequently to the question of viewers' *media* literacy.

How does this struggle over how to quantify the effects of realist medical drama play out in my example? Does the most gruesome episode of *House* make people scared of medicine? The patient with the enucleated eye and the swollen tongue continues to deteriorate: his testicles swell and rupture, and finally he is eviscerated by laser surgery gone wrong. What seems less memorable is that none of these things actually happen, even in the Dr. House's fictitious clinic: they turn out to be hallucinations experienced by House during a ketamine-induced dissociative coma. For a show whose protagonist's motto is, famously, "Everybody lies," *House* engages an interesting amount of investment in what in it is "real" – that is, plausible – and what is not – and then relinquishes these measures by using its realist mise en scene to present *unreal* and extreme patient events with such careful realism that viewers do not, even after being told that these particular events were hallucinations, differentiate between them and the more "accurate" symptoms and crises of the show's typical "actual" patient cases. Very unusually for the show, the patient's condition, being a figment of Dr. House's imagination, is never explained.

Viewers appear to have been disturbed by the episode not because the mystery goes unsolved but because the bodies represented, no matter how reassuringly we are later told they existed only in House's drugged imagination, look no less real than those of other patients in the show, and what happens to them might, plausibly, happen to any body subject to increased blood flow and the forces of physics. It is here, in the simple horror of the human body as vulnerable material object, that realism and reality collide. It is here, too, that television mediation of medicine escapes the rules of clinical realism.

This same escape from realism is evident in two other genres that appear at first to be diametrically opposed. *Diagnosis* and *American Horror Story* make very different rhetorical claims on prospective viewers. At the most bluntly obvious level, the first appears educational and serious, the second entertaining and escapist. I'll show that greater complexity is (unsurprisingly) at work in the appeal of each but will also show how medical subject matter is particularly active in both the persuasive effectiveness and the attractiveness of each. Unlike realist drama, both reality TV and genre horror draw attention, albeit in radically different ways, to their constructedness and contingency. In relinquishing verisimilitude, they both foreground representation and hence arguably engage more directly with the truths that are medicine's real material. In the Netflix non-fiction series *Diagnosis,* what we see is presented not only as plausible and possible but as having actually happened to the people on screen.

Reality

A seven-year-old girl, Sadie, has mysterious seizures. She is eventually diagnosed with Rasmussen's encephalitis, an inflammatory condition causing progressive damage to one side of her brain, marked by increasingly severe seizures and irreversible cognitive and motor damage. The indicated treatment is hemispherotomy, the surgical bisection of her brain with removal of the damaged half. This is non-fiction, presented in Netflix's program *Diagnosis*. Sadie's mother describes her response when the condition has been identified: "Once you Google Rasmussen's encephalitis it's pretty horrifying to read about" ("Second Opinions" 00:11:00). Her horror is different from the fear that *Diagnosis* purports to address by solving medical mysteries: as another patient on the show puts it, "Not knowing is the scariest thing in the world" ("Detective Work" 00:07:00). Fear is anticipatory; horror is reactive. Knowing can, Sadie's mother suggests, be worse than fearing.

In *Diagnosis*, physician Lisa Sanders (formerly a technical advisor on *House*) expands on cases from her long-running *New York Times* column (tag-line: "Diagnosis: Dr. Lisa Sanders on Hard-to-Solve Medical Mysteries"). Sanders frames her project in the first episode – "Diagnosis is the answer to the question, 'Doctor, what's wrong with me?'" – but her own role is more commentator than physician because *Times* readers, doctors or not, submit their own opinions, which are presented to the patient or, in this case, to her parents. Sanders calls this "crowdsourcing," an invitation to the audience to engage directly in the show's plot trajectory, at least as it emerges from the *New York Times* column. Even though the show is announced as "a documentary series for Netflix – with *Times* readers at the center," it is, strictly, *reality television* rather than documentary. Its events are not recorded as they happen by a bystander film maker; they are brought into being by the show itself, by the request for reader input, and the televised follow-up on this input. A comparable reality show might be the competition *American Idol*, where the winner is chosen based on viewers' texting – voting – their preferences. Each episode's narrative would be impossible without public participation.

But *Diagnosis* involves real patients with real conditions undergoing real treatment and, it turns out, not all episodes turn on a mystery diagnosis. In Sadie's case, the horrifying diagnosis has already been made, and the drastic surgery recommended. Sanders instead tries to crowdsource a second opinion, an alternative to hemispherotomy. The scary not-knowing is not the issue; the answer is one the family – and Dr. Sanders – want to avoid because they consider it too horrible. The surgery is framed as shocking not only because it so conceptually radical but also because success in halting the encephalitis can come at the cost of paralyzing the side of the body controlled by the removed, or disconnected, half of the brain, as well as unpredictable losses in visual, cognitive, and language ability.

Sadie's neurosurgeon wants the hemispherotomy to be done soon, to halt disease progression, but decision-making is delayed by the suspenseful – narratively compelling – search for alternatives. Audience resistance to the procedure is reinforced by the indirect evocation of horror at its imagined outcome: Sanders arranges for Sadie's mother to have a video call with a young man with Rasmussen's who had the surgery years before. We see him on the call, one side of his face noticeably paralyzed and distorted, and the camera cuts to Sadie's mother's own struggling face as she takes in his appearance and, we deduce, imagines her daughter looking this way as an adult. The young man's mother sees her seeing and acknowledges her reaction: "It's scary – but we didn't have another option."

But an alternative option *is* found, and a "new team of doctors" who recommend a less invasive procedure in which a responsive neurostimulation device (RNS), a kind of electrode, is implanted in Sadie's brain. We see this surgery itself, a sequence that at one time might have been shocking in its visual access to the child's opened skull, her living interior, but which has become quite familiar and is framed as being quite minor compared to the demonized version that appears to have been avoided. Instead, Sadie's mother cheerfully reports her child's sci-fi response to having the surgery: "She thinks it's cool that she's, like, a cyborg, because she has a computer chip in her brain" ("Second Opinions" 00:44:15). Unlike a singing competition, though, *Diagnosis* cannot wholly control its narrative. The format succeeds in finding Sadie an alternative treatment but cannot confirm that the treatment has been a success. That would take too long. Sadie's doctor reports at the end of the episode that she is doing well but "the road ahead is always a mystery" ("Second Opinions" 00:44:45). The scary not-knowing continues to haunt us.

Something else happens in this episode, though, a much longer-term masterplot concerning medical progress. The dread hemispherotomy is framed as an act where horror both emerges – as Sadie's mother realizes – and is temporarily foreclosed by the discovery of a less shocking (though maybe less effective) solution. Sadie's new neurologist implies that entities purified of horror by the veneer of clinical value and immediacy – the cutting-edge technology – may become horrifying (again) once they have been superseded by new technologies. What was once accepted medical practice is now indistinguishable from torture: "Hemispherotomy doesn't feel like a modern technique," she says. "It's really kind of *barbaric*." This dismissal led to a real-world controversy: the Brain Recovery Project, part of the Childhood Epilepsy Surgery Foundation, objected to the episode's stigmatization of hemispherotomy and the patients who have already undergone it (and indeed studies plausibly report that the procedure often has less debilitating outcomes than *Diagnosis* appears to suggest, especially when compared with the effects of Rasmussen's itself). Identifying the tension between narrative satisfaction and medical responsibility, they call the neurologist's words "a dramatic and sensational hook to the storyline."

Despite medical educators' use of its "cases," *House*, because classified as fiction, does not need disclaimers. *Diagnosis* does: "The following series is designed to entertain and inform – not provide medical advice." The irony is, of course, that the show exists only because "medical advice" is elicited not from medical experts but from the public at large and passed on to the show's subject patient. Despite presenting the conclusive answer of a secure diagnosis – a mystery solved, just as in *House* – as the cure for fear, *Diagnosis* cannot sustain its optimism. The diagnosis may be horrifying, and the doctor is as subject to anxiety as the patient. Dr. Sanders articulates her own fear, and its connection with horror, most vividly as she describes, and we see, the brain scan of a patient who is losing his memory: "Willie's MRI is really one of the scariest pictures I've ever seen. He has this big lesion at the base of his brain, and coming from that are these tendrils of white mist, like fingers. Those fingers represent a kind of inflammation and destruction ..., this creeping invasion of whatever this white stuff is" ("The Wisdom of the Crowd" 00:07:07). Beneath the clinical confidence of both *House*'s realism and *Diagnosis*'s reality is the body, in which human identity and its very situatedness within reality are threatened by creeping tendrils of white stuff. The horror genre has its own way of investigating such stuff.

The Real

Philosopher Slavoj Žižek illustrates the psychoanalytic concept of the Real, the foundation of horror as both affect and genre, by referring to what he calls the "parallax of neurobiology," the terrifyingly incommensurable dual perspective that the human, in all our particularity and significance, is also just bodily matter, or "stuff": "the realization that, when one looks behind the face into the skull, one discovers nothing, there is 'nobody home,' just stacks of brain-meat – it is almost impossible to tarry within this gap between meaning and the pure Real" (Žižek 21). Dr. Sanders, describing that MRI as we look at it with her, may give us a glimpse at this gap, but we do not tarry there. Medical imaging and diagnostic vocabulary quickly – and in her setting, rightly – move in to re-represent the "white mist" she has seen erasing her patient's mind. Horror stories instead invite us to stay a while and think about what we might glimpse.

This "Real" is the difficult fact that medicine and horror stories both have as their core content, the truth they both encounter and then, either through science and biotechnology or through narration and representation, recuperate into the manageable reality over here, on this safe side of that gap. Realism is fiction that attempts to resemble reality. Reality shows document not real life but real events brought into being with the intention of recording and broadcasting them. A different kind of realness is engaged in *American Horror Story*: the rift in reality (that is, what humans apprehend as real, the phenomenal world we experience as projected and internalized images – the imaginary – and describe in language – the symbolic), a wound or gap understood as trauma and undergone as horror. This is what psychoanalyst Jacques Lacan called "the Real," meaning a truth that is always unspeakable, beyond description, defined by the challenge it poses to all our efforts to order and control our selves and the world.

American Horror Story, in deliberately presenting and playing out a vast repertoire of existing horror tropes, does not itself generate horror so much as comment on how horror stories work. The Real, in Lacan's sense, is already digested by the show's representations – for instance, when Max becomes a kind of vampire, we are probably shocked but more by the show's efficient return from implausible clinical realism to the gothic than by the underlying terror that we are, beneath a thin (and, here, medicalized) veneer, just blood-thirsty predators or vulnerable prey. Nonetheless, the repertoire of tropes make clear how a biological or medical parallax underpins so many of the elements understood conventionally to generate horror. Two seasons of *American Horror Story* engage overtly medical plotlines: season 2, *Asylum*, explores inpatient psychiatry of the 1950s, and season 4, *Freak Show*, the performance of those with congenital anomalies in a 1930s show and the threat of collectors seeking specimens for a Mutter-like medical museum of curiosities. But in the first season, *Murder House*, a compendium of the sources of horror in a classic haunted house story, very few aspects do *not* correspond with the preoccupations of medicine. The house is owned, in the 1920s, by a surgeon, addicted to chloroform, who provided illegal abortions, and begins to perform Frankenstein-like experiments on fetal – and later adult – remains. The house's present-day owner and resident is a psychiatrist; his wife is mourning a miscarriage and soon becomes pregnant again. His teenage daughter self-harms and eventually overdoses; her best friend, one of her father's patients, is a high school shooter. The woman next door has a daughter with Down's Syndrome and cruelly hates her daughter for her difference. The house is haunted, then, by the pathologies of those who seek to control the Real, the stuff-ness of mortal human matter.

These stories draw the subject matter of health care out of medicine's disciplinary frameworks. The viewer is not expected to take the perspective of doctors or patients – or even, arguably, of any characters. Viewing horror, our structures of identification run deeper. Our bodies identify with those bodies onscreen, with their biochemical terrors and desires and their status as meat. We respond viscerally to the real inhuman substrata that both health care and storytelling struggle endlessly to make sense of and control.

The seeming realism in season 5's vaccination subplot, then, is a screen for the anxiety that in fact underlies all three of my examples. It is imaginable that an eye can explode from its socket, a living brain needs to be cut in half, and a child can be irrevocably damaged by a medical intervention (delivered or withheld). Each of these possibilities can be imagined with the reassuring structures of science-based health care to frame and explain them and, ideally, to mitigate their most terrifying effects. The catch is that imagining them in this way also draws them into the realm of plausibility – draws the unspeakable Real of our messy mortal bodies into the reality that demands of us decisions and actions rather than screaming and covering our eyes. For this reason, it seems that the honestly unrealistic representations of medicine and its contents offered by horror stories may be an undervalued site for exploring the real subject matter of health care.

Works cited

Barthes, Roland. "The Reality Effect." *The Rustle of Language*, translated by Richard Howard, Berkeley, CA: U of California Press, 1989, pp. 141–8.

Chung, Jae Eun, "Medical Dramas and Viewer Perception of Health: Testing Cultivation Effects." *Human Communication Research*, vol. 40, no. 3, 2014, pp. 333–49.

Childhood Epilepsy Surgery Foundation. "Our Response to Netflix *Diagnosis*." October 1, 2019. brainrecoveryproject.org/wp-content/uploads/2019/10/Official-Response_-Netflix-Diagnosis-Episode-2-1.pdf. Accessed April 30, 2021.

"Chutes and Ladders." *American Horror Story*. Created by Bryan Murphy and Brad Falchuk, season 5, episode 2, 20th Television (FX Networks), October 14, 2015.

"Detective Work." *Diagnosis*. Created by Scott Rudin and Lisa Sanders, season 1, episode 1, Netflix, August 16, 2019.

Diem, Susan J., John D. Lantos, and James A. Tulsky. "Cardiopulmonary Resuscitation on Television: Miracles and Misinformation." *New England Journal of Medicine*, vol. 334, June 13, 1996, pp. 1578–82.

Gerbner, George, and Larry Gross. "Living with Television: The Violence Profile." *Journal of Communication*, vol. 26, 1976, pp. 172–90.

Goodman, K. "Imagining Doctors: Medical Students and the TV Medical Drama." *Virtual Mentor*, vol. 9, 2007, pp. 182–7.

"Introducing *Diagnosis*, a New Show from the *Times* and Netflix." *New York Times*, July 22, 2019. www.nytimes.com/2019/07/22/magazine/diagnosis-tv-netflix-lisa-sanders.html. Accessed April 30, 2021.

Jauhar, Sandeep. "Magical Medicine on TV." *New York Times*, July 19, 2005. www.nytimes.com/2005/07/19/health/magical-medicine-on-tv.html. Accessed April 30, 2021.

Meyer, Michaela D. E., and Amanda L. Yermal, "Representing Illness in Medical Melodramas on Television: A Qualitative Content Analysis of Medical Diagnoses in *Grey's Anatomy*." *Qualitative Research Reports in Communication* vol. 22, 2021, pp. 22-29.

Mitrokostas, Sophia. "Doctors and Nurses Rate 10 Popular Medical Shows Based on Accuracy." *Insider*, April 6, 2020, www.insider.com/experts-reveal-the-least-and-most-accurate-medical-shows-2019-12. Accessed April 30, 2021.

"Mommy." *American Horror Story*. Created by Bryan Murphy and Brad Falchuk, season 5, episode 3, 20th Television (FX Networks), October 21, 2015.

"No Reason." *House, M.D.* Created by David Shore. Season 2, Episode 24. Heel and Toe Films / NBC Universal, May 23, 2006.

"Room Service." *American Horror Story*. Created by Bryan Murphy and Brad Falchuk, season 5, episode 5, 20th Television (FX Networks), November 4, 2015.

Sanders, Lisa. "This Little Girl's Seizures Won't Stop. Her Parents Need Your Advice." *New York Times*, October 11, 2018, www.nytimes.com/interactive/2018/10/11/magazine/netflix-diagnosis-series-sadie.html. Accessed April 30, 2021.

Serrone, Rosemarie O., Jordan A. Weinberg, Pamela W. Goslar, Erin P. Wilkinson, et al. "*Grey's Anatomy* Effect: Television Portrayal of Patients with Trauma May Cultivate Unrealistic Patient and Family Expectations after Injury." *Trauma Surgery and Acute Care Open*, vol. 3, 2018, doi: 10.1136.

"Second Opinions." *Diagnosis*. Created by Scott Rudin and Lisa Sanders, season 1, episode 2, Netflix, August 16, 2019.

Tian, Yan, and Jina H. Yoo. "Medical Drama Viewing and Medical Trust: A Moderated Mediation Approach." *Health Communication*, vol. 35, 2020, pp. 46–55.

Williams, Ruth, Lowri Evans, and Nora Talal Alshareef. "Using TV Dramas in Medical Education." *Education for Primary Care*, vol. 26, no. 1, 2015, pp. 48–9.

"The Wisdom of the Crowd." *Diagnosis*. Created by Scott Rudin and Lisa Sanders, season 1, episode 3, Netflix, August 16, 2019.

Witzel, Kai, Horst J. Koch, and Cornelia Kaminski. "Impact of Medical TV Shows on Preprocedural Fear of Surgical In-House Patients." *European Surgical Research*, vol. 58, 2017, pp. 121–7.

Žižek, Slavoj. *Interrogating the Real*. Edited by Rex Butler and Scott Stephens. London: Bloomsbury, 2013.

19

UNHEALTHY HORRORS

The biopolitical zombie in 21st-century film and television

Erik Larsen

Zombies hold a peculiar but prominent place in the contemporary pantheon of cinematic and televisual monsters. These decrepit creatures lurch endlessly onto our screens, usurping vampires, ghosts, and extraterrestrial invaders as the leading agents of dread. One of the most popular cable television shows in history – AMC's *The Walking Dead* (2010–2022) – evidences our continuing if not strengthening obsession with the monster. An immense number of zombie films and shows have been produced since 2001, a period often termed the "zombie renaissance" (Bishop 17). Many examples feature elaborate special effects and major Hollywood stars, including Brad Pitt (*World War Z* 2013), Woody Harrelson (*Zombieland* 2009), and Glenn Close (*The Girl with All the Gifts* 2016).

Hardly uniform in setting and genre, global zombie culture contains highly varied explorations of the monster. Most zombies appear stripped of personhood, speech, and thought, but some, for example the zombie protagonist of *Warm Bodies* (2013), express complex inner lives. Although many display signs of decay, the genre now includes dexterous monsters, more indicative of predatory vitality than creeping death, such as those stampeding through *World War Z* and *Train to Busan* (2016). While I neither dismiss this variety nor its rich interpretive implications, a common feature informs most recent zombie media: put simply, in the age of mass zombie culture, the zombies are conspicuously *unhealthy*.

In the last few decades, the genre has fixated on bodily disorder and pandemic disease, rendering the zombie explicable through biological and biomedical epistemologies. Increasingly, the figure expresses our fears of endemic health crises, genetic susceptibility, chronic disabling conditions, and infectious outbreaks in a globalized world. Some scholars argue that zombies stand in for our growing fears of senescent populations and neurological diseases, of disorders propagated as much from within as from without.[1] Modern televisual and cinematic zombies reflect both perceived challenges to health and the conceptual changes underpinning our obsession with health in the 21st century. More specifically, this changing monster illustrates our increasingly biological understanding of self and the degree to which we conceptualize our personal and social lives in terms of contemporary biomedicine.

And yet, focusing solely on their connections to health fails to elucidate why our media consistently represent zombies as lacking personhood. Whatever its specific medical connotation, the zombie's unhealthiness seems integrally linked with the absence of characteristics we

DOI: 10.4324/9781003007661-25

associate with the legal and social person. In most examples, the monster exhibits little or no evidence of thought, reason, and social awareness.

In many contemporary films and television series, this condition is highly contagious, resulting in apocalyptic violence. Expressing more than our individual fears of personal poor health, the zombie's spreading bodily disorder threatens us with the total and permanent collapse of political order. Equating political dysfunction with the diseased other, the genre reveals a troubling confluence of our social nightmares and medical concepts.

In what follows, I analyze a few prominent cinematic and televisual examples in order to elucidate a common assumption – the equation of self and personhood with the medicalized body – underpinning representations of the monster in 21st-century media. Investigating how this connection structures our fantasies of social collapse and political restoration, I consider specifically the role of contemporary biomedicine's emphasis on the molecular constituents of health as a paradigm reshaping our political fears. To begin, I briefly analyze the genre's cinematic self-reinvention around themes of health in the film inaugurating the zombie renaissance, Danny Boyle's *28 Days Later* (2002). Turning to television, I investigate how *The Walking Dead* series equates social order with health through its epic narrative of pandemic disease and political collapse.

In *Night of the Living Dead* (1968), George Romero reinvented the zombie for American movie audiences, transforming the monster into the apocalyptic flesh-eater we expect today. In *Night* and its two sequels, *Dawn of the Dead* (1978) and *Day of the Dead* (1985), the zombies are conspicuously fleshy beings; their decaying bodies and rapacious cannibalism are the traits of gratuitously physical creatures. The *Dead* trilogy began to visually link the zombie with our gross anatomy, opening the genre to its contemporary focus on biomedical selfhood. And yet, Romero's monsters function primarily as critical allegories – as reflections of American racism, consumerism, and militarism. They are physically grotesque in order to reveal Americans'

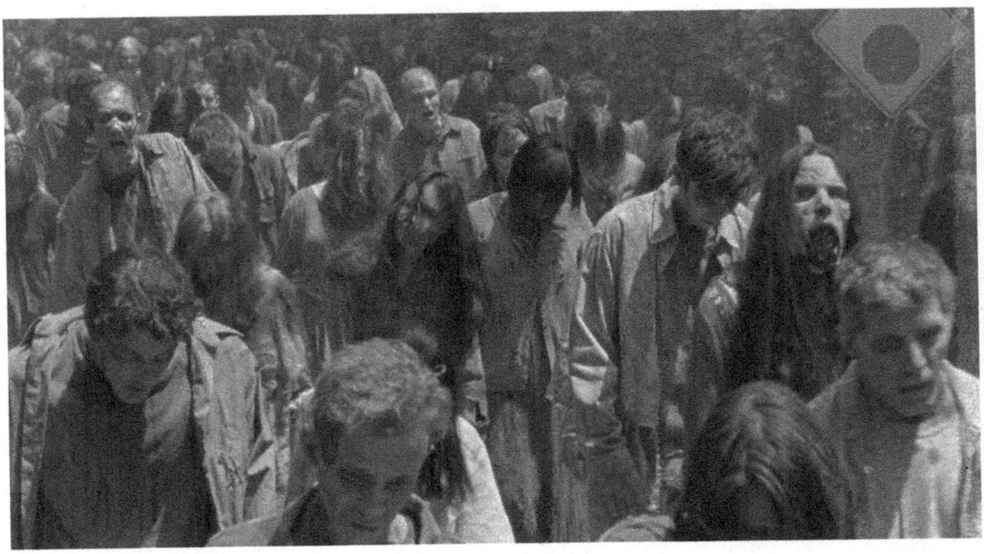

Figure 19.1 Wandering zombies in *The Walking Dead*

grotesque behavior and not to threaten us with disorders originating in our bodily tissues (Shaviro, "Contagious Allegories" 17–18).

In sharp contrast, most films of the zombie renaissance identify the monster as a thoroughly biomedical threat. One readily detects this shift in the opening scene of Danny Boyle's *28 Days Later*, in which animal rights activists break into a Cambridge primate research facility in order to free chimpanzees. A researcher (David Schneider) attempts to stop them, explaining that the animals are infected with the highly contagious Rage Virus. He justifies his experimentation by invoking its biomedical value: "In order to cure you must first understand." Despite his warning that the apes' blood and saliva carry the infection, the activists release a single chimp, which brutally bites and infects one of them, transforming her into a vicious zombie. Unlike Romero's lumbering and decaying creatures, these zombies seem possessed by frenetic energy and swiftness, attacking not to devour but to infect, which occurs in a matter of seconds. After the opening scene fades to black, an intertitle appears, informing the viewer that 28 days have passed – the 28 days in which the virus has spread, destroying all signs of social order in the UK.

While the *Dead* trilogy seemed uninterested in the material source for its zombie apocalypse, *28 Days* foregrounds a physical cause, rendering the threat intelligible through biomedical concepts. Prior to observing transmission and infection, the audience learns of its viral etiology from a scientific authority, and one whose warnings prove correct. The virus spreads through contact with common bodily fluids we associate with viral contamination. Minimal exposure to the eyes or mouth transmits the virus rapidly; in one scene, a single drop of blood falls into a character's open eye, infecting him in a matter of seconds. A common trope of the zombie renaissance, infection scenes like this one emphasize a relationship of physical, pathogenic cause and symptomatic effect.

Subsequent films strengthened the zombie's identification with communicable disease and biomedical frameworks. Whether the result of nefarious scientific experimentation or natural pathogens, films such as *Maggie* (2015), *Zombieland* (2009), *The Girl with All the Gifts* (2016), *Cargo* (2017), and *Train to Busan* (2016) render zombies as problems with biological origins, explanations, and effects. One popular example, *World War Z*, visualizes our fears of a rapidly spreading emergent virus. More so than *28 Days*, its zombies are athletically swift and predatory, infecting a host almost instantly. In *World War Z*, we watch as crowds transform swiftly into cascading walls of stampeding zombies. Although visually overwhelming, by situating the action within the unfolding apocalypse, the film offers hope for a biomedical cure. *World War Z* never doubts the efficacy of this approach, for it never questions the zombie's biological origins. Early in the film, a United Nation's epidemiologist identifies the plague as an emerging virus, recommending a search for patient zero. Relying on a loose understanding of evolutionary biology, and with the help of a WHO lab, Gerry Lane (Brad Pitt) eventually discovers a prophylactic treatment.

And yet, interpreting recent depictions of zombies merely as responses to infectious disease fails to convey how thoroughly biomedical concepts have redefined the genre. By imagining a virus originating in chimpanzees and transmitted through blood, *28 Days* invoked fears of the HIV pandemic and emerging zoonotic diseases, and anxieties about selfhood as we imagine it in 21st-century biomedicine. The film made tangible both the transferability of animal viruses to humans and the biological parity between species. Regarded in this light, its thematic interest in rage takes on a complex biological meaning; *28 Days* suggests that we are, like the chimps, genetically prone to anti-social behavior. Rage is literally in our blood, for we inherit our tragic flaw from intrinsic genetic structures. Thus, the chimp's bite – what brings about the apocalyptic downfall of civilization – signifies both viral transference and the long evolutionary history of transferred genes.

This tragic biologism may seem more the stuff of 19th-century naturalism than modern horror, but the film reflects popular acceptance of a new biomedical understanding of self. Released in 2002, one year before completion of the Human Genome Project, *28 Days* appeared in the midst of growing international interest in the molecular constituents of human life and disease. Nikolas Rose describes this "molecularization" in terms of a biomedical shift from large organ systems to the minutest elements of life – the genetic sequences, enzymes, proteins, and other basic materials of life (11–15). Developing since the 1960s, this paradigm shift has led, according to Rose, to a new medical ethos and culture of health (77–84). Beyond restoring function to ailing bodies and minds, as medicine has done for centuries, the new medicine aims to transform the limits of life itself (17). Genomic research promises both to detect the preconditions of many nightmarish diseases and to prevent them long before they are expressed, altering once fixed bodily limits (17–18). Within this paradigm, "mind is simply what the brain does. And mental pathology is simply the behavioral consequence of an identifiable and potentially correctible error or anomaly in some of those elements now identified as aspects of that organic brain" (192). Hardly the province of specialists, this increasingly biomolecular and biomedical understanding of human life informs how we conceptualize the self, its relationships, its problems, and their solutions (25–6).

Rose's description of a new medical ethos, one in which commercialized research and treatment offers to transform us from the molecular level up, might seem a far cry from the dystopic worlds of zombie media. Yet by redefining our sense of self, this paradigm has also transformed our fears. The more medical research investigates our molecular structures, the more it reveals our susceptibility to diseases that might, and likely will, profoundly alter body and mind. Although greater public understanding of molecular disease processes may inspire hope, this knowledge also creates the impression that we are all "asymptomatically or presymptomatically ill" (19). Due in part to modern biomedicine's success in prolonging life, many of us wonder when it will be our turn with cancer or Alzheimer's. Fear of susceptibility to disease is far from new (85–6), but this paradigm revisions and deepens this anxiety. We are, it seems, confronted constantly with mutation, infection, and degeneration, but these problems, and the biomedical knowledge developed to solve them, confront us with something more terrifying: these processes threaten to deform the entire self, leaving behind a damaged fragment of human life.

This fear – that everything human hinges on our protean, molecular biology – inspires the distinctive terror of the zombie renaissance. Thus, *28 Days* reimagines the zombie as a body stripped of self by contagious disease, but the film frames disease in terms of the mutating and flawed genetic structures we share with other life-forms. This and many subsequent examples imply that one becomes a zombie when a biological source alters the body's cellular machinery, damaging the "organic brain." If the paradigm described by Rose promises to improve us by unlocking our molecular structures, these films represent our terrified response to the dark possibilities of being remade from our tissues up. The "natural" vital stuff we are made of, they suggest, might make monsters of us all. Horror, it seems, no longer requires the supernatural – just a willingness to imagine the darkest aspects of the biomolecular self.

This existential threat to the individual reveals the dual but linked roles played by the monster in 21st-century imaginations: zombies realize our fears of bodily dysfunction, but for just this reason, they also threaten us with political collapse. Whether the result of spreading infection, genetic susceptibility, or nefarious experimentation, the damaged biological self is also a destroyed and destructive political subject. This trend should little surprise us; having linked the healthy self with proper functioning of biomolecular structures, we have begun to imagine deleterious physical changes as loss of self – the rational and ethical self upon which political order seems to rest.

Of course, nothing about the cultural linking of modern politics and health is new. For Michel Foucault, biopolitics emerged at the end of the 18th century when the European states began, in concert with the developing science of modern biology, to regard their subjects as fundamentally living beings (245). Around this time, traditional forms of political action – protecting, improving, and organizing the body politic – were reconceived in terms of the management of biological conditions. Biopolitics ignores the individual citizen, instead regarding life as a process operating between individuals or at the impersonal level of populations (249). Unlike the sovereign politics it replaced, biopolitics eschews waging direct violence against its subjects, for it creates national success by improving health and not by directly threatening subjects with death.

With its distinctive focus on biomedical threats, new zombie media continue this biopolitical conflation of health and politics. Although influenced by 21st-century medicine, the genre reflects many aspects of older biopolitical paradigms: it conflates illness with political disorder, reduces persons to the bodily dysfunction from which they suffer, and imagines the unhealthy as dangerous masses. In its simplest form, new zombie media follow this tradition with images of pervasive zombie crowds. Within the mass, the individual zombie, and all traces of the person it was, vanish into lurching or rushing waves of infection (see Figure 19.2).

Although simplifying Foucault's use of the term, these images crudely realize the biopolitical notion of the population (Schweitzer 177). They assume our participation in a paradigm that imagines politics as the improvement of biological life – life understood not as an individual phenomenon – but in terms of masses differentiated by criteria of health and sickness.

Despite this rich conceptual framework, much recent zombie scholarship takes its cue not from Foucault but from Italian philosopher Giorgio Agamben who argues that biopolitics

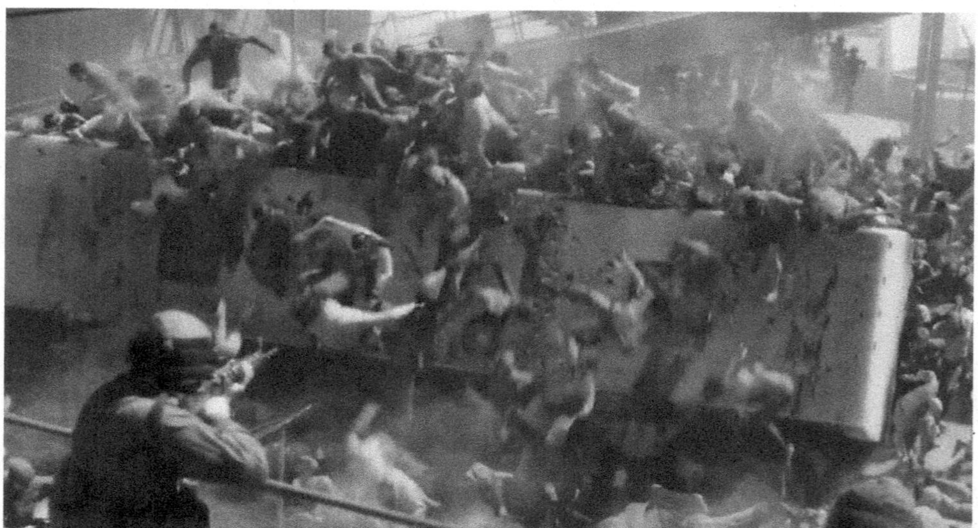

Figure 19.2 Zombies stampeding in *World War Z*

began when Greek political thought divided life into two categories: *zoē*, the natural or "bare life" shared by all creatures, including humans, and *bios*, the political life exclusive to humanity (1–8). By conceptually dividing the two, western political theory constituted politics in terms of an exclusion – the exclusion of bare life from the legal and social structures governing *bios*. This "inclusive exclusion," which politicizes bare life, inaugurates a practice of sanctioned extra-legal violence against those people classified as lacking political existence (8). Because they fall outside the sphere of law, these bare lives – like animal lives – may be killed but never murdered (82).

Scholarship informed by Agamben's work illuminates the nearly ubiquitous acceptance in new zombie media of extra-legal violence against the monster.[2] Like the many people who lack citizenship, or who we imagine to be incapable of political participation, the zombie is de facto excluded from legal protections; it may be killed individually or en masse, culled relentlessly but never murdered. And yet, applying Agamben's broad distinction between bare and political life to the genre may occlude health's defining role in new zombie media. Our acceptance of violence against zombies originates from their status as imagined non-persons *and* from the aggressive threat they represent to medically informed notions of health. The virtually universal depiction of violence waged *against* humans by zombies becomes legible through a biopolitics that, by equating health and political order, equates the unhealthy other with destruction. In other words, to fully decipher the genre's new biopolitical shift, one also requires Foucault's emphasis on health and populations, but refracted through 21st-century biomedical concerns. Zombies threaten with contagious violence because, as in Foucault's analysis, modern politics conceives of life as an unstable force operating through populations (Thacker 363); in this context, disability and disease occur not merely to individuals but threaten to enervate the population and thus, life itself. It follows that zombie media represent the ill or impaired as personifications of their conditions rather than persons with medical problems, for they signify nothing but waste or threat in the political imagination.

The Walking Dead makes this troubling biopolitical trope its singular focus over many seasons. The series probes our fears of biological selfhood, depicting the struggle for political order as a relentless battle with diseased masses. On a scene-by-scene basis, the show parrots many of the sensational visual elements made famous by its cinematic predecessors: eliciting our voyeuristic fascination, it dwells on images of grotesque zombie bodies, depicts gratuitous violence, and imagines a post-apocalyptic landscape (Figure 19.2). But while the series draws us into these cinematic moments, its serialized form builds a narrative that extends and deepens the political themes at work in films of the zombie renaissance. Set shortly after the zombie apocalypse has destroyed all traces of American government and society, *TWD* follows a small group of survivors struggling to form a sustainable and virtuous community. Led by former sheriff's deputy Rick Grimes (Andrew Lincoln), the small band encounters other groups, precipitating violent conflict or peaceful expansion of their community. Beyond moving the show's lumbering plot forward, these clashes reveal alternative political possibilities, exposing Rick's community to the best and worst of humanity. The series reflects, if not profoundly then consistently, on the uses and abuses of violence, the limits of inclusion, and the tension between survival and idealism.

This focus on conflicts within and between human communities has led some to interpret the show's zombies as a mere backdrop – the natural disaster out of which the political drama unfolds (Schweitzer 183–4). And yet, of the numerous threats to political order, the zombies are the ubiquitous, existential challenge to all forms of society. In addition to instigating the fall of American civilization and its resulting chaos, the monsters represent the persistent threat of a world devoid of political order. Crucially, the zombie scourge does not imperil humanity with extinction; far worse, *TWD* seems to suggest, is a reality dominated by damaged life than one silenced by total death. In contrast to its vibrant human characters, the series' zombies lack personal narratives, inner lives, and social intercourse, but this privation is integral, rather than peripheral to the show's political themes. Adjacent to its dramas of social formation lurks a life without politics – a kind of anti-political *polis* threatening to transform healthy humans into its newest citizens. The zombies, the series' most politically meaningful figures, indicate what life must possess to become political, or what deprives it of political order when lost.

As in many works of new zombie media, a biomedical explanation differentiates the series' zombies from the human community. In a telling departure from Kirkman's graphic novels, the televisual adaptation brings Rick's group to the CDC in the final episode of Season 1, where its one remaining scientist shares what little he knows about the plague. In a scene that functions as a brief lesson in neurobiology, Dr. Edwin Jenner (Noah Emmerich) projects the recording of a virtual MRI to illustrate synapses firing in the brain of an infected test subject. He explains to the puzzled group that "somewhere in all that organic wiring, all those ripples of light, is you, the thing that makes you unique and human." Soon the projection shows the infected brain going dark as the pathogen, which he describes as "invading the brain like meningitis," kills the subject. But this death gives birth to a new life, for the recording soon registers synapses firing again as the zombie awakens. Lacking an operative frontal cortex and "driven by mindless instinct," this damaged brain will, as Jenner forcefully observes, never resurrect its "human part." The show's representation of medical authority and imaging technology to demonstrate the pathogen's effects removes all doubt about the scourge's physical source.

Nothing like this scene, with its overt biomedical authority, imagery, and concepts appears elsewhere in the show, but its inclusion shapes our understanding of the entire crisis. Here, at the series' beginning, *TWD* equates the near total destruction of political order with bodily dysfunction on a cellular level. The scene assumes and reinforces a paradigm of biological selfhood resembling Rose's description of 21st-century biomedicine. For this CDC scientist, the brain's "organic wiring," and nothing more, produce the human person. Indeed, when viewed from Jenner's biomedical perspective, the zombies' violence might be seen as a medical problem like many others – one among many forms of anti-social behavior attributable to some neurological condition. This scene exposes the fears giving shape to the series' legions of monsters: as fully biological beings, governed by the whims of biomolecular processes, a minor shift in our bodily structures might rob us of selfhood.

The series employs a host of visual and rhetorical tropes to mark its zombies as categorically ill. Most basically, *TWD* forges this connection by representing its monsters as vectors of infectious disease. Because their drive to bite and consume healthy flesh functions as the vehicle for contamination, shots of "walkers," as they are called throughout the series, frequently focus on their teeth, which are bare due to decay of the lips and gums (Figure 19.3).

By emphasizing characteristics identified with spreading pathogens, *TWD*'s zombies, much like those of *World War Z*, personify infection more than they represent ill persons. And while the show identifies its monsters visually and titularly with death, seeming to grant them a supernatural element, their liminal status reflects the ambiguous vitality of many pathogens. When asked by Rick if the walkers are alive, Dr. Jenner responds with a question indicative of scientific indecision over the biological status of viruses: "you tell me?" Like viruses, the walkers are at once supremely active, driven ceaselessly to transform new hosts into copies of themselves (Vint, "Administering the Crisis"124) but also lack the dynamism and awareness we associate with life.The series deepens its thematic focus on health by telling narratives of illness that reflect anxieties surrounding 21st-century biomedicine. A far more gradual process than in *28 Days*, in *TWD* infection resembles the course of a terminal illness. Unless

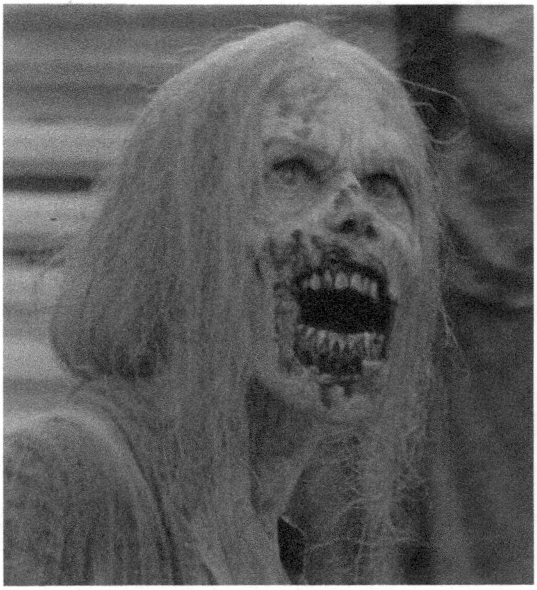

Figure 19.3 Walker with decayed mouth and lips

a bitten limb is quickly amputated, the pathogen gradually infiltrates the body, producing traditional symptoms of viral infection, including fever, weakness, and sweating. After a few days, the infected person dies, soon rising as a zombie. The show's infection scenes can be lengthy, creating dramatic moments resembling end-of-life scenes from any contemporary hospital drama. These moments encode the transition from human to zombie as one of health to disease. For Steven Shaviro, the series' fixation on these death scenes, and particularly on the anguished decisions of friends and family to terminate the life of the infected, reflect a culture preoccupied with end-of-life care issues ("Zombie Healthcare" 196). In a period in which biomedicine can preserve life after personhood has departed, *TWD* helps viewers explore the thorny moral decision to end a loved one's life. It can do this, Shaviro observes, because, in a significant departure from the graphic novel, the series imagines all humans to be pre-symptomatically infected with the pathogen (212). Like the various diseases and disabling conditions we anticipate developing at some point in our lives, the zombie plague seems coextensive with the body, as much a part of its structure as any other. Echoing our increasing acceptance of molecular and biomedical understandings of self, the show presents a world in which we are all "asymptomatically or pre-symptomatically ill" (Rose 19). By reimagining zombification as a process resembling degenerative brain disease, the *TWD* amplifies our deepest anxieties about some lurking flaw in our bodies that might render us nothing more than a set of "mindless instincts."

Beyond linking zombies to contemporary biomedical concerns, the series forges general negative associations with unhealthy life through its grotesque realization of the monsters. Virtually all pale, emaciated, and with mere wisps of ragged hair, the walkers resemble patients in the final stages of lengthy terminal illnesses (Figure 19.4). Many walkers bear graphic wounds, revealing internal organs in states of grotesque decomposition. Combining imagery of restlessness and disorder, *TWD*'s zombies concretize old and new senses of *disease*. Originally meaning a *lack of ease*, disease named a disruption to natural order and the destructive

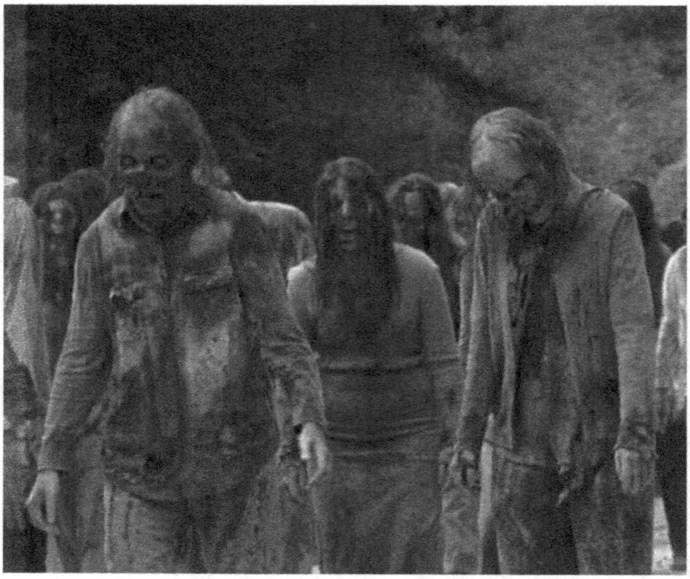

Figure 19.4 A horde of walkers

disorder or tension it produced. The walkers' endless wandering, eating, and grasping imply a similar unease or imbalance. Similarly, by visualizing zombies as mere collections of decaying and malfunctioning parts, *TWD* emphasizes the natural order they have lost. In numerous scenes, Rick's band easily smashes walkers into puddles of gore, revealing some inherent frailty or rottenness. Although the series represents its monsters as fundamentally enervated, this weakness inspires terror, for it threatens to propagate disorder and weakness throughout the body politic.

We hardly require Dr. Jenner's scientific presentation to conclude that walkers are cognitively impaired. Not a single walker displays signs of personal or social sentiment. Irreparably brain damaged, the walkers never learn, use tools, or strategize; in many episodes, they walk insipidly into danger and destruction. The series augments an impression of mental illness or mental disability by attiring its monsters in ragged and dirty clothing. Employing and emphasizing one of the genre's most tired tropes, *TWD* fills the screen with dragging feet and lurching steps. This caricature of motor disability becomes an indelible mark differentiating walkers from their human prey. Analyzing the show's obsession with dysfunctional bodies, Anna Mae Duane observes that its walkers are "the manifestation of disease and disability run amok" (242). As such, the series imagines a chasm separating the healthy from the unhealthy: "*The Walking Dead*, like other zombie narratives, repeatedly assures us that it's foolish to imagine any sort of continuum between physical health and repulsive decay. You are on one side of the equation or the other" (239).

This binary shapes the *TWD*'s political universe, building a series that equates a properly ordered body politic with bodily health. A few pivotal moments in the plot expose this underlying biopolitical ethos. Huddled in an abandoned barn in Season 5, Rick Grimes looks at his traumatized, hungry band and expresses a disturbing philosophy: "This is how we survive: We tell ourselves that we are the walking dead." Rick's pronouncement elevates survival to his guiding ideal, while hinting at the violence necessary to maintain it. Like the unsympathetic walkers, the group must live without moral commitments in order to kill and thus to live. Although Rick speaks of the walkers figuratively, the scene quickly reminds us that walkers are not simply grotesque expressions of our moral failings. Before the night is over, walkers attack the barn, forcing the group collectively to hold the door closed. In this moment, the community's struggle to maintain a literal partition between themselves and the walkers emphasizes the essential distinction between them. Ragged and violent, Rick's band may resemble zombies, but their collective resistance reveals, if nothing else, a capacity the walkers will never possess: the group can learn to improve individually and communally. This fact is born out when a stranger (Ross Marquand) appears the next morning, offering to guide them to Alexandria, the show's epitome of a civilized town. Eventually integrating with this community, Rick's band regains its moral compass and inaugurates a new political order that transforms the known human world. Indeed, in its numerous personal and group narratives of violence and redemption, *TWD* imagines virtually every person as capable of moral reintegration with the community. Walkers, on the other hand, will never heal, never reintegrate with society, and thus threaten political order per se. What differentiates the damage and disorder of one from the other is purely biological.

In as much as political order rests on securing and supporting healthy bodies, *TWD* treats the division between these bodies and the walkers as entirely literal and necessary. The barn door holding back the walkers is one of many physical partitions needed to separate the healthy from the unhealthy throughout the series. Alexandria's advantage over many other settlements consists, among other things, in its substantial steel wall (see Figure 19.5).

The groups within walled villages may be more or less accepting of each other, but without walls, health and any hope of civilization rapidly disintegrate. As in many cinematic examples, the need for physical barriers in *TWD* results from the zombie's persistent, violent threat of disease and chaos. Not merely figures of bare life, walkers appear as destructive infections because they reflect the threat of unhealthy populations in a modern biopolitical framework.

Along similar lines, and reflecting the biopolitical segmenting of life into populations, *TWD* envisions walkers as impersonal masses, even as it fixates on the personal narratives and struggles of its characters. Rarely does the camera focus on individual walkers, other than to emphasize

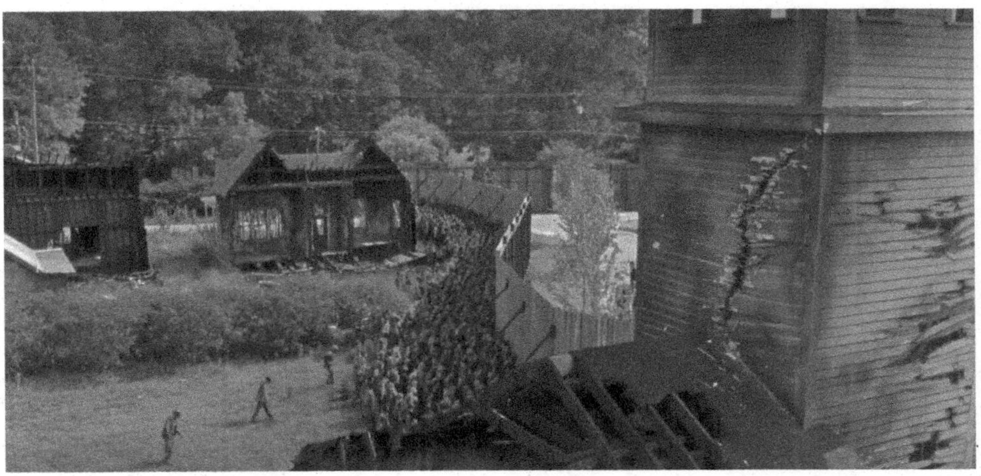

Figure 19.5 Alexandria's reinforced steel wall surrounded by walkers

their status as dysfunctional, contagious, and violent. As the series develops, long shots of moving masses become a common visual trope, one that subsumes walkers into populations defined by their danger to healthy life. Designated as "hordes," these lurching streams of bodies pose a constant danger to settlements, and must be lured away, lest they breach the walls and infect the healthy populations within (Figure 19.5). Over the course of many seasons, imagery of fortresses and diseased masses lose the sense of emergent novelty they might have conveyed in a feature-length film; by weaving these tropes into the fabric of its fictional reality, *TWD* normalizes the impersonal division of healthy from unhealthy, representing the extreme measures of pandemic biopolitics as the stuff of everyday life.

The same normalcy pervades the series' constant depiction of graphic violence waged against walkers. *TWD*'s unequivocal extermination of walkers indicates their status as life without political value. Not as passive as Agamben's bare life, but similarly positioned, walkers can be killed in the series but never murdered. The show assumes our acceptance of this unspoken rule, for it depicts the unhesitant killing of thousands of walkers while preaching the spiritual and social dangers of unchecked violence. Throughout the series, Morgan (Lennie James) undergoes a moral awakening, transforming him from merciless killer to peaceful guru. Carrying only a wooden staff to defend himself, Morgan abhors violence against the healthy, but he dispatches walkers without a second thought. Forced to engage in lethal violence to help save the community from the Saviors (a sadistic group), by Season Eight, he is a traumatized and confused figure. To assuage his guilt, a friend recommends that he return to his peaceful ways and use the sharp end of his stick on the dead and the round, non-lethal end on the living. In this and numerous examples, *TWD* explores how violence destroys personal lives and political order, while depicting violence against the dead as a necessary means for protecting both. Throughout the show, the uninitiated are instructed in specialized techniques for killing zombies, much as they are trained to perform basic life skills. What designates zombies as lives that may be killed in *TWD* – as life without political value – are their damaged bodies and brains. But the opposite point holds as well: the series designates a life as politically valuable, as warranting legal protection, when it consists of a supremely able body.

By interpreting the zombie renaissance as a reflection of our darkest biopolitical fantasies, I mean not to infer a link between contemporary medical practice and the genre's violent approach to disease and disability. My purpose is neither paranoiacally to imagine some insidious new eugenics nor to blame biomedicine for assumptions it never intended to support. Many healthcare workers labor diligently to know and treat their patients as persons; to these doctors and nurses, the patient is a complex self, a narrative, a history, but never a socially destructive disease. And yet, the contrast between our medical practice and our medicalized fictions should not lead us to dismiss the latter as meaningless entertainment. At the same time that television and film illustrate a strengthening conflation of disease and destruction, we increasingly accept a new paradigm of biomedicine – one that embroils the self in the body's vulnerable molecular structures. With what renders us legal and social persons so dependent on bodily function, how, indeed, could the stakes of health or its absence be greater?

The dramatic shift from Romero's zombies to our pervasive millennial monster hinges on many historical factors, but it indicates overwhelmingly the influence of biomedicine and health on our sense of political order. It is difficult to imagine how this seismic shift in the leading horror genre does not suggest or portend medical, economic, and political changes in our approach to those we label as healthy or unhealthy. For despite the best intentions of physicians, a society that maps the line between social order and chaos onto that between healthy and unhealthy populations will exist in a fraught relationship with both. Excluding the sick that it also attempts to heal, it fails to understand that "healthy" bodies inhabit a vital continuum with the "unhealthy," rendering the binary suspect. That the zombie renaissance makes policing this division one of its primary, perhaps unconscious goals becomes most apparent in *TWD*'s defining political moment. Having just defeated the Saviors, the group brutally enslaving their communities, Rick stands before his citizenry on a hilltop, overlooking a huge horde of walkers. He inaugurates a new age of political growth by condemning the Savior's false notion of community, but more importantly, by equating the future with healthy bodies: "We are life, that is death! And it's coming for us, unless we stand together! So go home. Then the work begins. The new world begins."

Notes

1 Recent scholarship indicative of this approach can be found in the collection, *The Walking Med: Zombies and the Medical Image*, which includes essays on geriatric populations, chemotherapy, anorexia, and many other health-related topics. Dahlia Schweitzer's *Going Viral: Zombies, Viruses, and the End of the World* explores the zombie's identification with apocalyptic pandemics.

2 Jon Stratton identifies the monster with our fears of invasion by displaced peoples and refugees (246–7). Sherryl Vint argues that zombies represent neoliberal fears of slipping from "the bios of being gainfully employed to the *zoē* of economically irrelevant biological life" ("Abject Posthumanism" 174). Travis Linnemann, Tyler Wall, and Edward Green connect the monster to bare life through examples of police violence that invoke zombies (333).

Works cited

Agamben, Giorgio. *Homo Sacer: Sovereign Power and Bare Life*. Translated by Daniel Heller-Roazen. Redwood City, CA: Stanford University Press, 1998.

Bishop, Kyle. "Dead Man Still Walking: Explaining the Zombie Renaissance." *Journal of Popular Film and Television*, vol. 37, no. 1, 2009, pp. 16–25.

Boon, Kevin. "The Zombie as Other: Mortality and the Monstrous in the Post-Nuclear Age." *Better off Dead: The Evolution of the Zombie as Post-Human*, edited by Deborah Christie and Sarah Juliet Lauro. New York: Fordham University Press, 2011, pp. 50–60.

Boyle, Danny, director. *28 Days Later*. DNA Films and British Film Council, 2002.

Darabont, Frank and Angela Kang, creators. *The Walking Dead*. American Movie Classics, 2010.

Dendle, Peter. "Zombie Movies and the Millennial Generation." *Better off Dead: The Evolution of the Zombie as Posthuman*, edited by Deborah Christie and Sarah Juliet Lauro. New York: Fordham University Press, 2011, pp. 163–74.

Duane, Anna Mae. "Dead *and* Disabled: The Crawling Monsters of *The Walking Dead*." *Zombie Theory: A Reader*, edited by Sarah Juliet Lauro. Minneapolis, MN: University of Minnesota Press, 2017, pp. 237–45.

Fleischer, Ruben, director. *Zombieland*. Columbia Pictures, 2009.

Forster, Marc, director. *World War Z*. Paramount Pictures, 2013.

Foucault, Michel. *"Society Must Be Defended" Lectures at the Collège de France, 1975-1976*. Translated by David Macey, Picador, 2003.

Hobson, Henry, director. *Maggie*. Grindstone Entertainment Group et al., 2015.

Howling, Ben and Yolanda Ramke, directors. *Cargo*. Umbrella Entertainment et al., 2017.

Levine, Jonathan, director. *Warm Bodies*. Mandeville Films and Make Movies, 2013.

Linnemann, Travis, Tyler Wall, and Edward Green. "The Walking Dead and the Killing State: Zombification and the Normalization of Police Violence." *Zombie Theory: A Reader*, edited by Sarah Juliet Lauro. Minneapolis, MN: University of Minnesota Press, 2017, pp. 332–51.

McCarthy, Colm, director. *The Girl with All the Gifts*. BFI Film Fund, 2016.

Romero, George, director. *Night of the Living Dead*. Image Ten, 1968.

Romero, George, director. *Dawn of the Dead*. Dawn Associated and Laurel Group, 1978.

Romero, George, director. *Day of the Dead*. United Film Distribution Company and Laurel Entertainment Inc., 1985.

Rose, Nikolas. *The Politics of Life Itself: Biomedicine, Power, and Subjectivity in the Twenty-First Century*. Princeton, NJ: Princeton University Press, 2007.
Schweitzer, Dahlia. *Going Viral: Zombies, Viruses, and the End of the World*. New Brunswick, NJ: Rutgers University Press, 2018.
Shaviro, Stephen. "Zombie Healthcare." *The Year's Work at the Zombie Research Center*. Bloomington, IN: Indiana University Press, 2014, pp. 193–226.
Shaviro, Stephen. "Contagious Allegories: George Romero."*Zombie Theory: A Reader*, edited by Sarah Juliet Lauro. Minneapolis, MN: University of Minnesota Press, 2017, pp. 7–19.
Stratton, Jon. "Trouble with Zombies: *Muselmänner*, Bare Life, and Displaced People." *Zombie Theory: A Reader*, edited by Sarah Juliet Lauro. Minneapolis, MN: University of Minnesota Press, 2017, pp. 246–70.
Thacker, Eugene. "Nekros; or, The Poetics of Biopolitics." *Zombie Theory: A Reader*, edited by Sarah Juliet Lauro. Minneapolis, MN: University of Minnesota Press, 2017, pp. 361–80.
Vint, Sherryl. "Administering the Crisis: Zombies and Public Health in the *28 Days Later* Comic Series." *The Walking Med: Zombies and the Medical Image*, edited by Lorenzo Servitje and Sherryl Vint. University Park, PA: Pennsylvania State University Press, 2016, pp. 123–44.
Vint, Sherryl. "Abject Posthumanism: Neoliberalism, Biopolitics, and Zombies." *Zombie Theory: A Reader*, edited by Sarah Juliet Lauro. Minneapolis, MN: University of Minnesota Press, 2017, pp. 171–81.
Yeon Sang-ho, director. *Train to Busan*. Next Entertainment World, 2016.

20

"THE CATEGORY IS *LIVE!*"

Transing care and the persistence of queer survival in F/X's *Pose*

JV Fuqua

Introduction

In July 1992, the body of LGBTQ trans rights activist Marsha P. Johnson was pulled from the Hudson River, near the Chelsea Piers in the West Village. The New York Police Department ruled her death a suicide, but supporters and family have continued to insist that she was a victim of transphobia and what writer Trudy has called, "(trans)misogynoir," the hatred of Black, trans, women.[1]

In August 2020, a few months into the Covid-19 pandemic, Johnson's family and friends gathered in her former hometown of Elizabeth, New Jersey, to announce the future site of the state's first public monument to an LGBTQ trans woman of color. The Marsha P. ("Pay It No Mind") Johnson memorial honors the work that she and her friend, Sylvia Rivera, did for homeless LGBTQ youth, sex workers, and others through forming the collective housing initiative, STAR (Street Transvestite Action Revolutionaries) House in New York City in 1970. In addition to the founding of STAR House, Johnson, Rivera, and Miss Major Griffin-Gracy fought tirelessly for LGBTQ rights from her involvement with the Gay Liberation Front, the Stonewall Rebellion in 1969, and the later formation of HIV/AIDS activist and outreach organizations.[2]

Johnson's death in 1992 and the public recognition of her contributions to LGBTQ political struggle and civil rights for, specifically, trans people of color frame my examination of the F/X series *Pose* (2018–). As one of television auteur Ryan Murphy's creations, it takes place in New York City's ballroom culture during the late 1980s through the early 1990s. The show focuses on the African American and Latinx LGBTQ and gender-expanding drag ball community that builds upon original work by Steven Canals, a bi-racial, gay, Bronx native and LGBTQ educator. The series is remarkable for several reasons including the critical acclaim it has received and the notoriety garnered by Murphy's brand.

Pose, as a generic hybrid combination of family dramedy and musical, centers around two threats to the characters' daily lives: HIV/AIDS and violence against trans women of color. The series looks back, with somewhat revisionist eyes, to the early years of HIV/AIDS, its ravages of the New York City LGBTQ community and its response with organizations such as Minority AIDS Task Force and Gay Men's Health Crisis and activist collectives like ACT University Press (AIDS Coalition to Unleash Power). Moreover, the series references specific places that

DOI: 10.4324/9781003007661-26

have been significant for the LGBTQ community in New York City including the Chelsea Piers, Times Square, the Harlem Ballroom scene, The Center (LGBTQ Community Center), and medical institutions such as the notorious St. Vincent Hospital "AIDS ward." In short, *Pose* looks back to the late 1980s and early 1990s informed by the losses and gains that shape contemporary LGBTQ lives. The paradox of visibility is that as trans lives become increasingly represented and public, violence against them increases. While it is impossible to determine causation, this correlation is undeniable.

This chapter focuses on the strategies that *Pose* uses in its representation of two public health crises that continue to disproportionately affect queer and trans communities of color: HIV/AIDS and transphobic, specifically transmisogynoir, violence. These strategies can be seen at the level of production, narrative, and reception. Passionately produced with obvious care by a host of trans and queer actors, writers, producers, and directors, *Pose* offers a captivating and critical re-visioning of queer and trans life from 1987 through the early 1990s in which daily survival is an act of collective resistance. While the violent deaths of, in particular, transwomen of color happen on almost a daily basis all over the world, it is not only the murders that are unjust, but as gender and sexuality theorist Cam Awkward-Rich clarifies, "everything that preceded the end" (2019). Thus, when I borrow the term "transing care" from feminist philosopher and queer studies theorist Hil Malatino (*Trans Care*, 7), I follow his lead as I critically embrace *Pose*; it is a unique series that dramatizes vibrant and necessary strategies of living, of care, that point to a "care ethics" that is not "White and Eurocentered, grounded in the colonial/modern gender system."[3] In the following sections, I will examine the industrial/production context for *Pose* with particular attention to queer, creative labors of care, the series' representation of networks of care in relation to HIV/AIDS and transphobic violence as public health crises, and the implications of the series in relation to the paradox of transvisibility.

Encoding trans care: trans labor as collective creativity

From the elaborate detail of each ballroom costume, to every judge's score, to every decision in the writer's room, queer and trans labor shapes the ways that *Pose* "shows up" for its creative collaborators as well as its audience. This form of queer investment, art, and industry is a form of community that is all about encoding care behind the camera and in front of it as well. For example, Janet Mock is not the only out trans writer or director on *Pose*; Silas Howard (*By Hook or By Crook*; *Transparent*) and Our Lady J (*Transparent*) have also directed, written, or produced episodes. In particular, Our Lady J, a classical pianist, composer, TV writer, producer, and performer has been integral and, to my mind, neglected as a major contributor to the show's success.[4] What interests me about the production context of *Pose* is the extent to which queer and, in particular, trans labor marks the program both as a particular kind of commodity but also because of its ties to a particular kind of *community*. Other LGBTQ people of color, such as co-producer Steven Canals, direct several episodes. And, when white gay men such as Ryan Murphy write and direct, they certainly do not operate without the support and criticism of the larger *Pose* team.

While the program depicts the complex, yet loosely affiliated houses and families of LGBTQ of color ballroom culture, it also is the case that the program is brought into being by different yet equally complex cultural industry networks and economy. However, a consideration of *Pose* from a purely political economic perspective has the potential to miss what I recognize as the affective investments in the show's production. In other words, it matters that the imaginations of LGBTQ folx are the ones, most significantly, both behind and in front of the camera, who are doing the creative work of *Pose*.[5] In other words, if the program centers around the competition among the various houses, their mothers and children, it is also dependent upon the care networks that are demonstrated throughout the show. It is this unique element, I argue, that gives *Pose* a difference in terms of production and its reception. One way to define this element is to say it is about demonstrative *care* that is encoded at the various levels of the program. By noting this, I mean to suggest that just as the houses and families demonstrate what can be called a trans politics of *networked care*, so the production/creative structure can also be understood as a *care network*.

The significance of the production of *Pose* as well as the industrial constraints placed upon trans actors is the subject of a *Variety* roundtable cover story and video interview with six trans artists: Laverne Cox (*Orange is the New Black*); Chaz Bono (*American Horror Story: Cult; American Horror Story: Roanoake*); Alexandra Billings (*Transparent*); Trace Lysette (*Transparent*); Jen Richards (*Her Story*; *I am Cait*; *Nashville*); and Brian Michael (*Queen Sugar*). *Variety* New York Bureau Chief and author Ramin Setoodeh conducted a roundtable video interview with these artists. He began the interview by asking Laverne Cox about her *TIME* Magazine cover from 2014 and the so-called "Transgender Tipping Point."

Setoodeh: "Do you feel like we're at a tipping point? Laverne, you were on the cover of *TIME* magazine four years ago, to signify your arrival as the first breakthrough transgender star."

> Laverne Cox: "There's been so much controversy from my last tipping-point moment, I'm not sure I would want to declare that. What I think is going on now that's really exciting for me, though, is I feel like *Pose* has changed the game. It's a shame that there's no one from the show here today. [Note: Creator Ryan Murphy would not allow any of the show's stars to participate, because he doesn't want them to do press around transgender-related issues.] I sat and watched the first episode and I just cried, because I knew this talent existed. It felt revolutionary. I said to myself, 'This proves that we can do the job, that we can lead shows, that we can write, that we can direct. We can tell our own stories, and it can be brilliant. This is going to change the game.'"[6]

The feeling that Cox describes about *Pose* changing the representational and trans labor game is crucial as the conversation among the actors focused on everything from the politics of casting to writing.[7]

Care, caregiving, caretaking have been identified as a feminine and also as an unseen form of, often, remunerated labor. Mostly unremunerated as an expected duty of love, stereotypically performed by women in the home, care and its histories and theories have been a central concern of women's studies for decades. It is beyond the scope of this chapter to offer a review of such scholarship; however, it is worth emphasizing that *caring* is more than feeling; it is *doing*. Perhaps that doing is for the self, as in Michel Foucault's *The Care of the Self* (1988), yet even in his theorizations of care, it is the care of the self *for others* that matters. Perhaps that doing, however, is also for others. By caring, I do not mean to signify mere attention to something. It is more like an investment – a psychic, an emotional, and a physical investment in a project, a politics, an individual, a community. It matters whose hands are turning and under which kinds of conditions. So, how can and under which circumstances should *caring*, as a mode of labor, as the production of a material thing such as a media text, be seen and recognized? In other words, how and why does *caring* matter?

The production context: who else besides the white, cis, gay guy gets to tell this story?

As a Ryan Murphy (*Popular*; *American Horror Story*; *Glee*) production that combines the writing and directing talents of Janet Mock, Steven Canals, Our Lady J, Jennie Livingston (*Paris is Burning*), Tina Mabry, Silas Howard, and many others, the program features over 50 trans characters each played by a trans actor. From the top down to the smallest, glittering rhinestone, *Pose* is a queer production about queer lives and communities.[8]

Moreover, in recent years, there has been a significant increase in core character, trans television representation from Netflix's *Orange is the New Black* (2013–2019) to Amazon Prime's *Transparent* (2014–2019) to web-based series such as *Her Story* (2016). I am focusing on *Pose* because of its inclusion of LGBTQ creative labor. I am focusing this chapter on *Pose* although *Transparent*'s use of LGBTQ writers, directors, and actors has also been very significant. However, the praise for *Transparent*'s use of trans actors and directors must be qualified because of sexual harassment charges brought against actor Jeffrey Tambor (who plays the transmatriarch, "Maura") by actor Trace Lysette.[9] Ater Lysette came forward, Tambor was fired from the show. Before his firing, Tambor had won two Emmys and a Golden Globe for his "Maura" role.

However, any analysis of *Pose* has to grapple with the significance of this program as a Murphy-Falchuk production. Indeed, this section's title refers to an observation that a friend of media scholar Alfred L. Martin made regarding the role of white men television production:

> A friend of mine often says of Hollywood, "sometimes it takes a white man" to get stories about people of color told. I believe her assertion is true. Concomitantly, it raises questions about the organization of the media industries and the capital whiteness and maleness holds within Hollywood. So, if it took a white gay man (Ryan Murphy) to tell the story of queers of color in 1980s New York (*Pose*) that took a specific and concerted effort to actually cast trans and queer people of color in the roles for a network engaged in courting white quality demographics (FX), how can scholars allegedly concerned with media images possibly ignore those factors when attempting to analyze the text?
>
> (*The Generic Closet* 73)

Yes, and, as Martin emphasizes, focusing on the image alone is and has always been, to my mind, inadequate. This multi-focused approach to the analyses of media texts has informed my research methodology since the early 1990s when I interviewed ABC network executives and Michael Malone, head writer of the soap opera *One Life to Live* (1968–2012), about its groundbreaking HIV/AIDS and gay teen (Ryan Phillippe) storyline.

Placed in the Black and Latinx ballroom culture of New York City, *Pose* focuses on the friendly, yet often intense and campy, rivalry among several "houses" including the House of Evangelista, the House of Abundance, House of Extravaganza, and the House of Wintour and the accompanying house mothers and their children. Composed of intergenerational, chosen bonds of kinship, each house functions as a family and endures typical struggles over rent, house chores, sibling rivalry, and basic day-to-day survival. As the characters experience AIDS-related deaths of friends and lovers, transphobic violence, and daily care routines for others who are HIV positive or recently diagnosed with AIDS, the program offers an important revisionary LGBTQ history. Informed by an intersectional feminist sensibility that radically challenges what it means to practice inclusion while experiencing exclusion, *Pose* offers queer community as a network of caretaking and survival.

Driven by hatred of women, hatred of "the feminine," racism, homophobia, and transphobia, the perpetrators of such acts from verbal harassment, to beatings, to murder are rarely, if ever, brought to justice. Families, by blood or by affinity and or an "infrapolitical ethics of care" (Malatino "Tough Breaks," 121) based upon community and collectivity such as Rivera's and Johnson's STAR House, emerge as ferociously protective structures within which lives may be protected, nurtured, and encouraged. As was made clear by the intersectional, activist interventions of Black Live Matter and Trans Lives Matter that seized public space and amplified rage at the indiscriminate disposal of Black and trans people of color during the summer of 2020, when the most victimized individuals among us are under threat, so are we all.

Racism, homophobia, misogynoir, and transmisogynoir represent intersectional threats to public health. In the midst of the Covid-19 crisis and in the wake of the Minneapolis police murder of George Floyd, the Brooklyn Liberation march coalesced the Black Lives Matter movement and trans liberation (Figure 20.1). Participants were encouraged to wear white as a tribute to the "Silent Parade, when the National Organization for Colored People (NAACP) assembled nearly 10,000 people in 1917, all wearing white and silently marching down Fifth Avenue to demand an end to violence against black people" (Patil). To underscore the significance of trans violence as a public health epidemic, the American Medical Association announced at its 2019 annual meeting that, "According to available tracking, fatal anti-transgender violence in the US is on the rise and most victims were black transgender women" (Euber).[10]

The 2020 protests for Black Trans Lives are connected to, not distinct from, the kinds of trans care that is evident in *Pose*. If both the representation and the public protests for trans lives can be understood as forms of what Malatino calls, "showing up for each other," then what? How do we make sense of the increase in television, film and web-based trans visibility while, on a daily basis, transwomen of color in particular are targeted, harassed, beaten, and or killed? Showing up with a crowd of 15,000 people, taking the streets in a silent march during a pandemic and showing up in a writer's room, on a set, behind or in front of a camera are all ways to do *care* work. Yet, these public forms of trans care work can have consequences. As media scholar Danielle Seid comments,

> Only a few years ago, a show like *Pose* might have seemed unimaginable for broadcast television. In 2014, *Orange Is the New Black* (Netflix, 2013-19) actress and activist Laverne Cox, hailed as a pioneer for trans people working in television, appeared on the cover of *TIME* Magazine as the face of the so-called "transgender tipping point." Cox and other trans celebrities raise the paradox of trans visibility – that is, what are the limits of trans visibility for effecting change? And at what costs to individuals does trans visibility come?
>
> *(2019)*

However, it is not only at the level of the text that this paradox can be understood. By what measuring system do we use to determine "progress"? It is surely the case that television representation does not prevent violence. Yet, this material, economic, and industrial difference in the production of *Pose* must not be underestimated. At all levels – production context, representation, and reception, *Pose* is a powerful statement to possibility, hope, and as Miss Candy might say, *ferocious survival.*[11]

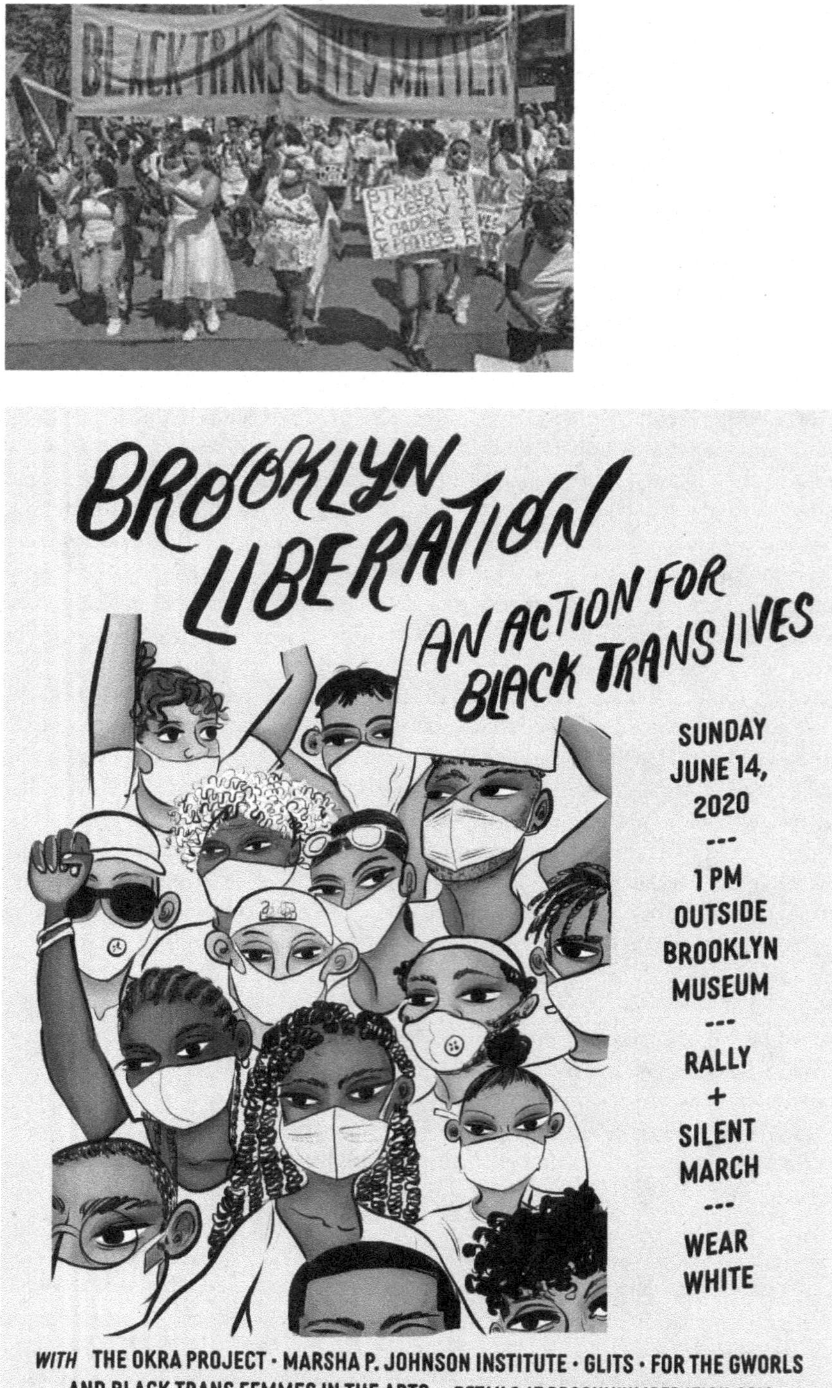

Figure 20.1 Black Trans Lives Matter Protest, June 14, 2020. Photo courtesy of Demetrius Freeman for the New York Times

> For now, busy with *Pose* and her recently-announced a multi-year deal, a first for a trans woman, [Janet] Mock has focused her energies on producing, writing, and directing. Her creative contributions on *Pose* emphasize hope, love, and community in the face of systemic violence.
>
> *(Seid 2019)*

Seid makes a crucial point about the production context out of which *Pose* emerges; it is one among several attributes that singles it out from the river of recent television, streaming, and web-based programs that focus on trans lives. The fact that Janet Mock, as a transwoman writer/author, musician and writer Our Lady J (transwoman, nonbinary), and over 50 trans actors that are playing trans characters are all deeply involved with the production of *Pose* makes it a challenge to say that the program is the sole responsibility of TV auteur, Murphy.

Yet, it is significant that Murphy and his writing-directing-producing partner Brad Falchuk share co-creator status with Steven Canals. While a screenwriting graduate student at UCLA, Canals, originally from the Bronx, wrote a screenplay based upon his response to Jennie Livingston's *Paris is Burning* (1990). Eventually, through Canals' persistence, he got the screenplay to Murphy and Falchuk. Then, through more persistence, *Pose* began to take shape.

As the past 20 years or so of production studies has taught us, it is imperative to take our examinations of the televisual text beyond the "text itself" to account for how "the text" comes to be. Of course, as students of cultural studies can tell you, Stuart Hall, Jane Feuer, John Fiske, Janice Radway, and Angela McRobbie among others, were engaged in what is now called "production studies" long before this area came into its own in the early 2000s.[12] And, more to the point, the rise of "queer production studies" builds upon the field of production studies to address

> the machinations of queer authorship as it is with the maneuvers of networks and their engagement with queerness and queer content. In particular, scholars have explored the ways the industrial production of queerness and queer-friendly audiences led to the production of queer content across media platforms, including network television, cable networks, films, and terrestrial and satellite radio networks…
>
> *(Martin, "Introduction: What is Queer," 4)*

Queer production studies attends to, as Martin says, "the many facets of queer production and the production of queerness" ("Introduction: What is Queer," 5). Thus, production studies and queer production studies account for the specificity of the text, its intertextual production, its intertextual circulation, and its reception. Recognizing that each facet of "the text" is connected to all the other aspects, Martin also encourages media scholars to engage in not only intertextual analyses but *intersectional* ones as well. In so doing, Martin challenges scholars to account for the multiple modes of not only production but also of the linkages among race, class, sexuality, and gender that create the conditions for the emergence of a given media text. Given that view, Murphy's status as a white, cis, gay male is one among several perhaps unequal features of the creation of *Pose*. Yet, how might we parse the significance of a "Murphy/Falchuk" enterprise from the production, circulation, and reception contexts of *Pose*? What are the conditions of visibility that brought Janet Mock, for example to *Pose* as the creative, writer/director power behind *Pose* and Murphy's Netflix series, *Hollywood* (2019). Mock, a transwoman, who began her writing career at *Marie Claire* and *People* magazine and has become well known for her memoir, *Redefining Realness: My Path to Womanhood, Identity, Love & So Much More* (2014). As an activist and advocate as well as a writer, director, and producer of

Pose, Mock has broken ground to be the first transgender woman of color to write and direct a television episode with the 2018 episode titled, "Love is the Message." In doing this, Mock made television history.[13]

Making trans care visible

One way of making trans care visible, as I have been describing, is to foreground who is behind the camera as well as to account for the stories that are being told. To emphasize the care behind the camera, it is helpful to acknowledge who makes what. Rather than listing the directors and writers for every episode (Wikipedia is a source for that), this examination focuses on three episodes, each of which involves Janet Mock, Our Lady J.

Foregrounding care, as something that can be rooted in chosen kin rather than biological connection, in the pilot episode, Blanca Evangelista (MJ Rodriguez) has founded her own house after a break with her mother, Elektra Abundance (Dominique Jackson). Blanca wanders through a park and finds Damon dancing for tips. She starts to talk to him, gives him advice, and asks him if he is hungry. She takes him to the diner which becomes a regular meeting space in the show. By the end of his meal, Blanca invites him to be part of her family and to come to live with her and her other children in their modest, in-need-of-repair, pre-war Harlem apartment. We understand Blanca's gesture to invite a young stranger into her home as an act of care and an extension of community. It is just one instance, but an important one, for setting the tone of care that the show continues to develop. While I would like the opportunity to discuss each episode of the series, I only have room for two.

This section examines an episode that Mock directed, "Love is the Message" (Season 1; Episode 6) that she and Murphy co-wrote and that Murphy directed and Mock-Murphy co-wrote, "Never Knew Love Like This" (Season 2; Episode 4). I have selected these two episodes not only because of the fact that "Love is the Message" is Mock's directorial debut but also because of the creative collaboration between Mock and Murphy. Another reason for this selection has to do with the representation of two of the show's main health-related issues: HIV/AIDS and transmisogynoir. Each of these issues has at its root the homophobic, transphobic, and racist ideologies of human disposability.

Beginning in 1987, *Pose* addresses several significant issues in relation to HIV/AIDS including:

- new anti-body testing services
- the rise of community service and educational organizations such as Gay Men's Health Crisis (GMHC) and Minority AIDS Task Force
- the early formation of AIDS Coalition to Unleash Power (ACT University Press) with its Monday night meetings at The Center (LGBTQ center in Greenwich Village)
- the homophobia endured by people living with AIDS (or dying from it, as the case may be) at St. Vincent Memorial Hospital's notorious "AIDS ward
- the role of lesbians in activism and caring for the ill
- the fear of sex and intimacy, early discourses around safer sex
- the Hart Island mass burials of people who died from AIDS
- the role of generation in educating youth
- the loss of a diminished if not eliminated embrace of liberated sexual desire and public sex
- the historic ACT University Press protest during mass at St. Patrick's Cathedral
- the constancy of death and funerals
- the ways that LGBTQ folx showed up for each other

The program addresses many more core issues wrought by HIV/AIDS that the program addresses than I have listed here. However, I will focus on "Love is the Message."[14]

In one of preceding episodes, "The Fever" (written by Mock), Pray Tell (MC of the balls) takes Damon (House of Evangelista), Ricky (House of Evangelista and Wintour), and Lil Papi Martinez-Evangelista (who identifies as heterosexual but who says that he "sometimes lets guys suck my dick for money") go to the public health clinic for HIV antibody tests. Damon contracts a sudden, high fever, one of the early telltale signs of HIV infection, and at Mother Blanca's insistence, he agrees to be tested. Ricky, Damon's lover, also concedes to take the test. Care is encoded at the levels of mise-en-scène and sound. Mock recounts in an interview that Murphy wanted her to direct what he considered to be the most "emotional" of that season's episodes.[15] That emotion, I argue, is carried by music, the *melos* in the family drama of the program.

The episode is structured around pairs of characters and culminates in a duet performed by Pray Tell and Blanca. Its opening sequence begins with Stan's wife, Patty (Kate Mara), and Angel (Indya Moore) sitting in a diner. This is the same diner in which Blanca buys homeless Damon a meal and invites him to live with her as one of her children. Patty and Angel have a frank conversation about Stan (Evan Peters), the man in both of their lives. Unfolding in the diner that is a gathering place in the series, they discuss quite frankly the details of Angel's and Stan's affair. Angel passes, and Patty is in disbelief when she discloses that she is a transwoman. Patty inappropriately asks probing questions about Angel's genitals. Angel informs her that her questions are not going to be answered (a stereotypical genital curiosity obsession).

After the title sequence, the next scene opens with a close-up of Costa's hands trying to grasp a plastic cup with a straw. Still in close-up, Pray Tell places his hands over Costa's and helps his ill lover bring the cup to his parched lips. In this minor moment, the significance of touch is emphasized. This intimate touch, seemingly trivial, contrasts with the avoidance of touch and care that is displayed through the nursing staff's avoidance of the patients on the AIDS ward. With the exception of Nurse Judy Kubrak (Sandra Bernhard), most of the other staff avoid contact and leave meal trays outside patient rooms. Pray Tell has learned that he is HIV+; he shares his results with Blanca, who has told him she is also HIV+. The soundtrack emphasizes his love for Costas as "Love is the Message" plays from a nearby boombox in the hospital room. The song continues as a bridge when the camera cuts to Pray Tell inside the ballroom as he calls categories as "Love is the Message" plays over and over. "Love is the Message," then both narratively and musically, functions as the affective stitch uniting the spaces of pain and of pleasure.[16]

In "Love is the Message," care is encoded in various ways both at the level of mise-en-scène and also through the musical soundtrack. Pray Tell makes a plan to bring some cheer to the doom and gloom of the AIDS ward. With Blanca's and Nurse Judy's help, he organizes an AIDS cabaret. As an intertextual reference to the scores of real-life Broadway fundraisers such Equity Fights AIDS, Broadway Cares, Visual AIDS, and the fictional "Nurses' Ball," that ABC television soap *General Hospital* held from 1994–2001, as part of the series' events.

The AIDS cabaret mise-en-scène evokes the pain and suffering of the patients in wheelchairs, with IV drips, medical gowns, grim fluorescent lighting, and stark furnishings. The patients resémble the most gaunt and sickly representations of the era, perhaps most strikingly if not problematically reminiscent of the photography of Nicholas Nixon. Nonetheless, the ward's recreational becomes a modest stage upon which Pray Tell, accompanied by Our Lady J on piano, sings Donny Hathaway's "For All We Know." He dedicates the song to Costas. Then, Blanca arrives and asks Our Lady J to play "Home" from the 1975 musical, *The Wiz*. Pray Tell joins her for a powerful duet. Mock, who personally selected this song, said that it is significant because a home is precisely what Blanca and the other mothers and fathers are building for their queer families. It is particularly poignant because they are performing this song of longing for people who, more than likely, perhaps never had homes or who will never go home again.

Mock has said that it is in this episode that Porter and Rodriguez get to unleash their voices.[17] Viewers who are familiar with Porter and Rodriguez most likely are aware of their status as "triple threats" – singers, actors, and dancers; however, it is this episode that reveals, through their performance, the intensity and power of their voices. In addition, then to touch, I want to emphasize voice and song as techniques of care as well: queer care made visible *and* audible.[18] This episode insists, through the repetition of "Love is the Message," that love and care is indeed the message.

AIDS and transviolence are common threads through each season and each episode of *Pose*. Yet, for this viewer the two most powerful episodes include "Love is the Message" and "Never Knew Love Like This." During 2018, the year that this episode aired on F/X, the Human Rights Campaign Foundation documented the violent deaths of at least 26 transgender people, most of them transwomen of color. Anti-trans violence is surely not a new phenomenon, however the paradox of increased media and activist visibility exists within a culture where trans and homophobia are nurtured and legitimated in the smallest family units and at the highest levels of government. Some forms of anti-trans stigma may include but are not limited to the following issues:

- lack of family acceptance
- hostile political climate
- cultural marginalization and conditional visibility
- exclusion from health care and social services
- unequal policing and criminal justice system
- barriers to legal identification
- racist and transphobic immigration policies (Mark 2018).

Merely refusing to be insulted, named, and obliterated becomes a mode of collective existence and survival. Thus, the seemingly modest acts of "showing up" (Malatino *Trans Care*, 5–6) for each other at bedsides, on city street, in houses of worship, in clinics, while waiting in line for a movie, or providing a meal to an acquaintance are all modes of care – necessary ones.

With the Mock-Murphy co-written and Murphy directed "Never Knew Love Like This," one of the core characters, Candy Ferocity (Angelica Ross) is murdered, a victim of transmisogynoir. After returning to sex work to help with living expenses with her mother and friend, Lulu Ferocity, Candy goes missing. Lulu and Blanca look for her at one of the "hotels on Grand Street," known for rentals-by-the-hour. Blanca leaves her home phone number with the manager; he later calls her to say that the housekeeper found Candy's body in a hotel room closet. Murphy has emphasized that he wanted viewers to get to know the characters, to have "fallen in love with the characters" in order to make Candy's murder all the more "earned," at least narratively and in the sense of story arcs: "We wanted to handle it [Candy's murder and funeral] in a way that felt responsible and not just gratuitous. In the first season, viewers probably didn't know the characters enough to be as invested as we wanted them to be for this particular narrative. We knew it would have more impact if the audience had already fallen in love with the characters, especially the one that would end up being a vehicle for this story" (Real).

As one of the most sassy and ferocious of the five transwomen of color who make up the most significant part of the show's central narrative, Candy's death is a cause of incredible sadness and shock. Viewers see the surviving friends, including Pray Tell who rarely had a kind word to say about Candy, struggling to get her body from the morgue. Not legal family, the friends have little power to get the coroner to release her body to them. Nurse Judy accompanies Candy's sisters and works some shame on the gay administrator at the morgue. He reluctantly releases her body to them and delivers Candy to the funeral home that has sadly become a regular and familiar space in *Pose*.

Trans care, then, is as much about holding and lifting up the living, one's queer mothers, fathers, brothers, and sisters, as it is about helping them move, with love, from this world to another. While Candy's memorial service unfolds, various of her friends approach the casket to say goodbye. Never one to be quiet, Candy's spirit comes to speak to Pray Tell, Angel, Lulu, Blanca, and Candy's estranged parents. When Candy visits Pray Tell, she asks him, "Why were you always such a bitch to me?" He replies, "You are unapologetic, loud, Black, femme, all the things I try to hide about myself when I go out into the real world. You are all of them. I guess I was just trying to protect you." Pray Tell recognizes, perhaps too late, that it is his own femininity that he has felt shame over, but that is precisely what, in Candy, he desires. Care as confrontation and reconciliation moves from each of the friends to the announcement from the emcee council that, in Candy's honor, they will offer a new category in lip synch, which they had previously and vehemently denied. "We're going to offer the new category at every ball and in Candy's honor we're going to call the category, Candy's Sweet Refrain," Pray Tell explains to the mourners.

As the pall bearers come forward and lift Candy's casket, the back wall of the memorial opens to reveal the ballroom. The linkage of mourning and celebration, much like a ballroom fantasy second-line parade, allows Candy to have her final performance. Her white casket with lavender lining is carried into the ballroom. As the crowd cheers, she rises from her casket. Decked out in Candy finery, she lip-synchs with an extraordinary performance of "Never Knew Love Like This" by Stephanie Mills. Candy commands the ballroom floor in a lush red dress, moving in ways that she never did in life. She moves around the dance floor and dances with her queer family, dances around the room, singing as a "free bird" as she called herself in the funeral home. Miss Candy, in death, earns the judges' highest scores, "10, 10, 10, 10, 10!"

In the following scene, Blanca walks down her apartment's long hallway carrying a bowl of macaroni and cheese. Elektra, Lulu, and Blanca's children are gathered around the dining room table, obviously grieving the loss of Candy. After a toast to Candy and dinner, Pray Tell and Blanca wash dishes and talk. Blanca had been encouraging Pray Tell to take AZT, one of the only approved drugs available at the time for treatment of HIV/AIDS.[19] The episodes ends with Blanca and Pray Tell make a toast, "To life," and take their AZT doses.

Care work is about the living. It is also about what the living *do*, how we respond to the losses we have endured. It is about continuing to make families of our own kinds of kin. It is about collaboration across difference. It is about telling our stories and about making our stories. We do this in front of and behind television cameras, on ballroom floors, in hospital rooms, as we fashion lives from ordinary objects, the remains of things that are no longer here. They remain, vibrant markers for ways forward into the arms of those who show up for us and who have held us against all odds.

Notes

1 While "misogynoir" was coined by Moya Bailey, "(trans)misogynoir" was first used by the writer and artist Trudy on *Gradient Lair*, a blog. See Bailey, *Misogynoir Transformed: Black Women's Digital Resistance*, New York University Press, 2021 and Trudy, *Gradient Lair*, www.gradientlair.com.

2 Miss Major continues her activism and advocacy at the age of 80. She moved her "House of GG", The Griffin-Gracy Historical Retreat and Educational Center", from San Francisco to Little Rock, Arkansas. The House of GG provides a place for trans folks to stay and receive various supportive services. For more information about Miss Major see, an animated documentary film, *Major!* (Ophelian, Annalise, 2015) and the forthcoming four-part, docu-series, *Trans in Trumpland*.

3 Lugones, Maria. 2007. "Heterosexualism and the Colonial/Modern Gender System." *Hypatia: A Journal of Feminist Philosophy* 22 (1): 186–209. (Cited in Malatino *Trans Care*, 7.)

4 I first became aware of the vast talents of Our Lady J while attending cabaret and other performances in New York City in the early 2000s. Along with performers such as Mx. Justin Vivian Bond, Our Lady J has been a recognizable and powerful force in the LGBTQ performance scene. As an out, HIV+, transwoman (and nonbinary), Our Lady J works as an advocate and an artist: "The whole point of my art is to create reflective surfaces so that people can have hope in their own journey of survival" (*Hollywood Reporter*, "How Our Lady J's Life Informs Her Art").

5 A word on language and why it matters. I use the inclusive term "folx" throughout this chapter. "Folx" is a gesture toward gender inclusivity such as the use of the term "Latinx."

6 The claim here that Murphy refused to allow actors, writers, directors connected to the show to speak on trans issues has been proved false, even though the rumor persists. Given the abundance of interviews that trans actors such as MJ Rodgriguez (Blanca Evangelista), Dominique Jackson (Elektra Abundance/Wintour); Indya Moore (Angel Evangelista), Angelica Ross (Candy Ferocity) have given in multiple media forms including *Entertainment Weekly*; *Jezebel*; *Refinery 29* and others, at the very least the *Variety* claim should be carefully examined. Mock and Our Lady J have also participated in media interviews and articles.

7 Martin, "Queer Business" (2018).

8 For a more detailed discussion on straight actors in LGBTQ roles see Martin, Alfred L., *The Generic Closet: Black Gayness and the Black-Cast Sitcom*. Bloomington: Indiana University Press, 2021.

9 Lysette is a transwoman. Or, as I prefer to say, Lysette is a woman.

10 This remark came from American Medical Association board member S. Bobby Mukkamala, MD. Euber, Julie, "American Medical Association: Transgender Deaths are an Epidemic," *Nonprofit Quarterly*, October 2, 2019.

11 Seid has noted that the character of Candy Ferocity (played powerfully by Angelica Ross) is based on Venus Extravaganza, from the House of Extravaganza, who was killed during the production of Jennie Livingston's documentary film, *Paris is Burning* (1991).

12 Obviously, a full consideration of *Pose* in relation to production studies is beyond the scope of this chapter. For more on production studies, see Caldwell, John Thornton, *Production Culture: Industrial Reflexivity and Critical Practice in Film and Television* (Durham: Duke University Press, 2008); Mayer, Vicki, Miranda J. Banks, and John Thornton Caldwell, eds. *Production Studies*, (New York: Routledge, 2009); Mayer, Vicki, *Below the Line: Producers and Production Studies in The New Television Economy*, (Durham: Duke University Press, 2011). For recent and welcomed attention to the labor of "queer" production, in relation to the pressing question of casting, the "writer's room," directing, and other media-industry related issues, see Martin, 2018, "Queer Production Studies").

13 By the end of the second season of Pose, Mock had directed three episodes, including "Love is the Message," Butterfly/Cocoon," and "In My Heels." She has been writer or co-writer on several other episodes. See Gimmell, Allie, "Janet Mock Wrote & Directed an Episode of *Pose* and Made TV History," *Teen Vogue*, July 9, 2018. www.teenvogue.com/story/janet-mock-wrote-directed-episode-of-pose-made-tv-history.

14 "Love is the Message" is also the first television episode directed by a transwoman of color.

15 Marine, Brooke. "Janet Mock's *Pose* Directorial Debut Proves She's a Natural Behind the Camera." *W*. July 7, 2018.

16 The classic 1973 disco song, "Love is the Message," recorded by MFSB (Mother Father Sister Brother) has its production roots in Philadelphia Sigma Sound Studios. The collective, MFSB, recorded under the label TSOP, "The Sound of Philadelphia." Artists affiliated with this label included Teddy Pendergrass, Harold Melvin & the Blue Notes, the Spinners, the Stylistics, and the O'Jays. See Nite, Norm N. *Rock On: The Illustrated Encyclopedia of Rock and Roll, 1964-1978*.

17 Ibid. I would like to note that MJ Rodriguez was Emmy-nominated for Outstanding Lead Actress in a drama series in 2021. She lost to Olivia Colman as Queen Elizabeth in *The Crown*.

18 Included in this episode, Candy and Angel visit a less than reputable source for the administration of silicone injections.

19 Azidothymidine, or AZT, was originally developed in the 1960s as a treatment for cancer. In the late 1980s, the FDA approved it for HIV/AIDS use. It was thought to slow the progression of the virus, however, many people taking the drug had severe side effects that hastened their deaths. It makes sense that Pray Tell expresses marked hesitancy about consuming AZT. Indeed, in a following episode, he has a dangerous reaction to the medication.

Works cited

Awkward-Rich, Cam. "Craft Capsule: Elegy." *Poets & Writers*, December 23, 2019. www.pw.org/content/craft_capsule_elegy. Accessed August 28, 2021.

Bailey, Moya. *Misogynoir Transformed: Black Women's Digital Resistance*. New York: New York University Press, 2021.

Caldwell, John Thornton. *Production Culture: Industrial Reflexivity and Critical Practice in Film and Television*. Durham, NC: Duke University Press, 2008.

Euber, Julie."American Medical Association: Transgender Deaths are an Epidemic."*Nonprofit Quarterly*, October 2, 2019, www.nonprofitquarterly.org/american--medical-association-transgender-deaths-are-an-epidemic. Accessed August 3, 2021.

Fuqua, Joy V. "There's a Queer in My Soap!: The AIDS/Homophobia Storyline of *One Life to Live*." *To Be Continued: Soap Operas Around the World*, edited by Robert C. Allen. New York and Abingdon: Routledge, 1995, pp. 199–212.

Gimmell, Allie. "Janet Mock Wrote & Directed an Episode of *Pose* and Made TV History." *Teen Vogue*, July 9, 2018, www.teenvogue.com/story/janet-mock-wrote-directed-episode-of-pose-made-tv-history. Accessed December 30, 2020.

"How Our Lady J's Life Informs Her Art." *Hollywood Reporter's Magic Hour*. June 12, 2019, www.youtube.com/watch?v=bJ4nhwonid4. Accessed December 30, 2020.

Lee, Mark. "Dismantling a Culture of Violence: Understanding Anti-Transgender Violence and Ending the Crisis." Human Rights Campaign Foundation, 2020.

Lugones, Maria. "Heterosexualism and the Colonial/Modern Gender System."*Hypatia: A Journal of Feminist Philosophy*, vol. 22, no. 1, 2007, pp. 186–209.

Major! Directed by Annalise Ophelian. What Do We Want Films, 2015.

Malatino, Hil. "Tough Breaks: Trans Rage and the Cultivation of Resilience," *Hypatia*, Vol. 34, No. 1, Winter 2019, pp. 121–40.

Malatino, Hil. *Trans Care*. Minneapolis, MN: University of Minnesota Press, 2020.

Marine, Brooke. "Janet Mock's *Pose* Directorial Debut Proves She's a Natural Behind the Camera," *W.*, July 7, 2018. www.wmagazine.com/story/janet-mock-interview-pose-directorial-debut. Accessed August 15, 2021.

Mark, Lee. "Dismantling a Culture of Violence: Understanding Anti-Transgender Violence & Ending the Crisis." HRC Foundation, 2018. http://hrc-prod-requests.=3-us-west-2.amazonaws.com. Accessed August 28, 2021.

Martin, Alfred L. Jr., "Introduction: what is Queer Production Studies: Why is Queer Production Studies?"*Journal of Film and Video*, Vol. 70, No. 3–4, 2018, pp. 3–7.

Martin, Alfred L. Jr., *The Generic Closet: Black Gayness and the Black-Cast Sitcom*. Bloomington, IN: Indiana University Press, 2021.

Mayer, Vicki. *Below the Line: Producers and Production Studies in the New Television Economy*. Durham, NC: Duke University Press, 2011.

Mayer, Vicki, Miranda J. Banks, and John Thornton Caldwell, eds. *Production Studies*. Durham, NC: Duke University Press, 2009.

Mukkamala, S. Bobby, and Julie Euber. "American Medical Association: Transgender Deaths are an Epidemic," *Nonprofit Quarterly*, vol. 2, October 2019.

Nite, Norm. *Rock On: The Illustrated Encyclopedia of Rock and Roll, 1964-1978*. New York: Thomas Y. Crowell Company, 1974.

Patil, Anushka. "How a March for Black Trans Lives Became a Huge Event." *New York Times*, June 15, 2020, www.nytimes.com/2020/06/15/nyregion/brooklyn-black-trans-parade.html. Accessed August 28, 2021.

Real, Evan. "Nothing has Changed: Why *Pose* Puts Its Spotlight on Violence Against Trans Women of Color." *Hollywood Reporter*, July 9, 2019, www.hollywoodreporter.com/live-feed/pose-death-explained-ryan-murphy-janet-mock-violence-trans-women-color-1223057. Accessed December 20, 2020.

Seid, Danielle. "Television Is Burning: Revolutionary Queer & Trans Representation on TV." *FlowJournal*, September 16, 2019, www.flowjournal.org/2019/09/television-is-burning/. Accessed December 20, 2020.

PART VI

Comics

"What 'cha doing?"

"Oh, hey Comics. I'm writing about what you can bring to the health humanities."

The above is the opening exchange of MK Czerwiec's contribution to this section, aptly titled: **"Comics and the health humanities."** In graphic form, she addresses the complexity and multiplicity of health humanities as well as their reliance on stories to achieve the goal of improving health for people on a broad scale. Czerwiec illustrates what comics do that a written or oral story cannot do – simultaneously representing multiple, often conflicting realities and making visible the invisible elements of illness and health, such as rendering in line and color both physical pain *and* psychic pain in the same panel.

In the past decade, comics and graphic narratives have become a popular form for telling stories of illness, impairment, and injury in a medium that artfully combines words and images. In his chapter, Williams, who coined the term "graphic medicine," focuses specifically on autobiographical comics and graphic novels and reminds us that the medium, with its radical tradition of irony and humor, can render even the most tragic conditions engaging – even entertaining. In his essay, **"Mad world-building: comics and OCD,"** Williams explores how obsessive-compulsive disorder (OCD) is portrayed in comics, and how artists, including himself, have found novel ways of characterizing the disorder and conveying the experience of living with it.

That disorder also figures in Sathyaraj Venkatsen's discussion and analysis of several graphic works that explore non-western complementary and alternative medicine (CAM) in the third chapter, **"'I found balance': complementary and alternative medicine in selected graphic medical narratives."** The selected texts underscore both the collective and individual benefits of CAM practices and include various philosophies of health, illness, and well-being as well as specific health interventions such as yoga and meditation.

Finally, Lisa Diedrich explores the multi-modal form of graphic medicine as a means for articulating the illness politics and care practices that emerged out of the response to HIV/AIDS in her chapter, **"Drawing health activism: illness politics and practices of care in graphic AIDS narratives."** She focuses on a selection of hybrid verbal and visual narratives: from the beginning of the pandemic in the 1980s to the quite recent publication Czerwiec's *Taking Turns* (2017), which recounts her own experience as a nurse working in an AIDS unit in Chicago.

DOI: 10.4324/9781003007661-27

21
COMICS AND THE HEALTH HUMANITIES

MK Czerwiec

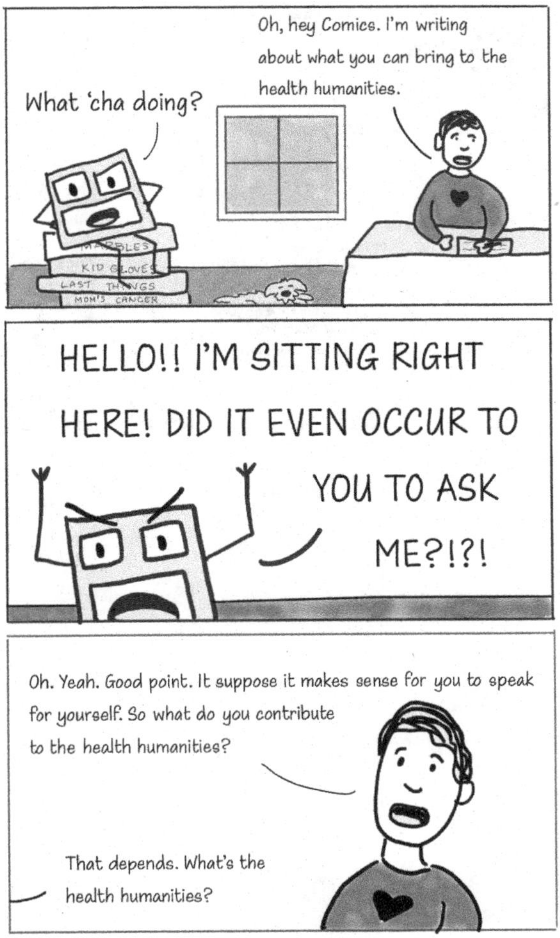
What 'cha doing?
Oh, hey Comics. I'm writing about what you can bring to the health humanities.
MOM'S CANCER
HELLO!! I'M SITTING RIGHT HERE! DID IT EVEN OCCUR TO YOU TO ASK ME?!?!
Oh. Yeah. Good point. It suppose it makes sense for you to speak for yourself. So what do you contribute to the health humanities?
That depends. What's the health humanities?

Figure 21.1 Part 1

DOI: 10.4324/9781003007661-28

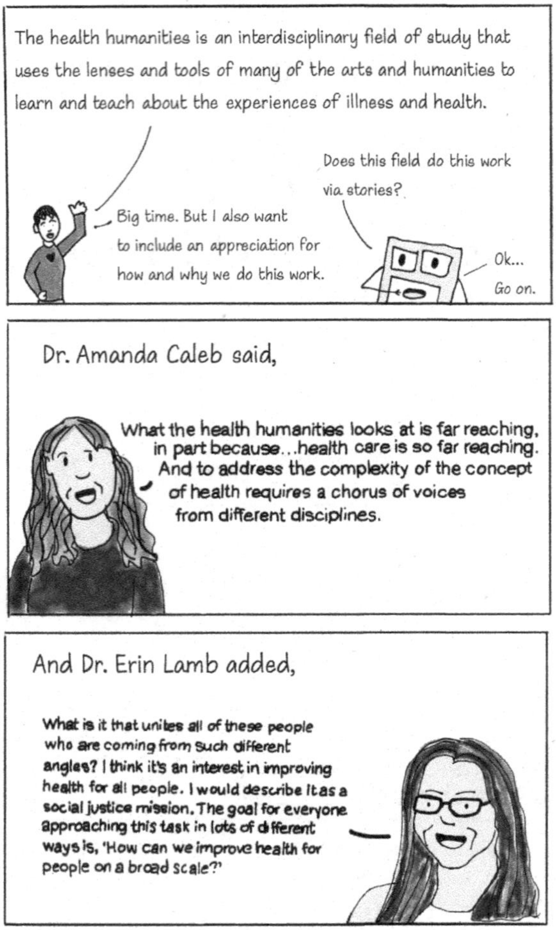
The health humanities is an interdisciplinary field of study that uses the lenses and tools of many of the arts and humanities to learn and teach about the experiences of illness and health.
Does this field do this work via stories?
Big time. But I also want to include an appreciation for how and why we do this work.
Ok... Go on.
Dr. Amanda Caleb said,
What the health humanities looks at is far reaching, in part because...health care is so far reaching. And to address the complexity of the concept of health requires a chorus of voices from different disciplines.
And Dr. Erin Lamb added,
What is it that unites all of these people who are coming from such different angles? I think it's an interest in improving health for all people. I would describe it as a social justice mission. The goal for everyone approaching this task in lots of different ways is, 'How can we improve health for people on a broad scale?'

Figure 21.2 Part 2

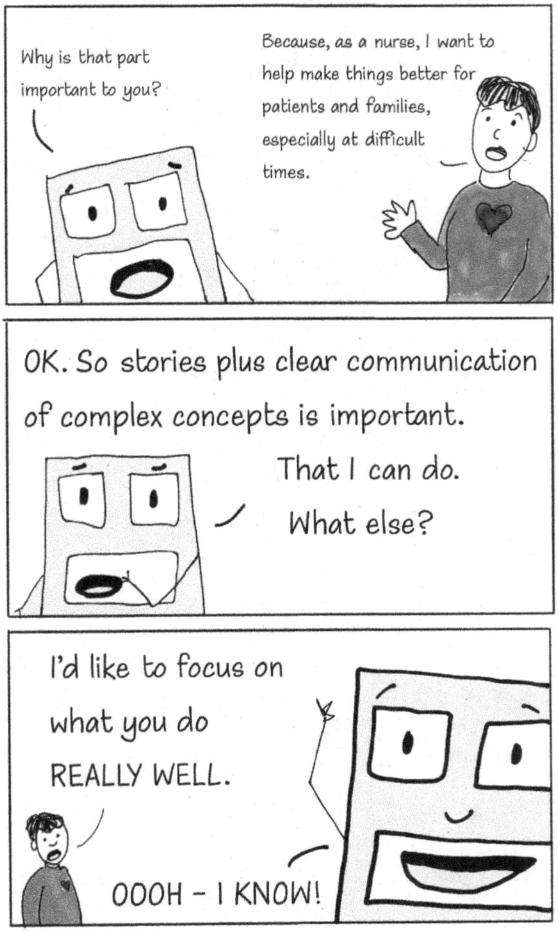
Why is that part important to you?
Because, as a nurse, I want to help make things better for patients and families, especially at difficult times.
OK. So stories plus clear communication of complex concepts is important.
That I can do. What else?
I'd like to focus on what you do REALLY WELL.
OOOH – I KNOW!

Figure 21.3 Part 3

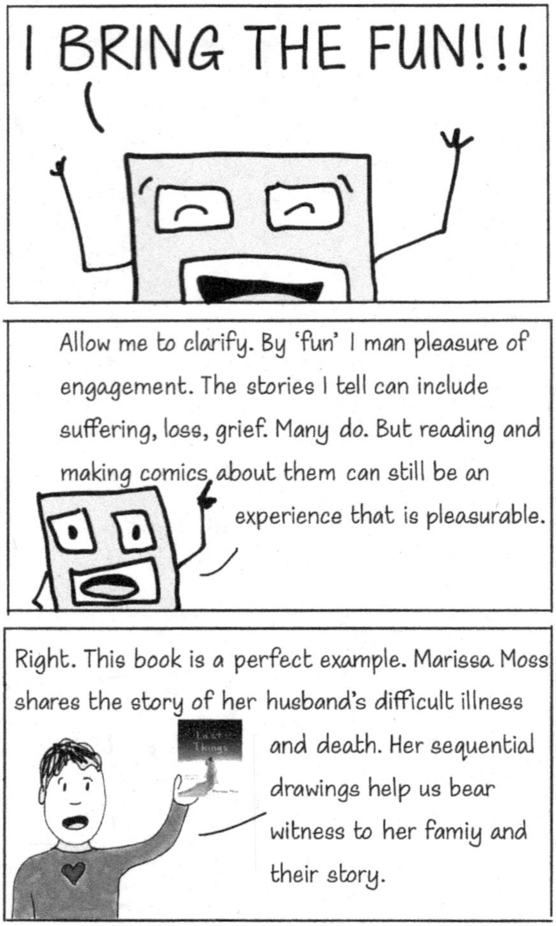

Figure 21.4 Part 4

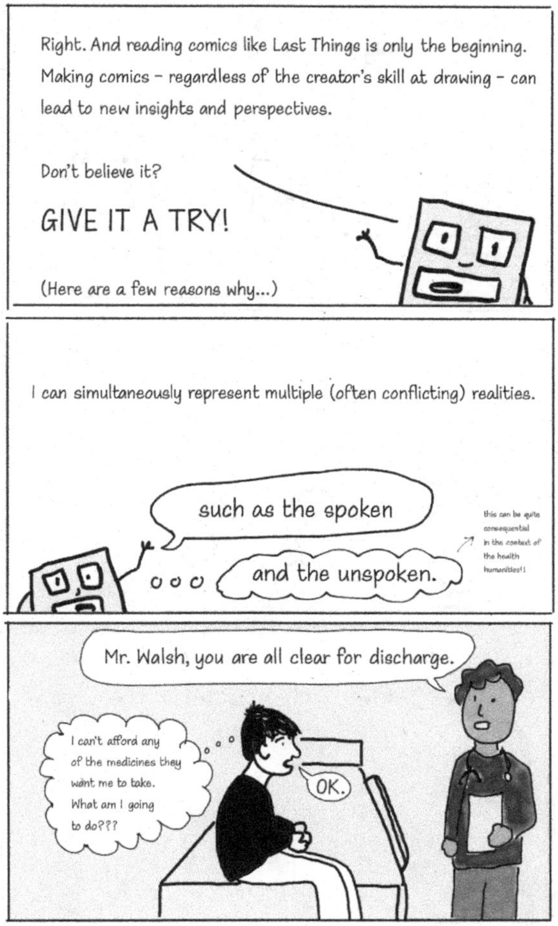
Right. And reading comics like Last Things is only the beginning. Making comics – regardless of the creator's skill at drawing – can lead to new insights and perspectives.
Don't believe it?
GIVE IT A TRY!
(Here are a few reasons why...)
I can simultaneously represent multiple (often conflicting) realities.
such as the spoken
and the unspoken.
this can be quite consequential in the context of the health humanities!!
Mr. Walsh, you are all clear for discharge.
I can't afford any of the medicines they want me to take. What am I going to do???
OK.

Figure 21.5 Part 5

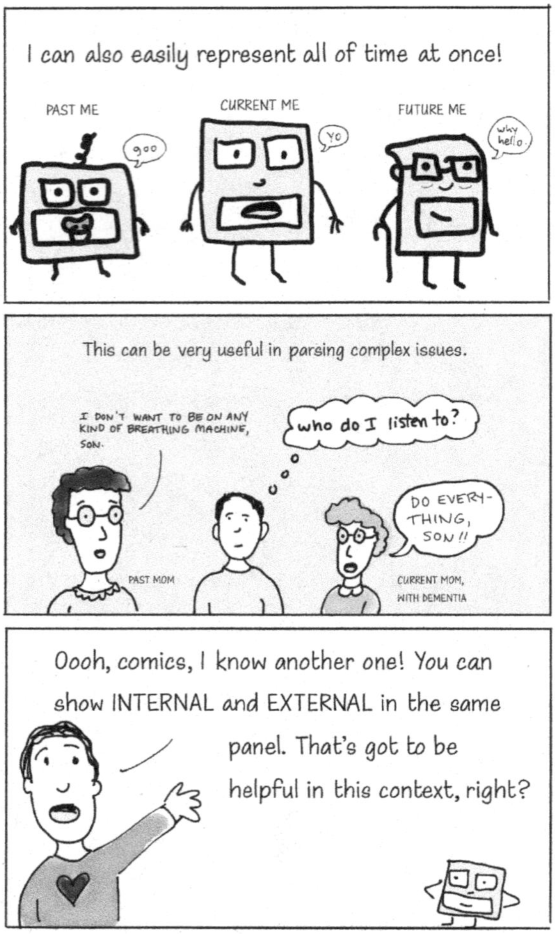
I can also easily represent all of time at once!
PAST ME
goo
CURRENT ME
yo
FUTURE ME
why hello.
This can be very useful in parsing complex issues.
I DON'T WANT TO BE ON ANY KIND OF BREATHING MACHINE, SON.
who do I listen to?
DO EVERY-THING, SON!!
PAST MOM
CURRENT MOM, WITH DEMENTIA
Oooh, comics, I know another one! You can show INTERNAL and EXTERNAL in the same panel. That's got to be helpful in this context, right?

Figure 21.6 Part 6

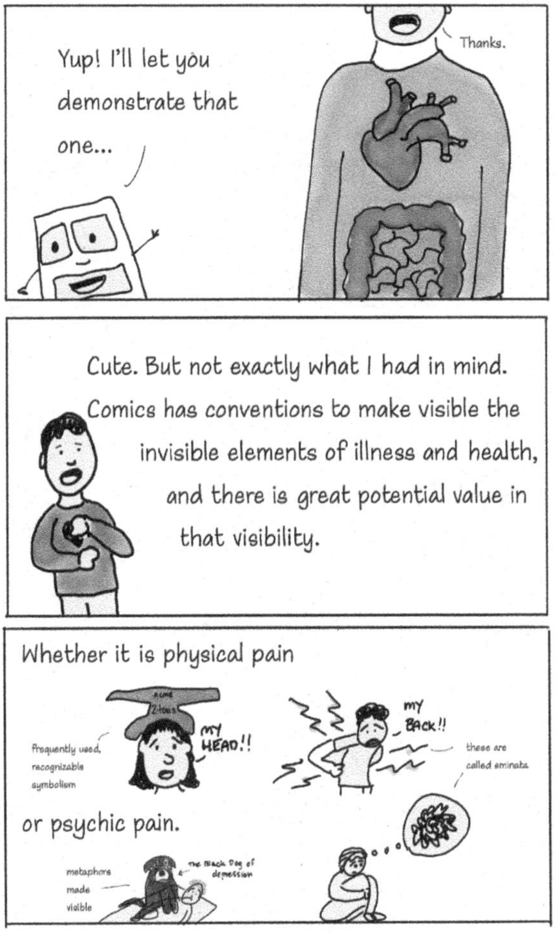
Yup! I'll let you demonstrate that one...
Thanks.
Cute. But not exactly what I had in mind. Comics has conventions to make visible the invisible elements of illness and health, and there is great potential value in that visibility.
Whether it is physical pain
Frequently used, recognizable symbolism
MY HEAD!!
MY BACK!!
these are called eminata
or psychic pain.
metaphors made visible
The Black Dog of depression

Figure 21.7 Part 7

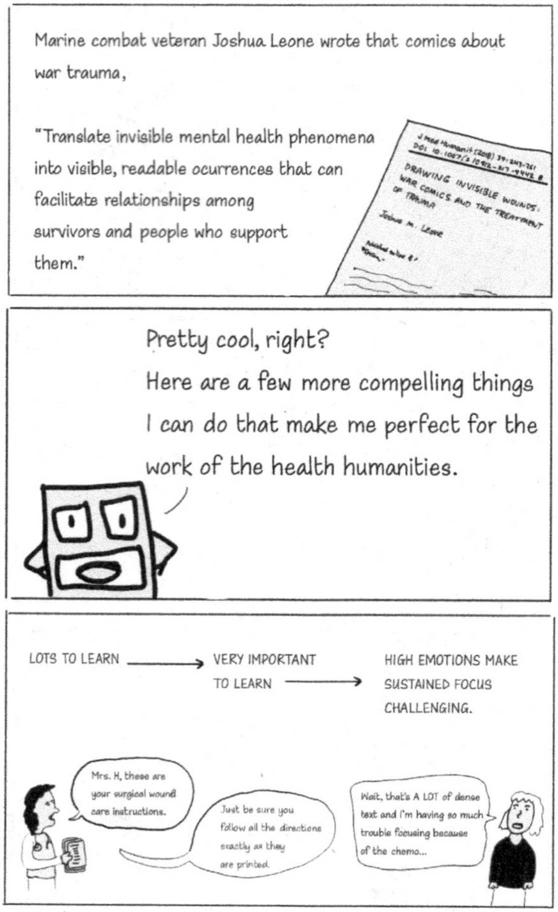

Figure 21.8 Part 8

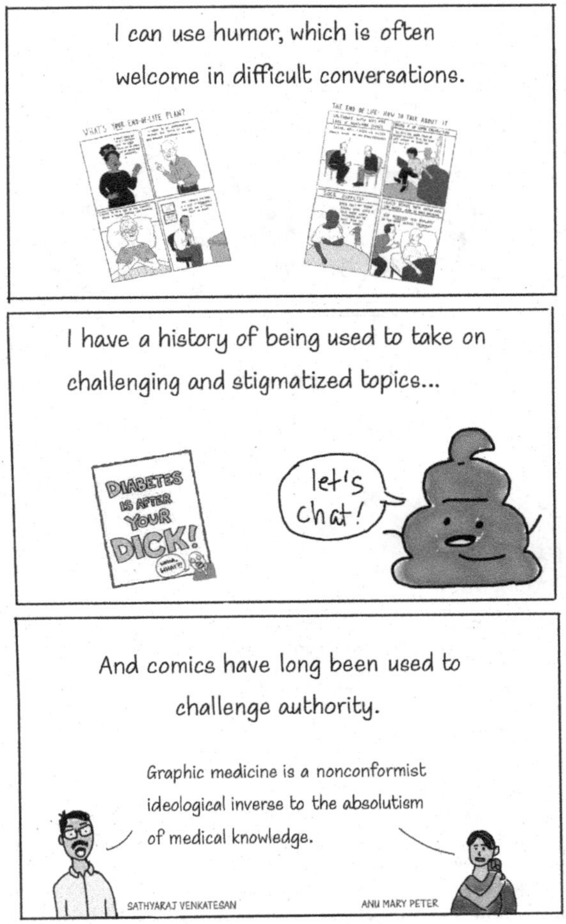
I can use humor, which is often welcome in difficult conversations.
I have a history of being used to take on challenging and stigmatized topics...
DIABETES IS AFTER YOUR DICK!
let's chat!
And comics have long been used to challenge authority.
Graphic medicine is a nonconformist ideological inverse to the absolutism of medical knowledge.
SATHYARAJ VENKATESAN
ANU MARY PETER

Figure 21.9 Part 9

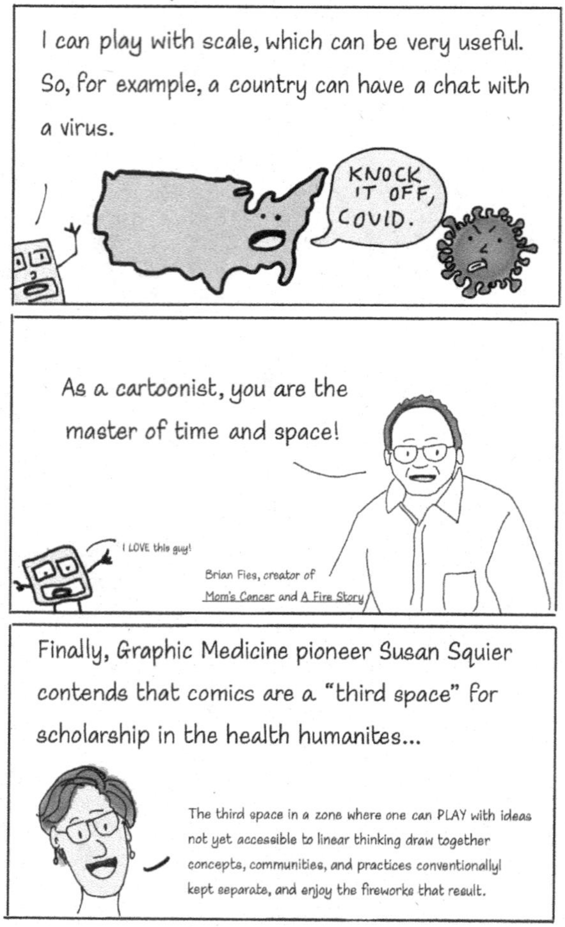
I can play with scale, which can be very useful. So, for example, a country can have a chat with a virus.
KNOCK IT OFF, COVID.
As a cartoonist, you are the master of time and space!
I LOVE this guy!
Brian Fies, creator of Mom's Cancer and A Fire Story
Finally, Graphic Medicine pioneer Susan Squier contends that comics are a "third space" for scholarship in the health humanites...
The third space in a zone where one can PLAY with ideas not yet accessible to linear thinking draw together concepts, communities, and practices conventionallyl kept separate, and enjoy the fireworks that result.

Figure 21.10 Part 10

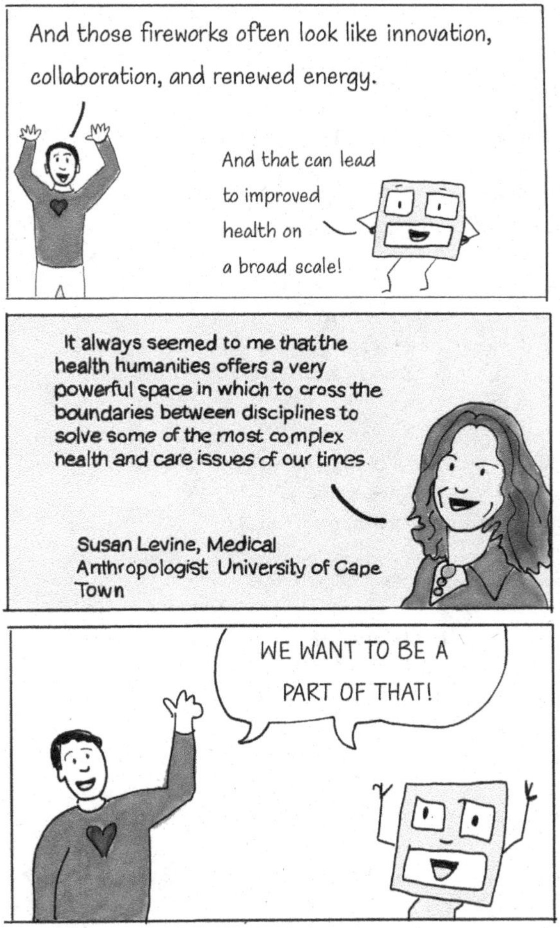
And those fireworks often look like innovation, collaboration, and renewed energy.
And that can lead to improved health on a broad scale!
It always seemed to me that the health humanities offers a very powerful space in which to cross the boundaries between disciplines to solve some of the most complex health and care issues of our times.
Susan Levine, Medical Anthropologist University of Cape Town
WE WANT TO BE A PART OF THAT!

Figure 21.11 Part 11

References

Caleb, Amanda. "Episode 1: What Is the Health Humanities?" Misericordia Digital Commons, Misericordia University, Sept. 20, 2020, digitalcommons.misericordia.edu/health_humanist/1/.

Fies, Brian. "Techniques and Tools of Storytelling." Workshop at the Comics and Medicine Conference: Spaces of Care, Riverside, CA, July 18, 2015.

Flake, Emily. "What's Your End of Life Plan" and "The End of Life: How to Talk About It." Included in the exhibit, "Death Panels: Comics That Help Us Face End of Life", 53rd Street New York Public Library, October 27 - November 3, 2018.

Lamb, Erin. "Episode 1: What Is the Health Humanities?" Misericordia Digital Commons, Misericordia University , Sept. 20, 2020, digitalcommons.misericordia.edu/health_humanist/1/.

Leamy, Cathy. "Diabetes Is after Your Dick!" Metrokitty, 2012.

Leone, Joshua M. "Drawing Invisible Wounds: War Comics and the Treatment of Trauma." Journal of Medical Humanities, vol. 39, no. 3, 2017, pp. 243–261., doi:10.1007/s10912-017-9442-8.

Susan, Levine, and Steve Reid. Medicine and the Arts: Humanising Healthcare. University of Cape Town via Futurelearn, www.futurelearn.com/courses/medicine-and-the-arts

Moss, Marissa. Last Things, a Graphic Memoir of Loss and Love.: Marissa Moss. Conari Press, 2017.

Squier, Susan M. "Graphic Medicine in the University." The Hastings Center Report, vol. 45, no. 3, 2015, pp. 19–22., www.jstor.org/stable/44158959. Accessed Dec. 20, 2020.

Squier, Susan M. "Comics and Graphic Medicine as a Third Space for the Health Humanities." The Routledge Companion to Health Humanities, 2020, pp. 60–65., doi:10.4324/9780429469060-11.

Venkatesan, Sathyaraj, and Anu Mary Peter. "Towards a Theory of Graphic Medicine." Rupkatha Journal on Interdisciplinary Studies in Humanities, July 20, 2019, rupkatha.com/V11/n2/v11n208.pdf.

Figure 21.12 Part 12

Works cited

Caleb, Amanda. 'Episode 1: What is the Health Humanities?' Misericodria Digital Commons. Dallas, PA: Misericordia University, Sept 20, 2020, digitalcommons.misericordia.edu/health_humanist/1/.

Fies, Brian. 'Techniques and Tools of Storytelling.' Workshop at the comics and medicine conference: Spaces of care, Riverside, CA, July 18, 2015.

Flake, Emily. 'What's Your End of Life Plan' and 'The End of Life: How to Talk About It.' Included in the exhibit, 'Death Panels: Comics that Help Us Face End of Life', 53rd Street New York Public Library October 27–November 3, 2018.

Lamb, Erin. 'Episode 1: What is the Health Humanities?' Misericodria Digital Commons. Dallas, PA: Misericordia University, Sept 20, 2020, digitalcommons.misericordia.edu/health_humanist/1/.

Leamy, Cathy. 'Diabetes Is after Your Dick!' Metrokitty, 2012.

Leone, Joshua M. Drawing Invisible Wounds: War Comics and the Treatment of Trauma.' *Journal of Medical Humanities*, vol. 39, no. 3, 2017, pp. 243–61, doe: 101007/s10912-017-9442-8.

Moss, Marissa. *Last Things, a Graphic Memoir of Loss and Love*. Newburyport, MA: Conari Press, 2017.

Squier, Susan M. 'Graphic Medicine in the University.' The Hastings Center Report, vol. 45, no 3, 2015, pp. 19–22, www.jstor.org.stable/44158959. Accessed December 20, 2020.

Squier, Susan M. 'Comics and Graphic Medicine as a Third Space for the Health Humanities.' in *The Routledge Companion to Health Humanities*, edited by Paul Crawford, Brian Brown, and Andrea Charise. New York and Abingdon: Routledge, 2020, pp. 60–5.

Susan, Levine, and Steve Reid, Medicine and the Arts: Humanising Healthcare. University of Cape Town via Futurelearn, www.futurelearn.com/courses/medicine-and-the-arts.

Venkatesan, Sathyaraj, and Anu Mary Peter. 'Towards a Theory of Graphic Medicine.' *Rupkatha Journal on Interdisciplinary Studies in Humanities*, July 20, 2019, rupkatha.com/v11/n2/v11n208.pdf.

22
MAD WORLD-BUILDING
Comics and OCD

Ian Williams

Introduction

Comics artists have been self-imaging their illnesses since 1972 when Justin Green produced what is possibly the first substantial illness memoir in comic form: *Binky Brown Meets the Holy Virgin Mary*. This groundbreaking comic portrayed Green's struggles with an undiagnosed mental condition that he referred to as an "obsessional neurosis." In the 50 years since, the publishing industry has seen a remarkable growth in autobiographical comics and graphic novels, and, due in part to broadsheet reviews and academic interest, comics memoirs have become a respected medium for the telling and study of stories of illness and trauma. The analysis of these comic book stories, sometimes known as *graphic pathographies,* has burgeoned over the last decade into a thriving field of scholarship and practice called *graphic medicine* (Williams, "Comics and the Iconography" 116).

One of Green's expectations in producing *Binky Brown* was that he would exorcise his mental turmoil by telling his story. Although he did not know it at the time, he suffered from a religious form of Obsessive Compulsive Disorder (OCD); this diagnosis was made much later, and the condition was not well understood at the time (Figure 22.1). If Green had been living in the digital age, he would have no doubt trawled the internet, first for a diagnosis and then for information on the condition. The information "out there" – written, visual, aural, oral, and memetic – would have likely influenced the way that Green experienced and portrayed his illness, but in his pre-internet world, with no health insurance and so no access to mental health care, the cartoonist (like many artists before him) recorded his unnamed condition as best he could based on his own perceptual experiences. Because of this, the work remains a stand-out example of unmediated graphic self-storytelling, describing the mental purgatory of OCD in its purest form and largely uninfluenced by cultural stereotypes of the condition.

Or is it? Let's look at that last sentence again. Although Green had did not have a label for his condition, he and his illness were still a product of his upbringing in a Jewish-Catholic home, educated by rigidly demanding nuns and indoctrinated with then prevalent doctrines of sin-and-damnation and the culture of his times. In the absence of a psychiatric diagnosis, Green constructed the story around ideas of Catholic guilt and rendered it in a drawing style that is clearly influenced by contemporaries such as R. Crumb. Autobiography in comics was in its infancy, and Green evidently seized on this opportunity to create, if not the first, then the

DOI: 10.4324/9781003007661-29

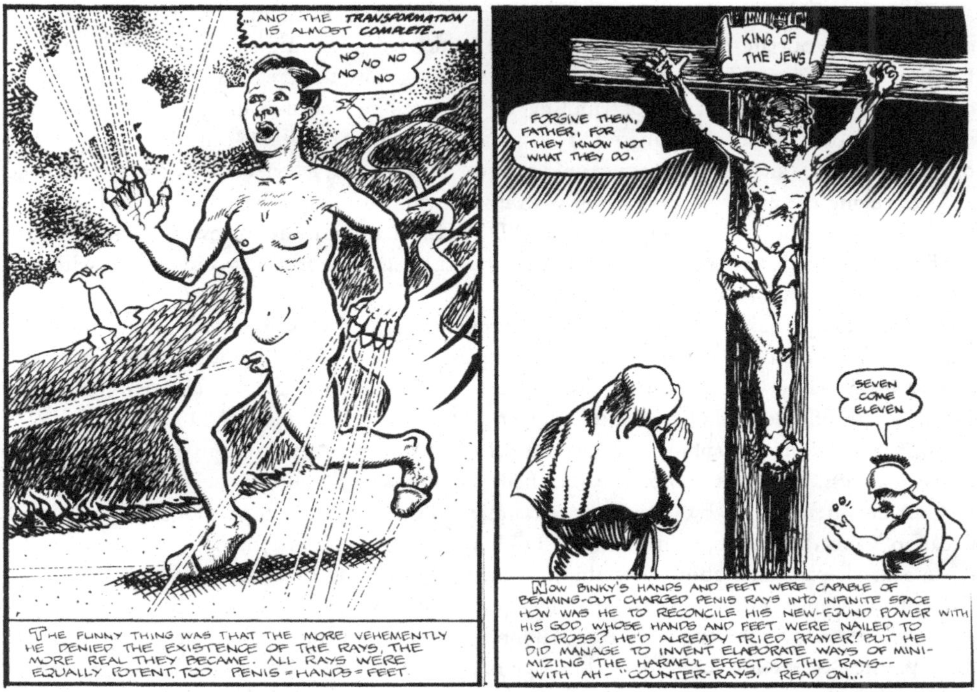
...AND THE TRANSFORMATION IS ALMOST COMPLETE...
NO NO NO NO NO
THE FUNNY THING WAS THAT THE MORE VEHEMENTLY HE DENIED THE EXISTENCE OF THE RAYS, THE MORE REAL THEY BECAME. ALL RAYS WERE EQUALLY POTENT, TOO PENIS = HANDS = FEET
KING OF THE JEWS
FORGIVE THEM, FATHER, FOR THEY KNOW NOT WHAT THEY DO.
SEVEN COME ELEVEN
NOW BINKY'S HANDS AND FEET WERE CAPABLE OF BEAMING-OUT CHARGED PENIS RAYS INTO INFINITE SPACE HOW WAS HE TO RECONCILE HIS NEW-FOUND POWER WITH HIS GOD, WHOSE HANDS AND FEET WERE NAILED TO A CROSS? HE'D ALREADY TRIED PRAYER! BUT HE DID MANAGE TO INVENT ELABORATE WAYS OF MINI-MIZING THE HARMFUL EFFECT OF THE RAYS-- WITH AH- "COUNTER-RAYS." READ ON...

Figure 22.1 Justin Green, *Binky Brown Sampler*, Last Gasp, 1995, p. 42

first *substantial* comics memoir, and comics, like any media, are constructed, edited, influenced, and received through the lens of the dominant societal value at the time of their making. As disabilities scholar Lennard Davis attests, no disease exists outside of its cultural context (12).

Debate continues as to whether OCD is a disease, or what is termed a *disease entity* (Davis 21). It is a mental condition characterized by repeated intrusive thoughts (obsessions) and the need to perform certain routines repeatedly (compulsions), causing distress and impairing general functioning. There is generally a realization that the thoughts or routines do not make sense, the person retains a degree of insight, but at the same time, he might consider himself insane. People throughout history have displayed neurotic or obsessional traits that have often been labelled retrospectively as OCD including Samuel Johnson, Charles Darwin, and St Ignatius of Loyola, but the diagnosis is a modern one. The nature of OCD seems woven into the very fabric of our culture, taking the themes of the anxiety and suffering it causes from common concerns or moral panics of the day. Thus, in the 18th century, someone riven with anxiety about sin, blasphemy, and eternal damnation might have been said to be suffering from "scrupulosity," a proto-OCD condition, while someone suffering with this condition today, particularly in the United Kingdom, might worry that he is, unconsciously, a pedophile or might be thought by others to be one or falsely accused of being one, mainly because he finds the thought utterly repugnant.

The comics form, with its radical tradition of irony and self-deprecating humor, can render the most tragic of conditions digestible for the interested reader. Not that comics have to be funny: many autobiographical comics are tragic and dark, dealing with the most unfunny of subject matter – sexual abuse, the death of children, and cancer – yet these works retain the ability to engage the readers and draw them in, even entertain them, if that word could be considered appropriate, in ways that might be a harder sell in traditional prose. In this chapter, I will look at how OCD is portrayed in comics, asking how the creators of comics might be creating new knowledge and contributing to the bank of available images and stories that inform our collective ideas of illness and healthcare, what Sander Gilman calls the "iconography of illness" (1988), and how they are finding novel ways of characterizing this protean menace and conveying the experience of living with it. The protagonists in these stories are not "a bit OCD," and the clue to their reality is in the "D" of the acronym; their lives are disordered and blighted by their obsessions and compulsions, and they struggle to find a way to live with this *thing* – and with themselves.

OCD is often characterized as an anxiety problem caused by over-activity in the amygdala, that part of the brain concerned with the processing of memory and emotion. It is commonly treated in the same way that anxiety is treated: with antidepressants and cognitive behavioral therapy, both of which can be effective. But, in addition, I believe that OCD has a special relationship with *media,* morphing and feeding off news stories and cultural memes. It is a post-modern illness, concerned with the internalization of societal rules. The public perception of OCD is often shaped by popular entertainment such as television programs about "OCD Cleaners," and the phrase, "I'm a bit OCD," has become a modern cliché, usually indicating the speaker is particular about something or other. The reality of living with the actual condition is the cause of much manifest suffering: a hellish web of virally-proliferating thoughts and propositions which can paralyze the sufferer in agonizing doubt or else drive her to repeat futile physical or mental activities in the hope of satisfying or defeating the entity that seems to control her very soul. It is no wonder, then, that OCD has been historically linked to religion, that those afflicted have worried about demonic possession or that some cartoonists choose to visually embody the condition as a creature, taunting and vexing its miserable host. Comics artists are able to use their inventive graphic skills to relate to others what it is like to live which this particular form of madness.

I am using the word *madness* here as a form of "psychiatric contention," Helen Spandler's term that refers to the way that dominant ideas, practices, and polices in mental health have been challenged and critiqued by psychiatric service users, survivors and their allies, supporters, and social movements, including the Mad movement (127). Making comics or zines about one's own mental health can be a form of protest against the prevailing medical hierarchy's categorization and othering, re-writing the patient information circulated by experts who tell patients what it is they are experiencing. From early adolescence, I suffered debilitating OCD, which afflicted me throughout my teenage years, followed me through medical school and into my years working as a junior doctor, before finally settling somewhat in my mid-thirties. It was many years before I sought help or told anyone about my problems, which is typical of those who experience the condition, and eventually I came to terms with it by writing and drawing a graphic novel about my experiences: *The Bad Doctor* (2014) – a fictional work that contains autobiographical elements. When the book was published, I thought I would never work in health care again, that I would be thought by my colleagues to be insane, but, to my surprise, I received a lot of warm feedback, and the book was highly commended in the British Medical Association Book Awards.

OCD as a condition of exaggerated self-monitoring: comics as self-representation

OCD is *ego-dystonic* in that aspects of individuals' thoughts, impulses, and preoccupations are repugnant, distressing, and at odds with the rest of their personality; this is reflected in the comic work that I consider here. The general theme of all these works is the suffering and torment of an overactive and overwrought mind, one that seems to churn out obscenities. The subject is forced to keep his or her thoughts and actions in check so as not to contravene the "rules" that the illness has set for them. The experience of OCD, therefore, is one of exaggerated self-monitoring and self-regulation (Davis 14); the person with OCD is often preoccupied with a constant evaluation of his or her own worth, morals, character, attractiveness, position in society, and public persona (14).

As OCD is linked to eating disorders and body dysmorphophobia, issues of body image are often important, and the distortion of self-image is common. Ideas of contamination by dirt, disease, toxins, ideas, or spiritual entities are also frequent, so the boundaries of the body become unclear. The visual-verbal medium of comics is ideal for representing such perceptual vexations, demonstrating how intricately mental states are bound up with lived bodily experience and an embodied sense of self (Koch 2016). Emanations may project from the body. In *Binky Brown*, for example, our protagonist senses invisible "pecker rays" that emerge from his penis and from all elongated appendages. Like powerful lasers, they project for an infinite distance, contaminating any religious icons that they hit with sacrilegious sexual vibes. Binky has to keep not only his mind in constant check, blocking out sinful thoughts as they arise with the repeated chant "Noyatin" (not a sin) but also his bodily alignments and orientation.

Binky Brown is a graphic confession, a self-flagellation in which the author lays down his darkest and most blasphemous thoughts in ink and on paper for the entertainment of the reader. Feminist scholar Leigh Gilmore (2001) highlights western autobiography's debt to the religious tradition of confession, "a practice that institutionalizes penance and penalty as self-expression" (14). *I'm Crazy*, an autobiographical work by Canadian comics artist Adam Bourret (2009), also has an intensely confessional flavor to it with the author spilling his most unspeakable worries – that he is a racist or that he will rape his sister who has Down's syndrome. Like *Binky Brown*, bodily changes also feature in which branches and foliage grow out of Adam's body, and he is fixed to the spot by tree roots growing out of his anus (Figure 22.2). The vegetal roots and branches are metaphors for Adam's "crazy thoughts" (np). They tear him to pieces, as they escape his body, paralyzing him and rendering him a victim and useless, neither plant nor animal and unable to function as a regular human being. He is exposed to the world's judgment and hanged like a criminal from a gibbet.

Roots, branches, and pecker rays bring to mind ideas of universal connectedness so beloved of certain spiritual traditions. My OCD, like Green's, focused on religion, and my adolescent mind was bound up in ideas of luck, spiritual contamination, and magic. When I began work on *The Bad Doctor*, I also began to experiment with images that reflected my experience of the condition. In one such work, I painted my adolescent self in bed, constrained by a psychic frame of virally proliferating thoughts with a structure based on the Sefirot of the Kabbalah (Figure 22.3). In the end, I used a slightly different version of the drawing as part of a series of tableaux in *The Bad Doctor*.

Our motives, I suspect, are often opaque to ourselves, but there seems to be an aspect of performance in what I have done, and I suspect that in rendering my OCD with a series of images that I was trying to own it – to transform it from a stigmatizing mental defect and source of shame into something of a creative mystery and beauty. An autobiographical artist has a chance to examine and rework his body and mind and thus the *self*. The reconstructed graphic self is an icon, placed in a world that reflects the author's and the artist's perceptions – a mad world perhaps, which reflects his concerns and is peppered with motifs that echo his obsessions. Media scholar Lisa El Refaie describes how "producing multiple drawn versions of the self entails an

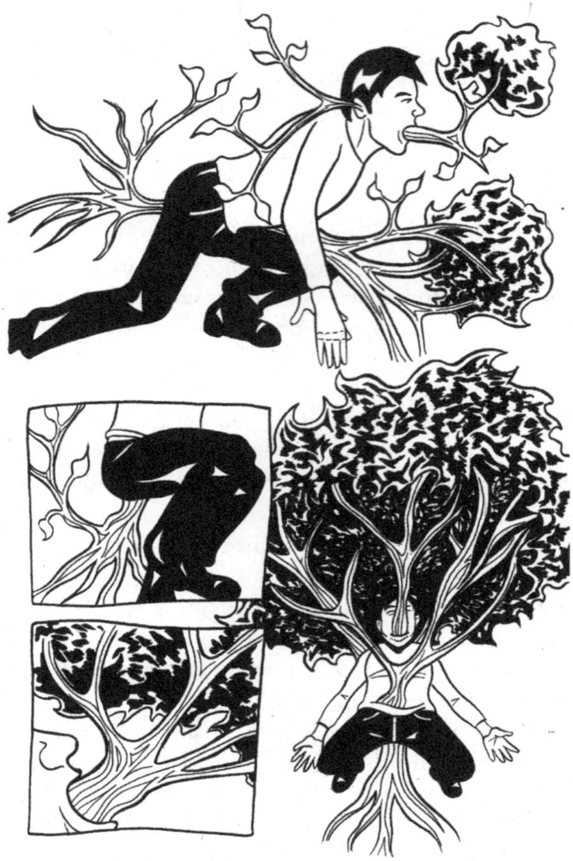

Figure 22.2 Adam Bourret, *I'm Crazy*, self-published, 2009, no page numbers

explicit engagement with physicality," and she uses the term "pictorial embodiment" in order "to capture the different ways in which graphic memoirists' sense of self is linked with the act of visually representing their bodily identities" (8). English and media scholar Gillian Whitlock refers to these self-representations as "autobiographical avatars" (971), which brings to mind the world of gaming, where players reconstruct a fantastical, sometimes somewhat idealized, version of themselves to play onscreen. In some cases, this reconstruction of the self, or healing, seems to be an intention in the making of the work. In his introduction to *Binky Brown*, Green announced to his readers that the work was not "intended solely for your entertainment, but also to purge myself of the compulsive neurosis which I have served since I officially left Catholicism on Halloween, 1958" (1995, 10).

I met Justin Green in 2015, and he told me that he had continued to suffer from OCD long after making *Binky Brown* and long after receiving his diagnosis which, to be fair, is hardly surprising. OCD is a complex neuropsychological and cultural problem, and making a comic is not going to make it disappear altogether. Indeed, in his preface to the 1995 reprint of *Binky Brown*, Green says that he "continues [his] nomadic search for mental peace, aware that before the inevitable punch-line dooms [him] to silence there may never be complete fulfilment" (1995, 8).

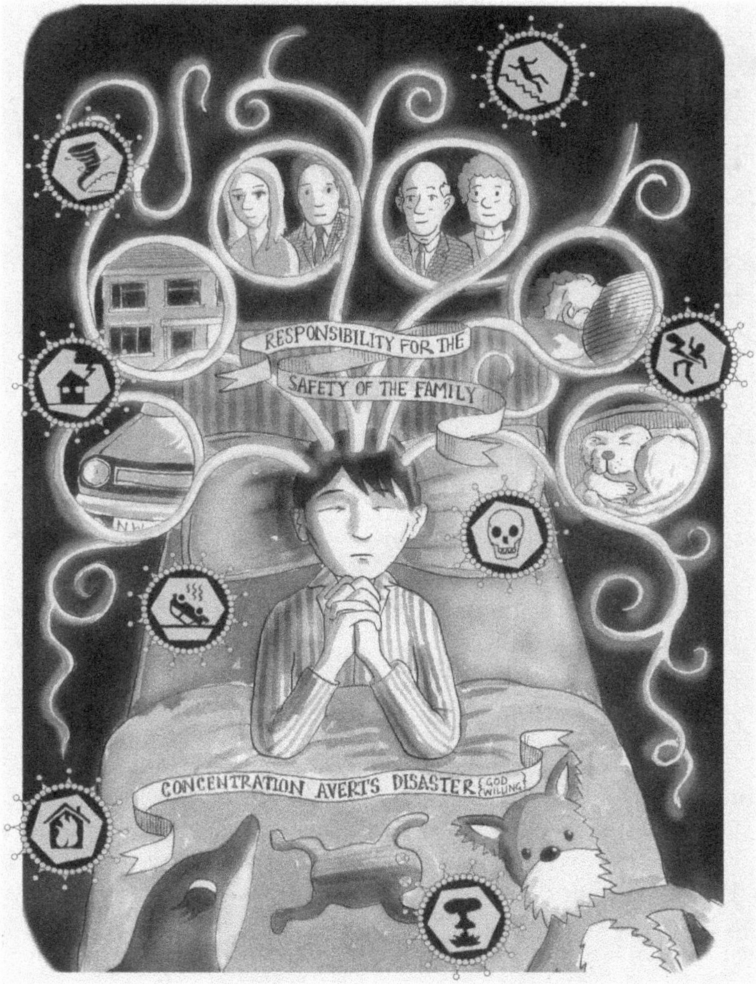
RESPONSIBILITY FOR THE
SAFETY OF THE FAMILY
CONCENTRATION AVERTS DISASTER
GOD WILLING

Figure 22.3 Ian Williams, *The Bad Doctor*, Myriad Editions, 2014, p. 57

OCD as a problem of doubt: comics as truth

In *A Condition of Doubt: the Meanings of Hypochondria*, scholar Catherine Belling outlines the history of the eponymous condition – the constant fear that a serious physical disease is present despite doctors' failure to find corroborating objective evidence (84). This sad condition can be a feature of OCD, and indeed, the term hypochondriac was sometimes applied to male patients with OCD (female patients being hysterics) (Cooke 283). That constant, gnawing doubt that hypochondriacs feel despite reassurance is the same repetitive doubt that forms the core of many peoples' OCD (Findberg 7) – doubt about one's motives, character, morals, and unconscious desires. A good friend of mine, a very mild-mannered cartoonist, spent his adolescence in perpetual doubt over whether he might be a latent murderer. He experienced violent intrusive images of murder that were so repugnant and distressing to him that he doubted his own moral makeup. He has not murdered anyone thus far, but there is, I suppose, still time.

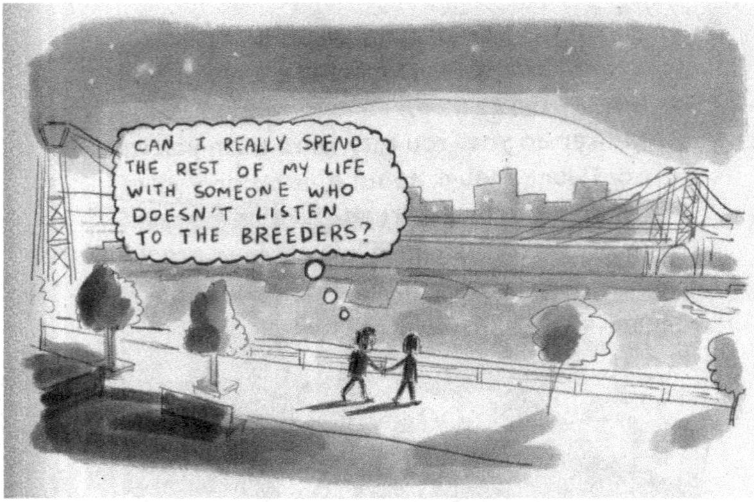
CAN I REALLY SPEND THE REST OF MY LIFE WITH SOMEONE WHO DOESN'T LISTEN TO THE BREEDERS?

Figure 22.4 Jason Adam Katzenstein, *Everything Is An Emergency*, Harper, 2020, p. 133

In *Everything Is an Emergency* (2020), Jason Adam Katzenstein, a cartoonist for *Mad Magazine* and the *New Yorker*, touches on the common theme for obsessional doubt: relationships (Figure 22.4). "Am I with the right person? Do I love them enough? Is this how it's supposed to feel? How do other people feel? Would we be better off apart? Is this healthy or codependent? Am I slowly ruining my partners life? Am I making a mistake? Can I love? Can I be loved?" (132). An already anxious child, Jason is traumatized at an early age by his parents' divorce and their subsequent new relationships. His world had been dismantled. It is not surprising, perhaps, that one of the themes of his OCD is his relationships with significant others. He is also obsessed with dirt and contamination and with inadvertently causing harm to others. Katzenstein illustrates the circular nature of his recurring doubts and anxieties by drawing himself with a record player on his head which voices his fears.

Alison Bechdel, winner of a MacArthur Genius Award,, illustrates the malignant doubt of OCD in her classic "autography," *Fun Home* (2006) which tells the story of her childhood and adolescence growing up in the eponymous **fun**eral home which is run by her undertaker and interior designer father. The story also tells of her father's untimely death, possibly by suicide, and of her realization that she is queer. Bechdel, a meticulous chronicler of her own life, sees her propensity to autobiography as a compulsion (140). Although her OCD encompasses counting, negotiating invisible negative forces, arranging objects, and a complex bedtime ritual, pervasive doubt is clearly demonstrated in her adolescent diaries. Bechdel became a compulsive diarist when her OCD was already established. As she lays down the mundane happenings of each day, she experiences a "sort of epistemological crisis" (141): how did she know that the things she was writing were absolutely, objectively *true*? She begins to pepper the text with the minutely lettered phrase, "I think," between her comments. Not satisfied that these "I thinks" are enough to satisfy her doubts, she begins to re-ink them repeatedly fortifying them until they are blots (142). Typically, however, feeding the monster makes it stronger, and Bechdel's doubts expand. To save time she creates a shorthand version of "I think": a curvy circumflex, which becomes an "amulet, warding off evil from [her] subjects" (142). Soon she is drawing this caret sign over whole entries. This is an example of how the logic of obsessionality defies the real world rules of science – people with OCD worry that they will cause harm by stray thoughts or bring disaster by not carrying out a particular compulsive ritual. They may not wholly believe these things, a degree of insight delineates OCD from psychosis, but magical thinking abounds nonetheless. So little surprise then, if the rules of the objective world are flexible, how is one to trust one's own perceptions and beliefs?

Bechdel's doubts about the veracity of her diary entries echo a broader concern that has dogged the autobiographical genre since its inception: is it all true? Worn down by her anxiety, she concludes that "all [she] could speak for was [her] own perceptions, and perhaps not even those" (141). "Is it autobiography if parts of it are not true?" asks comics guru and "Accidental Professor" Lynda Barry in the Introduction to *One Hundred Demons* (2017). "Is it fiction if parts of it are?" Barry's solution to these questions is to term her books "autobifictionography." The comic strip, with its hybrid, visual-verbal nature, is so obviously constructed, drawing attention to its own artificiality, that there is little need for the artist to make any grand claims for truth, yet the perceived honesty of what is portrayed serves to convince the reader of the emotional, if not the literal, truth of what is being shown. Charles Hatfield calls this effect "ironic authentication" (125). As Bechdel suggests, and as anyone with OCD can attest, it is difficult to know what absolute truth is, and, as Gilmore points out, conversations about truth telling, "salutary as they are, can be inimical to the ways in which some writers bring trauma stories into language" (14). Maybe this willingness to be loose with the facts in the name of making a good story explains, at least in part, why autobiographical comics have proved so popular over the last couple of decades.

OCD as creativity: comics as a therapy

Much has been written about the supposed link between mental illness and creativity (e.g. Jamieson 1989, Rothenberg 1990, Andreason and Glick 1988), but most writing seems to concentrate on the effect of mental illness *on* creativity. The mad, inspired artist is a hackneyed cliché. In his book *Strong Imagination – Madness, Creativity and Human Nature* (2001), Daniel Nettle describes how personality traits for psychoticism aids creativity, how the persistent elevated mood of hypomania allows increased production of work, and how schyzotypy aids divergent and original thinking. Little, however, has been written about mental illness *as* creativity, and I wonder why this should be. What is the difference between the complex theatre of delusional thinking, detailed in biro or email by a patient with psychosis and a short fantasy story by a creative writing undergraduate? Creativity and psychosis, Rothenburg suggests, are very close in terms of thought process, but creativity is *deliberate and healthy thinking*, and psychosis is not (36). Does creativity have to be deliberate, intentional? I am thinking about the actual mental processes that are integral to the disease – that pattern of circular thinking and novel associations that may be caused by depression. Is that creativity? The OCD mind is on overdrive and, unbidden, cannot help but construct vast tableaux of horrific narratives, hung with webs of overvalued ideas and rendered with fear. I have spent an awful lot of time and energy on my own OCD, and when I have tried to turn the neural networks of virally proliferating thoughts into drawings, I find that the art falls significantly short of the complexity of interconnected associations that my mind has constructed. I may still get there: I envisage the thought processes of OCD as some kind of humongous branching tree of possibilities and pathways, made out of the thinnest individual wires, that would need great effort to construct. OCD is exhausting, and, for the most part, materially unproductive, but does a project have to have a tangible product, to be "creative," or can it be wholly destructive? Conceptual artists might argue for the latter.

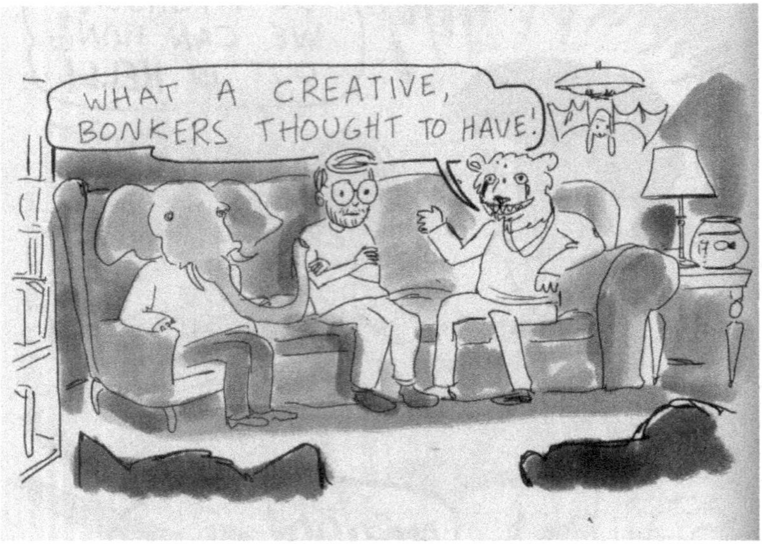

Figure 22.5 Jason Adam Katzenstein, *Everything Is An Emergency*, Harper, 2020, p. 206

Creativity, suggests Rothenburg, is very positively valued (3) and involves the production of something that is both *new* and truly valuable (5). That is one definition, and it may be true that mental illness will tend to distort and destroy the positive value of the product in any area, but it has also led to an awful lot of good comics. The question, "what is creativity," is surely as knotty as the similar question, "what is art?" or, indeed, "what is truth?" Jason Adam Katzenstein draws links between his illness and his creative process, seeing his snowballing anxious thinking as analogous to the way he comes up with jokes for the *New Yorker* magazine (185) (Figure 22.5). The way that one anxious thought seems to extrapolate to another, with tenuously related possible calamities, mirrors the way he manages to make surreal connections between otherwise unrelated comedic elements: "It's not that I need to be anxious to make art, but that the way my thoughts spiral can lead me towards creative conclusions and anxious ones." He also feels that his illness is possibly related to being creative (as well as the other way round): "One tactic I learned in therapy is to call my distressing thoughts a product of my 'creative brain'" (183).

Like madness, the making of good art requires a certain loosening of logic and meaning. In comics, as in painting, poetry or songwriting, the viewer, listener or reader must be allowed some room for her own interpretation and insertion of her own experiences. Just as artfully vague song lyrics invite poetic interpretation, the decoding of a comic involves audience participation – the reader turns the staccato series of drawings separated by white spaces or gutters (where the movement and action occur) into something more like a lived experience, animated in the mind (McCloud 68). Madness may exist in the human species because it is an extreme form of normal human cognition, and the extreme forms produce both good and bad outcomes (Nettle 159). Most people with mental illness are unproductive. Those who lay their thoughts down in writing, emails, blogs, and complaints to politicians might find themselves dismissed, ignored, and ridiculed, or their output used as evidence against them, but there is a significant place in the culture market for outsider art, shamanic storytelling, and the music of Daniel Johnston, who also produced visual art and comic books. Insanity is surely a relative concept, a social construct which is culturally specific, and the promotion of the products depends upon marketing, context, contemporary relevance, privilege and perceived aesthetic value that can also be linked to notoriety or fame. Most treatises on madness and creativity published in English are situated within a western, capitalist worldview and written by white people. The supposed link also presents researchers with a difficult subject to quantify: science tends to assume that all creative output is equal when, of course, it is not (Zara 14), and the concept of mental illness is itself protean, varying from the definitions found in the Diagnostic and Statistical Manual of Mental Disorders (itself a contentious publication) via a myriad of professional-or-self-identified states, to a label applied by governments or institutions to those who do not share their aims and views.

Storytelling and healing have been linked since ancient times, and the disclosure of one's story forms part of the psychotherapeutic treatment of trauma. Herman (1997) suggests that "given the 'iconic' visual nature of traumatic memories, creating pictures may represent the most effective initial approach to these 'indelible images'" (178). I have written elsewhere about graphic autobiography as "auto-therapy" (Williams, "Autography as Auto-Therapy"). Justin Green's making of *Binky Brown Meets the Holy Virgin Mary* was, by definition, a self-styled effort at self-exorcism, based possibly on a romantic, though traditionally understandable, notion of catharsis. Moreover, the making of comics is being used in the treatment of mental distress. At the Center For Cartoon Studies in White River Junction, Vermont, the faculty works with members of the Veterans Association to turn the ex-soldiers' traumatic experiences into graphic narrative. "Comics," says CCS Faculty member and cartoonist James Sturm, "are a therapeutic blowtorch and so far we have only lit a few cigarettes with them" (Personal correspondence 2016).

The comics form is complex, compact, and well suited for those of a visual disposition to rebuild their fractured world. As Alison Mitchell states: "planes of reality can coexist in the diegetic space of a comic – daily life, fantasy, spirit world, dream-space, myth, historical past, allegory, metaphor, metonym" (258), which is ideal to illustrate the perceptual dynamics and thought processes or of OCD. In his masterful graphic novel, *The Nao of Brown* (2012), Glynn Dillon shows his protagonist, Nao, slumped over her desk having completed her daily therapeutic "homework," which she uses to try to combat her OCD. As well as writing out her intrusive violent fantasies, Nao also draws her fear of uncontrollably stabbing a pregnant woman with a pen (Figure 22.6). She is able to draw like this, of course, because Dillon is an expert draughtsman: this page serves as a brilliant meta-example of therapeutic storytelling.

Conclusion

There are other works I could have mentioned in this essay, but space prevents it: Hannah Eaton's *Naming Monsters* and John Porcellino's *Map of My Heart* are both graphic novels which allude to, without naming, OCD. *Stand Up to OCD* (Wood and Fletcher, 2019) is a self-help comic book, aimed at teenagers, in which the condition is anthropomorphized as a nasty looking reptilian creature. Artist Lily Williams publishes web comics about her OCD on her website, and many other cartoonists have drawn their condition and posted the work online, thus garnering feedback and affirmation and, perhaps, creating therapeutic bubbles or communities in the process. Comics are good at broadcasting the voices of those who might not otherwise be heard – queer folks, people with disabilities, and the mentally ill or "mad" – demographics who get 'othered' by the political classes and mainstream media. This, incidentally, is an example of the "autobiographical paradox" (Gilmore 19) in which the unusual or unrepresentative life becomes representative.

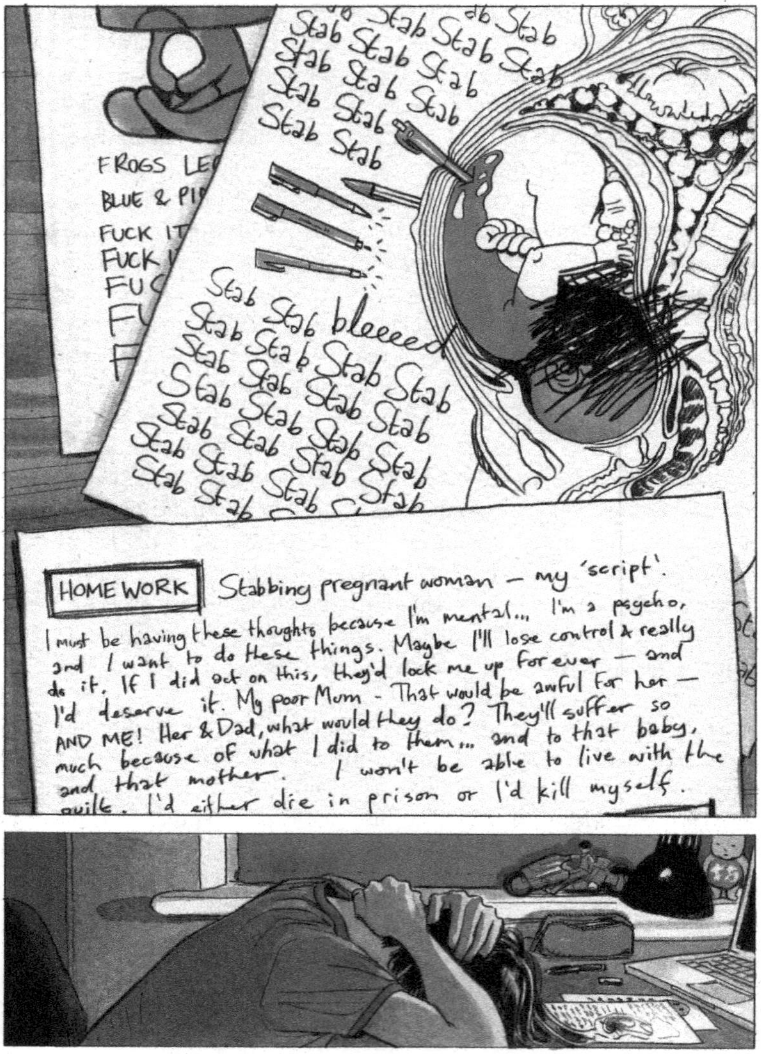

Figure 22.6 Glyn Dillon, *The Nao of Brown*, Self Made Hero, 2012, p. 121

In summary, authors of graphic memoirs of OCD depict their conditions and their experiences, creating valuable new knowledge, which informs the iconography of illness, and influencing the way that others think of or experience the condition. The comics medium is a powerful tool which, in skilled hands, can create intensely absorbing narratives through which the reader enters into the world of the author, creating empathic bonds between the two. The multiple planes of reality, coexistent in the panels of the comic, can mirror the novel perceptions of OCD sufferers, and the creatively "bonkers" thinking that builds their mad world. However, how much one can understand another's psyche remains open to question, and, given that for me at least, OCD at its worst was a kind of living hell, so why would anyone *want* to enter the author's mind? Readers do, however, gain insight into the condition, and one of my particular interests in comics is what healthcare professionals might glean from reading them. Their attractive and inventive artwork makes them, I think, more enjoyable to consume than prose memoirs or depictions of the disease. Making a comic about one's illness is a way of meditating on and objectifying the condition. It is perhaps a form of therapy; although, to be honest, I could only make the book after I was better. At the height of the illness, I was too anxious and too disordered to make any work about it. There are also, of course, risks associated with putting oneself "out there," whatever the medium, but aside from the occasional acid comment on social media, I have found my own autobiographical performance to be, on the whole, deeply rewarding. I found my voice in comics and making a story out of my experiences allowed me to shed the shame associated with this troublesome condition.

Works cited

Andreasen, Nancy C. and Ira D. Glick. "Bipolar Affective Disorder and Creativity: Implications and Clinical Management," *Comprehensive Psychiatry*, vol. 29, 1988, pp. 207–17.

Barry, Lynda. *One! Hundred! Demons!* Drawn and Quarterly, 2017.

Bechdel, Alison. *Fun Home – a Family Tragicomic.* London: Jonathan Cape, 2006.

Belling, Catherine. *A Condition of Doubt – The Meanings of Hypochondria.* Oxford: Oxford University Press, 2012.

Bourret, Adam. *I'm Crazy.* Self-published, 2009.

Cooke, Alistair. "Hypochondria: The Layman's Specialty." The 1972 Lloyd-Roberts Lecture. *Journal of the Royal College of Physicians of London*, vol. 7, 1973, pp. 277–96.

Davis, Lennard. *Obsession.* Chicago: University of Chicago Press, 2008.

Dillon, Glyn. *The Nao of Brown.* London: Self Made Hero, 2012.

Eaton, Hannah. *Naming Monsters.* Brighton: Myriad Editions, 2013.

El Refaie, Elizabeth.*Autobiographical Comics – Life Writing In Pictures.* Jackson, MS: University Press of Mississippi, 2012.

Findberg, Naomi, Donaello Marazziti, and Dan J. Stein, eds. *Obsessive Compulsive Disorder: A Practical Guide.* London: Dunnitz, 2001.

Galvin, Margaret. "Thinking Through Thea: Alison Bechdel's Representations of Disability."*Disability in Comic Books and Graphic Narratives*, edited by Chris Foss et al., London: Palgrave Macmillan, 2016, pp. 187–202.

Gilman, Sander. *Disease and Representation: Images of Illness from Madness to AIDS.* Ithaca, N.Y.: Cornell University Press, 1988.

Gilmore, Leigh. *The Limits of Autobiography – Trauma and Testimony.* Ithaca, N.Y.: Cornell University Press, 2001.

Green, Justin. 1972. "Binky Brown Meets the Holy Virgin Mary." *Justin Green's Binky Brown Sampler*, edited by J. Green. San Francisco, CA: Last Gasp, 1995.

Green, Justin. *Binky Brown Meets The Holy Virgin Mary.* San Francisco, CA: McSweeney's, 2009.

Green, Michael and Kimberly Myers. "Graphic Medicine: Use of Comics in Medical Education and Patient Care." *British Medical Journal*, vol. 340, 2010, p. c863.

Hatfield, Charles. *Alternative Comics – An Emerging Literature.* Jackson, MS: University Press of Mississippi 2005.

Herman, Judith Lewis. *Trauma and Recovery.* New York: Basic Books, 1997.

Jamieson, Kay R. "Mood Disorders and Patterns of Creativity in British Writers and Artists." *Psychiatry*, vol. 52, 1989, pp. 125–34.

Katzenstein, Jason Adam. *Everything Is An Emergency.* New York: Harper Perennial, 2020.

Koch, Kristina Maria. "When You Have No Voice You Don't Exist"?: Envisioning Disability in David Small's Stitches." *Disability in Comic Books and Graphic Narratives*, edited by C. Foss, J. W. Gray, and Z. Whalen. London. Palgrave Macmillan, 2016, p. 29.

McCloud, Scott. *Understanding Comics.* New York: Harper Collins, 1993.

Mitchell, Alison. "Distributed Identity: Networking Image Fragments in Graphic Memoirs." *Studies in Comics*, vol. 1, 2010, pp. 197–211.

Nettle, Daniel. *Strong Imagination – Madness, Creativity and Human Nature.* Oxford: Oxford University Press, 2001.

Porcellino, John. *Map of My Heart*. Montreal: Drawn and Quarterly, 2010.
Rothenberg, Albert. *Creativity and Madness: New Findings and Old Stereotypes*. Baltimore, MD: Johns Hopkins University Press, 1990.
Spandler, Helen. "Grafting Psychiatric Contention through Single Panel Cartoons." *Pathographics: Narrative, Aestherics, Contention, Community*, edited by S. M. Squier and I. M. Kruger-Furhoff. University Park, PA: Penn State Press, 2020, p. 127.
Williams, Ian. "Autography as Auto-Therapy: Psychic Pain and the Graphic Memoir. *Journal of Medical Humanities*, vol. 32, 2011, pp. 353–66.
Williams, Ian. *The Bad Doctor*. Brighton: Myriad Editions, 2014.
Williams, Ian. "Comics and the Iconography of Illness." *Graphic Medicine Manifesto*, edited by Czerwiec, Williams et al. University Park, PA: Penn State Press, 2015, pp. 115–42.
Williams, Lily. O.C.D. Comics. https://lilywilliamsart.com/portfolio/ocdcomics/
Whitlock, Gillian. "Autographics: The Seeing 'I' of Comics." *MFS Modern Fiction Studies*, vol. 52, no. 4, Winter 2006, pp. 965–79.
Wood, Kelly and Fletcher, Douglas. *Stand Up to OCD!* London: Jessica Kingsley Publishers, 2019.
Zara, Christopher. *Tortured Artists*. Avon, MA: Adams Media, 2012.

23

"I FOUND BALANCE"

Complementary and alternative medicine in selected graphic medical narratives

Sathyaraj Venkatesan

In her review of John Porcellino's autobiographical comic, *The Hospital Suite* (2014), Hannah, a reader for the social cataloging website *Goodreads,* observes that "questionable medical and cult choices are made while disregarding everything science has to say." John Porcellino's memoir, *The Hospital Suite* concerns his illness during the 1990s and early 2000s and how he seeks solace in Buddhist philosophy and alternative medical practices. Hannah's response to the alternative and complementary health interventions in *The Hospital Suite* captures a common attitude about non-western complementary and alternative medicine (hereafter CAM). Although the use of non-western medical practices has dramatically risen in recent times, skepticism toward these methodologies is still prevalent. Unlike the reductionist and biomedical approach of diagnosis and treatment, CAM treats the patient-experience as paramount and is predicated on the interrelationship of body, mind, and spirit. Graphic medicine, a productive intersection of comics and health care, is one of the sites that examines complex and nuanced issues related to alternative and traditional medicine. In addition to explicit descriptions of CAM practices, graphic medical narratives also express their philosophies of health/illness/wellbeing through symbols, images, and conceits.

The present chapter investigates non-western medical practices, modes of healing, and philosophies of health/wellbeing through a close reading of Ellen Forney's *Marbles: Mania, Depression, Michelangelo, and Me* (2012) (hereafter *Marbles*) and Glyn Dillon's *The Nao of Brown* (2012), concentrating on the practices of yoga[1] and meditation and the use of symbols such as yin yang as non-medical health interventions. In addition to providing both theoretical and historical background on the practices associated with CAM, this chapter foregrounds various types and expressions of CAM, demonstrating how the selected texts both underscore the collective/individual benefits of CAM and also expand the boundaries of health, medicine and treatment.

Introduction to CAM

Before addressing graphic medicine's engagement with CAM, it may be instructive to consider basic and pertinent questions such as: what is CAM? why is it increasingly used in recent times? and what are the dominant attitudes toward it? CAM as a medical concept is "a collection

DOI: 10.4324/9781003007661-30

of disparate healing practices" (Ruggie 3). Given the wide range of interventional types, the National Center for Complementary and Alternative Medicine (NCCAM) has grouped CAM into five domains: mind–body interventions (for example, yoga); alternative systems of medical practice (for example, herbal and homeopathic medicines); manual healing methods (for example, chiropractic); pharmacological and biological treatments (for example, Neural therapy); and energy therapies (for example, reiki, healing touch, polarity therapy) (Ruggie 4–6). While some practices are self-administered such as prayers and meditation, others are institutionalized systems such as massage therapy and yoga. Put differently, CAM is not a monolithic phenomenon but rather encompasses an assortment of health therapies and practices shaped by divergent philosophies and epistemologies. It is holistic, natural, and patient-centered and typically constructed in opposition to the mainstream medical paradigm, specifically western/allopathic medicine, which merely focuses on diagnosis and treatment.

Challenging the reductionist and dualistic (mind versus body) biomedical approach toward health and disease conditions, CAM sits at the nexus of the metaphysical and the empirical with its emphasis on patient-centered experience. For Mary Ruggie, Harvard sociologist, CAM is a "social transformation" (xiii) of health care which "poses huge challenges not only to the dominance of biomedicine, but also to the fruits of dominance – status and power in decision making about health care and in the livelihood of physicians" (13). Ironically, the reductionism of biomedicine is amplified by the Human Genome project, which reduces every disease condition to genetic and molecular levels at the expense of the role of larger than life forces such as the environment and phenotypic traits. As opposed to the dominant medical paradigm, which segregates disease from the suffering body and attempts to implement a cure through diagnosis and treatment procedures (even at the level of molecular level), CAM unites mind, body, and world with an emphasis on self-care and wellness. As such, it goes well beyond simply eliminating symptoms and treating the sufferer. As Foss rightly observes, CAM is "a concept of medicine as a science of the human person and insists on an understanding of disease as something that involves a systematic dislocation of the whole person, not just of the body" (126). That is, CAM at once embraces the environment and self-healing values as well as existential, personal and communal needs in the process of healing and curing the sufferer. Moreover, CAM is not just a method or a protocol but a way of healthy living drawing on various philosophical schools of thought. Elaborating on the diversified conceptual and philosophical frameworks of CAM, Ruggie maintains that "Each therapy has its own practices and products, practitioners make recommendations based on the particular approach to healing found in their field of practice and practitioners within the same field may differ in their interpretation of the information they have about any one patient" (9). Although the binary of CAM versus western allopathic mainstream medicine is encouraged, "there are deep divisions within both 'communities' as well as 'between them'" (9), as Ruggie notes in *Marginal to Mainstream*.

A number of factors account for an increased interest in CAM. These include structural and cultural changes in health care; the transformation in authority relations between doctors and patients; over-medicalization; the search for a meaningful understanding of one's existential and disease conditions; patient autonomy; and dissatisfaction with the current biomedical system. However, despite the dramatic increase in the use of CAM such as the rise of integrative medicine clinics, CAM typically receives mixed reactions. Citing Gale and McHale, Brosnan et al. sum up the dominant attitude thus: "CAM is dismissed as 'quackery' by some, while others ardently defend it based on their own experiences of use" (1). In 1998, Phil Fontanarosa and George Lundberg would declare that "there is no alternative medicine" and further contend that there is "only scientifically proven, evidence-based medicine supported by solid data or unproven medicine, for which data is lacking" (1618).

Graphic medicine: an overview

As an interdisciplinary field, graphic medicine refers to the "intersection of the medium of comics and the discourse of healthcare" (Czerwiec et al. 1). It combines the principles of narrative medicine with an exploration of the visual systems of comic art and seeks to represent psychosomatic conditions. In practice, graphic medicine encompasses the use of visuals in the education of patients and healthcare professionals as well as the creation and reading of comics about the illness experience from a wide-range of perspectives and scholarly inquiry. As such, graphic medicine provides a way to analyze "different traditions to regain those forgotten dimensions of health and illness and to see what a postmodern culture can retain or even take as a starting point for a new understanding" (Mordacci and Sobel 37). Often biographical or autobiographical, graphic medicine as a subfield of health humanities combines "subjective feelings and perception with objective representation" (Czerweic 19). In so doing, it disrupts the normative approaches of comprehending and visualizing illness and disease. Put differently, in giving prominence to the experiences of patients, caregivers, and physicians, graphic medicine unfolds "unvoiced relationships, unarticulated emotions, unspoken possibilities and even unacknowledged alternative perspectives" (Squier 130), which are often overlooked by the traditional healthcare, diagnostic and treatment systems.

Unlike verbal texts, graphic medicine combines the affordances of word and image. Comics also invests in six meaning-making elements as identified by Bill Cope and Mary Kalantzis: "Linguistic Meaning, Visual Meaning, Audio Meaning, Gestural Meaning, Spatial Meaning, and the Multimodal patterns of meaning that relate the first five modes of meaning to each other" (7). Besides such multimodal affordances, the visual economy, a near-universal language of lines, sequentiality, balloons, and panels also convey the "unsettling worries and concerns that may be difficult to articulate through words alone" (Squier 128). Furthermore, it bears witness to how minds and bodies exist in space and time, and thus facilitates our understanding of others' experience better than that available in words alone. This is not to argue for comics exceptionalism but to highlight how its intrinsic nature (sequentiality, multimodality etc.) is befitting and apposite to enunciate the conventional and extraordinary, differences and homogeneity, banal and uncommon, and binaries and non-dualisms.

Texts and contexts: *Marbles* and *The Nao of Brown*

Ellen Forney's acutely personal and visually dynamic graphic memoir, *Marbles* (2012), documents her four years of struggle with and effects of bipolar disorder in her life. While *Marbles* concerns Forney's ricocheting between mania and depressive conditions, it also chronicles a tale of "long pharmacopic trek towards balance," as Alison Bechdel notes (*Marbles* n.p). Upon diagnosis, it is the effect of tranquilizers and medication on her creativity that terrifies Forney: "art was my blood, my heart, my life. I'd always been terrified at the thought of going blind, but what if I couldn't even think creatively?" (24). In the process of finding balance and stability, Forney offers a visceral delineation of the healing powers of CAM. Accordingly, she not only lays bare the processes of rehabilitation and self-recovery but also deploys conceits and symbols such as yin yang. *Marbles*, for instance, opens with Forney referencing white-light energy traveling through her body, suggestive of *kundalini*. *Kundalini* refers to a vital unrealized force within us which unfolds through seven *chakras* or energy centers.

Glyn Dillon's fictional *The Nao of Brown* concerns Nao, a half-Japanese girl, suffering from obsessive compulsive disorder (OCD). Plagued by distressing mental rituals, Nao endures violent morbid obsessions and homicidal and intrusive thoughts of violence toward others. As a part of her struggle to advance her career, she works part-time at a designer vinyl toy shop and searches for the love of her life. As OCD is closely linked with depression, Nao combats her destructive feelings with the repeated invocation of "Mum thinks I'm good" as well as reminding herself that other people don't think she is a horrible monster capable of murdering children. What unites these two, otherwise disparate texts is not only the portrayal of challenging mental conditions but also their exploration of a range of CAM practices.

Graphic medical texts present CAM in mixed ways – negative, ambivalent, or positive. While some texts foreground the positive benefits of CAM, others imagine it as creating harm. For instance, David B's *Epileptic* presents a negative impact of alternative medicine on Jean-Christophe and his family, while John Porcellino in *Hospital Suite* turns to self-administered practices such as prayers, meditation, and alternative treatments such as acupuncture and naturopathy to treat his multiple ailments including abdominal pains, OCD, and hyperacusis. Porcellino also pursues well-being enhancement practices such as yoga, psychotherapy, and Buddhism. In the appendix section of the book, for instance, Porcellino introduces "Zen Stories," which are often used during meditation to facilitate non-reasoning, "Heart Sutra" scriptures of the Mahayana tradition of Buddhism and part of the *Prajnaparamita Sutras*, which offers a metaphysical apparatus to cope with his diseased condition. In fact, his alternative practices help him realize the emptiness of life, different psychological states, and more importantly, reflect on the transient nature of life itself. Furthermore, they also help him to segue into imaginative mindfulness, which allows him to disown the static past and attend on the present.

"I found balance": yoga and balancing the poles

Forney's *Marbles* foregrounds the healing benefits of CAM. In fact, the memoir is steeped in philosophies of yoga – its techniques, symbols, conceits and images. Based in Indian philosophy, yoga (approximately 3,000 years old) means 'union' and involves a mix of breathing (*pranayama*), meditation techniques, physical poses/movements (*asanas*) and moral practices. In practice, yoga enhances the capacities of body and mind, helps discover spiritual essence and higher conscious states of the human being, augments emotional wellbeing, and promotes balance. Most important, yoga is at once a physical, ethical, moral, and philosophical practice which aims at cultivating a focused state of mind and ethics of self-care. Such a lifelong work on one's body and mind not only requires *abhyasa* but also *vairagyam*. When practiced together, they can minimize and even eliminate perturbations of the mind and body. While *abhyasa* refers to self-disciplined practice, *vairagyam* alludes to detachment/surrender. Within the framework of yoga, surrender is not weakness but discipline toward the life forces/divinity/laws of nature, which results in a positive self-appraisal, mindfulness, and harmony. Forney's *Marbles* dramatizes many of these principles of yoga in explicit and positive ways.

Forney is introduced to yoga by her psychiatrist, Karen. At the outset, Karen admits that finding a right set of medicines to treat Forney's bipolar disorder condition will be "a long process of trying different things before finding what works" (25). In one interaction, Karen cites some studies and asks Forney whether she has ever tried yoga. Although Forney initially deems yoga as a "wishy-washy non-competitive new age stretching fad" (26), she eventually and grudgingly pursues it one year after diagnosis. Despite "feeling graceless," "weak," and hating her yoga teacher (110), Forney forces herself to attend one yoga class per week. In a comic-within-comic titled, "Wednesday Morning Yoga," she subtly mocks yoga's spiritual tendencies, and the sequence ends with Forney smoking a cigarette (125–6). In some instances, she also uses the yoga center as a venue for crying and "secretly revealing her insides" (125). However, Forney's skepticism about yoga changes to a new acceptance over time.

During Forney's classes, her instructor emphasizes breathing exercises *pranayama*, which reliably facilitates the opening up of subtle channels of mind and body. In one of the pages, Forney illustrates five different yoga postures – *Surya Namaskar* (Sun Salutation), *Balasana* (Child's pose), *Sethubandhasana* (Bridge pose), *Shavasana, Pranayama* and *Vajrasana* – and annotates each *asana* (posture) while performing them. For instance, while performing *Balasana,* Forney correlates the posture to her curling up when she experiences depression ("Curling inside was familiar") (110). Initially, Forney pursues yoga as a mere physical activity ("my neighbour told me yoga was 'slimming'") (110), as a milder alternative to the energy guzzling, "rigorous" and "competitive" (110) activities such as swimming and as a "good" way "to spend time with other people" (110). Having said that, she eventually experiences inner peace, and, in a self-portrait titled "peace mission" (111), readers see a meditative and self-indulgent Forney with ear plugs. Much later, Forney integrates yoga into the circle of her life activities. In minute jottings, Forney links her self-identity to yoga, treats it as a therapy and plans on attending more workshops/retreats. That is, she soon realizes the positive benefits of yoga including its assured ways to improve mindfulness, self-control, and pacification.

Elsewhere, describing her condition, Forney observes that "my mood swings weren't extreme, but it was a struggle to keep myself grounded" (173), and, in her journal, she mentions "crying, curled in a ball under a blanket on the rug - - calmed down and did some alternate nostril breathing" (174). In one of her intensely restless, anxious, and "emotionally bowled" moments, visually expressed as untethered balloons in the wind (176), Forney practices alternate nostril breathing called *Nadi Sodhana Pranayama* (174), a dynamic technique for relaxation and calming the mind. *Nadi* refers to the energy channel, and *sodhana* means purification. *Yogis* consider it to be one of the superior ways to calm the nervous system and achieve mental discipline. *Pranayama* commences with an exhalation and an inhalation through the left nostril, followed by a full breath through the right with the whole pattern repeated several times. Forney resorts to this breathing practice to experience the harmony of body and mind and oneness of mind and breath. In fact, Forney presents a detailed diagram and clear instructions in a "do it yourself (DIY)" format and notes that "these faces are reversed so it's like you're looking into a mirror" so that readers are not confused (174). The six elliptical images of Forney with closed eyes illustrate the ancient adage, "When the breath wanders the mind is unsteady. But when the breath is calmed, the mind too will be still" (Svatmarama 5).

Frequently adjusting western allopathic medications and yoga, Forney eventually finds peace through investing in multiple techniques of yoga. After class, she writes in her journal: "I am so at peace. . . is this what it's like to practice yoga all the time?" (186). Finding herself neither "manicky" (186) nor depressed, she frames her yoga experience positively with terms such as "blissed-out," "beautiful," "magical," "good, "and "so cute" (186). Elsewhere, she characterizes her change as, "I can feel myself . . . healing" (186) and reassures the readers' of the benefits of yoga. She soon finds the much desired stability and meaning in her life, and she expresses the sense of balance, wholeness, and self-realization ("finally after four years . . . I found balance") by balancing on one leg on a yoga mat (197). In fact, her mission to find balance and gain stability, "balancing the dark with the light without comprising either" (29), augurs well with the project and broader aims of yoga itself. Much later, Forney also introduces the idea of *vairagyam* or philosophical detachment and surrender. Elaborating on the word 'surrender' lest the reader misinterprets it as weakness, Forney explains: "not meaning defeat, but acceptance, recognition, release – like floating down a river" (195). Put differently, 'surrender' in the context of yoga implies serving oneself to a higher purpose and a dedicated resolve. In practicing *vairagyam*, Forney fashions and forges a philosophical self and affirms the integrity of herself.

Toward the end of the memoir, Forney realizes that the best way to deal with her bipolar condition is to evolve a "multifaceted treatment plan" (229) which includes medicines, proper diet, blood tests, swimming, and yoga. It takes several years for her to balance both Western biomedicine and CAM, especially yoga, into her regimen. In her non-fictional statement, *Rock Steady*, she describes different ways of dealing with bipolar disorder as SMEDMERTS: Sleep, Meds, Eat, Doctor, Mindfulness, Exercise, Routine, and Support system. In addition, she introduces an inventory of self-care techniques such as meditation, journal writing, mantras, and music.

In her attempt to find stillness, purpose, and quietude of mind, Forney accepts and experiences the positive benefits of yoga. It helps her to minimize her pre-diagnostic habit of regularly smoking marijuana and frequent masturbation. While there are several medical reports and articles that demonstrate how meditation and yoga calms and makes one less stressful, Forney's *Marbles* is a visual testament about its benefits.

"Balancing the dark with the light": yin yang and other symbols

Reinforcing the distributive nature of mind and body, Forney imaginatively deploys a range of symbols which not only embody non-western, non-(bio)medical perspectives but also convey the fullness of an Eastern perspective and way of life. For instance, there is the Laughing Buddha which symbolizes good luck and prosperity; the third eye which alludes to non-dualistic thinking; the magic lamp which suggests the pinnacle of illumination and self-sacrifice; and the diamond that represents the oriental understanding of elemental alchemy (earth, air, water, fire). All these symbols articulate a non-western worldview of mind–body balance, spiritual entitlement, liberation, and mindfulness.

Among such symbols, yin yang emerges as the most important symbol in *Marbles*. Although its philosophy and its implications are available in the *I Ching/Yijing* ("Book of Changes"), yin yang, in simple terms, refers to the complementarity between two seemingly different fundamental forces. As an icon of familiar dualities such as light and dark, good-bad, well-ill, male-female, sun-moon, and water-fire, yin yang is a metaphorical and metaphysical abstraction of wholeness, entirety, and dynamism. Subscribing to the idea and ideal of duality, yin yang celebrates the essential integration of oppositions and the need to transcend them. It is commonly represented as a black dot in white background and vice versa and is called *T'ai chi* (or *Taiji*) or Supreme Ultimate.

Forney represents a divided self that yearns for oneness and balance through a separated yin and yang. Using dark and light/black and white, Forney reinforces her struggle for wholeness and balance through the visual language of yin yang. She conveys her new found affirmation with a drawing of a pair of black and white hands joined together. In the language of yin yang, Forney articulates the positive accommodation of her bipolarity: "for better & worse, bipolar disorder is an important part of who I am and how I think" (226). She realizes life's constant dynamic and brings together her poles of mania and depression for greater creative force. Put differently, yin yang functions as a deep structure, as an explanatory account, and as a health metaphor to diagram her inner desires and to convey mutual exclusivity and non-oppositional duality.

"The circle of life": OCD, Enso and *The Nao of Brown*

Dillion's graphic narrative, *The Nao of Brown*, extensively deploys multiple CAM-related practices particularly meditation to alleviate Nao's OCD experiences. As a rapidly increasing efficacious application, meditation (*dhyana*) is "a type of mind-body complementary medicine" (Mayo Clinic). As a typical CAM procedure, meditation involves restoration of balance to the individual and "members of the family or community," "specific places" or "sacred groves" (Bodeker and Burford 11). Nao, the protagonist in *The Nao of Brown,* suffers from violent obsessions, and her compulsions take the form of unseen mental rituals. Her OCD experience involves the constant fear and guilt of hurting someone; for instance, she confesses to her boyfriend, Gregory Pope, that, "IF I'm left alone with kids...or anyone smaller, or weaker than me...I get anxious. I'm worried I'll ***hurt*** them" (167) (italics and bold in original). In medical terms, Nao suffers from morbid obsessions, which include "intrusive unpleasant thoughts, unceasing doubt, guilt fears of being insane, and crushing anxiety" (Penzel). In fact, the presence of a pen or knife increases her violent thoughts, and she requires either internal or external validation that she is a good person. Against such a background, it is Nao's meditation as opposed to medication that assuages her.

As a Hafu (a half English and a half Japanese), Nao uses Eastern cultural symbols and the philosophies of Enso, Buddhism, and itchi to externalize, mitigate, and explain her illness experience. Nao's mentors, Nagarjuna and Ray (an art teacher at the Buddhist Center), teach her to quiet her mind through philosophical deliberations and Enso (the ink drawn circle). As a Zen symbol, Enso symbolizes "enlightenment," refinement and "an expression of the 'moment'" (28). In particular, Ray introduces the art work Thangkas, painting on silk or cotton to depict a Buddhist deity or scene, to his students while discussing the story of Palden Lhamo ("Glorious Goddess") or Shri Devi, a wrathful protector. Similarly, the long-eared and closed-eye Buddha at the Buddhist Center which Nao visits also cultivates in her a sense of tranquility and mindfulness. Although Nao acknowledges that she is not a devout Buddhist ("I don't call myself a Buddhist") (26), she visits the Center to mitigate her violent thoughts.

Likewise, the Japanese animation series, Itchi, whose faces are predominantly circular also liberates Nao from her morbid thoughts, providing a sense of quietude and peacefulness. When Nao learns that itchi facilitates control over her thoughts, she begins to draw them. In fact, she falls in love with Gregory because his face resembles an itchi character called Nothing. This image of a circle provides Nao with the sense of completion partly because she believes in the philosophy of Enso. Rooted in the Japanese and the Tibetan traditions of calligraphy and painting, Enso is a Zen Buddhist philosophy, which involves drawing a circle on paper with ink/paint brush in a single stroke. Such a method is a way of achieving *samaai,* the unification or absorption of the individual with the highest reality. Therefore, it is no surprise that an aspiring cartoonist and troubled OCD patient derives healing from the symbol of Enso. Interestingly, inspired by the Enso displayed in Nao's drawing room, Gregory also has an epiphany. When Nao explains the philosophy of Enso, Gregory associates the symbol with his washing machines, also circular in shape, and later, he shares a dream with Nao. In Gregory's dream, Nao appears as a Japanese Thangka and then changes into "Llkiyo...rising up out of a ***washing machine***" (106) (bold in original). Although Nao practices drawing the symbol of Enso religiously, she does not attain, at least in the beginning, the philosophical liberation that the symbol signifies.

To conclude, meditation not only facilitates Nao reaching a point of spiritual oneness with herself but also helps her find individual authenticity. Although her thoughts occasionally meander, she assures the readers that she knows "exactly where to look for solutions" (200). If yoga facilitates Forney's coming to terms with herself, it is Zen inspired Buddhist meditations that aid Nao in identifying the causes of her bondage and suffering. Toward the end, Nao understands that "[t]houghts don't really need to be kept in check," (196) just our attachment to them. Nao soon realizes the fundamental proposition of Buddhist philosophy; that is, the cause of suffering is found in the (sensory) attachment. As Nagarjuna makes it clear: "The experience is not the problem, it's the ***attachment*** to it" (197) (bold and italics in original). Further, the practice of meditation and its insights tranquilize Nao's mind and provide her with a confidence to focus on the "now." More importantly, it enables her "not to remain a prisoner to a fixed psychic configuration that is usually paralyzing and painful" (Malabou 45). As readers, we witness Nao's silent sitting (one of the four meditation poses in Buddhism) in multiple pages toward the end of the narrative. Finally, the Enso that she paints with her son contains no stroke of agitation which was present in almost all of her earlier paintings, signifying a general state of accomplishment, inner calm, and concentration (*dharana*). In short, meditation, as a healthcare intervention "heals" Nao in the original sense of the word, that is, "to make whole."

Coda

Complementary and alternative medicine refers to a broad range of health practices, taking different forms in different settings and embracing a variety of practices including meditation, acupuncture, massage, tai chi, yoga, and even drinking green tea. Central to CAM is the use of non-dominant and non-allopathic health philosophies, practices, and knowledge systems for the wellbeing and holistic improvement of the suffering person. Given the multiple perspectives and genres that constitute graphic medicine, it is not surprising that graphic medicine presents a wide variety of attitudes toward CAM. Predominant responses toward CAM in graphic medical narratives include indifference, ambivalence, and support. In *Marbles,* Forney not only confirms how CAM serves as an adjunctive practice but also ratifies how CAM shares the goal of health and healing of a medical treatment. Forney finds peace of mind, a sense of self-control, and definitive growth of her analytical individuality in yoga. As a (non)pharmacological effect on the human mind and body, CAM in *Nao of Brown* is imagined as a prophylactic and cathartic practice. Nao, the protagonist, through meditation finds individual authenticity and inner reflexivity, traits that resonate through the discourses of CAM and mind-body. Beyond being a mere health intervention, CAM in graphic medicine also appears as abstract tropes, as spiritual exercise, and as a way of life. While these tropes and symbols (for instance, yin and yang in *Marbles*) convey the abstract philosophical grammar of CAM, for Porcellino, CAM constitutes a way of life and a healthy foundation for human action. Put together, both *Marbles* and *Nao of Brown*, the chosen texts in this study, attest to the positive and therapeutic benefits of CAM practices particularly meditation/yoga.

Note

1 The foundational and the most important textual source of yoga is *Yoga Sutras* (aphorisms on yoga) written by Patanjali. As a collection of 196 Sanskrit *sutras* (aphorisms), *Yoga Sutras* concerns with nature of mind, inner peace, and methods toward steadiness of mind. Yoga predominantly focuses on healing as opposed to curing: while healing implies an intervention at the level of body-mind-spirit, curing suggests mere elimination or management of one's disease condition.

Works cited

Baer, Hans A. "The Work of Andrew Weil and Deepak Chopra: Two Holistic Health/New Age Gurus: A Critique of the Holistic Health/New Age Movements." *Medical Anthropology Quarterly*, vol. 17, no. 2, 2003, pp. 233–50.

Bechdel, Alison. "Marbles." 2020. www.penguinrandomhouse.com/books/308184/marbles-by-ellen-forney/.

Bodeker, Gerard, and Gemma Burford. *Traditional, Complementary and Alternative Medicine: Policy and Public Health Perspectives*. London: Imperial College Press, 2006.

Brosnan, Caragh, et al. "Introduction:Complementary and Alternative Medicine: Knowledge Production and Social Transformation." *Complementary and Alternative Medicine: Knowledge Production and Social Transformation,* edited by Caragh Brosnan, Pia Vuolanto, and Jenny-Ann Brodin Danell. London: Palgrave Macmillan, 2018, pp. 1–29.

Cope, Bill, and Mary Kalantzis. "Introduction: Multiliteracies: The Beginnings of an Idea." *Multiliteracies: Literacy Learning and the Design of Social Futures,* edited by Bill Cope and Mary Kalantzis. New York and Abingdon: Routledge, 2000, pp. 3–8.

Czerwiec, M. K., et al., editors. *Graphic Medicine Manifesto*. University Park, PA: The Pennsylvania State University Press, 2015.

Dillon, Glyn. *The Nao of Brown*. London: SelfMadeHero, 2012.

Fontanarosa, Phil B. and George D. Lundberg, "Alternative Medicine Meets Science." *Journal of the American Medical Association*, vol. 280, no. 18, 1998, pp. 1618–19.

Forney, Ellen. *Marbles: Mania, Depression, Michelangelo, & Me: A Graphic Memoir*. London: Penguin, 2012.

Foss, Laurence. *The End of Modern Medicine: Biomedical Science under a Microscope*. Albany, N.Y.: SUNY Press, 2002.

Hannah. Comment on the Post "The Hospital Suite", *Goodreads,* December 17, 2015. www.goodreads.com/en/book/show/20613690.

Malabou, Catherine. *Ontology of the Accident: An Essay on Destructive Plasticity*. Translated by Carolyn Shread. Cambridge: Polity Press, 2012.

Mayo Clinic. www.mayoclinic.org/tests-procedures/meditation/in-depth/meditation/art-20045858. Accessed August 3, 2021.

Mordacci, Roberto and Richard Sobel. "Health: A Comprehensive Concept." *Hasting Center Report*, vol. 28, no. 1, 1998, pp. 34–7.

Penzel, Fred. "How I Treat OCD Killer Thoughts: Treating Violent Obsessions."*International OCD Foundation*, https://iocdf.org/expert-opinions/expert-opinion-violent-obsessions/.

Ruggie, Mary. *Marginal to Mainstream: Alternative Medicine in America*. Cambridge: Cambridge Unversity Press, 2004.

Squier, Susan M. "Literature and Medicine, Future Tense: Making it Graphic."*Literature and Medicine*, vol. 27, no. 1, 2009, pp. 124–52.

Svatmarama. *Hatha Yoga Pradipika*. Translated by Becherer Elsy and Hans Ulrich Reiker. Detroit: MI: The Aquarian Press, 1992.

Walter, Suzan. "Holistic Health." *American Holistic Health Association*, May 21, 2020. ahha.org/selfhelp-articles/holistic-health.

24

DRAWING HEALTH ACTIVISM

Illness politics and practices of care in graphic AIDS narratives

Lisa Diedrich

In recent years, comics and graphic narratives have become a popular, innovative form for telling stories in a medium that artfully combines words and images. One exciting sub-field of the form is graphic medicine, which explores the conjuncture between comics, health care, and experiences of illness, trauma, and disability. The scholarly, educational, and clinical impact of graphic medicine has already been significant. Coined by general practitioner and comics artist, Ian Williams in 2007, the phrase *graphic medicine* is a "handy term to denote the role comics can play in the study and delivery of healthcare" ("Why Graphic Medicine"). For Williams, the term suggests how comics can deliver a kind of medicine with healing effects. Increasingly, comics and graphic narratives have become important resources for communicating a range of ethical and clinical issues related to the experience of illness, and this hybrid verbal/visual form helps healthcare practitioners, patients, families, and caregivers creatively reimagine the boundaries of health, illness, life, and death.

In this chapter, I explore this multi-modal form as a means for articulating the illness politics and practices of care that emerged out of the response to AIDS as represented in a selection of hybrid verbal and visual narratives from the 1980s to the present, including: Cindy Patton and Janis Kelly's *Making It: A Woman's Guide to Sex in the Age of AIDS* (1987); Alison Bechdel's comic strip *Dykes to Watch Out For* (1983–2008); Jaime Cortez's online comic *Sexile* (2004);and MK Czerwiec's graphic memoir *Taking Turns: Stories from HIV/AIDS Care Unit 371* (2017). Patton and Kelly's guide to safer sex for women incorporated comics drawn by Bechdel in the style and tone of her comic strip, *Dykes to Watch Out For*, and Bechdel's strip, which began its long-syndicated run in 1983, dealt occasionally with safer sex, AIDS activism, and other forms of health activism. *Sexile* is an HIV-prevention publication created with the AIDS Project Los Angeles and Gay Men's Health Crisis of New York and features the story of and interviews with Adela Vázquez, a Cuban transgender person and AIDS activist who came to the United States as part of the Mariel boatlift in 1980. *Taking Turns* draws on Czerwiec's own experience as a nurse working in an AIDS unit in Chicago, as well as on her interviews with other practitioners and patients on the unit. All of these graphic narratives document the intimate relationship between sexual politics and illness politics, and through formal experimentation and mixed methods, the texts give shape to particular experiences and events of AIDS in history and, more generally, to what I have called the conjunction illness-thought-activism in time (Diedrich 2016). I argue that these eclectic graphic AIDS narratives depict a multiplicity of practices of

DOI: 10.4324/9781003007661-31

care, art, and politics. They show how graphic narratives – a capacious, multi-modal form – can make visible certain experiences that might otherwise remain on the margins, acting as an antidote to stigmatizing images of sexuality and illness.

Sex, health, and community: *Making It*

In 1987, Firebrand Books, a small feminist press, published *Making It*, a 30-page safer sex resource printed back-to-back with a Spanish translation.[1] Along with Bechdel's illustrations, the text includes first-person testimony from women on sex, drugs, support groups, and activism. The guide provides advice that is pragmatic and non-judgmental; even 30 years later, the tone and recommendations hold up as smart in relation to sexual politics, public health, and community organizing. And, although the singular "woman" of the title is a product of its time, the non-identarian, practice-based approach to sex and sexual health would prove medically and politically prescient. What is apparent from the people and institutions involved in this collaboration is the importance of lesbian, feminist, and anti-racist activism in creating the conditions of possibility for AIDS activism. At the time of its publication, Patton (1987) had already made the argument that safer sex activism was continuous not discontinuous with earlier forms of gay liberation politics, and indeed, *Making It* demonstrates how feminist health activism and alternative publishing projects born out of earlier liberation movements created a foundation for AIDS activism and a network of politically savvy AIDS activists and queer cultural workers.

Bechdel's brief biography included in *Making It* touts her as an "obsessive observer of the women's community," capturing well her work in the 1980s. In an email interview, I asked Bechdel how she came to work on this particular project and about the relationship between her work on *Making It* and her *Dykes to Watch Out For* strip. She noted that she had been drawing *DTWOF* for years before *Making It*, publishing her first cartoons in the feminist monthly *WomaNews* in 1983.[2] "That's where Nancy Bereano, who was in the process of founding Firebrand Books, first saw them," Bechdel wrote. "She invited me to do a collection of *DTWOF* for Firebrand, and that was published in the fall of 1986." *Making It* was a commission that also came from Bereano. Bechdel admitted that she was a "little reluctant about the project," because, as she joked, "drawing heterosexuals seemed a bit of a stretch for me at the time!" She recalls that Bereano encouraged her to do the project, even "sending [her] condoms in the mail," so she could figure out how to draw them, having "never seen one in [her] life!" (Figure 24.1).

"Making Condoms Fun" is one of the sections in the pamphlet, and it encourages verbal and visual – we might even say graphic – play as part of sex: "If you like to talk dirty, add the condom to your verbal games. Find images that make the condom part of sex instead of an interruption" (12), the text instructs. Bechdel's drawings of a woman blowing up a condom like a balloon while her male partner waits with an impatient and unamused look on his face and of a woman on her own putting a condom on a very large vegetable in her lap humorously puncture some of the earnestness surrounding not only safer sex but also sex in general. The concept and practice of "making it" wasn't just about having more sex but about making it better and more fun through safer sex play and creativity.

Another key lesson of *Making It* is that safer sex is not about identity categories but about practices. Emerging first in LGBTQ community-based safer sex initiatives like *Making It*, this distinction between sexual identity and practice would eventually influence the nascent projects of queer theory and politics as well as mainstream epidemiological and public health studies into how HIV is spread and the best interventions for preventing its spread.[3] The section, "Sex for

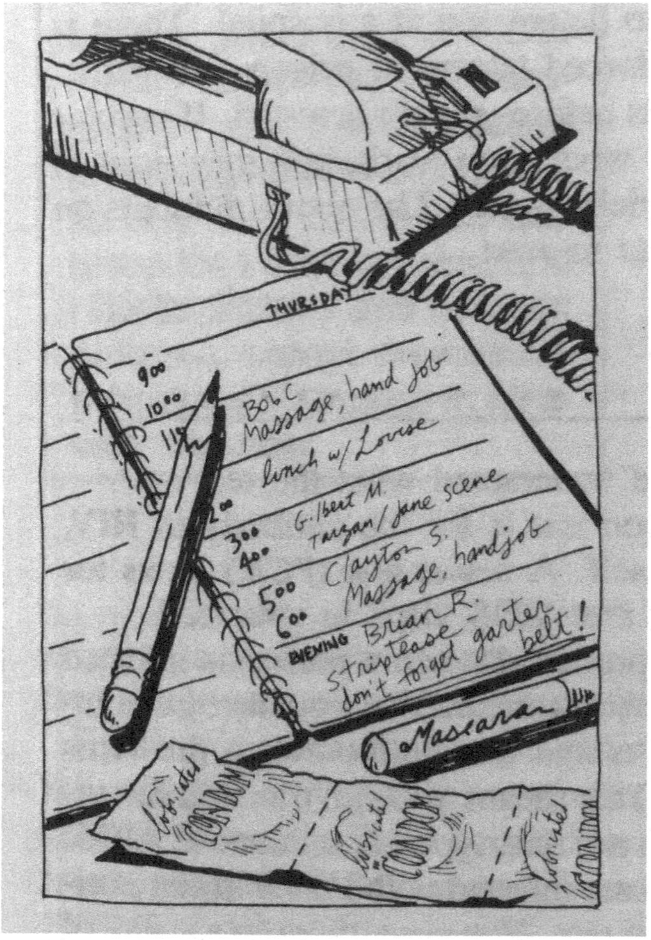

Figure 24.1 Alison Bechdel recalls that Nancy Bereano, founder of Firebrand Books, sent her condoms in the mail so she could figure out how to draw them

Source: Detail from p. 17 of *Making It*. Reprinted by permission of the artist

Lesbians and Bisexuals," begins with the fact that "[m]any lesbians have the misconception that AIDS is not their problem," but immediately and emphatically challenges this misconception by explaining that "*risk comes from what you do, not how you label yourself*" (15; emphasis in original). The cartoon accompanying this section humorously clarifies the point about the important difference between sexual identities and practices. Bechdel draws two women in conversation: one with an insouciant look on her face who says, "So **what** if I sleep with a **man** now and then? I **still** identify myself as a **lesbian!**" Her companion responds pointedly: "I don't care if you identify yourself as an **anti-nuclear macrobiotic foot-fetishist!** It's who you have **sex** with that **counts!**" (15; emphasis in original). *Making It* makes clear that lesbians can and do have sex with men, and men who don't identify as gay or bisexual can and do have sex with both men and women. The pamphlet also makes clear that people aren't always entirely truthful about their sexual lives and thus encourages "[l]earning to feel good about safer sex" with the support of friends and through participation in "rap groups" (16), a continuation of the feminist practice of consciousness raising.

One rap group activity that Patton and Kelly recommend is the ranking exercise in which participants are handed cards with examples of a variety of explicit sexual practices, and they must organize the activities in order from "most safe" to "most dangerous" in terms of HIV transmission. The authors explain that this sounds easier than it is in practice, and, more importantly, they note that uncertainty often leads to frank discussions about what is safe, what isn't, and how best to practice safer sex. The exercise creates a framework in which people can learn to talk about risk, preparing and informing them to talk about and practice safer sex with their partners. Bechdel's cartoon of a rap group doing the ranking exercise is illustrative of both the frank talk about sex that emerges out of such activities and the surprising things we can learn from others and about ourselves. It also shows yet again why the multi-modal approach to safer sex instruction works well. Bechdel's cartoon works on multiple levels. The group is diverse in terms of physical appearance, race, and age, allowing readers to see themselves represented in the cartoon. The image also encourages an identification with the rap group itself – that is, with the process of learning and teaching together as a practice of freedom. That *Making It* was published as a cheap pamphlet, including both comics and humor to draw readers into a serious discussion of safer sex increases the likelihood of wider circulation and readership of important public health information.

Cartoons as antidote: *Dykes to Watch Out For*

In her "Cartoonist's Introduction" to *The Essential Dykes to Watch Out For*, Alison Bechdel describes arriving in New York City in 1981, having just finished college and recently come out. We flashback to the scene of her queer arrival: Olivia Newton-John's "Physical"[4] is the soundtrack welcoming her to the city and more specifically to The Duchess, a lesbian bar in the Village. We first see Alison outside of The Duchess looking startled, as if she can't quite comprehend what she is apprehending – apprehension here meaning both graspable and anxiety-provoking (x). The arrival scene is redolent with desire and a sense of possibility, both sexual and political; although, as Bechdel illustrates, the political possibilities are not immediately apparent to the young Alison.

The top tier of the following page includes three small panels, beginning with Alison walking through the door of The Duchess, still looking apprehensive (ix). This is followed by a close-up of narrator/cartoonist Alison in her archive in the present, describing her initial impression of her arrival in New York City and presenting a historical genealogy of queer New York: "The underground scene of the fifties, the revolutionary ferment of the sixties, the radical gay and lesbian counterculture of the seventies…it was all over by the time I showed up" (xi). The next panel returns to the scene at the Duchess in 1981 with an awkward Alison spilling her drink as a dancing woman backs into her, confirming the impression that Alison has arrived too late for liberation politics. The middle of the page contains a single, large horizontal panel of a stoned Alison drawing in her sketchbook and sharing a bong with her girlfriend and her girlfriend's father. A caption between the top and middle tiers states: "I was adrift that summer, aimless, lost, at sixes and sevens. In short, bewildered" (xi). The newly-elected Ronald Reagan appears twice in this panel – first, in a headline in the newspaper Alison's girlfriend is reading and second, as the unnamed and rather innocuous-sounding referent in a caption at the bottom right of the panel that reads: "…But some absurd old actor seemed to be running the country" (xi).[5]

The bottom tier of two panels punctures the feeling of aimlessness with a haunting reminder of another queer arrival to New York City in 1981: the AIDS virus. The first panel covers two-thirds of the bottom of the page and is the only panel in the entire two-page spread that does not contain an image of Alison, either as cartoonist introducing the collection of *Dykes to Watch Out For* strips or as Alison becoming a cartoonist. It includes an image of *The New York Times* dated Friday, July 3, 1981, and folded open to page A20. Prominently featured on the page is the headline, "Sing out on the 4th!" with the music and lyrics to the *Star-Spangled Banner* below. Next to this advertisement is the now-infamous first article ever published in *The New York Times* about the illness that would later come to be known as AIDS. Bechdel re-draws the article's headline, "Rare Cancer Seen in 41 Homosexuals."

The panel reminds us that this first article in *The Times* was buried deep inside the paper rather than on the front page, and highlighting the headline, Bechdel renders how the article was primarily concerned with reassuring "nonhomosexuals" that there appeared to be no danger to them of contagion (Altman). I've read the article many times, yet until I saw Bechdel's redrawing of the page, I'd never seen the full-page layout and its juxtaposition with the *Star-Spangled Banner* music and lyrics as part of an advertisement for Independence Bank.[6] Bechdel's redrawing of the page captures the strange juxtaposition, making us look anew at the placement of the article in the newspaper and giving us an eerie sense of how this moment might have felt for some readers but not for others. Her one addition – the words "With Spirit" under "The Star-Spangled Banner" heading and in the same cursive script – works as a critique of the thoughtlessness – even cruelty – of the page layout and figures as a sign of the battle with many losses to come. On top of the drawn newspaper, Bechdel has placed a caption that reads, "The tidal wave of AIDS hadn't hit yet." A second caption in the panel reads, "For all we knew, it was really morning in America," which is clearly another reference to Reagan, echoing his 1984 campaign ad "Morning in America." Reading the caption aloud, we might hear what is foreshadowed on the page: *mourning* in America, a structure of feeling also gestured to visually by the partially visible drawing of an angel in Alison's sketchbook. The final panel on the page shows our cartoonist back in the archive, telling us that "as the months wore on, I started to wake up," and returning the bong of the middle panel to a file drawer labeled 1981, as if to say: after 1981, getting high was no longer the antidote for feeling bewildered.

Bechdel now wakes up in relation to the lesbian and proto-queer politics of the 1980s through her desire to find a form that captures "this unruly pageant, the sheer plenitude of it all" (xii). She discovers there is "plenty of revolutionary ferment still afoot" and that she wants to be "part of this insurrection" (xii). Her awakening is as much political as it is formal. Bechdel depicts a head-spinning Alison, both as she takes in the pageant and plenitude of lesbian politics and culture and, on the next page, as she realizes the possibility that emerges out of her decision to start drawing women in their many shapes and forms (masculine, feminine, nonbinary), which would become the characters for her long-running cartoon *DTWOF*, syndicated in alternative newspapers (xii–xiii) (Figure 24.2). Bechdel's portraits of a twisting, double-headed avatar of herself also suggests the formal doubling and torqueing that comes out of her recognition that she wasn't "a writer **or** an artist" (xiii) but "a writer **and** an artist!" (xiv). This is a *keyimage*[7] for Bechdel's queer vision and form (combining word and image, past and present, feminine and masculine, art and politics). Alison's eyes on the head on the left look tired, even closed (she could be asleep), whereas her eyes on the right are popped open and huge: the image literalizes her awakening.

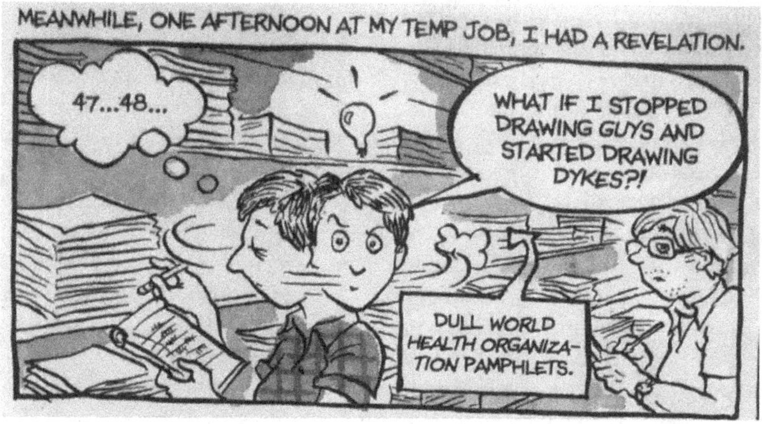

Figure 24.2 Bechdel's portraits of a twisting, double-headed Alison also suggests the formal doubling and torqueing that comes out of her recognition that she wasn't "a writer **or** an artist" (xiii) but "a writer **and** an artist!" (xiv). Panel from THE ESSENTIAL DYKES TO WATCH OUT FOR by Alison Bechdel

Source:

Trans-everything: *Sexile*

The twisting, double-headed Alison breaks the fourth wall of the panel to make eye contact with and speak to the reader: "What if I stopped drawing guys and started drawing dykes?!" Next to Alison's torqueing head is a caption that reads, "Dull World Health Organization Pamphlets" with an arrow pointing to a stack of pamphlets on the shelf behind her. In a single panel, Bechdel verbally and visually connects her awakening about the political and aesthetic transformation of her art with the possibility of creating new modes of communication about health activism. A similar motivation and sense of transformative possibility is at work in the creation of the HIV-prevention publication *Sexile*. Written, drawn, and lettered by Mexican-American artist and cultural worker, Jaime Cortez, *Sexile* is, like Bechdel's work, far from a "Dull World Health Organization Pamphlet." Cortez came up with the project after he conducted multiple interviews with transgender AIDS activist Adela Vázquez. He opens with a vivid image of her: "The life of Adela Vázquez is trans-everything – transnational, transgendered, transformative and fully transfixing" (vii).

By presenting Adela's trans-everything life in a digital comic, Cortez shows that comics as a medium are themselves transformative and fully transfixing. In his foreword, editor Patrick "Pato" Hebert anticipates a question from readers about form, asking, "Why a comic book when so many pressing issues about AIDS are worthy of our resources?" (iv). Answering his own question and linking art, politics, and wellness, Hebert asserts:

> In order to reinvigorate prevention, we must continue to innovate our concepts and modalities. AIDS service agencies can learn much by listening to Adela and the very communities that prevention efforts seek to assist. With more people living with HIV than ever before, and communities of color disproportionately affected, we need nothing less than holistic, dynamic approaches to wellness.
>
> *(iv)*

As a medium, comics has the potential to convey knowledge not only about HIV transmission and safer sex but also about the interconnected histories of LGBTQ activism, illness politics, and practices of care that have emerged out of communities of color in the U.S. and beyond. In its presentation of public health information, *Sexile*'s "holistic, dynamic" approach is more evocative and less pragmatic than *Making It*. If *Making It* uses comics to illustrate information and generate a sense of community through the presentation of practices of safer sex and the use of humor, *Sexile* offers Adela's story as an exemplary yet relatable personal narrative framed by a context that is both geographically broad and historically deep. Here I draw on Paul Farmer's (2004) anthropological public health method of telling "exemplary stories" to understand how structural violence operates to constrain people's choices in relation to maintaining health and wellbeing, as well as how individuals and communities nonetheless find ways to resist structural violence in their everyday lives.

Vázquez's personal story is nested within what Hebert calls "compelling meta histories, two that were front page news as the United States stumbled into the 1980's, and a third that unfolded with much less visibility" (iv). The two front-page news stories are both arrival stories: the first, the arrival of approximately 130,000 Cuban refugees to the U.S. as part of the Mariel Boatlift in 1980 and the second, the arrival of AIDS around the same time,[8] which as we know from Bechdel's *Essential Dykes to Watch Out For*, was not immediately a front-page story. The third, less prominent but still significant, meta history that Hebert identifies is "transgender organizing and theorizing" that was also emerging in the early 1980s (iv). These meta histories create a conjuncture in which illness politics, racial politics, and sexual politics are intertwined. Not unlike Bechdel's story of her arrival in New York City along with the AIDS virus, Adela's personal story is a portal into this meta historical conjuncture, and the term "sexile" linguistically suggests both an emergent identity category as well as a social and cultural disposition born out of displacement.[9] Cortez literalizes the concept in his drawing of the word "sexile" in and as the water under the boat that transports Adela to the U.S. from Cuba.[10] The caption, in Adela's words, reads: "On May 13, 1980, I left Cuba forever" (31). While *Sexile* shows how Adela's escape from Cuba made her becoming-woman and indeed becoming-Adela possible, the passage is also marked by loss, including the loss of a supportive family environment and what Hebert describes as the "manifold ways [Adela] had embodied and enacted a rich gender in Cuba."[11] Yet, as with *Making It* and *DTWOF*, the tone of *Sexile* is not portentous but often self-deprecating and campy.

"Not to brag, but my birth was revolutionary" (3). Adela's statement opens *Sexile*, and the full-page black-and-white image that accompanies it is a re-drawing of a newsreel still of the victorious Cuban revolutionaries led by Fidel Castro and Che Guevara, arriving in Havana and being cheered on by onlookers. Adela explains that she was born in November 1958, at the same time that the rebels were making their way across Cuba, "kicking ass from East to West" (4). Like Bechdel, Cortez reproduces other media to capture the complexity of the historico-political moment into which Adela is born. Despite the feelings of hope that bloomed for many in Cuba during Adela's and the revolutionary government's early years, we soon learn about how the spirit of the times was in fact not so revolutionary when it came to sexual politics. The political contradictions are contained in a single page depicting a young Adela[12] in Cuba and an older Adela recalling her life in Cuba in her interview with Cortez (Figure 24.3).

We first see 15-year-old Adela getting a "hit of girl power" by performing in the school drag pageant (10). At the top of the page are three elongated, rectangular panels, presenting different views of Adela's performance. In the panel on the left, we see her headless body from behind, framing the pageant audience between her strong, curvy legs, which dominate the panel. The top middle panel shows Adela at the center of the stage flanked by two other drag

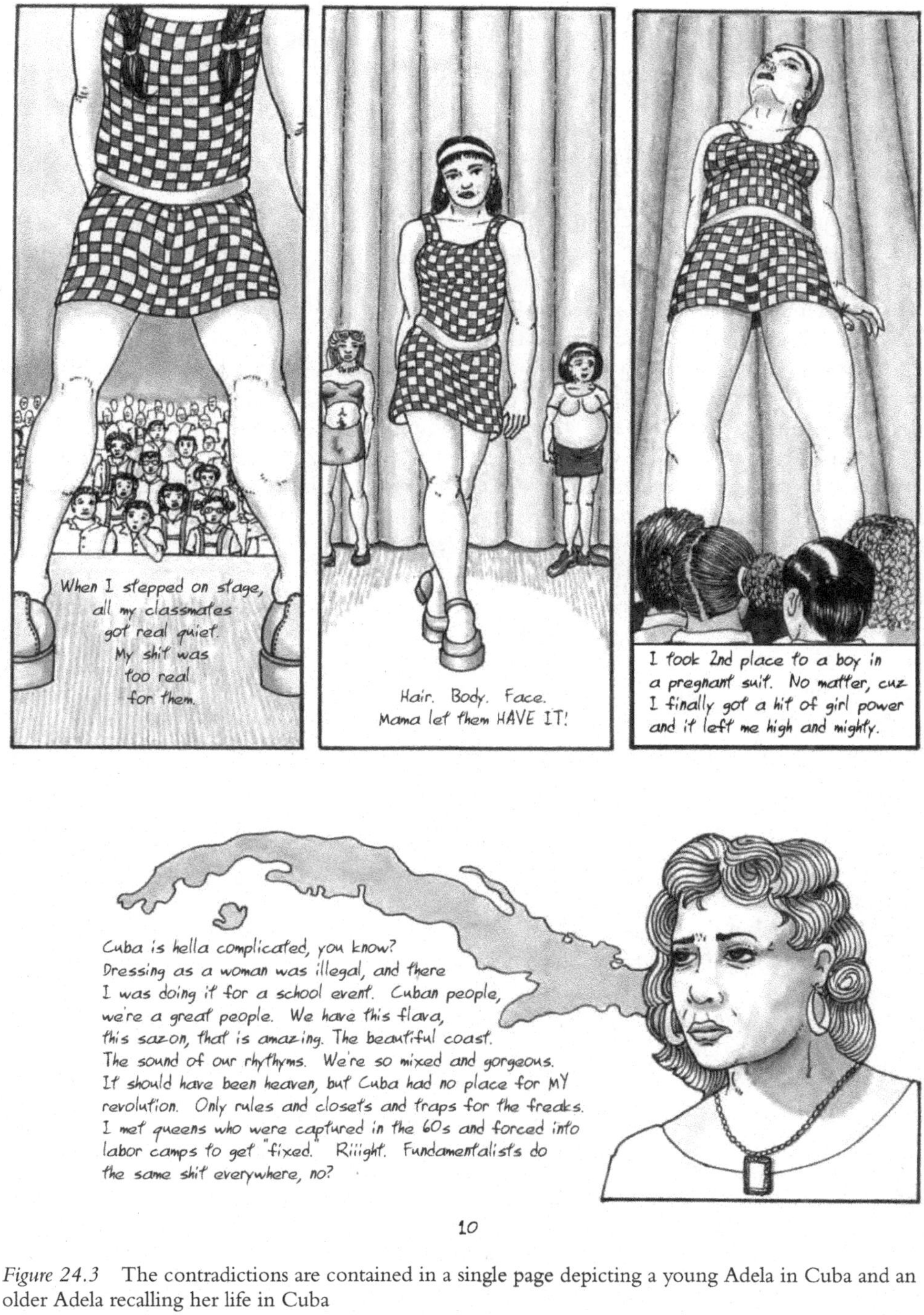

Figure 24.3 The contradictions are contained in a single page depicting a young Adela in Cuba and an older Adela recalling her life in Cuba

Source: Cortez, *Sexile*, p. 10. Reprinted by permission of the artist.

performers in the background. In a spotlight, she strides forward confidently and fabulously. In the top right panel, we are now in the audience looking up at her as she stands at the edge of the stage, exuding sensuality and exuberantly holding her head "high and mighty" (10). Below these panels, Cortez has drawn Adela in the present with an outline of Cuba behind her, as she explains, "Cuba is complicated, you know? Dressing as a woman was illegal, and there I was doing it for a school event" (10). With a sorrowful expression, Adela recalls the missed opportunity for Cuba and the predicament for people like her at that time: "It should have been heaven, but Cuba had no place for MY revolution. Only rules and closets and traps for the freaks. I met queens who were captured in the 60s and forced into labor camps to get 'fixed'" (10). Adela manages to escape this ideological cure and, after a harrowing transit to the U.S. on her own, is fortuitous to be sponsored by Rolando Victoria, the "most bitchy, hilarious, faggoty faggot ever" (45), who helps her settle into a new life in America.

Adela is especially lucky that Rolando is a nurse. When she explains to him that she has had to be treated for gonorrhea, Rolando tells her, "From now on Chiclet, you use a condom **every time** you gonna fuck" (47) (Figure 24.4). Adela is dismissive of this advice, but Rolando describes what he has seen at the hospital where he works: "Queens. Young queens. They're coming into the hospital sick. They get crazy exotic cancers and infections and then they die." Cortez renders the last four words – "and then they die" – in smaller lettering, as if Rolando whispers them, seemingly in shock, not quite believing what he has seen. In the background of the middle panel, at the center of the page, Cortez has drawn a ghost-like man dying in a hospital bed, creating a holy trinity with Rolando's talking head on either side of the spectral image as he describes the "horrible, painful deaths" that he has witnessed (47). This, then, is how AIDS first appears in the text, through the witnessing of deaths by a queer Cuban nurse as well as his advice on how to survive.

In the next panel, Rolando explains to Adela that he thinks the disease is transmitted sexually. When Adela tries to make a joke about getting pregnant and starting a family, Rolando becomes very angry, yelling that this is not a joke and insisting that Adela always use condoms. This page provides a glimpse into the early years of the AIDS epidemic in the U.S., showing both the terrifying emergence of the disease in the LGBTQ community, as well as how members of the community took care of their own and advocated for practices of safer sex from the start. Rolando doesn't tell Adela not to have sex; rather, he provides her with information about how to have sex safely, advice that helps her survive the AIDS crisis and inspires her to become an activist. Many in the LGBTQ community do not survive this period, including Rolando. His death is communicated via a completely black page with only a single hand-lettered sentence: "Rolando eventually drank himself to death" (51). The burnout from caring for so many sick and dying and the trauma of witnessing to the AIDS crisis became too much to bear for Rolando and many other queer healthcare workers.

Drawing comics as care: *Taking Turns*

I conclude with a brief discussion of another story of a queer nurse caring for people with AIDS, MK Czerwiec's *Taking Turns*. Czerwiec's graphic narrative recounts the philosophy and practices of a clinical unit dedicated to the care of people with AIDS (PWAs) in Chicago during the early 1990s. Czerwiec explains that Unit 371 looked and felt different from other units – Broadway show posters and patients' artwork covered the walls of the art therapy room (18–19); there was a kitchen that was always open with healthy and delicious food available for patients and staff; and there was a sense of camaraderie between patients and staff (22). The ethos of the unit came from its founders – doctors David Blatt and David Moore, who were gay and saw the clinic as an opportunity to "take care of our own people" (26). Patient advocacy was an

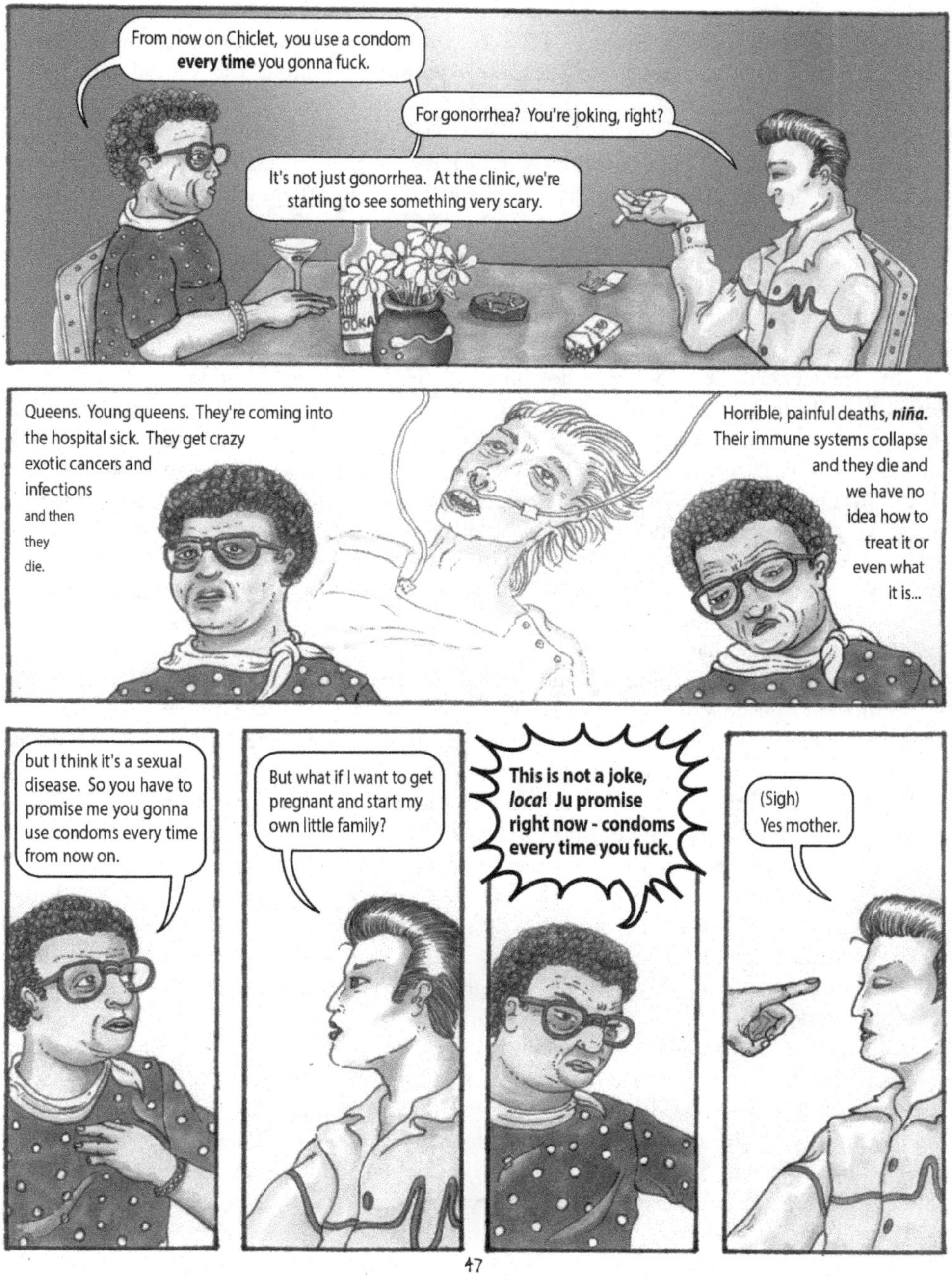
From now on Chiclet, you use a condom **every time** you gonna fuck.
For gonorrhea? You're joking, right?
It's not just gonorrhea. At the clinic, we're starting to see something very scary.
Queens. Young queens. They're coming into the hospital sick. They get crazy exotic cancers and infections and then they die.
Horrible, painful deaths, ***niña.*** Their immune systems collapse and they die and we have no idea how to treat it or even what it is...
but I think it's a sexual disease. So you have to promise me you gonna use condoms every time from now on.
But what if I want to get pregnant and start my own little family?
This is not a joke, *loca*! Ju promise right now - condoms every time you fuck.
(Sigh) Yes mother.
47

Figure 24.4 This page provides a glimpse into the early years of the AIDS epidemic in the U.S. Source: Cortez, *Sexile*, p. 47. Reprinted by permission of the artist.

important aspect of their practices of doctoring, as well as the radical empathy that the AIDS crisis generated among many in the LGBTQ community, a response that we see in all the texts I have analyzed in this chapter. Czerwiec's title expresses this ethos of care on the unit: "we are just people taking turns being sick," as Dr. Blatt says (30).

The unit's ethos of care can also be seen in what Chris Haen, a social worker on the unit, describes as the "very diffuse boundaries" (90) between staff and patients. For example, staff were encouraged to sit on patients' beds and touch and hug them. Because so many people with AIDS had been treated as pariahs, even by health care professionals, the staff on unit 371 went "in the other direction" (22), as an antidote to the stigmatization people with AIDS experienced. When MK becomes especially close to one of her patients, Tim, an artist, she worries that their friendship crosses a professional line. When he learns MK is also an artist, Tim invites her to his studio and suggests they create a piece together. Art becomes a practice of care between them, breaking down boundaries between nurse and patient and creating intimacy and connection beyond the space and time of the clinic and even into the future. The art object they imagined and planned together, which Czerwiec completes on her own after Tim's death, is a triptych of painted wooden boards depicting a paintbrush painting a star that replicates a tattoo on Tim's arm that Czerwiec had sketched one night in the clinic. This image visually echoes the epigraph to *Taking Turns*, a quotation from poet Marie Howe: "All art holds the knowledge that we're both living and dying at the same time. Art can hold it." By documenting the process by which they came to create art together and by re-drawing the object Czerwiec makes after Tim's death, the graphic narrative *Taking Turns* is a work of art that holds the knowledge that we're both living and dying at the same time.

The unit's art therapy program and art space, described as its heart, helps patients and practitioners to create "an alternative emotional vocabulary" (51). Yet, the image with which I want to end this chapter is not one made in the art room but made after the unit closes, and it functions as a passageway in the text and real life. Czerwiec chronicles the arrival of protease inhibitors and the excitement and relief of finally having a treatment for HIV/AIDS that transformed it from a death sentence to a chronic condition for those with access to the new drug therapies. As a result of these successful treatments, the AIDS unit closes in 1999, which as Czerwiec notes, was a cause for celebration but left her feeling miserable and "ashamed for feeling miserable" (165). Echoing Bechdel's aesthetic and political revelation in *DTWOF*, Czerwiec explains that neither painting nor writing felt adequate to document the complexity of her feelings about what she had lived through – both the trauma of AIDS and the incredible caring response from so many in the gay community (Figure 24.5). At the end of the penultimate chapter of *Taking Turns,* just after the AIDS unit has closed and as the millennium turns, Czerwiec illustrates how she had to find a "new way," and in a series of four panels across the page, she draws herself drawing her first comic. In the first panel, we see Czerwiec from behind, sitting in front of a blank white piece of paper. Once she draws herself on the page, the crude representation stands in for the artist in the remaining panels. Below each panel is a thought balloon, and in the words, the concept of a comic takes shape in a series of steps: 1. "Maybe I'll just draw myself." 2. "I'll put a box around it." 3. "Another box and it's a comic. Like Lynda Barry." The final panel shows a completed comic with Czerwiec's realization that it contains both sadness and hope. This comic within a comic depicts the emergence of the comic we are reading, Czerwiec's becoming Comic Nurse, and graphic medicine as a formal way out. Both word and image, both sadness and hope, both nurse and artist – both/and doubled and torqued as practice of care of the self and others.

The comics and graphic narratives I have explored in this essay document the illness politics and practices of care that emerged with the AIDS crisis. I end with Czerwiec's image of drawing

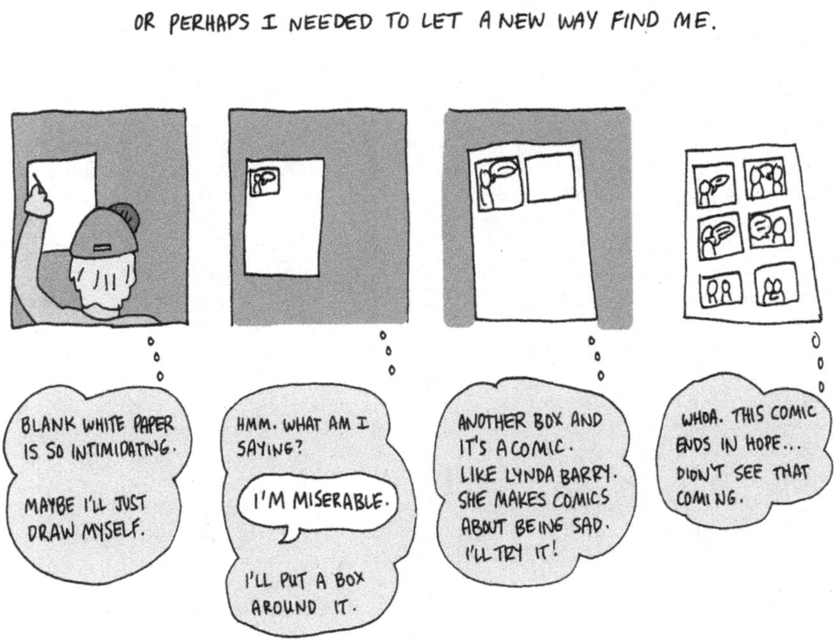

Figure 24.5 Czerwiec shows how she had to let a "new way" find her for documenting her experiences on the AIDS unit

Source: Czerwiec, *Taking Turns*, p. 166. Reprinted by permission of the artist.

her first comic because that image captures on a meta-formal level another theme across these works: the importance of finding a form capacious enough to capture the AIDS crisis and the responses to it in the LGBTQ community. My analysis also provides a portal into questions of why and how form matters. The essay moves from a safer sex guide, in which comics are merely illustrative and add a humorous component to the written text, to works that ask the question of why and how comics can be an effective and innovative form for communicating information about public health and health activism, and, finally, to a text that participates explicitly in the enactment of the project of graphic medicine. The project of graphic medicine emerges historically, then, in conjunction with the AIDS crisis and as itself a practice of care.

Acknowledgments

Thanks to Alison Bechdel, Jaime Cortez, Pato Hebert, and MK Czerwiec for giving permission to use images from their work in this chapter. I am also incredibly grateful for their generosity in responding to my queries and offering feedback on my work. Thanks also to Tess Jones and Les Friedman for their helpful feedback and vision for this book.

Notes

1 The first pamphlet in the series was *Words to the Wise: Writer's Guide to Feminist and Lesbian Periodicals and Publishers* by Andrea Fleck Clardy published in spring 1986. Firebrand Books was founded by Nancy Bereano in 1984 and published lesbian and feminist literary fiction, poetry, and nonfiction until 2000.

2 Personal email communication with Alison Bechdel on June 5, 2019.
3 See, for example, UNAIDS, Policy Brief: "HIV and Sex Between Men" (2006).
4 Curious, I checked to see when Olivia Newton-John's "Physical" was released, and sure enough, it was 1981. Had Bechdel noted this song in one of her diaries? Was it really playing when she first walked into The Duchess?
5 "Reagan Reversing Many U.S. Policies" by Howell Raines is one of the articles on the front page of *The New York Times* on July 3, 1981, discussing how the Reagan Administration "has quietly set about accomplishing a sweeping reversal of policy and practice in the way the Government deals with business and individual citizens." Raines writes that the administration has "lifted restrictions on business while playing down the Government's activist role as a protector of workers, consumers and minorities" and attempted "to modify the network of laws and reforms put into place as a result of the Watergate scandals, the civil rights movement of the 1960's and the environmental movement of the 1970's." A stoned Alison and the reference to "some old actor" in the same panel as this article suggests a certain cluelessness about the concerted efforts to undermine and undo the social changes and expansion of rights that the activism of the 1960s and 1970s had brought about. And, this is the political climate into which AIDS would arrive.
6 The film *Longtime Companion* (1990) deals explicitly with the piece in the *Times* and begins on the date July 3, 1981, showing various characters picking up copies of *The New York Times*, reading the paper, discovering the article, alerting others to the article, and reading it out loud to others over the phone, in bed, and at the beach on Fire Island for the July 4 weekend. Blondie's version of "The Tide Is High" is the soundtrack for the opening scene that accentuates healthy male bodies and desire. Although the scene doesn't show the page itself, we do see a reference to July 4 in an ad on the back side of the paper one of the men reads. Much of the article is read out loud in a fascinating image of how newspapers help create a sense of imagined community between people who might not otherwise know each other, as described by Benedict Anderson (1983).
7 For a project called *Keywords and Keyimages in Graphic Medicine*, Briana Martino and I have coined the term *keyimage* to indicate the significance of images, separate from and in relation to words, in articulating a visual vocabulary of culture and society. In formulating this concept, we are of course drawing on the work of Raymond Williams (1976).
8 As Pato Hebert noted in a comment on a draft of this essay, we now know that AIDS did not "arrive" in the U.S. in 1981, and thus his Foreword is somewhat dated in the context of what we know now about the virus's history. For a discussion of the longer history of HIV/AIDS in the U.S., see Kerr (2016). Although I appreciate Hebert's concern about accurately presenting the history of HIV, I am also interested in analyzing the verbal and visual narrative trope of arrival as it functions in graphic AIDS narratives.
9 In his introduction, Jaime Cortez explains why he chose *Sexile* for the title: "I first saw the word used as the title to a beautiful essay on immigration and HIV by Pedro Bustos [Aguilar, 2003], who informed me that it was coined by the Puerto Rican academic Manolo Guzman [1997]. Guzman used the term to describe the state of people who had been cast out from the prickly bosom of their birth cultures and families. Sexile the word is full of longing, awareness, invention and displacement" (vii).
10 For an analysis of images of water and boats in *Sexile*, see Kaur (2021). Using Gloria Anzaldúa's concept of borderlands as creating a third space, Kaur argues that "Cortez employs water as a proxy for the borderlands throughout the text; each time Adela is depicted as immersed in water, she is pondering and entering the third space" (7).
11 Personal email communication with Pato Hebert on April 17, 2021. Hebert notes that while we may read Adela's transition across the sea as " 'the' transition of her gender as well," it may also be the case that "she was enacting trans in multiple ways all along." Thanks to Hebert for his incredibly insightful comments on *Sexile* and my analysis.
12 I have chosen not to use Adela's deadname or male pronouns even when discussing her adolescence and period prior to her becoming-woman through hormones and surgery.

Works cited

Aguilar, Pedro Bustos. "Sexilio." *Corpus*, vol. 1, no. 1, Spring 2003, pp. 47–52.

Altman, Lawrence K. "Rare Cancer Seen in 41 Homosexuals." *The New York Times*, July 3, 1981, p. A20. www.nytimes.com/1981/07/03/us/rare-cancer-seen-in-41-homosexuals.html. Accessed July 13, 2021.

Anderson, Benedict. *Imagined Communities: Reflections on the Origin and Spread of Nationalism*. London and New York: Verso, 1983.
Bechdel, Alison. "Cartoonist's Introduction." *The Essential Dykes to Watch Out For*, Boston and New York: Houghton Mifflin Harcourt, 2008, pp. vii–xviii.
Clardy, Andrea Fleck. *Words to the Wise: A Writer's Guide to Feminist and Lesbian Periodicals and Publishers*. Ithaca, New York: Firebrand Books, 1986.
Cortez, Jaime. *Sexile*. Los Angeles and New York: The Institute for Gay Men's Health, 2004.
Czerwiec, MK. *Taking Turns: Stories from HIV/AIDS Care Unit 371*. University Park, PA: Penn State Press, 2017.
Diedrich, Lisa. *Indirect Action: Schizophrenia, Epilepsy, AIDS, and the Course of Health Activism*. Minneapolis, MN: University of Minnesota Press, 2016.
Farmer, Paul. *Pathologies of Power: Health, Human Rights, and the New War on the Poor*. Berkeley, CA: University of California Press, 2004.
Guzmán, Manuel. "Pa la Escuelita con mucho cuidao y por la orillita: A Journey Throught the Contested Terrains of the Nation and Sexual Orientation." *Puerto Rican Jam: Essays on Culture and Politics*, edited by Frances Negrón-Muntaner and Ramón Grosfoguel, Minneapolis, MN: University of Minnesota Press, 1997, pp. 209–28.
Kaur, Guneet. "Community Narrative as Borderlands Praxis: Anzaldúa's *Mestiza* Consciousness as Explored in Cortez's *Sexile*." *Journal of Medical Humanities*, February 15, 2021. https://doi.org/10.1007/s10912-021-09678-2.
Kerr, Theodore (Ted). "AIDS 1969: HIV, History, and Race." *Drain Magazine*, vol. 13, no. 2, 2016, http://drainmag.com/aids-1969-hiv-history-and-race/. Accessed June 3, 2021.
Patton, Cindy. *Sex and Germs: The Politics of AIDS*. Boston, MA: South End Press, 1985.
Patton, Cindy and Janis Kelly. *Making It: A Woman's Guide to Sex in the Age of AIDS*. Ithaca, New York: Firebrand Books, 1987.
Raines, Howell. "Reagan Reversing Many U.S. Policies. *The New York Times*, July 3, 1981, p. A1. www.nytimes.com/1981/07/03/us/reagan-reversing-many-us-policies.html. Accessed July 13, 2021.
UNAIDS. Policy Brief: "HIV and Sex Between Men," August 2006, pp. 1–4, www.unaids.org/sites/default/files/media_asset/jc1269-policybrief-msm_en_0.pdf. Accessed July 13, 2021.
Williams, Ian. "Why Graphic Medicine?" 2007, www.graphicmedicine.org/why-graphic-medicine/. Accessed July 23, 2020.
Williams, Raymond. *Keywords: A Vocabulary of Culture and Society*. New York: Oxford University Press, 1976.

PART VII

Apps, devices, and wearables

"There's an app for that." Most of us are familiar with the incredible variety of computer software applications that can be downloaded to our mobile devices. And most of us use them, perhaps even rely on them, to negotiate and enrich our daily lives. However, the contributors to this section introduce us to the ways in which individuals and industries are pushing the boundaries of creative expression, psychiatric surveillance, and data-driven health care with the hard- and software we seek out to better our lives.

There is, as Gillian Andrews and Lorenzo Servitje note in **"On mediating women in *Unsane* spaces,"** no shortage of films that represent and reinforce American cultural anxieties about psychiatric power. Many narratives distill the dread of institutional confinement, evil providers, and barbaric technologies such as ECT and psychosurgery. Stephen Soderbergh's 2018 film, *Unsane,* adds to the sub-genre of psychiatric thrillers set in gruesome asylums, but as Andrews and Servitje argue, it is also something else: a film that reflects on the medical implications and technological dimensions of the sexual, emotional, and physical harassment of women. Soderbergh manifests this critique through a unique deployment and representation of mobile media by shooting the movie exclusively on an iPhone 7.

In the second chapter, **"Black sites in the matrix: digital psychiatric power and racialized technologies,"** Olivia Banner begins by citing the dire warnings of mental health professionals on the emotional, psychological, and spiritual toll of the coronavirus pandemic. Conversely, messages from the informatics, teletherapy, and digital psychiatric industries optimistically greeted what they believed to be the transformative moment that they had been awaiting. *Finally,* the pandemic's enforced increase in the use of digital tools would enable vulnerable populations, already underserved, to engage with mental health professionals, and *finally,* professionals reluctant to use these tools would be compelled to do so. Banner questions how digital ecosystems will actually serve the "vulnerable." To illustrate, she discusses a short film, *Blaxites* (2017), that dramatizes issues of racialization and digitalization of psychiatry by introducing questions about surveillance, consent, and power.

In the third chapter, **"Mobile health and its problems: the case of hearing and communication apps,"** Nicole Matthews describes how health and well-being apps such as the ones she, as a person with single-sided deafness, might use to find social settings in which to have a quiet conversation, are increasingly a growth market during the period of the

DOI: 10.4324/9781003007661-32

coronavirus pandemic. Matthews argues that while the pitch of mobile media is to offer handy solutions to social challenges and daily problems, they shape the ways we imagine, organize, and understand our identities, our bodies, and the environments through which they move.

In the final chapter of this section, **"Data visualization and digital contact tracing technology: emerging forms of health media,"** Kirsten Ostherr moves from the micro – the personal – to the macro – the global – to explore how "big data" has fundamentally transformed the role of digital media in health care. Here, she focuses on data visualization, a component of visual health communication that shapes meaning in the social and financial ecosystems of global digital health, and its use in the Covid-19 pandemic. She pays special attention to the visual health surveillance logic of digital contact tracing technology (DCTT), demonstrating how the pandemic pushed a rationale for developing DCTTs even as technologists and epidemiologists were acknowledging their failure to perform the tasks they were designed to complete.

25

ON MEDIATING WOMEN IN *UNSANE* SPACES

Gillian Andrews and Lorenzo Servitje

Introduction

No shortage of films manifest American cultural anxieties about psychiatric power: the medicalization of social deviance, the afterlives of hysteria's sordid history, and the hegemony of for-profit healthcare. Of this archive, a smaller set of influential films concern the more institutional, potentially coercive, and punitive capacities of psychiatry – be they based on sordid histories of medicine or mythologized fictions in the public imagination. Spanning different genres and eras, we might recall everything from Anatole Litvak's radical *The Snake Pit* (1948), *Girl, Interrupted* (1999), through *Shutter Island* (2010). But, perhaps Miloš Forman's *One Flew Over the Cuckoo's Nest* (1975) remains the touchstone in the dramatized critique of inpatient psychiatric treatment. A product of the culture of deinstitutionalization, it distills the dread of confinement, nefarious and dehumanizing providers, and disquieting technologies (tranquilizers, psychosurgery, ECT). All under the under the carceral sterility – white coats, walls, pills, and restraints – of a hospital milieu that does anything but allay unquiet minds.

In this tradition, Stephen Soderbergh's *Unsane* (2018) is ostensibly an asylum, psychiatric thriller. The typical conventions we expect are all here: the questionable sanity of the protagonist; tamer versions of Nurse Ratched-esque antagonists; an undercover journalist posing as a patient a la Nellie Bly;[1] and that aggressively administered shot of Thorazine. Even the culturally vilified ECT makes a perverse appearance, a trope we see early as the first asylum film, *The Snake Pit* (1944) and more recently in Aronofsky's *Requiem for a Dream* (2000) – figured as a coercive and punitive means to control woman's unquiet minds. But *Unsane* does more than rehash the conventions of the genre populated by the dozens of movies with "asylum" in their title. Produced and released in the wake of the #MeToo moment, the film reflects on the medical implications and technological dimensions of the sexual, emotional, and physical harassment of women. Soderbergh manifests this critique through a unique deployment and representation of mobile media – specifically, the mediation between its depiction within the film in the hands of the protagonist, Sawyer, and its role in the filmmaking process in the hands of Soderbergh, who filmed *Unsane* exclusively on an iPhone 7.

Unsane (2018) documents the involuntary psychiatric commitment of Sawyer Valentini (Claire Foy). Sawyer seeks support for post-traumatic stress symptoms, which she developed after being victimized by a stalker: she presents as hypervigilant and experiences intrusive

DOI: 10.4324/9781003007661-33

hallucinations, seeing her stalker everywhere, including in the faces of men who are not him. After what she believed to be a standard therapy appointment, Sawyer finds herself tricked into consenting to an extended stay in a psychiatric facility via paperwork that her therapist insists is routine. The horror intensifies as she starts to believe her stalker has infiltrated the staff, just as she simultaneously learns that the hospital could be knowingly detaining her unfairly to charge her insurance as much as possible. While there is only a brief period for Sawyer and the audience (six minutes) where her sanity is in question, the corrupt medical staff do not believe that the new hire, "George Shaw," is really David Strine (Joshua Leonard) – Sawyer's stalker. The hospital's administration clearly has a financial motive, and with the unwitting help of dismissive and inattentive medical staff, Strine gaslights Sawyer into thinking she has lost touch with reality. Sawyer's anger and frustration create conflict and justifies a longer stay, working in the hospital's financial favor. Sawyer eventually tricks Strine into helping her escape and kills him, but only after he has murdered several people including her mother. Six months later, Sawyer is seemingly recovered and receives a promotion at her new job. However, the film concludes with Sawyer believing she sees Strine; she moves to threaten him with a knife before realizing that this time she was once again hallucinating him – briefly exhibiting again the paranoid symptoms the Highland Creek clinicians diagnosed.

The modern smartphone, specifically the Apple iPhone 7, is part of this story. Sawyer is a tech-savvy protagonist who takes advantage of many technological safety precautions, but Soderbergh highlights that the affordances of the smartphone with respect to safety and security against gendered violence – documentation, constant contact, and safety apps – mediate but don't resolve structural sexism. Soderbergh's use of the smartphone as a filmic and digital medium, constructing Sawyer's narrative with the medium that fails to protect her, draws our attention to what the technology itself obscures. Similarly, *Unsane*'s visions of enabling structural inequality and failed female solidarity – including many female characters who enable Sawyer's victimization – demonstrate that addressing the true complexities of gender bias in health care can be revealed in conversation with, rather than be obscured by, the surface horror narrative of victim versus identifiable male attacker. Because harassment and stalking so frequently result in health-related consequences and because institutions like medicine have naturalized and at times still remain stalwart in labeling women as irrational and histrionic (Sojo et al. 2587; Sweet 857–8), it is necessary to be attentive to the way gendered harassment influences diagnosis and treatment especially in the business and systems of mental health care.

Missed opportunities, obfuscated mediums, and reinscribed messages

Unsane has yet to be an object of sustained inquiry in health humanities and film studies scholarship, but it did garner significant attention in reviews. It was met with mixed responses from critics, but what the vast majority have in common is their attention to three dimensions of the film: the fact that Soderbergh filmed *Unsane* on an iPhone 7; the representation of gaslighting women; and the film's focus on the capitalist corruption of mental health. While only the lattermost seems explicitly relevant to a health humanities reading of the film, this chapter suggests that the film's production with and representation of the smartphone, its depiction of gendered psychological manipulation, and its villainization of institutional psychiatry together inform how the film mediates medicine. In short, it documents how health systems can co-produce and mediate structural inequalities, all the while ascribing responsibility to individuals and the capacities of innovative technology – be they pharmacological or digitally communicative.

It is not difficult to notice there is something unique about *Unsane*'s aesthetics. The film is grainy; it is not lit for optimal clarity and color, and the perspectives have an uncanny quality to them – they look similar to the videos we have filmed and viewed on mobile media, distancing the film from expected cinematic polish. At the same time, because of the publicity surrounding Soderbergh's use of mobile media cinematography, the novelty of the iPhone format has dominated critical responses to *Unsane* and obfuscated its complex connections to Sawyer's story. Richard Brody of *The New Yorker*, for example, dismissed the plot of the film as "a story of plain and conventional simplicity" that provides a vehicle for Soderbergh's "inspired iPhone experiment" (Brody). Brody's assessment assumes *Unsane*'s narrative is merely another iteration of the asylum/psychiatric thriller. By dismissing this as "a furious movie that signifies nothing but the irrepressible vitality of the cinema itself," (Brody) critics isolate the iPhone outside the narrative – a tool for filmmaking – from the iPhone within the narrative – a tool for harassment and stalking – while at the same time for self-defense against these invasions. In reviews which do address the narrative in more detail, narrative still often takes a back-seat to Soderbergh's directorial mode. Tasha Robinson at *The Verge* praised the plot, mainly the early sections of the film, but also says of the quality of the iPhone format: "audiences may feel like they're in the same position as Sawyer, though, being gaslighted over the huge gap between what they'll see onscreen and what Soderbergh is telling them they're seeing" (Robinson). This association is catchy but problematically over-simplifies gaslighting, a serious and often-gendered experience, as a way to criticize Soderbergh's mobile media filmmaking. Robinson's review highlights that even when considered in tandem, *Unsane*'s exploration of harassment and its relationship to mobile media have been glossed over in favor of discussions about quality, some of which harmfully perpetuate minimizing women's experiences rather than exploring how *Unsane* can help us think critically about them.

Part of the reason for missing one aspect of the film vis-à-vis mobile media is the fact that the mobile phone itself has become an integral component to our habitus, what Bourdieu characterizes as the interplay between free will and social structures that become internalized in individual dispositions and practices (6; Abeele, De Wolf, and Ling 7). Like our everyday lives, the phone is at once integral and prosaic. In *Unsane*, likewise, the smartphone seems to occupy a quotidian or strictly functional role. In its assumed role as an instrument, it's easy to disregard how the smartphone capacitates and crystallizes social structures that influence behaviors, beliefs, and subjectivity. Zara Dinnen characterizes such obfuscation as "the digital banal": the way we don't notice our becoming with digital media (4). How our phones are requisite prosthetic memory for everything from our bank account, to our parents phone number; how we use its camera to remember information we could write down. We use it to get directions; get picked up from shared riding services; we use it to give our friends our ETA, or a location to meet us. More black boxed algorithms and proprietary data gathering seem to read our minds when we search the web or address for an item or location we were just texting or talking about. We use these functions the same way we use the phone to take selfies for posting online. Everyday life develops within this new mobile digital infrastructure, becoming a habit, becoming part of us – a habitus. Of course, this does not come without a cost, beyond of course, the complaint that "smart phones are too much with us" inasmuch as they detract from "real" social interactions. Perhaps of more concern is how all this data is "leaky," made available through loopholes in terms and conditions and flawed securities, creating new intimacies and risks (Chun and Friedland 3). The smart phone is, in a sense, a technocultural infrastructure for contemporary subjectivity. These capacities and effects are rendered less visible over time; they become digitally banal.

The taken-for-grantedness of the smartphone in everyday life and in media is not unlike the way media form itself is taken for granted, especially in medical humanities work or pedagogy. Therese Jones convincingly articulates this problem with respect to form and health-related content: "the content itself is likely not explored through the methodologies of literary criticism or media studies but is often used to exemplify something… The aesthetics of a short story or film are bypassed for the examination of clinical or bioethical content" (35). While reviews of *Unsane* have the opposite problem (not considering the film's form critically in relation to its content), Jones's incisive assessment of some interpretive tendencies within the medical and health humanities reminds us to remain attentive to the medium so that we might best parse its messages, to borrow phrasing from Marshall McLuhan. To understand the significance of the film's implementation of mobile media beyond its mere novelty, we must examine how mobile media operates in the film itself, in concert with mobile media's role in its production.

Cell phone slippage: phones as both risk and risk mitigation

By framing Sawyer's life through a voyeuristic lens before any narrative conflict arises, Soderbergh builds the film's plot and themes of observation and stalking into its aesthetics. Many of the film's formal qualities mimic modes of modern surveillance, such as long-distance observation, webcams, security cameras, and phone cameras, by virtue of being filmed on an iPhone 7. During the opening credits, the audience tracks Sawyer as she walks to her office building (Figure 25.1). The point of view shot, interrupted by out of focus plants and buildings, evokes the infamous i-camera of 80s slasher like *Friday the 13th* where the audience is aligned with the point of view of the villain lying in wait. Soderbergh uses this "stalker shot" whenever Sawyer is entering or exiting institutional settings, namely her office and the behavioral health hospital. As soon as she enters a building, the surveillant cinematography continues intermittently in other forms. The first scene, for example, places Sawyer in the center of a mildly hemispheric fisheye lens at face-height. This perspective, especially in terms of camera placement, mimics a webcam on top of/in a monitor. While the first shot is ambiguous in

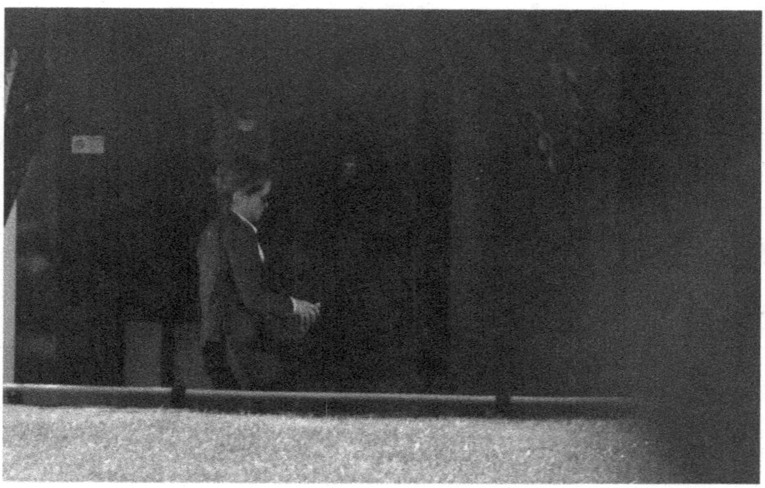

Figure 25.1 (00:06:59) Cinematographically stalking Sawyer

terms of viewer positionality – are we supposed to be seeing through the stalker's eyes directly or a digital recording of such an action? – the webcam shot clearly evokes digital mediation, less in terms of communication and more in terms of surveillance. Indeed, the iPhone aesthetic of the film as a whole leaves the "stalker shots" open to the interpretation that we are actually seeing diegetic recordings of Sawyer produced by her stalker. The cinematography, here, underscores the dangers of surveillance technologies used to safeguard people from crime in general and more specifically women from harassment, stalking, and rape, highlighting that technologies like smartphones can be used to track and spy on victims.[2]

As the slippage between footage within the diegesis[3] (made by the stalker) and footage beyond the diegesis (made by Soderbergh) causes uncertainty within the viewer and reveals important information about Sawyer's situation as a victim of stalking, so too does it reveal conceptual slippages in how we think about health and mobile media. Phones can be a tool of self-defense for women against harassment and assault (whether it be safety apps, phone calls to 911, calling a friend while walking home, or *pretending* to call a friend to escape an uncomfortable situation), but the voyeuristic associations of these shots highlight that the modern smartphone is also a networked device that leaves users vulnerable to surveillance, loss of privacy, and cyberstalking. This is a particularly concerning "affordance" for women: smartphones used to document sex acts have affected the genre of "revenge porn," where private moments become tools for public shaming and effectively tarnishing their online curated, digital subjectivity. In this way, these devices are, according to Wendy Hui Kyong Chun and Sarah Friedland, "leaky." In the case of revenge porn and related "slut-shaming," the new media of Web 2.0 concretized in the smartphone "transforms the consequences of the endemic publicity of the internet." This is an effect, they contend, "of its technological, social, and political infrastructures – into user-induced accidents. It blames the user – her habits of leaking – for systemic vulnerabilities, glossing over the ways in which our promiscuous machines routinely work through an alleged 'leaking' that undermines the separation of the personal and the networked" (Chun and Friedland 3). If the smartphones' digital seep disproportionately blames women for public consequences of their revealed sexual behaviors, we might make a similar assessment of medicine and health: biomedicalized neoliberal culture (Clarke et al. 162), prevalent in responsibilitization,[4] including the self-defense measures of the phone listed above. This is especially the case in relation to increased technical innovation and especially relevant to the rise of the digital healthcare metonymic with the smartphone.

Unsane expands this conversation about the dual affordances of mobile media by framing the role of the smartphone in Sawyer's double victimization – being stalked and gaslit, whilst confined to a hospital where her stalker manages to get hired – as indicative of the broader systemic issues of sexism, toxic masculinity, risk, and self-perception that affect women's mental health. *Unsane*'s backstory, narrated with remarkable narrative economy, is provided halfway through the film; considering the brief length of this flashback (approximately a four-minute sequence in a 97-minute film), the smartphone plays a noticeably large role in contouring Sawyer's trauma. The audience learns these details after Strine, while posing as hospital staff, intentionally replaces her prescribed mood stabilizer with a high dose of amphetamine. This maleficence leads to Sawyer's consequential psychotic break and justifies extending her stay. Following that traumatic experience and in a moment of despondency, she opens up to Nate (Jay Pharoah), an undercover journalist who feigns an opiate addiction to investigate Highland Creek. Sawyer confesses that she wanted to be this "renegade medical student that was able to pinpoint all the disease the old, traditional doctors couldn't see." She admits, however, that she didn't have the drive or follow through, but still wanted to "do something, so [she] volunteered at a hospice" (00:53:51).

Enter David Strine, son of a dying man that Sawyer tended to: "He was nice, you know. Quiet, uncomfortable and I felt bad. How do you spend two hours a week talking to your father who doesn't even recognize you." At the funeral, Sawyer's voiceover continues, "So, while I was fantasizing about being the savior who would pull his father back to clarity," the camera cuts to a close up of their respective hands next to each other and she continues, "David was having his own fantasies" (00:54:53). Preying on Sawyer's sympathy as he grasps her hand, Strine whispers, "He would have wanted us to be together." Sawyer's politeness and pity for Strine triggers his persistent pursuit and stalking. He declares his love is "pure" and perpetual in the face of rejection, an assumption that follows the mythologized narrative of masculine conquest, ever-present in media representations. Social scientists have documented how "the core dynamic in relational stalking – persistence in seeking a relationship in the face of continuing rejection – mirrors in the extreme the dogged pursuit of 'true love' idealized in the culture and media" (Emerson, Ferris, and Gardner 292; Lippman 412). Unlike films where this persistent pursuit plot falls into romantic drama (*Love, Actually*) or comedy (*Something About Mary*), *Unsane* attests to the pernicious, lasting sequelae this myth has on women's mental health – and how, despite her best efforts in averting risk, Sawyer is ultimately driven into an even more precarious situation.

Sawyer's smartphone occupies a significant amount of narrative volume during this short sequence, while the compressed time puts into sharp relief the facility by which Sawyer's compassion triggers obsession, pursuit, and intrusion. After Strine's father's funeral, Sawyer receives a spectacular arrangement of flowers, along with a note: "Sawyer – You are always on my mind. I love you always and forever. Xxxxxx – David" (00:54:52). Her co-workers marvel at the gesture while Sawyer maintains shreds of composure, despite being visibly troubled, while the camera slowly zooms out. Only the audience sees this distress. The sequence continues with an aggressive cut, punctuated by taut music: a close-up of Sawyer's hands holding her phone in a dark room, simulating our own perspective of checking a text message late at night (Figure 25.2). Strident notes from the soundtrack's score match the phone's vibrations. Sawyer doesn't even unlock her phone, paralyzed by the deluge of eleven messages, one every second. The perpetual contact the smartphone affords as technology facilitating an always-on

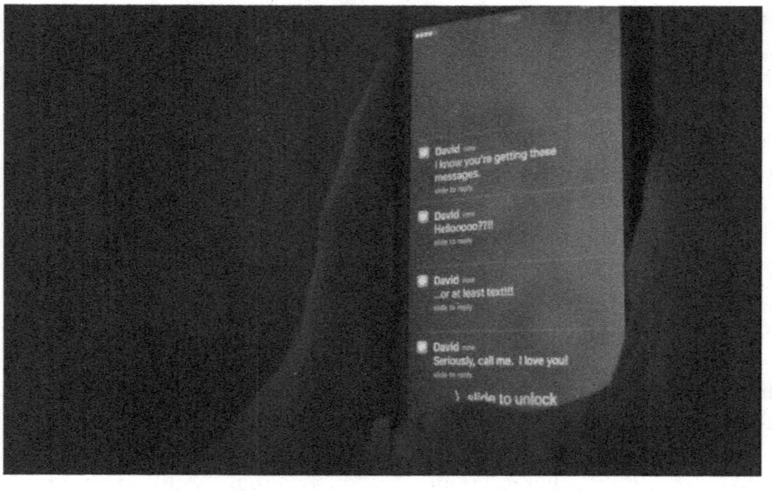

Figure 25.2 (00:55:13) Text bombed

culture allows for this kind of harassment and perpetual pursuit. But this technology also offers protection against this kind of harassment, which Sawyer utilizes. When the texts stop, Sawyer goes to her contact record and taps "block this caller" (00:55:30). The following morning she checks her phone with a sigh of relief, finding no new messages from Strine; she goes about her morning, taking a shower, putting on makeup. Relief is fleeting, and the score strikes a hard chord as she finds a brand new blue dress laid on her bed. Blocking unwanted communication, it seems, only escalates persistent pursuit to stalking, breaking, and entering. The next scene shows her filing a restraining order, and the next, consulting a police detective on home and personal safety, Soderbergh's quick cutting between these moments highlighting the urgency of the actions. Sawyer does all the right things afforded to her as a white woman of privilege and means, including technological protections. And yet, under the constraints of patriarchy and individualism, these efforts fall short of protecting her from Strine and from processing the trauma he effects.

In its brevity, this initial backstory rivals some of the more violent scenes. This narrative economy is meaningful in terms of unwanted pursuit stemming from toxic masculinity and structural sexism: so quickly and so easily does Sawyer become Strine's object of pernicious infatuation. *Unsane*, through its depiction of gaslighting in a psychiatric institution corrupted by profit, fraud, and malpractice, demonstrates the way in which toxic masculinity is facilitated and facilitates other injurious social structures. Strine is ultimately able to play out his fantasy by controlling the freedom, mental health, and movement of his victim because he capitalizes on a corrupt health system that relegates Sawyer to a stereotype of irrational and hysterical women – a systematic construction of women's minds in bodies that justifies paternal medical control of their brains and bodies.

These flashbacks are integral to the film's exposure of the smartphone's metonymic relationship to the larger structures of neoliberalism and patriarchy that induce Sawyer's subsequent and PTSD-resonant traumatization by means of institutionalization. The smartphone facilitates victim-blaming in cases of stalking, harassment, and assault, where the only solution is that women have to adopt new ways of living and socializing in the world. The onus falls on women to exercise individual risk reduction and discipline (Shelby 1097; Mason and Magnet 111; Harris and Woodlock 531). After filing a restraining order, the audience becomes familiar with what inculcated Sawyer's hypervigilance, a symptom that comes to bear beyond David Strine himself. A police detective (Matt Damon) instructs Sawyer on *The Gift of Fear*, a system of risk reduction that rivals the kind of tradecraft required for clandestine espionage. The scene begins with a brief montage of the detective assessing Sawyer's house from different angles, a voiceover bridges to their conversation inside her home.

The detective's monologue is worth quoting in its entirety (0:56:10–0:58:39), as the amount of uninterrupted, life-altering imperatives hyperbolizes the burden (both logistic and psychological) imposed on women to rape/harass/stalk-proof their lives (Figure 25.3).

> Let's talk about Sawyer Valentini, Boston, year zero. I would swap the terrace doors out for a steel-core door. Um, update your dead bolts. Uh, I want to talk to you about situational awareness, okay? Where's the nearest police station? Where's the nearest fire station? These are things that should always be right on the tip of your tongue. Yeah, parking…Um, I know you have parking in the rear of the building with the back entrance. I'm gonna ask you not to use that anymore. I know it's convenient, but I would advocate selling your car and using a ride service. If you can't or won't do that, uh, I would say park on the street, preferably under a light source.

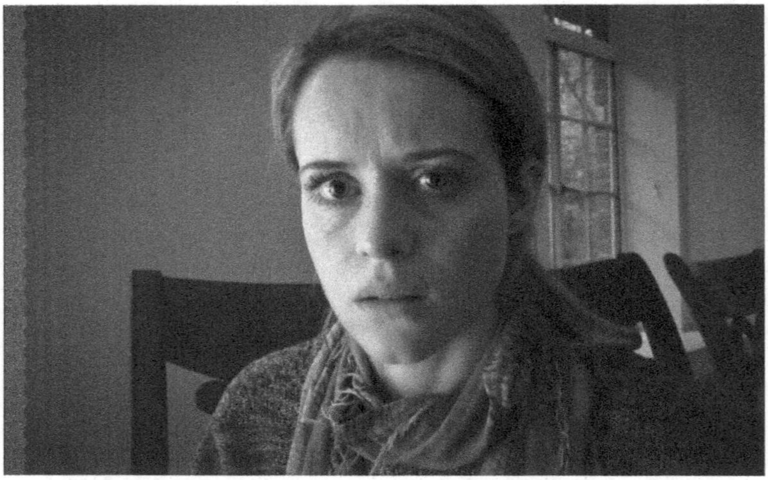

Figure 25.3 (00:57:35, 00:57:54) "Let's talk about Sawyer Valentini"

As the monologue continues, the shots transition between him inspecting her home and his face-to-face meeting with Sawyer. During this exchange we see Damon at a distance, across the table that sits between him and Sawyer, as if viewing him from Sawyer's point of view. Sawyer, on the other hand, we see in close-up shots of her face as she looks increasingly distressed – rather than comforted – by his words. As he continues, amongst the myriad of responsibilities that must become Sawyer's new normal, his concluding point crystalizes the entangled dangers of mobile, digital, and social media – the technoscape of ubiquitous computing:

> And come back and walk through this courtyard here where people can see you. With your keys in your hand, by the way. You want your keys always in your hand. You don't want to be digging around in your purse in the dark for your keys. Um, and I'll talk to you about and help you with a go-bag. You know, just cash, credit cards, uh, change of clothes, flashlight, charger, that kind of thing. A firearm, if you're open to that idea of purchasing or registering a firearm and learning how to use it. Think about altering your routine. Uh, when you go to work, when you leave work, um, that kind of thing. How about social media? Are you on any social media accounts?

The shot cuts back to Sawyer's overwhelmed face, as she responds that she is on Facebook *but* that her "account's private, so" – he interrupts:

> Right. Okay, that's no good, because he'd be able to, you know, figure out a friend of yours from marching band or a sorority sister and go get photos from them, create a bogus account and then try to friend you that way. Your friends know your e-mail. Just… That's enough. Just delete the Facebook today. Um, and then talk to your friends, you know. Be open about this. Inform them what's going on. Tell them not to mention you. Don't tag you on Instagram. You know, uh, um...You know, baby showers or, you know, Chardonnay date with the girls. You know, whatever it is, if there's someone taking a picture, you do whatever you can to get out of it, all right? *And think of your cell phone as your enemy.*

The cell phone indexes persons – their habits, relations, locations – and their leaky data, a concern that is, indeed, inescapable in the era of ubiquitous computing. Images taken with cell phones include metadata, often global positioning or GPS coordinates. It does not take much sleuthing or degrees of separation for Sawyer's stalker to reconnect. In the criminology and gender violence literature, this form of abuse is known as "technology-facilitated abuse," "technology facilitated stalking," and "digital coercive control" (Harris and Woodlock 532).[5] This is not even to mention the troves of "snoopware" available that empower stalkers to spy on their victim, or "creepware," which facilitates interpersonal attacks by creating spoofed phone, or sms "bombing," among other nefarious features (Fitz-Gibbon et al. 19; Roundy et al. 626; Valentino-DeVries). The discomforting associations surrounding mobile media, originally prompted by the silent, potentially-diegetic stalker shots at the opening of the film, are broken down here and explained in horrifying detail as a justification for self-surveillance. The detective's dismissive attitude toward Sawyer's concerns and interjections, his rote repetition of this overwhelming regimen, and his casual sexism (assuming that "baby showers or, you know, Chardonnay dates with the girls" are the core of Sawyer's social life) all produce an undercurrent of uncomfortable paternalism in the scene, highlighting that this form of self-defense functions clearly within established patriarchal power structures, reducing Sawyer's risk rather than challenging the systems which rendered her vulnerable. It is significant that Soderbergh cast Matt Damon to deliver this speech, as he is historically known for his persona as an unthreatening "good guy next door" in films like *Good Will Hunting* (Jacobs). This strategic casting choice heightens the discomforting nature of his condescending attitude; by subverting audience expectations about the gentle, supportive male character audiences might expect to see Matt Damon play, Soderbergh highlights that male responses to stalking and domestic violence are often shockingly callous.

In these flashbacks, Soderbergh breaks down and explicitly depicts the conflicting logics surrounding technological vulnerability that he foreshadows early in the film. At each stage of Sawyer's original traumatic experiences, whether it be the inciting events with Strine, or the initial response with the detective in which she is still visibly shaken, phones and technology are central, but their significance is always in flux. For years, the modern smartphone has been positioned as an interventional technology that women can use to protect against rape, harassment, and stalking. The problem with these technologies is twofold. First, they don't account for how the mobile phone can provide affordances for pathological behaviors of toxic masculinity, such as the software detailed above or the litany of dangers the detective cautions against. Second, the alluring promise that mobile technologies will empower women with the tools and resilience to fend off harassment, attacks, or stalking is at best a band aid. These instances of "techno-physical feminism" can reify the constructions of women as fragile and in need of protection. Moreover, and in line with *Unsane*, the aspirations of mobile media qua technofix "embraces a form of individual, self-optimizing empowerment that fails to challenge the structural misogynistic logics that facilitate sexual violence" (Shelby 1090). The smartphone, then, in Sawyer's flashbacks draws attention to structural problems related to women's health (physical and mental) in the face of toxic masculinity and the trauma it engenders: smartphones and their broader technoscape meditate but don't resolve sexism or misogyny.

Uncopable, uncanny measures, and media

Despite the advice we later hear Sawyer receiving from the Detective in the establishing flashbacks, at the opening of *Unsane*, Sawyer is practicing a different kind of self-defense: the performance of an affable calm and the leveraging of her privilege as a well-educated white woman. We meet Sawyer in her everyday office milieu, where Soderbergh quickly establishes that she is assertive, perspicacious, and excellent at her job. The narrative opens with Sawyer on the phone, telling a customer not to take their frustration out on her and that they "are quite within their rights to take [their] business to another bank and another analyst may interpret the data more to their liking but they'll be doing a bad job." She hangs up, her co-worker staring in amazement. "I hope he likes vinegar more than he likes honey – " (0:03:29). Sawyer corrects her: "She." This clarification subtly introduces a hint of sexism, even between the two women. Without much time to reflect on the meaning of such an interjection, the next shot (over Sawyer's shoulder) catches a nondescript man walking in the background and turning the corner. Cut to an expression of alarm in a close up of Sawyer's face as she pushes her chair out to get a better look at him. While there appears to be no threat, this hypervigilance is the first sign of Sawyer's trauma that the audience is privy to. Despite this moment of concern, Sawyer almost immediately calmly leaves to meet with her boss (Marc Kudisch), who praises her hard work and performance. Whatever affirmation these accolades might have had vanishes when the conversation shifts, and he attempts to convince Sawyer to attend a conference with him, with clearly sexual implications. Sawyer adeptly navigates the awkward invitation; she needs "a little more experience" (0:05:24). When he responds that he could "help her with that," she more firmly rejects the proposal, saying, "I should get back to work" with a tone so final that her boss simply agrees awkwardly. Soderbergh here begins to develop a complex characterization of Sawyer: attuned to sexism in the workplace, she at once displays signs of hypervigilance provoked by the possibility of Strine's presence, while also demonstrating the ability to navigate compromising professional encounters with other men, assertively and with decorum. The unflappable self-presentation only breaks, allowing the audience to see her true thoughts, when she leaves the room and, with her back to him, pulls a disgusted face at her boss's behavior.

In subsequent scenes, the mobile phone belays that this front is one of Sawyer's primary coping mechanisms: performed sanguinity. Speaking to her mother via video chat during her lunch break, Sawyer asserts how well she's doing (0:06:00). Facetime demands this in a way that phone and text conversations do not, the multimedia format and synchronicity providing a virtual co-presence and immediacy, a portability of care (Alinejad 2). Her mother cannot only hear her tone of voice but also see the facial nonverbal cues that telegraph affect. Sawyer has to tell *and* show her mother that she is doing well. Her boss is "great," and "he has really high standards and he's really demanding, but when he says you got something right, you know you got it right" – a harsh contrast to the preceding scene the audience was privy to. Providing more insight into Sawyer's personal history, her mother complains about Sawyer moving "450 miles away." Sawyer chides her mother not to "do that," and reminds her that the job was a "fantastic opportunity," and that she "could not say no." She further attempts to comfort her mother, "Everything is great and [she] couldn't be happier," closing with "Besides, you know what an impulsive girl, I am."

The film has established, and maintains throughout, that Sawyer is far from impulsive; when not triggered by the imagined or real presence of David Strine, she is perceptive and circumspect. During the Facetime call, Sawyer can see herself performing sanguinity. The mirroring is doubled, mediated through the box that shows her own live video feed and reflected in the screen's glass. This shot draws attention to itself as hypermediated: the compilation of various media forms re-presented through Facetime (video and audio) and to the mobile phone itself as media device. When she hangs up the call the digital presence she performs for her mother disappears, yet the reflection of her own resigned face remains like a mirror. The lingering reflection suggests a self-awareness to her actions as she looks at herself, an acknowledgement of the trauma that still exists beneath her insistence to others that she is doing well. Her forced smile, now, a frown; she slumps. Soderbergh visualizes this process through multiple cuts: a high angled medium shot, intimating a sense of vulnerability; a cut to a close-up, expressively rendering her dysphoria, as the audience sits uncomfortably with Sawyer in her feelings, perhaps with an inkling of what's driving them. This exposition presents a complicated picture of Sawyer's steadfastness in response to her trauma. However well-adjusted Sawyer really is at this moment, it is not enough to mitigate the trauma-intrusive hallucination that occurs in the proceeding sequence.

Unsane's exposition concludes with the inciting event that sets in motion the asylum thriller plot, occasioned by the facilitating technology of her mobile phone. After Sawyer's check-in with her mother, we observe her on a Tinder date (0:07:25), which follows a set of now somewhat generic conventions: walking into the bar, she checks her phone, looks for her date; the awkward double take from phone to stranger at the bar, the sharing of shots, her date, Jesse, a bit charmingly befuddled. The scene is filmed with a slightly-low angle shot, not mimicking exactly but still indexing its production from a phone, placed horizontally on the bar, capturing their encounter. The visual foregrounding of alcohol in the shot intimates the risk of the interaction – meeting a stranger while lowering her inhibitions, a recipe for "you should have been more careful," that victim-blaming refrain all too familiar to most women and which Matt Damon's detective would echo. Sawyer's confidence exuberant, she cuts, from the playful banter, to the chase: "Promise me one thing, Jesse, tonight is going to go how you want it to go. But afterwards, you don't call me, you don't contact me, it's like we never met." Back at Sawyer's apartment, a back lit close up of the couple kissing shows the briefest of moments when they break and look into each other's eyes. The intimacy and eroticism of the moment vanishes, as we observe Sawyers eyes-widening, rapidly pushing herself away from her date onto the floor as she screams "Fuck!..No!" Sawyer experiences an intrusive hallucination associated with PTSD (00:09:36),[6] seeing her stalker's everywhere, seeing his face on other men. This is certainly attributed to her individual response to trauma, but when read structurally, like the film's other elements of uncanny multiplicity, it signals systemic problems. Soon, the audience will observe how Sawyer is algorithmically coaxed from cultural sexism to concrete institution.

Sawyer's panic is temporarily quelled by ingesting an anxiolytic. It becomes clear, in this moment of reckoning, that self-empowerment, even with psychopharmacologic support, falls short of returning her to any kind of normalcy in the face of trauma. In fact, after the briefest of repose, rather than pursuing a psychiatric and psychopharmacological remedy, Sawyer sits down at her computer and types "support groups for victims of stalking" in the search engine. The results do not lead her to the National Center for Victims of Crime's Stalking Resource Center, Safehope, or Victimconnect.org.[7] Instead, the top of the search foregrounds a paid advertisement for "Highland Creek Behavioral Health." She clicks; the scene transitions to her driving to the clinic. There is certainly the basic plot of Highland Creek's insurance fraud, which the undercover investigative journalist intimates is a pervasive practice; however, it is necessary to consider this inciting event in terms of the structural – and, more specifically, the algorithmic – determinants that put her there.

This convenient search result is a key moment in the film's critique of corporatized mental health, specifically the way in which it is systemically imbricated in the contemporary technoscape of ubiquitous computing and digital health. Olivia Banner has documented how patient support groups, narratives, and other mediations online have become datasets of value from which surplus labor of the ill is harvested (Banner 13). Search algorithms, likewise, have their own "coaxed affordances," in this case reinforcing "certain structures of social, political, and economic capital," and in some cases direct which support groups or blogs users

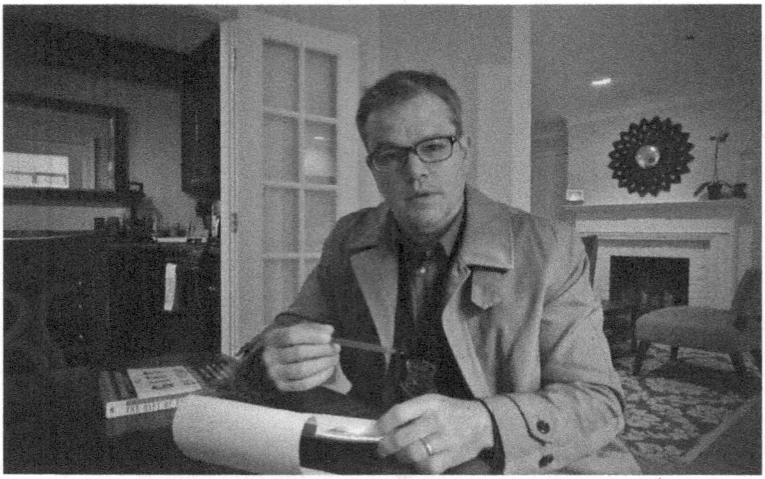

Figure 25.4 (00:10:18) Coaxed affordances

encounter (19, 108) (Figure 25.4). Though there is no representation of Sawyer's experience being aggregated and monetized through analytics, her ensnarement into corporatized health care when she seeks out peer-support through a search engine emblematizes the injurious effects of what Banner calls "communicative biocapitalism."

In our contemporary technoscape of communicative capitalism, where phones mediate so much of our connection with the rest of the world, they have likewise fallen into neoliberal logics of self-determination and individualism. Metonymic to (at once representation and a part/property of) the larger network of ubiquitous computing – that links to desktops, cloud servers, social media, wearable devices, and medical devices – they also function as what Foucault notably characterizes as "technologies of the self" (225). They mediate, record, and actualize various operations that individuals use to act on their body, mind, and soul to improve, account, and confess themselves. They have become an essential tool for self-fashioning and formations of contemporary subjectivity (Gill and Orgad 1315; Luthar and Pušnik 2–4). Moreover, in the inflection of "digital health," mobile technologies, almost always mediated through the smartphone, have offered individuals the means to " 'take control' over their health via contributing to and harnessing online information and engaging in self-monitoring and self-care practices using digital technologies." Many of these apps, and their extension into health, self-tracking and monitoring are strongly gendered (Lupton 611–12). In this way they form, as mentioned above, part of our digital, leaky, habitus.

Just as phones within the diegesis of *Unsane* expose the ways that technology can mediate but not resolve structural issues, the use of an iPhone to capture these scenes assists in exposing these oppressions. Some moments in *Unsane* feature a more exaggerated digital aesthetic, but the iPhone format is clear throughout the film. As noted earlier, the effect of the iPhone on the color and quality of the film has been levied as a critique by some reviewers (Robinson), but this compromise in quality comes with one significant side-effect: the audience can visibly recognize that this was filmed on a phone. While this might be a criticism in relation to the film's cinematic polish, it also results in a product that evokes subtle associations with our digital lives and online self-expression. In many cases, these associations with recognizable forms of digital communication inform the audience's readings of Sawyer's emotional state.

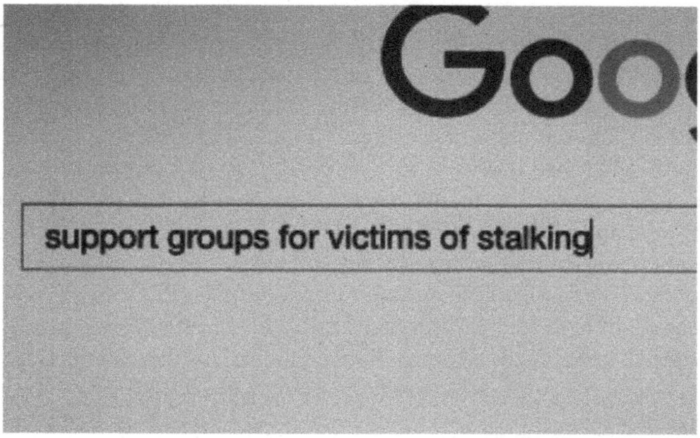

Figure 25.5 (00:11:13) "Well, rationally I know this is my neuroses colluding with my imagination to manifest my worst fears. But I'm not rational"

Early in *Unsane* these digital associations promote a stable, emotional connection between Sawyer and the audience. During her first encounter with a therapist – one which will ultimately lead to her confinement – Sawyer talks with immense emotional vulnerability about her stalking and subsequent trauma. Soderbergh films this scene head-on with the camera capturing Sawyer at face height in a medium-close up shot, looking almost into the lens as she confides her deepest secrets (Figure 25.6). Unlike the scene where Sawyer performed sanguinity for her mother, where we saw multiple reflections of her from a high, tilted angle, this shot is uncluttered and direct. With the phone absent and a listener who she thinks she can trust, we see Sawyer confessing the trauma that she has been hiding. While within the diegesis Sawyer may be talking to her therapist – occasionally seen in reverse-shots – to the viewer it appears that she is speaking directly to us. While the absence of a phone within the film facilitates the dropping of Sawyer's performance, the continued presence of the aesthetic of iPhone-as-camera evokes associations with vlogging (video blogging) and other online forms of self-expression. Vlogging and other forms of expressing personal experiences online form "intimate publics" (Hjorth and Lim 478), where mobile media blurs the lines between online and offline worlds and becomes a key tool for facilitating intimacy. In his analysis of YouTube vlogging and bereavement, Gibson notes that "bereavement vlogs function as online support groups; they tap into a need to be expressive about sadness and find others who know what it means in an ordinary, everyday way. The internal world of hidden sorrow is recast back into the social world through the bereavement vlog" (642). Here, the audience's voyeuristic view of Sawyer is turned on its head as she shares her trauma with us in a visual digital register that evokes one that viewers are likely to recognize: a digital vlog.

This connection – which feels not unlike the support group that Sawyer was originally seeking before she was algorithmically directed to this therapist – is soon subverted by the therapist's medicalized response and Sawyer's subsequent commitment. This identifiable vlogging format in the therapist's office encourages the audience to view the moment as intimate, but it is also a moment that anchors Sawyer's level-headedness and sanity. The unwavering, level camera angle looks unflinchingly at Sawyer's suffering, but she also looks unflinchingly back (at both the audience and the therapist), demonstrating confidence and self-awareness as well as vulnerability. Once within Highland Creek, however, the affordances of iPhone filming take on a new significance. Within this space, Sawyer's assertive confidence is rendered futile, the world no longer responds to her leveraging of privilege as she expects. In this latter section of the film, Soderbergh deviates from cinematic norms not to evoke a comfortingly recognizable aesthetic like the vlog format but to subvert the visual norms of polished Hollywood filmmaking in a way that extends the distinctly off-kilter world to the viewer.

The disquieting uncertainty of *Unsane* is related to the initial ambiguity about Sawyer's mental state and the generic conventions of the asylum genre evident in films like *Shutter Island* (2010), but the iPhone's use in achieving this atmosphere elevates *Unsane*. One review that stands out at amongst the others is Laura Kremmel's in *Gothic Studies,* where she contends, "the iPhone create[s] the confused sense of reality/unreality that so troubles the audience and that sets this aside from other asylum horror films" (Kremmel 157). This confusion is distinctly uncanny in nature, rendering the space of the asylum at once familiar and confusing. Once within the asylum, Soderbergh's color balancing alternately exaggerates blue and yellow-brown hues, connoting an atmosphere that is alternately (and conflictingly) sterile and dirty, distant and claustrophobic. Combined with the often-low lighting, the iPhone's resolution also becomes grainy and muddied. Where the dark, gritty aesthetic of the iPhone's camera errs unsettlingly close to true crime videos taken on phones and featured on the news, Soderbergh's editing and framing adds an air of off-kilter unreality; Highland Creek is at once painted as familiar and other. While some critics cite these effects as criticisms of the iPhone format, they are actually instrumental in creating the atmosphere within the asylum. In their conflicting affects, the iPhone aesthetics begin to render the space of Highland Creek uncanny; eerie and unsettling.

This uncanny atmosphere is heightened during confrontations with Strine, when Sawyer truly begins to question her surroundings. When Sawyer first sees him, she – and perhaps for a short while the audience – questions her sanity. This scene occurs when she is receiving her daily medication and encounters Strine posing as an orderly. As he offers her medication, Soderbergh cuts to a reverse-shot of Sawyer's face where Strine's hand hovers in the foreground of the frame, his presence infringing threateningly on Sawyer within the frame as the audience sees her reaction. The subsequent exchange is filmed as a shot-reverse-shot sequence, but one that is uneven and off-kilter. Sawyer is filmed from a slightly side-angle, looking up at her attacker who is framed as slightly above as well as to the side of the frame (Figure 25.6). However, rather than pairing these shots with corresponding shots of Strine from the same side of the 180-degree line,[8] the intercut shots of Strine are head-on and uncomfortably close, his face almost filling the screen as he looks down at Sawyer and at the camera.

By offsetting this exchange with inconsistent eyelines, Soderbergh uses the flexibility and maneuverability of the iPhone to subvert the audience's expectation, resulting in a disconcerting filmic product. Strine's gaze is direct and threatening for the audience as well as Sawyer, in contrast to the connection viewers felt with Sawyer's direct "vlogging"-esque address in her therapy session; that honest emotional expression has been replaced by the medicalized (and medicated) unreality of Highland Creek, which sparks fear in both Sawyer and the viewer alike. Now crowded in the frame and confined in the narrative, she can no longer leverage her privilege to challenge her abuse. This atmosphere reflects Sawyer's horror at her confinement and her individual abuse at Strine's hands alike, conflating the individual and systematic harms she is experiencing. In re-orienting the affordances of the iPhone from enabling emotional vulnerability to reflecting uncanny disconnection, Soderbergh makes Sawyer's mental state visible in recognizable digital aesthetics; he also demonstrates the complicity of mobile technology in her suffering. The horror of Sawyer's situation is recognizably filtered through, and enabled by, the iPhone-as-artefact in Soderbergh's hands. This makes mobile media key in the creation of Sawyer's suffering both within and outside the diegesis of the film, as a tool of stalking and a

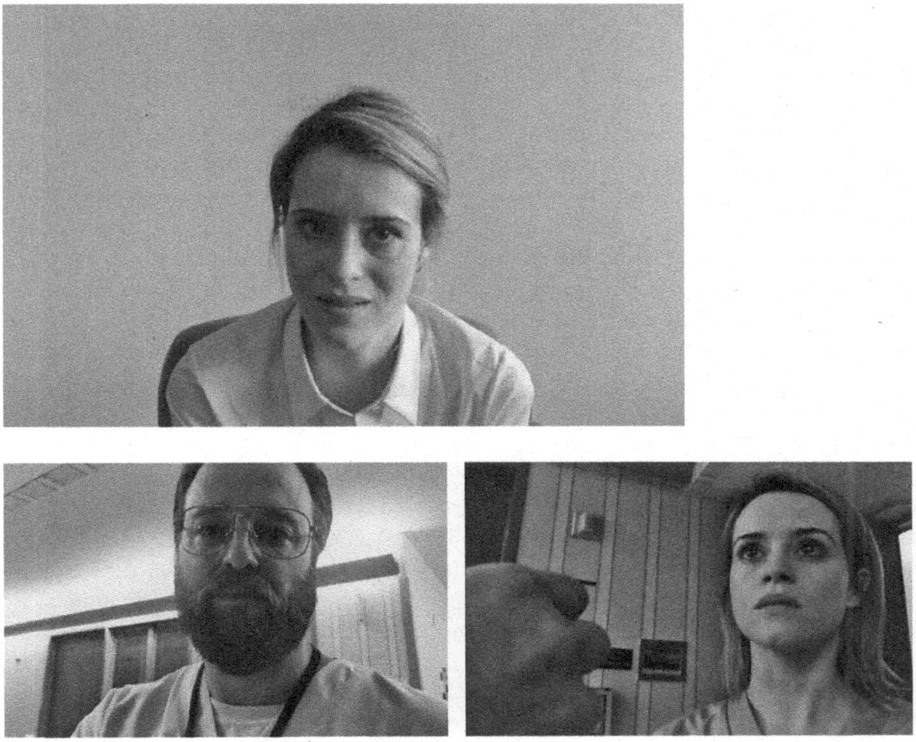

Figure 25.6 (00:33:17, 00:33:25) "You can't be anywhere near me"

tool of narrative creation. In doing so, the phones' digital aesthetic becomes a powerful tool for producing – and reading – *Unsane,* rather than merely a novel auteur experiment or a shortcoming which undermines the final product.

Reading for *Unsane* structures and an unresolved closure

While *Unsane* focuses much of its exploration on Strine himself and on Sawyer's uncertain fears, Soderbergh highlights the structural problems which allow, and in many cases facilitate, Strine's harassment of Sawyer at Highland Creek. Indeed, the horror of Sawyer's experiences begins before Strine is introduced as an employee, when Sawyer is misled by the intake counselor about what the "standard forms" she signs actually mean, is refused answers to her questions by the receptionist, and is spoken over by multiple nurses during her intake. Nate's investigative reporting later reveals that this procedure is relatively standard at Highland Creek to generate more profit from the insurance payments of involuntarily committed patients, but it is unclear which (if any) of these initial characters are knowingly complicit in unnecessary and traumatizing medical response for economic gain. Later, however, it is obvious that numerous characters are consciously facilitating this economic scheme: the sleazy and distracted doctor; the hospital administrators who lie to and subtly threaten her mother to stop investigating. Importantly, Soderbergh makes clear that the oppressive forces within Highland Creek are not *only* patriarchal. Throughout *Unsane,* women are at the heart of Sawyer's confinement, and she is mistreated by her therapist, the receptionist, the head nurse, the hospital administrator, who are all women likely driven by their economic benefit from her situation. While Strine may be the classical villain of *Unsane,* he is only able to conduct his campaign of terror against Sawyer because the medicalized system allows him to; firstly by falsely committing her, and secondly by dismissing her concerns about Strine in favor of ensuring she stays longer in their facility. Gendered violence and torment are hidden and facilitated, at least in part, for economic gain.

Here, Soderbergh highlights the multiple oppressions contributing to Sawyer's suffering at the hands of the medical system. The transition from her confidence and privilege as a white woman in the opening scene where she confidently shuts down her boss's advantage, to her treatment in the facility is a shock for both the viewer and Sawyer's privileged sensibilities. In several scenes once she is at the facility, she tries to use her privilege and confidence in the same way she did with her boss, to escape. She performs sanguinity, once again, to her doctor (who is just as sleazy as her boss) and the nurses. Once this approach doesn't work, she tries calling the police and asking to be rescued, but this also fails. Highland Creek systematically rejects and disassembles the defense mechanisms and performances she used in the outside world to cope with her trauma and achieve her goals, leaving her more vulnerable. The ways in which she navigated patriarchal aggressions no longer function when combined with the erasure of her voice as a patient and a system in which she is a tool for economic gain.

Soderbergh highlights the pervasive power of these oppressive systems in the latter part of *Unsane,* when he shows that even Sawyer – a survivor of gendered violence – is not immune to the corrupting influence of these oppressive systems. At the close of the film, she manipulates Strine into kidnapping her fellow patient, Violet (Juno Temple), because Sawyer knows that Violet has a knife. Sawyer convinces Strine to do this by saying that he needs to sexually assault Violet to gain experience to be with Sawyer. Strine ultimately kills Violet as Sawyer watches through the window in the door and finally escapes. Under the impossible conditions of her confinement and torment by Strine, Sawyer is forced to place another woman in danger of sexual assault, which almost occurs, and ultimately causes her death. The betrayal of female solidarity seen in the many women who work at Highland Creek and refuse to help Sawyer despite her impassioned pleas about Strine is replicated by Sawyer in how she treats Violet. Focusing solely on Strine as a villain is tantamount to suggesting that addressing Sawyer's safety and trauma properly is the solution to what ails *Unsane*. Likewise, solely calling out the whitewashing, gaslighting, and corrupt care providers and administrators – psychiatrist, nurses, intake counselors – limits the film's potential for health humanistic inquiry. *Unsane* does more than document neoliberal logics at work. A critical reading of the film suggests blaming the staff, clinic, or organizations is merely a band aid to the larger cultural and social structures and institutions (the culture and social body enmeshed with the innumerable health systems) that catalyze the gender violence and harassment that Sawyer experiences, and which she, eventually, is forced to participate in.

Attending to the film's complex media specificity – film, mobile, social, and digital media – makes *Unsane* well-suited to health humanist inquiry in the form of structural competency. Following the work of Metzel and Harris on structural competency in medicine, Banner's theorization of communicative biocapitalism takes this a step further in identifying how media technologies are shaped by structural racism. Instead of reading for individual experience and empathy, she proposes *reading for structures*: "textual readings that elucidate how ideologies of race, gender, and disability inform social, political, economic and institutional structures, which then inform health and illness" (Banner 27). *Unsane*'s most resonant dimension in this vein is structural sexism, a social determinant of health made widely visible in the wake of #MeToo. The medical sociology literature on gender inequality and health has documented the health consequences of harassment, perceived gender discrimination and systematic gender inequality.

Drawing on Kreiger's ecosocial theory of social epidemiology, Patricia Homan demonstrates that women exposed to structural sexism experience more chronic health conditions, worse self-rated health, and worse physical functioning. She suggests that structural sexism operates through a variety of pathways to harm women's health: "reduced access to material resources, goods, and services; exposure to violence, harassment, or unsafe working conditions; perceived discrimination; low subjective social status; increased stress; reduced psychosocial resources such as self-esteem, mastery, sense of control, autonomy, coping resources, and social support; and inadequate healthcare quality or access" (Homan 507).

The conclusion of *Unsane* suggests that Sawyer will be subject to these long-term health impacts following her experiences not only with Strine, but with the structural exploitation and oppression within Highland Creek that exacerbated his power to harm her. In the final scene, while at a restaurant with a friend, Sawyer thinks that she sees Strine at a neighboring table and approaches the man with a knife. Unlike in the asylum, Soderbergh reveals this moment to be a trauma-induced hallucination. In a tense close-up of her face, brief flashes of Strine's face (shots that viewers will recognize from within Highland Creek) intercut the shot of Sawyer approaching the man, demonstrating the link between her traumatic experiences within the asylum (not beforehand) and this paranoid behavior: Highland Creek has helped to re-produce the very symptoms of trauma that it claimed it could allay. Realizing her mistake as the man turns around, Sawyer drops the knife and flees the restaurant, the camera ending on a final shot of her looking fearfully into the lens. While she escaped the asylum and killed Strine, *Unsane* ends on a scene which anchors the long-term psychological and health consequences that are going to follow to Sawyer. While it is not useful to attempt to diagnose a fictional character like Sawyer, it is clear that the narrative of *Unsane* ends with her experiencing increased stress and worsened trauma and anxiety symptoms, which have the potential to put women in danger of further social and health-related problems, as Homan notes. Indeed, within *Unsane* these consequences and health outcomes are compounded by Sawyer's disastrous experiences with psychological and health care, likely undermining (or at least rendering traumatic) any attempts at seeking further care for these ensuing symptoms. The horror highlighted at the close of *Unsane* is not just the threat of Strine as an individual, now deceased, but rather the long-term health consequences that structural sexism have wrought on Sawyer by further exposing her to his stalking; the smartphone at once revealer, inhibitor, and catalyst. *Unsane* therefore leaves attentive viewers better equipped to navigate the triangulation of for-profit healthcare, patriarchal power, and the digital dissemination of communicative biocapitalism that come to bear on health, especially for women; all facilitated by the smartphones in our pockets.

Notes

1 The pen name for the American journalist Elizabeth Cochrane Searman, most famous for her *New York World* article "Ten Days in the Madhouse," where she described "the hysteric's hyper-female, hyper-expressive body" and exposed the inhumane conditions of the Women's Lunatic Asylum on Roosevelt's Island in 1887 (Lutes 13).

2 Beyond the behavioral sciences and criminological literature, this phenomena has been well-established across disciplines and emerged as an interdisciplinary field itself, generating edited collections and special issues. See Dubrosky and Magnet's *Feminist Surveillance Studies* (2015), Boyle and Rathnayake's "#HimToo and the Networking of Misogyny in the Age of #MeToo," and Shelby's "Techno-Physical Feminism: Anti-rape Technology, Gender, and Corporeal Surveillance," among others.

3 A film's diegesis is the world of a film. If music plays from a radio seen on screen, heard by the characters, it is part of the film's diegesis and therefore it is diegetic sound. Music on the soundtrack which is not heard by characters and only by the audience does not exist within the diegesis of the film, meaning it is non-diegetic sound.

4 The biopolitcal and critical theory literature is vast, including scholars such as Jasbir Puar, Deborah Lupton, Nikolas Rose, and Michel Foucault.

5 The terms are sometimes used interchangeably, discretized, or contested (Harris and Woodlock 533).

6 While the DSM-V does not include hallucinations as a symptom of PTSD, nor are we formally attempting to diagnose the fictional Sawyer, visual and intrusive hallucinations have been widely documented in both psychological and psychiatric literature. The phenomenological crossover between hallucination, intrusive memory, and "flashbacks" as a phenomena and terminology that is used broadly was observed at least as early as Ehlers and Stiel's widely cited "Maintenance of Intrusive Memories in Posttraumatic Stress Disorder" of the then extant research (Ehlers and Stiel 219). See also Geddes, Ehlers, Freeman's more recent review of the literature surrounding trauma and hallucinations (602).

7 These are amongst the top results generated from an observational run of the same terms through Google.com (December 25, 2020).

8 The 180-degree line or 180-degree rule is a filmmaking practice where, to preserve continuity, a conversation between characters is shot from the same side. If you visualize a line being drawn directly between two characters speaking, cameras are only placed on one side of them (one 180-degree section of the room). By observing the 180-degree rule, each character remains facing the same way in resulting footage, and remains oriented in relation to the other characters.

Works cited

Abeele, Mariek Vanden, Ralf De Wolf, and Rich Ling. "Mobile Media and Social Space: How Anytime, Anyplace Connectivity Structures Everyday Life." *Media and Communication,* vol. 6, no. 2, 2018, pp. 5–14.

Alinejad, Donya. "Careful Co-Presence: The Transnational Mediation of Emotional Intimacy." *Social Media and Society,* vol. 5, no. 2, 2019, pp. 1–11.

Banner, Olivia. *Communicative Biocapitalism: The Voice of the Patient in Digital Health and the Health Humanities.* Ann Arbor, MI: University of Michigan Press, 2017.

Bourdieu, Pierre. *Distinction: A Social Critique of the Judgement of Taste.* London: Routledge & Kegan Paul, 1984.

Boyle, Karen, and Chamil Rathnayake. "#HimToo and the Networking of Misogyny in the Age of #MeToo." *Feminist Media Studies,* vol. 20, no. 8, 2020, pp. 1259–77.

Brody, Richard. "Steven Soderbergh's Inspired iPhone Experiment in 'Unsane.'" *New Yorker,* March 27, 2018. www.newyorker.com/culture/richard-brody/steven-soderberghs-inspired-iphone-experiment-in-unsane. Accessed 28 October 2020.

Chun, Wendy Hui Kyong, and Sarah Friedland. "Habits of Leaking: Of Sluts and Network Cards." *Differences: A Journal of Feminist Cultural Studies,* vol. 26, no. 2, 2015, pp. 1–28.

Clarke, Adele E., et al. "Biomedicalization: Technoscientific Transformations of Health, Illness, and U.S. Biomedicine." *American Sociological Review,* vol. 68, no. 2, 2003, pp. 161–94.

Dinnen, Zara. *The Digital Banal: New Media and American Literature and Culture.* New York: Columbia University Press, 2018.

Dubrofsky, Rachel E., and Shoshana Amielle Magnet, editors.*Feminist Surveillance Studies.* Durham, NC: Duke University Press, 2015.

Ehlers, Anke, and Regina Stiel. "Maintenance of Intrusive Memories in Posttraumatic Stress Disorder: A Cognitive Approach." *Behavioural and Cognitive Psychotherapy,* vol. 23, no. 3, 1995, pp. 217–45.

Emerson, Robert M., Kerry O. Ferris, and Carol Brooks Gardner. "On Being Stalked." *Social Problems,* vol. 45, no. 3, 1998, pp. 289–314.

Fitz-Gibbon, Kate, Sandra Walklate, Jude McCulloch, and Jane Maree Maher. *Intimate Partner Violence, Risk and Security: Securing Women's Lives in a Global World.* New York and Abingdon: Routledge, 2020.

Foucault, Michel. *Ethics: Subjectivity, and Truth.* Edited by Paul Rabinow. New York: New Press, 1997.

Geddes, Georgina, Anke Ehlers, and Daniel Freeman. "Hallucinations in the Months after a Trauma: An Investigation of the Role of Cognitive Processing of a Physical Assault in the Occurrence of Hallucinatory Experiences." *Psychiatry Research,* vol. 246, 2016, pp. 601–5.

Gibson, Margaret. "YouTube and Bereavement Vlogging: Emotional Exchange between Strangers." *Journal of Sociology,* vol. 52, no. 4, 2016, pp. 631–45.

Gill, Rosalind, and Shani Orgad. "The Shifting Terrain of Sex and Power: From the 'Sexualization of Culture' to #MeToo." *Sexualities,* vol. 21, no. 8, 2018, pp. 1313–24.

Harris, Bridget A., and Delanie Woodlock. "Digital Coercive Control: Insights from Two Landmark Domestic Violence Studies." *British Journal of Criminology*, vol. 59, no. 3, 2019, pp. 530–50.

Hjorth, Larissa, and Sun Sun Lim. "Mobile Intimacy in an Age of Affective Mobile Media." *Feminist Media Studies*, vol. 12, no. 4, 2012, pp. 477–84.

Homan, Patricia. "Structural Sexism and Health in the United States: A New Perspective on Health Inequality and the Gender System." *American Sociological Review*, vol. 84, no. 3, 2019, pp. 486–516.

Jacobs, Matthew. "How Weinstein and the Hollywood Machine Created 'Good Guy' Matt Damon." *Huff Post,* March 4, 2018, www.huffpost.com/entry/matt-damon-harvey-weinstein-good-guy-image_n_5a9477c5e4b01f65f5994a29. Accessed June 29, 2021.

Jones, Therese. "'Oh, the Humanity(Ies)!': Dissent, Democracy and Danger." *Medicine, Health and the Arts: Approaches to the Medical Humanities*, edited by Sam Goodman, Victoria Bates, and Alan Bleakley. New York and Abingdon: Routledge, 2014, pp. 27–38.

Kremmel, Laura. "Review of *Unsane,* Directed by Steven Soderbergh." *The Irish Journal of Gothic and Horror Studies*, vol. 17, 2018, pp. 154–7.

Lippman, Julia R. "I Did It Because I Never Stopped Loving You: The Effects of Media Portrayals of Persistent Pursuit on Beliefs about Stalking." *Communication Research*, vol. 43, no. 3, 2018, pp. 394–421.

Luthar, Breda, and Maruša Pušnik. "Intimate Media and Technological Nature of Sociality." *New Media and Society*, vol. 23, no. 5, 2021. https://doi.org/10.1177/1461444820912387.

Lupton, Deborah. "Apps as Artefacts: Towards a Critical Perspective on Mobile Health and Medical Apps." *Societies*, vol. 4, no. 4, 2014, pp. 606–22.

Lutes, Jean Marie. *Front-Page Girls: Women Journalists in American Culture and Fiction, 1880–1930.* Ithaca, N.Y.: Cornell University Press, 2006.

Mason, Corinne, and Shoshanna Magnet. "Surveillance Studies and Violence Against Women." *Surveillance and Society*, vol. 10, no. 2, 2012, pp. 105–18.

Martinez, Inmaculada J., Juan Miguel Aguado, and Iolanda Tortajada. "Managing the Unbalanced: Gendered Mobile Appropriation, Identity Boundaries and Social Role Coordination." *Feminist Media Studies*, vol. 12, no. 4, 2012, pp. 506–16.

Puar, Jasbir K. *The Right to Maim.* Durham, NC: Duke University Press, 2017.

Robinson, Tasha. "Steven Soderbergh's All-iPhone Movie *Unsane* Makes a Poor Showing for the iPhone 7." *The Verge,* March 23, 2018, www.theverge.com/2018/3/23/17156978/unsane-movie-review-iphone-7-steven-soderbergh-claire-foy. Accessed October 28, 2020.

Rose, Nicholas. *The Politics of Life Itself: Biomedicine, Power, and Subjectivity in the Twenty-First Century.* Princeton, NJ: Princeton University Press, 2007.

Rosenhan, David. L. "On Being Sane in Insane Places." *Science*, vol. 179, no. 4070, 1973, pp. 250–8.

Roundy, Kevin A., et al. "The Many Kinds of Creepware Used for Interpersonal Attacks." *Proceedings – IEEE Symposium on Security and Privacy*, vol. 2020, May, no. 63, 2020, pp. 626–43.

Shelby, Renee Marie. "Techno-Physical Feminism: Anti-Rape Technology, Gender, and Corporeal Violence." *Feminist Media Studies*, vol. 20, no. 8, 2020, pp. 1088–1109.

Sojo, Victor, et al. "The #MeToo Movement: An Opportunity in Public Health?" *The Lancet*, vol. 391, 2018, pp. 2587–9.

Sweet, Paige L. "The Sociology of Gaslighting." *American Sociological Review*, vol. 84, no. 5, 2019, pp. 851–75.

Unsane. Directed by Steven Soderbergh, performances by Claire Foy and Matt Damon. Bleecker Street, 2018.

Valentino-DeVries, Jennifer. "Hundreds of Apps Can Empower Stalkers to Track Their Victims." *New York Times,* May 19, 2018, www.nytimes.com/2018/05/19/technology/phone-apps-stalking.html. Accessed 3 November 2020.

26

BLACK SITES IN THE MATRIX

Digital psychiatric power and racialized technologies

Olivia Banner

In late summer 2020, as the United States continued its mangled approach to the coronavirus pandemic and deaths continued to tick up, mental health experts sounded alarms about how prolonged isolation during grief would contribute to people's mental states. Three psychiatrists authored a Viewpoint for the Journal of the American Medical Association (JAMA), writing, "A second wave of devastation is imminent, attributable to mental health consequences of Covid-19. The magnitude of this second wave is likely to overwhelm the already frayed mental health system, leading to access problems, particularly for the most vulnerable persons" (Simon, Saxe, and Marmar). Those most vulnerable, its authors noted, would disproportionately be "Black and Hispanic individuals, older adults, lower socioeconomic groups of all races and ethnicities, and health care workers." The rest of the viewpoint elaborated ways to address this devastation focused primarily on strengthening social and community support networks. The only mention of digital tools made in the article concerned using video calls to put grieving family members in touch with each other.

When considered against the discourse of the mental health industries during the pandemic, however, the differences in emphasis on digital tools are striking. For the informatics, teletherapy, and digital psychiatry industries, the mantra around the novel coronavirus and its associated lockdown orders has been that the pandemic serves (finally!) as the catalyst for the digital transformation that these industries have been awaiting. *Finally*, the pandemic forces a reckoning with the increased access that digital tools have all along been ready to provide. *Finally,* the pandemic's increase in use of these tools will allow vulnerable populations, some of them already underserved by the mental health professions, to engage with mental health professionals. *Finally*, professionals reluctant to use digital tools will be forced to do so.

In neither of these two professional domains are questions about big data and structural digital ecosystems that this article will raise front and center in light of the caring professions' heightened attention to the racism and inequality made evident in the Covid pandemic as well as its overlapping with social activism against racist policing. Below, I illuminate issues about vulnerable populations within big data ecosystems that structure digital networks. How do digital ecosystems, which operate through buying and selling data in markets primed to intensify existing inequalities, recalibrate what it means to be "vulnerable"? The thorny questions about the nexus of technology and psychiatry may not, at first glance, seem relevant to clinicians and those directly providing care to people in distress, especially in light of how

DOI: 10.4324/9781003007661-34

pandemic isolation requirements made computers a professional life-saving device. In order to make what might seem to be abstract issues regarding big data and Artificial Intelligence (AI) more immediate, I bring those abstractions home in a discussion of a short film that illuminates them through narrative means.

Underlying this chapter's three sections is a concern with shifting how we view what Michel Foucault termed "psychiatric power." Since the 1960s, anti-psychiatry thinkers and activists have contested the mental asylum as the seat of psychiatry's oppression. However, for Foucault, the psychiatrist–patient relationship is itself where power is exercised: psychiatry legitimates the professional's discursive and institutional capacities to discipline the person into a patient subject to psychiatry's interpretation of their relationship and, ultimately, to psychiatry's diagnoses of madness (Foucault). I propose that we consider digital psychiatry and teletherapy as new players in the scene of disciplinary power. When joined to digital networked technologies, psychiatric practices, both research and clinical, enter patients as well as their care professionals into big data ecosystems. These ecosystems connect previously walled off arenas of professional practice and daily life that intensify vulnerabilities. I propose that practitioners and the psychiatric professions broadly need to rethink what "vulnerable populations" means in the era of big data.

In what follows, I present three domains for digital psychiatry: research, its clinical manifestations, and a cultural response to it. The first section summarizes large-scale trends and initiatives in federally sponsored research. The second summarizes consumer-facing apps. The third investigates a short film that thematizes some of these developments by illustrating them through a Black woman's experience of mental health care via digital technologies. I connect these three areas to illuminate how digital psychiatry changes psychiatric power by joining it to technological power, and what this means for those made most vulnerable by social inequalities.

NIMH's RDoC matrix and professional power

In 2010, just as the American Psychiatric Association (APA) announced the fifth revision of the *Diagnostic and Statistical Manual* (DSM), the National Institute of Mental Health initiated a new research and funding stream called the Research Domain Criteria Project (RDoC) (Jeste; Insel). The RDoC established a "matrix" of affects, which would allow data gathered from new technologies to be integrated with data from genomics and neuroscience for the aim of advancing new discoveries in brain function and mental health. The matrix breaks behavior and affect down into domains – "valences," "social processes," "cognitive systems," and others – as well as "units of analysis," categories of data gathered from digital tools, assessments, genetic studies, and neuroimaging (NIMH). By reformulating psychiatric knowledge in relation to the biological and neurological sciences, the RDoC intends to overcome the ongoing issue that the subjective (i.e., nonscientific) nature of psychiatry's diagnoses have posed for research into their supposed biological causes. The RDoC reframes psychiatry as a subset of neuroscience and decouples the clinic from research. Although its announcement on the heels of the DSM-5's publication seemed an intended usurpation of psychiatry's bible, a quickly arranged follow up press release, co-signed by NIMH's director and the APA's president, explained this delinking (Insel and Lieberman). In the clinic, psychiatrists would continue using the DSM, which serves its practical purposes, among them insurance reimbursement. Researchers, using the RDoC, would build a new neuroscience of mental illness.

Psychiatrists have critiqued the RDoC as divorced from clinical needs (Pickersgill). Certainly the RDoC "domain" categories seem foreign to psychiatry's more familiar language of emotions, affects, and behaviors. Understood, however, as an initiative with the goal of "precision psychiatry" – that is, the development of tailored psychiatric medications or, perhaps, simply the capacity to spur additional pharmaceutical research – the RDoC clarifies itself as very much divorced from the needs of the clinic. As Dorte Bemme, Natassia Brenman, and Beth Semel put it, "[T]he emergent knowledge practices of digital phenotyping are part of a burgeoning digital psychiatry that crafts an alternate future no longer reliant on shared linguistic constructs, symptom recall, interpersonal rapport, or the clinic as a separate sphere and infrastructure" (Bemme, Brenman, and Semel). Indeed, the envisioned future is one that realizes the dream of biopsychiatry, where treatment of people in distress could perhaps be accomplished without any professional consultation at all. Instead, data gathered from wearables, DNA testing, and fMRIs will be enough to match a patient to a pharmaceutical salve.

Also arising here are older contests among professional domains. NIMH's project shifts psychiatric expertise away from clinicians to researchers—from psychiatrists to neuroscientists. At the same time, the project intends to help shore up the flagging legitimacy of psychiatry, whose continued shifting diagnoses, as evidenced in contests over the DSM's fifth revision, are an ongoing source of illegitimacy. Martin Pickersgill argues that the incoherence and unfamiliarity of this matrix signals its true intention: to intervene in the "epistemology of psychiatry" (Pickersgill 615).

An additional site of contestation continues to pressure the psychiatric project more generally, and I contextualize the RDoC in relation to this ongoing interrogation: challenges mounted by populations psychiatry pathologizes. Although the early 1970s activism featured more direct disruption of APA conferences – in 1970, gay rights activists disrupted the annual conference, and at the 1969 annual conference, Black psychiatrists demanded measures toward an anti-racist psychiatry – today communities of mutual aid and mutual care continue to propose alternatives to state-sanctioned psychiatry and its institutions specifically because of their racist and often heterosexist practices, and because mental health care is intertwined with carceral logics. By moving away from the DSM, with its racist, homophobic-saturated histories, neuroscientific psychiatry counters the counter-discourse. In constructing a future where cell phone data, rather than a psychiatrist, combined with neuroimaging and DNA testing can "diagnose" a person in distress, the RDoC breaks with all of psychiatry's pasts, including those most explicitly marked by psychiatry's direct role in oppression. The abstract and neutral language of the matrix is disengaged from valences loaded with cultural meanings. A future of diagnosis based on data gathering tools rather than the individual, subjective psychiatrist who draws on a diagnostic manual constructed by a (subjective) committee of humans gathered to review and update psychiatric diagnoses positions itself as developing out of objective, neutral technologies. I would argue that this data turn in psychiatric diagnosis allows the impression that a digital psychiatry is no longer imbued with psychiatry's racist, heteropatriarchal, and sanist pasts. While data is never raw, and technology is never neutral, the cultural framing of data as bias-free imbues it with the aura of objectivity and scientism that psychiatry is so often criticized as lacking. As in other professional venues, such as judicial sentencing, HR departments, and welfare work that are turning to digital technologies for their presumed neutrality, the data and digitalized turn beckons to psychiatry as a means of exculpation before its critics.

The ultimate goal of the RDoC – to usher in "precision psychiatry" – sounds like a positive development away from those pasts as well, for a psychiatry modulated to respond to individuals rather than the "group categories" of diagnoses seems to center on tailoring to individual biological and biochemical substrates. Yet as Anthony Hatch has so compellingly shown in *Silent Cells: The Secret Drugging of America* (2019), it would be naive not to assume that precision psychiatry will be used to develop new forms of "technocorrections" – that is, psychotropics to sedate the incarcerated population of the United States. Into what contexts of psychiatric power will such new medicines enter? Forensic psychiatrists are working to align neuropsychiatry with risk assessment algorithms in order to create a disciplinary field with the obfuscatory name of AI neuroprediction (Tortora et al. 220). Everything we know so far about cell phone data collection and about AI algorithms for judicial sentencing warns that law enforcement will use it to aid the carceral state in its goal of creating new prisoners. Defense Advanced Research Projects Agency (DARPA), the research arm of the US Department of Defense, is involved in researching veterans' mental health through passive collection of wearable data (see Bickford). For some populations, there will be choice. For others there will be domination, coercion, and force.

The app economy, participatory culture, and shifting cultures of expertise

In these same years, health entrepreneurs and academic researchers have explored the affordances of networked technologies for providing care. I demarcate three types of mental healthcare apps: apps for self-care; apps for group support; and apps for professional care providers and their patients. Of the first two types, many employ cognitive behavioral therapy principles of reframing thought patterns. For example, Koko was a support-group app that, in its first version, allowed anonymous members to post messages about problems and receive feedback from other users about reframing their "negative" patterns of thinking. Other developments include automated therapy chatbots such as Tess and Woebot. The first has been deployed in corporate contexts; large corporations view chatbots as first-level mental health interventions for struggling employees that can also help them fulfil legal requirements for mental health coverage parity. The second, Woebot, is a consumer-facing chatbot with multiple options of access, including through Facebook Messenger. Apps that serve as virtual platforms for communication between therapists and clients are that third category, for example, BetterHelp and Talkspace. Both enable text messaging between therapist and user. These therapy apps differ in terms of their technological features, but they share promotional rhetoric that claims they make therapy accessible to more people.

Each of these therapy apps has generated concern about their data practices. Woebot, for example, maintains a Facebook Messenger feature. Messenger is notoriously the worst privacy offender: among its most egregious violations of people's privacy was accessing the microphone on users' cell phones to record audio without users' consent. Although the makers of Woebot claim that the messaging in a client/bot session is private, privacy advocates argue this is not true because Facebook's profit model banks on mining its users' data (McMahon). TalkSpace, another popular teletherapy app offered by many large corporations to their employees, was recently exposed as monitoring supposedly confidential therapist/client sessions. When questioned about this, TalkSpace executives referred to an automated algorithm that might flag a session if a therapist referred a client to cannabis (Hill and Krolik). Even if this is true (the therapist in question said she shared with a client a link to an anxiety worksheet), it provokes questions about the principles behind such flagging. Cannabis, the use of which has been decriminalized in some states, is also culturally racialized, and, where criminalized, enforcement of those laws harms racialized communities disproportionately. In any event, major psychiatric professional organizations have intervened, when and how they can, once these privacy infringements are brought to their attention. These various data exposures in digital psychiatric contexts happen because app makers are entrepreneurs, not psychiatrists. Just as the RDoC reframes psychiatric power within the neurosciences, teletherapy by app places a new so-called "expert" in the mix: the technology entrepreneur whose expertise is data markets, not psychiatric care.

Teletherapy apps enter another networked mediated arena where participatory culture challenges professional expertise: cultures of podcasting and YouTube. Some critics argue that YouTube, like other platforms where communities of people who share affiliations communicate, has aided in destigmatizing mental illness. More recently, with Google's purchase of YouTube, newly instituted algorithmic sorting, and Google's capacity to integrate data from its linked online services (such as a user's Google Account), YouTube has become highly monetized. Teletherapy apps enter this media monetized sphere through sponsorships of influential YouTubers, whose monetizing strategies intersect with their performance of identity through self-branding culture's emphasis on "authenticity" (see Banet-Weiser). A controversy around BetterHelp, a teletherapy platform, illuminates how this rhetoric of authenticity underpins both influencers' and therapy apps' corporate marketing strategies. Advertised heavily in podcasts and YouTube, BetterHelp "sponsored" a number of YouTube influencers in return for talking about BetterHelp in their content. When some users of BetterHelp, referred to the service through online advertising, had unsatisfying experiences with therapists, they began to post online accusing the company of hiring unlicensed people in the role of therapists.

Specific YouTubers caught up in this controversy because of their BetterHelp sponsorship – including Philip DeFranco, Shane Dawson, and Bobby Burns – are all white, and many are also queer. Their internet celebrity is bound up with their performances of coming out online, where public performances of personal struggles with stigma lend the aura of "authenticity" to their brands. In other words, by publicly struggling with and ultimately refusing cultural stigmas, influencers build their brands and their YouTube market power. Thus, a connection to a therapy app criticized as inauthentic, its services potentially more damaging than therapeutic, threatens to harm their audience appeal.

Media studies scholars argue that self-branding culture privileges the same people privileged in the offline world: white, wealthy, and male – and it also favors those who pursue, in their branding strategies, middle-class normativity (Marwick; Pham). By the end of the 20th century, the act of seeing a therapist was saturated with white middle-class normativity, even if mental illness still carries stigmas. I argue that, as self-branding culture and its opportunities for self-monetization favor those who are privileged and those who perform characteristics of the privileged, the opportunities for influencers of color to monetize through therapy app sponsorship are distinctly different from those of white influences. But especially, in light of psychiatry's history of racism, whose narration of such experiences does a therapy app corporation view as revenue-generating for therapy itself?

Psychiatric-technological power within racializing health care systems

A short film, *Blaxites* (dir. Josh Lyon, 2017; available at www.sscqueens.org/projects/screening-surveillance/blaxites), produced by Surveillance Studies Centre at Queen's University, uses narrative to bring into high relief the issues around racialization and the digitalization of psychiatry, introducing questions about hidden audiences, coerced consent, and racialized power differentials.

Blaxites begins with a Black female college student, Jai (Joy Mwandemange), concentrating on her smart phone screen as she responds to social media posts from family and friends, using a breathing app ("WellBreathe") to calm her breathing and pulse, and communicating with its automated Siri-like feature, called Zola, to place an order to refill her Lorazepam prescription. Zola informs Jai that the refill was denied and makes an emergency appointment for Jai with her doctor. At the appointment, her doctor tells Jai the system flagged her as noncompliant because of a social media post where she is drinking a glass of wine. The only option available to her, if she wants to refill the prescription after a 15-day wait, is to wear a tracking device that will monitor her blood alcohol levels; with no other option in sight, and desperate for the medication, she accepts. As she sobs in frustration, her friend Karl, who has opted-out of all electronic devices, leads her to an underground group that provides her with medication. When, after 15 days, Jai returns to the doctor's office for her refill, the doctor says that the device recorded Lorazepam in her system, and she is now blocked from accessing further care. Outside his office, Jai freaks out and scatters her underground medication in a puddle of water. The film ends as Jai, collapsing to the sidewalk, deletes all of the apps from her phone, including the WellBreathe app, as she follows Karl in "opting-out." The screen fades to black, and the viewer is left without knowing whether Jai will be able to obtain care. What is the future for a young Black girl who uses an unofficial method to obtain needed medications – when she "opt outs" – if the state-sanctioned way to obtain medication requires opting-in?

Although labeled "science fiction," *Blaxites* draws from contemporary technology and developments in medicine and media so faithfully that there is little futuristic about it. Wellness programs *are* using tracking devices and health insurance companies *are* denying claims based on claimants' social media posts. The film also subtly highlights the differences between how a Black woman experiences her technology versus a white man: Karl is able to exercise free choice and opt-out, while Jai's anxiety, heightened by the pressure, as a Black woman, that she feels to succeed at college, makes it such that she cannot opt-out. Additionally, Karl does not consider that providing Jai access to a mutual-aid group which could provide her with medication would jeopardize her access to state-provided care. In other words, systemic racism makes a Black woman's college experience more stressful than that of a white man; this pressure contributes to the Black woman relying on state-sanctioned treatments; Karl can opt-out of surveillance, but Jai cannot.

As a Black disabled woman, Jai is the most targeted by state and social practices of surveillance and tracking. *Blaxites* astutely dramatizes what Patricia Hill Collins named, in her 1989 *Black Feminist Thought*, as the matrix of domination. In Collins's conceptualization, race, gender, and class are interlocking systems of oppression, with Black women situated at the bottom of their mesh. Disability studies has added, to Collins's original formulation, the axis of ability – a Black *disabled* woman is situated within interlocking structures of race, gender, class, and *ability*, all of which make her a target for monitoring, discipline, and punishment. These are "black sites": spaces in which the state suspends a citizen's rights and spaces that must "go dark" to provide care outside the state's sanctioned venues. When her doctor enforces the health system's regulations of increased surveillance, the power his medical license grants to him – the ability to conduct "psychiatric power" within the clinical relationship – here joins to the power society (and the medical system) has granted to digital technologies – the ability to exercise power, via surveillance. It is Black disabled women who bear the full weight of this matrix of domination that is enabled by the cleaving of psychiatric to technological power.

How do Black lives matter in the matrix?

What conclusions might healthcare practitioners arrive at by examining the developments in digital psychiatry, teletherapy, and the cultural responses to these ecosystems holistically, as forming a symbiosis of cultural, political, economic, and social responses to digital psychiatry? What happens in the black sites that extend between the matrix of domination and the matrix of the RDoC? What if the RDoC matrix is an expression of the matrix of domination?

I do not have firm answers to these questions. But, one avenue for exploration might be located, again, in Collins's foundational text of Black feminist thought. After elaborating on the explanatory power of the matrix of domination, Collins asks where feminists might theorize ruptures to these systems, and she foregrounds the situated knowledges of Black women as a method for developing new epistemologies in the struggle against oppression. One response, then, to the homonymic matrix – the potential for the RDoC matrix to interlock with the matrix of domination – would be to turn to Black women's knowledge of, epistemologies for, and organizing around Black mental distress. In this time of Black Lives Matter, reconstituting mental health care *away* from state institutions that endanger Black lives has become a priority for the movement (see Khan-Cullors).

Mental health care provided through digital means exacerbates the possibilities that vulnerable people will be harmed through the use and misuse of their data. This makes well-meaning seeming apps like Ayana, a new entry into the therapy app market that brings together patients of color with therapists of color, a potentially less sanguine development than it at first appears (see Elassar). This will continue to be an ongoing tension as clinicians seek to care for, rather than do harm to, people seeking their care.

Works cited

Banet-Weiser, Sarah. *AuthenticTM: The Politics of Ambivalence in a Brand Culture.* New York: New York University Press, 2012.

Bemme, Dorte, Natassia Brenman, and Beth Semel. "The Subjects of Digital Psychiatry." Somatosphere, October 13, 2020, http://somatosphere.net/2020/subjects-of-digital-psychiatry.html/. Accessed October 23, 2020.

Bickford, Andrew. *Chemical Superheroes: Pharmacological Superheroes in the US Military.* Durham, NC: Duke University Press, 2020.

Collins, Patricia Hill. *Black Feminist Thought: Knowledge, Consciousness, and the Politics of Empowerment.* New York and Abingdon: Routledge, 2002.

Elassar, Alaa. "This App Connects Black People with Therapists of Color." CNN, July 19, 2020. www.cnn.com/2020/07/19/health/ayana-therapy-app-black-people-of-color-trnd/index.html. Accessed October 23, 2020.

Foucault, Michel. *Psychiatric Power: Lectures at the College de France, 1973–1974.* Macmillan, 2008.

Hatch, Anthony. *Silent Cells: The Secret Drugging of America.* Minneapolis, MN: University of Minnesota Press, 2019.

Hill, Kashmir, and Aaron Krolik. "At Talkspace, Start-Up Culture Collides with Mental Health Concerns." *New York Times*, August 7, 2020, www.nytimes.com/2020/08/07/technology/talkspace.html. Accessed October 23, 2020.

Insel, Thomas. "Transforming Diagnosis." NIMH, April 29, 2013, www.nimh.nih.gov/about/directors/thomas-insel/blog/2013/transforming-diagnosis.shtml.

Insel, Thomas, and Jeffrey Lieberman. "DSM-5 and RDoC: Shared Interests." American Psychiatric Association, May 14, 2013, Release No. 13-37.

Jeste, Dilip. "A Message from APA President Dilip Jeste, M.D., on DSM-5." *Psychiatric News*, December 1, 2012, https://psychnews.org/files/DSM-message.pdf.

Khan-Cullors, Patrisse. *When They Call You a Terrorist: A Black Lives Matter Memoir.* New York: St. Martin's Press, 2018.

Marwick, Alice E.*Status Update: Celebrity, Publicity, and Branding in the Social Media Age.* New Haven, CN: Yale University Press, 2013.

McMahon, Ciarán. "What the Research Really Suggests about That Facebook Chatbot Therapist." *Slate*, July 18, 2017, https://slate.com/technology/2017/07/what-research-says-about-woebot-the-facebook-chatbot-therapist.html. Accessed October 23, 2020.

NIMH. "RDoC Matrix." 2020, www.nimh.nih.gov/research/research-funded-by-nimh/rdoc/constructs/rdoc-matrix.shtml. Accessed October 23, 2020.

Pham, Minh-Ha T. *Asians Wear Clothes on the Internet: Race, Gender, and the Work of Personal Style Blogging*. Durham, NC: Duke University Press, 2015.

Pickersgill, Martin. 2018. "Psychiatry and the Sociology of Novelty: Negotiating the US National Institute of Mental Health 'Research Domain Criteria' (RDoC)." *Science, Technology, and Human Values*, vol. 44, no. 4, 2018, pp. 612–33.

Pickersgill, Martin. "Digitising Psychiatry?: Sociotechnical Expectations, Performative Nominalism and Biomedical Virtue in (digital) Psychiatric Praxis." *Sociology of Health and Illness*, vol. 41, no. S1, 2019, pp. 16–30.

Simon, Naomi M., Glenn N. Saxe, and Charles R. Marmar. 2020. "Mental Health Disorders Related to COVID-19–Related Deaths." *JAMA*, vol. 324, no. 15, 2020, pp. 1493–4.

Tortora, Leda, et al. "Neuroprediction and A.I. in Forensic Psychiatry and Criminal Justice: A Neurolaw Perspective." *Frontiers in Psychology*, vol. 11, 2020, p. 220.

27

MOBILE HEALTH AND ITS PROBLEMS

The case of hearing and communication apps

Nicole Matthews

I'm sitting at a table in the café nearest to my office, waiting for my pot of tea to arrive. The building is brand spanking new and pretty fancy: shiny terrazzo floors, deep blue wall tiles, and a light-drenched multi-story atrium. This place is popular with university students, their teachers and people visiting the community organizations that have their headquarters here. I can – just – hear the buzz of lively talk between colleagues as they stand in the queue to order over the clattering of trays and the hiss of the coffee machine. There's another line of people waiting by the gleaming side counter for take-away lattes and espressos, hovering watchfully so they don't miss their name called out over the many sounds reverberating around this big open space. High heels clip up the wooden stairs; lift doors open and close as older folk, research volunteers, head to the lab at the top of the building; toddlers whine as their mothers lead them into the audiology clinic next door. I'm lucky I've got the time to wait for table service – there's no way I could do take-away here. I have single-sided deafness, scarcely noticeable in more acoustically friendly environments, but in this venue, my cuppa would be cold before I'd realize my order was waiting for me. Ironically, this noisy café is located in what has been dubbed, "The Hearing Hub," a space bringing together clinics, researchers and advocacy organizations working with and for deaf and hard of hearing people.

My central case study in this chapter is a mobile phone app designed to navigate – or perhaps avoid – just this kind of environment. SoundPrint, described as "Yelp for noise," crowdsources readings of the ambient sound in cafés, bars, and restaurants to help its users, seeking enjoyable places for lunch dates and nights out, "find their quiet." I'm interested in using this app – and hearing and communication apps more broadly – to counter the idea that mobile media simply offer handy solutions to pre-existing problems out there in the world. Rather, I'll argue, mobile media – including what has been called mHealth – shape the ways in which we imagine, organize, and understand our identities, our bodies, and the environments they move through.

What counts as "health" often seem to be self-evident. But critical health studies scholarship has shown that health can be understood in very different ways. For example, health is often seen as a feature of individual bodies rather than springing from the interaction between those bodies and particular physical, economic or social environments. Media play an important role in framing and reframing the ways we imagine and enact categories like "health," a process the

DOI: 10.4324/9781003007661-35

comparative media studies scholar Mack Hagood has described as "biomediation" (Hagood). Hagood underscores that a range of media – from medical equipment like ultrasound to popular forms like television – represent and shape the body, diagnosing, screening, treating, and defining what counts as 'normalcy.' Hearing and communication apps are particularly interesting to use as a route into this process because the problems they set out to solve are so evidently politically laden. Such apps work at the boundaries of ideas about communication, language, disability, equality, and health. The very categories through which they are described on the app store are weighted with meaning, conveying assumptions and silences that I want to unpack here.

Health, hearing apps, and the problems they set out to solve

Health and wellbeing apps, particularly "patient-centric" apps, are a growth market, only increasing in value during the period of the coronavirus pandemic (*PR Newswire*). Rising rates of chronic disease and the increasing penetration of smart phones in the majority world have been seen as drivers of this growth market. mHealth – the use of mobile media such as phone apps and wearables as a tool for health and wellbeing – can be understood as offering technological solutions to a wide range of social, economic, and political problems. From the perspective of health professionals, mobile health provides, variously, a way of staying in touch with difficult to reach patients, promoting preventative health behaviors, enhancing patient compliance with doctors' instructions and communicating between professionals and patients, as well as managing patient data (Lupton "The Diverse Domains," "Apps as Artefacts"; Kenner; Paglialonga, Pinciroli and Tognola). mHealth is also widely viewed as a route to trimming the cost of providing health services (Levina; Hunn; Valente and Amlani; Zeng). Popular accounts of these technologies suggest that that digital media will empower health service users to manage their own health conditions and create new communities sharing important information (Topol). Media studies scholars have also pointed out that apps and wearables offer rich pickings, gathering biometric data for both research and profit for a range of actors (Van Djick and Poell; Couldry and Mejias).

In the area of hearing, mobile apps and hearables have been understood as threatening the oligopolistic and vertically integrated hearing aid industry, dominated by five global companies making 90 percent of all hearing aids (Seelman and Werner; Hunn; Oliver). The industry has featured "high margins, considerable barriers to entry, limited power among suppliers and lack of substitutes" (Keppeler, cited in Seelman and Werner). While personal sound amplification technologies – such as hunting earpieces – have long been available commercially, changes in regulation within the United States in 2017 to allow over-the-counter sales of amplification devices for people with mild to moderate hearing loss have created new markets (not to mention a blizzard of TV and newspaper ads touting them) (Zeng; Oliver). The role and status of hearing health professionals like audiologists are shifting in the midst of these changes. Where in the past hearing aids were a stigmatized technology associated with old age and disability and reluctantly used by those under the sign of a medical diagnosis of "hearing impairment" or "hearing loss," increasingly mainstream communication tech, such as earbuds, are converging with hearing aids. Music, audio, and phone calls can be streamed to Bluetooth enabled hearing aids as easily as wireless headphones. A new market has been created for hearables – earbuds with in-built sensors which are in effect a two-way "smart wearable human-computer interface" (Hagood, "Here Active Listening" 278). Hearables are now an increasing share of the mHealth market (Gilmore; Hagood, *Hush: Media*; Llamas, Ubrani and Shirer), gathering biometric data from their wearers. This kind of data, drawn from both wearables and apps, is seen as so commodifiable that it has been described as "the new oil" by many observers (Couldry and Mejias).

If the hearing device industry teeters between biomedical and consumer driven understandings of hearing technologies, what it means to be hard of hearing can also be understood from quite different perspectives. Biomedical framings of individual "hearing loss" and "hearing impairment" are the dominant understandings deployed by audiologists, speech pathologists, and other health professionals. Experiences of differential hearing are framed as health problems with medical, technological or, for some progressive audiologists, bio-psycho-social solutions. However, culturally Deaf communities have viewed the experience of "Deafhood" very differently, as about shared languages, culture, and pride. This perspective, like the social model of disability, refuses to see Deafness as any kind of biomedical deficit or impairmen, but rather as a route to "Deaf gain" (e.g., Baumann and Murray; Paul and Moores). Rather than individual divergent bodies, Deaf perspectives focus on questions of access, rights, and equality, enabled particularly through access to sign languages for communication. Like the social model of disability, this understanding turns away from a focus on bodies (Mitchell and Snyder) and indeed the language of health toward the social, economic and communicative environments where embodied differences come to make a difference. Hearing and communication apps, then, exist at the junction of very different ways of understanding hearing, hearing loss, and hearing and amplification technologies. Apps and hearables are at the nexus of mainstream consumer technologies and high-cost assistive devices. The tools they offer can be understood within the framework of "health" or as about communication, access, and equality.

Paglialonga and her colleagues offer a helpful taxonomy of what they describe as "hearing health" apps, categorising them into four groups – apps that seek to deliver information and education; those that can be used for screening; those that are used for intervention and rehabilitation' and finally assistive tools (Paglialonga, Pinciroli, and Tognola). I am particularly interested to explore those "patient-centric" apps that Paglialonga describes as "intervention and rehabilitation" and "assistive tools" and apps that hover around the outer boundaries of these two categories. The former category include the apps and devices that Hagood calls "orphic media" – white noise generators, recordings of nature, and apps that filter sound – each of which "promise to help users… remain unaffected in changeable, stressful, and distracting environments, sonically fabricating microspaces of freedom for the pursuit of happiness" (*Hush: Media* 3). Assistive tools include the live captioning apps of Google Live Transcribe, Ava, and Otter. These applications address a market of hard of hearing and deaf people amongst a wide range of other users. Others in this same category include apps like Audiofix, which enhances sound within video; Musixmatch which offers the lyrics to music videos as synchronized captions; Sonic Cloud, which enhances the audio on phone calls; and Ear Machine, like iPhone's native accessibility apps, allowing a mobile to be used as a microphone (for more examples Childress).

I would suggest that these apps offer a clear example of a process evident in many other contexts where media and health come together: the important work done by categorization. Hearing and communication apps are particularly interesting because they often choose to avoid the category of "health." The location of hearing and communication apps between biomedical, consumer, and cultural frames is perhaps best indicated by the ways in which they are categorized on the app store. The hearing and communication apps mentioned above are located variously under "entertainment," "music," "photos and video," "productivity," "utility," and "social networking" with only Ear Machine amongst the apps listed here – funded by the US National Institute of Health – labeled as a "health and fitness" app. The case study of hearing and communication apps, then, shows how deploying – and choosing not to deploy – the category of "health" does political work.

To unpack this, I want to use an approach from a different area of health – health policy – political theorist Carol Bacchi's "what is the problem represented to be" (WPR) method. Rather than seeing health policy as addressing pre-existing social problems, Bacchi suggests that problems are constituted by policy even as that those problems are addressed. She suggests that "every policy proposal contains within it an implicit representation of what the problem is represented to be" (1). Following this approach, she notes, "taken-for-granted categories and concepts – "drugs," "addiction," "crime," "youth," "skill," "human capital," "wellbeing" – become things to interrogate" (1). The WPR method asks us to excavate the underpinning assumptions that support a particular understanding of a "problem," the silences that ensue from that formulation and the effects of that way of imagining the "problem." The critical health studies literature on apps has suggested some important directions here. Critical health and digital media studies have identified three ways in which the problem of health is formulated in most mobile health apps. Apps tend to focus on individuals taking responsibility for their own health; most encourage users to gather and reflect on quantitative data about themselves; and underpinning many apps is a vision of health as a secular moral goal.

Many writers have emphasized the ways in which mobile technologies address the individual as a choosing subject (Kao and Liebovitz; Levina; Lupton, "Apps as Artifacts"; Rich and Miah; Van Dijck and Poell). mHealth in particular fits neatly with and emerges from an emphasis on individuals managing and taking responsibility for their own health. This is a particular mode of what Rabinow and Rose, drawing on Foucault, have called "biopower" – that is, ways of managing the health of the population "at a distance" by encouraging individuals to work on themselves, drawing on the authorized truths of experts disseminated in health communication and health promotion campaigns (Rabinow and Rose). This focus on individual self-management is typical of neoliberal ways of governing populations. Managing the risks of being healthy, rather than being seen as the responsibility of government, is devolved to individuals – as is the responsibility if things go wrong.

Secondly, as part of this self-monitoring process, health apps frequently prompt users to quantify themselves, dwelling upon how many hours they have spent sleeping or staring at the screen of their phones or how many miles they've walked or run. Deborah Lupton, analyzing what has been called "the quantified self" notes that such "self-tracking … [conforms] to cultural expectations concerning the importance of self-awareness, reflection and taking responsibility for managing, governing oneself and improving one's life chances" ("The Diverse Domains" 115). Thirdly, health apps neatly fit within what has been called "healthism" (Lupton, "Apps as Artifacts"), a term used to describe a constant preoccupation with an always unfinished project of self-improvement aiming toward health and wellness (Cheek). This perspective produces the sense of health as manageable and controllable and views efforts to improve it as morally valuable (Lupton, "Apps as Artifacts").

Some recent scholarship on health apps illustrates how this way of casting the problem of health works and some of its possible effects. Alison Kenner, for example, in her case study of asthma apps, points out that despite the GPS affordances of contemporary phones, many health apps choose not to integrate mapping and environmental information. The app developers Kenner spoke to acknowledged the possibility of incorporating into their apps pollen counts, weather information, or other environmental variables that might impact on asthmatics' day to day health. Nonetheless, developers ultimately conceptualized the problem of the app as users' "low health literacy and non-adherence" to medication (517) and focussed on encouraging compliance to doctors' instructions. Kenner points out that this way of framing the problem of asthma ignores the wider potential of "collective, place-based approaches to global environmental health problems" (511). Here assumptions that individuals are responsible for their own health and that rectifying deficiencies in individual behavior – especially compliance to medication – are the easiest if not the only route to improved health and wellbeing.

Dylan Mulvin demonstrates a similar problem formation – a focus on individuals managing themselves – in his recent work on night mode settings on mobile phones. The introduction of night modes by phone developers acknowledges the trouble many people have getting enough sleep and underscores the potential role of technologized environments – the blue screens of ubiquitous phones – in creating these difficulties. In this sense, the incorporation of night modes in phones indicates a move beyond a focus on individuals and their biomedical conditions in understanding sleep difficulties. However, as Mulvin points out, this focus on individual practices of using media technologies as both a cause of and solution to such difficulties displaces or ignores the wider social conditions producing sleeplessness – precarious, flexible, and shift work, for instance. The conclusion Mulvin comes to in relation to night modes echoes many of the wider critiques of health apps from media studies: individualized, technological solutions to health problems produce silences around the wider social and economic determinants of health. Marina Levina offers a particularly pessimistic account of mHealth when she says "an increased focus on consumer empowerment through technology disrupts a political engagement with health as an issue of socioeconomic inequality" (559).

SoundPrint: reframing the problem of hearing by mapping soundscapes

I want to explore in more detail the way mobile media and their marketing both set up particular problems and address them by considering the case study of the app SoundPrint. This app is interesting, in part, because it draws on an increasingly common way of representing the "problem" of hearing and communication. It evokes the idea that everyone's hearing is unique – a notion increasingly used to market hearables, hearing devices, and other hardware that can be tailored to their wearer's individual hearing profile. Although this approach sidesteps understandings of bodily differences as deficits, common within biomedicine, this way of imagining the "problem" of differences in hearing fits very nicely within a broader trend toward healthism where individuals are urged to work on and improve their health and wellbeing. More importantly, SoundPrint also offers an opportunity to respond to Bacchi's exhortation to think through how dominant problem formations "can be questioned, disrupted, and replaced" (9). This app suggests some lines along which those disruptions in the space of hearing and communication might take place. It does this by shifting attention from individuals and their diverse hearing experiences toward the environments in which those individuals might be harmed or, alternatively, might flourish.

The app was launched in early 2018 in North America and given a special mention in *Time Magazine*'s "Best Inventions of 2019." It aims to collect and share information about the noise levels in cafes, bars and restaurants. The description of SoundPrint on the app's website – "like Yelp for Noise" – invokes the consumer who "wants to find [a] quiet place in a restaurant, bar [or] coffee shop… where you can actually hear your date, colleague or partner." The app empowers others – consumer-reviewers – to help identify those quiet places. It has a search function, which includes both a "quiet list" for particular cities in the United States and a map, dotted with venues labelled on a traffic light schema as quiet (green), moderate (yellow) or loud (red). iPhone users (but not those in the Android environment) can also measure the loudness of a venue they are visiting with the app's decibel meter. The "problem" addressed in SoundPrint, then, is not that of "hearing impairment" or "hearing loss" but of excessively noisy venues.

In the "About" section of the app its founder, Gregory Scott, credits his hearing loss with inspiring a desire to find quiet bars and restaurant to meet friends, socialize, and eat. He describes SoundPrint as "born for the hearing-impaired community" though he notes "even those with typical hearing can benefit." However, this information is tucked away in "about SoundPrint" in the settings menu, and the main page doesn't foreground deafness, "hearing loss," or "hearing impairment" in its text or iconography. On the app store, SoundPrint is not classified as a "medical" or "health and wellness" app but as a utility. The imagery on its website – smiling people, young, middle-aged and older, chatting and interacting in atmospheric settings – foregrounds the social world of leisure and pleasure rather than individual bodies or biomedicine. Amongst the gallery of photos that greet the visitor to the app's website all but one include human figures, but these shots are very much of both people *and* places. The clusters of diners, tranquil readers, or people leaning against a bar take up less than half of each frame, the remainder filled with expanses of warm wooden paneling, long tables, rough-textured brick and stone walls, and glinting rows of wine glasses. This imagery signals that the app is as much about places as about the people who use them.

The name and the icon of SoundPrint invokes a familiar metaphor: a simplified blue and white illustration of a fingerprint with an outline of an ear within it. Other technology developers in the hearing space over the past few years have regularly made this comparison between hearing and the fingerprints so famous for their variety and their uniqueness. Cochlear, for example, recently developed a Chrome plug-in called HearPrint which aims to calibrate online content to its users' hearing. The website for the plug-in stresses "our hearing is as unique as our fingerprint… everybody hears the world differently." German start-up, Mimi Hearing Technologies, uses very similar iconography and language and the notion of the "earprint" in its Mimi Music app, which employs the data from an app-based hearing test to tweak users' streamed music (Matthews). This metaphor of the fingerprint replaces the language of deficit like "hearing loss" with the language of diversity, sidelining a biomedical framework, and foregrounding services and experiences tailored to the individual. Increasingly prevalent in commercial, community, and even activist contexts, this language of diversity functions as an alternative to the language of health or indeed disability (Hamraie; Friedner and Weingarten; Friedner). Both disability and critical race studies scholars have long noted the problems of this notion of "diversity" – especially its use to side-step questions of power, exclusion, and inequality (e.g. Puwar; Friedner and Weingarten; Hamraie).

While the fingerprint iconography of the app's name points us toward diversity rather than deficit, marketing materials frame the app as, in part, about preventative hearing health. With its decibel meter to gauge excessive noise, SoundPrint is one amongst a wide range of apps which aim to prevent hearing loss by allowing people to avoid or ameliorate loud environments. This dimension of the app does foreground the idea of hearing loss as deficit. SoundPrint presents the preventative health dimensions of their apps in the description on the app store as helping users "practice safe hearing." Their September 2019 blog proudly announces that they have been selected by the World Health Organization as a member of the World Hearing Forum. The blogpost ends with the statement that the company are "looking forward to contributing to helping the world prevent hearing loss." Elsewhere we find an article entitled, "How noise levels affect your long term health." Here, like other decibel measuring apps, the app's developers focus on the problems and difficulties associated with hearing loss. However, this dimension of hearing health is an undertone to the app rather than its main focus, which is rather upon the pleasure of social interaction in quiet places.

Ideas about pleasure, social life, and connection with family and friends are central to the way hearing devices like cochlear implants and hearing aids are sold. Advertisements regularly frame acquired hearing impairment through the lens of social isolation. To lose your hearing is to lose connection to other people, in this telling. In perhaps the most overt form of this kind of marketing, device manufacturer Cochlear has developed a short film, "Does Love Last Forever," which offers vignettes of a married couple interacting over a sequence of decades – a film which serves as a narrativized hearing test. Viewers with more acute hearing will realize that the couple, despite their sometimes cranky facial expressions, are constant in their affections, while those with trouble hearing dialogue over the sounds of boiling kettles, clanking cutlery, and rain on the roof may end the film thinking that the couple fell out of love. This kind of marketing for hearing devices presents the social world as a desired space but also a space of deficits and loss – only to be avoided through techno-medical solutions. The "problem" in Cochlear's film is not the noisy restaurant where, in the final scenes of the film, the couple struggle to communicate. Rather, the problem is individual hearing loss, which requires individual technological solutions. SoundPrint, in contrast, presents social connection as not only desirable but also attainable through the medium of collective action.

SoundPrint, in some respects, fits within Hagood's conception of orphic media, with its question to "find quiet," and indeed perhaps plays into what Hagood calls contemporary "sensory intolerances" (*Hush: Media* 4). However, it does so not through producing an individual technologized bubble of quietness but through collaborative, social methods – by using the information on the crowd-sourced quiet list for each city. Quite distinctly from the personalized hearing apps discussed by Hagood, SoundPrint acknowledges more boldly the environmental conditions in which people communicate or struggle to do so. This app recognizes that moving through urban spaces can be hazardous to individual wellbeing but points toward social and architectural, rather than techno-medical, strategies for avoiding these hazards.

The US Deaf University, Gallaudet, where the language of instruction is American Sign Language, has pioneered the idea that social spaces might help or hinder communication. Architects developing new spaces on campus have acknowledged the connections between physical environments and communication by developing the notion of DeafSpace. Corridors are wider and progress with ramps rather than steps to allow colleagues and students to sign while walking; large spaces with mezzanine levels are configured to take advantage of "sensory reach" – the ability of signers to communicate over long distances, and illumination is diffuse to avoid harsh backlighting that will render signed conversations more difficult to read (Edwards and Harold; Dangermond Keane Architecture). The idea of DeafSpace acknowledges the links between culture, communication, and space. However this connection between communicative modalities and space has been less attended to in the case of hearing and hard of hearing people, aside from narrowly framed building regulations around acoustics (Ng et al.; Gatehouse, Naylor, and Elberling). SoundPrint, unusually, focusses on this "problem" of "auditory ecologies" (Ng), not as a problem of individual deficient bodies but as one of particular places and the interaction of bodies within them. This framing moves beyond the individualizing focus of many health and wellbeing apps.

Like many health apps, SoundPrint involves quantification, but not of individual users and their activities – their daily step count, calories consumed or even the number of hours they've spent listening to headphones. Instead SoundPrint quantifies the noise level in environments through which the app user moves. A central functional element of the app, at least in the IoS environment, is its soundcheck – 15-second long readings of the volume of noise in a particular venue. One of the critiques made of the self-tracking and self-monitoring so common in digital health and wellbeing apps is the ways in which personal data, gathered by devices and their users, becomes a commodity. This data is extracted from bodies, it has been argued, just as natural resources are extracted from deep underground, as if data is simply produced as a by-product of peoples' activities (Couldry and Meijas). However, in the case of SoundPrint, data produced from in urban environments are more environmental rather than personal.

SoundPrint's users are primarily framed as consumers. However, in some respects, people using this app to measure and share the loudness of different venues are also acting like citizen scientists, or as Jennifer Gabrys calls them "citizen sensors." In talking through the implications of citizen science, Gabrys suggests that citizenship should not be thought of as a pre-existing legal or immigration status. Rather she suggests, it should be understood as a form of subject-ivity – a way of being "citizenly," in this case, emerging through the use of digitized sensing technologies. Such uses of sensing technologies to evaluate environments, she and her colleague Helen Pritchard suggest, produce new forms of collectivity.

This is not to make over-the-top claims for crowd-sourcing data. In their discussion of a participatory project monitoring environmental pollution, Pritchard and Gabrys note the ameliorative politics of citizen sensing. This kind of monitoring in their case study was used as an attempt to work around the agonistic politics of the fracking of natural gas. "Citizen sensing," they suggest "often promises a relatively friction-free form of empowerment" (358). The objective act of measuring in a quantifiable format offers an apparent step away from political challenges and tensions. It's interesting to reflect on whether SoundPrint's politics can be understood similarly. As I have noted, the way the app is framed evokes a set of shared concerns for quiet spaces that points toward the common interests of hard of hearing people and others. In moving beyond individual technological solutions and in invoking an alliance of hard of hearing people, sympathetic venue owners, and more broadly lovers of quiet, the app steps away from the kinds of individual techno-medical solutions so often offered by mHealth. However, in framing its mission through the uncontroversial language of consumerism and leisure, diversity, and commonality, like the citizen-science projects described by Pritchard and Gabrys, SoundPrint seeks to sidestep political conflicts over identities, equality, access, and resources.

Conclusion

This chapter unpacks the "problems" that mobile health apps set out to address. Much of mHealth presents health as a problem of individual biomedical deficits that can be tackled through better information, more effective communication with practitioners, greater compliance with medication – broadly more effective self-monitoring and self-management. This way of presenting health problems largely sidelines the social, environmental, and economic determinants of health. Many companies, although by no means all, frame and market hearing and communication apps in similar ways. Apps that screen or rehabilitate hearing generally accept a biomedical frame. Some others, such as decibel meters apps, acknowledge the potentially hazardous impact of toxic environments – especially loud noise – in producing bodily damage. Usually, however, individual app users are presented as responsible for identifying those hazards and addressing them. In the case of apps that monitor the length of time headphones are worn and the volume of the music played on them, the user is also understood as the unwitting instigator of hearing damage.

SoundPrint points out ways in which the "problem" of hearing and communication might be framed otherwise. Like a number of other hearing apps and plug-ins, it imagines users not as deficient but as diverse – a point made visually through the use of the fingerprint as a metaphor. Along with this evocation of diversity comes a focus less on the biomedical frame and more on the pleasure of individually tailored media (Hagood, *Hush: Media*). This diversity framing, I would suggest, is an increasingly common way of trying to market assistive and utility apps to the widest possible audience (Gilmore). Both critical race and disability studies scholars have pointed to some of the pitfalls here. The "feel good" language of diversity can obscure a terrain of power, 'eras[ing] difference, or … present[ing] difference as easily surmountable' (Friedner and Weingarten).

Perhaps more significantly, SoundPrint, unlike many health and wellness apps, turns away from the quantification and monitoring of individual bodies, toward crowd-sourced measurements of environments. Its focus on the way communication difficulties are produced by spaces rather than the particularities of individual bodies is a very different framing of a "problem" which is normally described in terms of individual "hearing loss." Its mission – "to educate venue owners on how to optimize the noise level to create a more pleasant atmosphere for patrons"– recalls Alan Roulstone hope for 'technology giving scope to the rehabilitation of environments' (94).

In the case of my noisy local café, critical – even quantifiable – feedback from patrons might encourage the proprietors to install acoustic paneling, purchase some soft furniture or even just add a computer screen that allows the caffeine-deprived folks waiting in line to see, even if they can't hear, when their latte is ready. Until that happens, I'll only be visiting that particular venue when I meet my Deaf friends for a chat in sign language where terrible acoustics won't interrupt the flow of the conversation.

Acknowledgments

Many thanks to my colleagues in the Interiors and Mobiles research groups at Macquarie University – Karen Pearlman, Julie-Anne Long, Jeannine Baker, Peter Doyle, Willa McDonald, Kate Rossmanith, Jane Simon, Denis Crowdy, Andrew Alter, and Yuji Sone – for their feedback on early drafts of this chapter.

Works cited

Bacchi, Carol. "Problematizations in Health Policy: Questioning How 'Problems' Are Constituted in Policies." *Sage Open*, June 1, 2016, pp. 1–16.

Baumann, H-Dirkson L. and Joseph J. Murray, eds. *Deaf Gain: Raising the Stakes for Human Diversity*. Minneapolis, MN: University of Minnesota Press, 2014.

Cheek, Julianne. "Healthism: A New Conservatism?" *Qualitative Health Research*. vol. 18, no. 7, 2008, pp. 974–82.

Childress, Tina. *Apps for Kids (and Adults) with Hearing Loss*. https://docs.google.com/spreadsheets/d/1jBcMgGGKgUY2myJz8749IIZIWFwjlxBUjcy35SnahPo/edit?hl=en_US&hl=en_US#gid=0. Accessed August 1, 2020.

Couldry, Nick and Ulises A. Mejias. "Data Colonialism: Rethinking Big Data's Relation to the Contemporary Subject." *Television & New Media*, vol. 20, no. 4, 2019, pp. 336–49.

Dangermond Keane Architecture. "Campus Design and Planning: DeafSpace Gallaudet University." Gallaudet University, www.gallaudet.edu/campus-design-and-planning/deafspace. Accessed August 1, 2020.

Edwards, Claire and Gill Harold. "DeafSpace and the Principles of Universal Design." *Disability and Rehabilitation*, vol. 36, no.16, 2014, pp. 1350–9.

Friedner, Michelle. "How the Disabled Body Unites the National Body: Disability as 'Feel Good' Diversity in Urban India." *Contemporary South Asia*, vol. 25, no. 4, 2017, pp. 347–63.

Friedner, Michelle and Karen Weingarten. "Disability as Diversity: A New Biopolitics."*Somatosphere*, May 23, 2016, http://somatosphere.net/2016/05/disability-as-diversity-a-new-biopolitics.html

Gabrys, Jennifer. "Programming Environments: Environmentality and Citizen Sensing in the Smart City." *Environment and Planning D: Society and Space*, no. 32, 2014, pp. 30–48.

Gatehouse, Stuart, Graham Naylor, and Clous Elberling. "Benefits from Hearing Aids in Relation to the Interaction between the User and the Environment." *International Journal of Audiology*, no. 42, sup.1, 2003, pp. 77–85.

Gilmore, James N. "Design for Everyone: Apple AirPods and the Mediation of Accessibility." *Critical Studies in Media Communication*, vol. 36, no. 5, 2019, pp. 482–94.

Grundy Quinn, Fabian Held, and Lisa Bero. "A Social Network Analysis of the Financial Links Backing Health and Fitness Apps." *American Journal of Public Health,* vol. 17. no. 11, 2017, pp. 1783–8.

Hagood, Mack. "Here Active Listening System: Sound Technologies and the Personalization of Listening." *Appified: Culture in the Age of Apps*, edited by Jeremy Wade Morris and Sarah Murray. Ann Arbor, MI: University of Michigan Press, 2018, pp. 276–85.

Hagood, Mack. *Hush: Media and Sonic Self-Control.* Duke University Press, 2019.

Hamraie, Aimi. "Universal Design and the Problem of 'Post-Disability' Ideology." *Design and Culture,* vol. 8, no. 3, 2016, pp. 285–309.

Hunn, Nick. "Hearables the New Wearables". *Wearable Technologies*. April 4, 2014, *www.wearable-technologies.com/2014/04/hearables-the-new-wearables/*.

Kao, Cheng-Kai and David M. Liebovitz. "Consumer Mobile Health Apps: Current State, Barriers, and Future Directions." *Physical Medicine and Rehabilitation*, vol. 9, 2017, pp. S106–S115.

Kenner, Alison. "Asthma on the Move: How Mobile Apps Remediate Risk for Disease management." *Health, Risk & Society*, vol. 17, no. 7–8, 2016, pp. 510–29.

Levina, Marina. "Disrupt or Die: Mobile Health and Disruptive Innovation as Body Politics." *Television and New Media*, vol. 18, no. 6, 2017, pp. 548–64.

Llamas, Ramon, Jitesh Ubrani, and Michael Shirer. "Worldwide Wearables Shipments Surge 94.6% in 3Q." *Businesswire*, December 9, 2019, www.businesswire.com/news/home/20191209005097/en/.

Lupton, Deborah. "Apps as Artefacts: Towards a Critical Perspective on Mobile Health and Medical Apps." *Societies*, vol. 4, no. 4, 2014, pp. 606–22.

Lupton, Deborah. "The Diverse Domains of Quantified Selves: Self-tracking Modes and Dataveillance." *Economy and Society*, vol. 45, no. 1, 2016, pp. 101–22.

Matthews, Nicole. "Commodifying Diversity in the Marketing of a Digital Hearing Start-up" *Television and New Media*, vol. 23, April 2021, n.p.

Mitchell, David and Sharon Snyder. "Re-engaging the Body: Disability Studies and the Resistance to Embodiment." *Public Culture*, vol. 13, no. 3, 2001, pp. 367–90.

Mulvin, Dylan. "Media Prophylaxis: Night Modes and the Politics of Preventing Harm." *Information & Culture: A Journal of History*, vol. 53, no. 2, 2018, pp. 175–202.

Ng, Stella L., Shanon Phelan, MaryAnn Leonard, and Jason A. Galsterk. "Qualitative Case Study of Smartphone-Connected Hearing Aids: Influences on Patients, Clinicians, and Patient–Clinician Interactions." *Journal of American Academic Audiologists*, vol. 28, 2017, pp. 506–21.

Oliver, Suzanne. "Hearing Aids Are Getting Smarter." *Wall Street Journal*, September 15, 2019, www.wsj.com/articles/hearing-aids-are-getting-smarter-11568599441.

Paglialonga, Alessia, Francesco Pinciroli and Gabriella Tognola. "The ALFA4 Hearing Model (At-a-Glance Labeling for Features of Apps for Hearing Health Care) to Characterize Mobile Apps for Hearing Health Care." *American Journal of Audiology*, vol. 26, 2017, pp. 408–25.

Paul, Peter and Donald Moores, eds. *Deaf Epistemologies: Multiple Perspectives on the Acquisition of Knowledge*. Washington, D.C.: Gaudellet Press, 2012.

PR Newswire Europe. "Patient Centric Healthcare App Market to Reach USD 64.33 Bn, Globally, by 2027 at 37.2% CAGR: Allied Market Research." September 15, 2020. www.prnewswire.com/news-releases/patient-centric-healthcare-app-market-to-reach-usd-64-33-bn-globally-by-2027-at-37-2-cagr-allied-market-research-301130891.html

Pritchard, Helen and Jennifer Gabrys. "From Citizen Sensing to Collective Monitoring: Working through the Perceptive and Affective Problematics of Environmental Pollution." *GeoHumanities*, vol. 2, no. 2, 2016, pp. 354–71.

Puwar, Nirmal. *Space Invaders: Race, Gender and Bodies out of Place*. Berg, 2004.

Rabinow, Paul and Nikolas Rose. "Biopower Today." *BioSocieties,* vol. 1, 2006, pp. 195–217.

Rich, Emma and Andy Miah. "Understanding Digital Health as Public Pedagogy: A Critical Framework." *Societies,* vol. 4, no. 2, 2014, pp. 296–315.

Roulstone, Alan. *Disability and Technology*. New York and Abingdon: Routledge, 2016.

Seelman, Katherine D. and Roye Werner. "Technology Transfer of Hearing Aids to Low and Middle Income Countries: Policy and Market Factors." *Disability and Rehabilitation: Assistive Technology*, vol. 9, no. 5, 2014, pp. 399–407.
Topol, Eric. *The Patient Will See You Now*. New York: Basic Books, 2016.
Valente, Michael and Amyn Amlani. "Cost as a Barrier to Hearing Aid Adoption." *Journal of Otolaryngogology – Head and Neck Surgery*, vol. 43, no. 7, 2017, pp. 647–8.
Van Dijck, Jose and Thomas Poell. "Understanding the Promises and Premises of Online Health Platforms." *Big Data and Society*, vol. 3, no. 1, 2016, pp. 1–11.
Zeng, Fan-gang. "A New Landscape for Hearing Aids." *The Hearing Journal*, vol. 70, no. 12, 2017, p. 6.

28

DATA VISUALIZATION AND DIGITAL CONTACT TRACING TECHNOLOGY

Emerging forms of health media

Kirsten Ostherr

Introduction

The emergence of "big data" in the early 2010s was a much-hyped phenomenon that would reshape many industries, including health care (Mayer-Schönberger and Cukier). A notable consequence of this development was the fundamental transformation of the role of digital media in health care. While computational technology had a growing presence in medicine since the 1960s (Reiser; Greene), the rise of "big data" made screen-based computational media – that is, electronic technologies for representing, transmitting, storing, and retrieving information – essential tools for clinicians and patients. The availability of extremely large and complex health and medical data sets that were constructed through novel uses of sensors and other forms of passive data capture led to the emergence of new fields of research and new models of patient care, including personalized and precision medicine (Jameson and Longo), which were built upon computational approaches to health. However, the resulting phenomenon of "data-driven medicine" (Shah and Tenenbaum) required an interface between the vast, quantitative repositories of numbers and code and the human users who were supposed to interpret and act upon the discoveries that these datasets claimed to enable. This demand for a translational interface gave rise to a widespread embrace of data visualizations in health care (Shneiderman).

In simple terms, data visualizations are "the presentation of data in a pictorial or graphical format" (SAS Institute Inc.) such as bar graphs, tables, maps, column charts, pie charts, timelines, scatter plots, and so forth. Many researchers and technologists link the need for data visualization tools to the limited capacities of human cognition to comprehend and make sense of information at the scale and complexity of big data, noting that visual and moving images are easier for the human brain to process than "poring over spreadsheets or reports" (SAS Institute Inc.). Moreover, data visualization is often linked to a new type of computationally mediated storytelling – an implicit acknowledgement that scientific representations of data are not merely technical apparatuses but are also rhetorical devices, as the promotional materials of one company claim: "As the 'age of Big Data' kicks into high-gear, visualization is an increasingly key tool to make sense of the trillions of rows of data generated every day. Data visualization helps

DOI: 10.4324/9781003007661-36

to tell stories by curating data into a form easier to understand, highlighting the trends and outliers. A good visualization tells a story, removing the noise from data and highlighting the useful information" (Tableau Software LLC).

Data visualization is now an integral component of visual health communication that shapes meaning in the social and financial ecosystems of global digital health across high, middle, and low income settings, appearing on mobile health apps as digital dashboards in hospital emergency services, in field logistics, and as scorecards for measuring progress toward health outcomes goals (Aung et al.; Christen et al.). For this reason, data visualization merits examination as a unique form of representation, that is, as a form of media. Indeed, the software company Tableau describes data visualization as a technologically-mediated aesthetic form: "Our eyes are drawn to colors and patterns. We can quickly identify red from blue, square from circle. Our culture is visual, including everything from art and advertisements to TV and movies. Data visualization is another form of visual art that grabs our interest and keeps our eyes on the message" (Tableau Software LLC). In this description, the company makes clear that data visualization tools simultaneously present and interpret information, an assertion also made by scholars in media studies and science and technology studies (de Chadarevian and Hopwood). Yet, in many health science applications, data visualizations occupy an elevated evidentiary status, functioning as ostensibly neutral and transparent depictions of data, particularly as compared to qualitative forms of evidence, whose reliability may be more likely called into question (Pauwels).

Mobile visualization tools became particularly important for Covid-19 field data collection and management (Ahmed et al.), and their narrative utility was quickly grasped by users beyond the domains of public health and government, as ordinary citizens monitored the evolution of the Covid-19 pandemic in near real-time. This chapter examines the impact of data visualizations on health by exploring their use in the Covid-19 pandemic with special attention to the visual health surveillance logic of digital contact tracing technology (DCTT). I will show how data visualization shaped a technological determinist rationale for developing DCTTs, even as many technologists and epidemiologists acknowledged the persistent failure of DCTTs to perform the tasks they were designed to complete. Testing was meant to produce a representation of the numbers of infections and was a primary data source for the majority of Covid visualizations (in addition to hospitalization and mortality data). Tracing was meant to control the spread of disease and theoretically, by connecting the dots across geographic rendering of cases, would layer causality on top of incidence data maps. Testing and tracing were meant to be the linked foundations for public health response to infectious disease outbreaks (Contreras et al.). Yet, the operational and societal challenges faced by these entwined efforts in the context of Covid-19 resulted in flawed data sets and visualizations that obscured the gaps in testing and tracing, thereby constructing misleading narratives of contagion and control that reproduced existing racial health disparities. The framing of Covid as a technological and data problem produced results that have distorted our understanding of the crisis itself as well as limiting our framing of potentially effective interventions. This chapter will describe the role of data visualization in the pandemic and present several examples, followed by a discussion of DCTT, to illuminate the sociotechnical dimensions of these approaches in representing health and illness and the limitations they reveal in data-driven healthcare.

Data visualizations: seeing with technology

In a paper from a recent colloquium sponsored by the National Academy of Sciences (2019), a team of researchers described the demand for new literacies in the age of big data, placing the interpretive challenges of data visualizations in the historical lineage of media studies. The report stated: "The invention of the printing press created a mandate for universal textual literacy; the need to manipulate many large numbers created a need for mathematical literacy; and the ubiquity and importance of photography, film, and digital drawing tools posed a need for visual literacy. Analogously, the increasing availability of large datasets, the importance of understanding them, and the utility of data visualizations to inform data-driven decision making pose a need for universal data visualization literacy" (Börner et al.). The researchers went on to describe the disjunction between the widespread use of data visualizations and the low "dataviz" literacy of the general public, leading to simultaneous dependence upon and misinterpretation of the significance of these images.

Like other forms of health media, health data visualizations play a profound role in shaping the ways that clinicians and patients see and make meaning about health and disease. Yet, unlike some other forms of health media, data visualization appears both as an end product of efforts to make research findings accessible and as an integral component of the process for exploring data and making new discoveries. In this way, data visualization fits into a history of scientific discovery through visualization. For example, early 20th-century scientists used the cinematograph as a tool of discovery in their laboratories, incorporating cinematic representation into the very design and documentation of experiments that used microscopic close-ups, time-lapse, and slow motion to reveal the secrets of cell embryogenesis and other processes impossible to observe with the naked human eye (Landecker; Gaycken; Beckman; Ostherr, "Animating Informatics"). The entwined evolution of scientific research with techniques of cinematography and animation has been discussed by film scholars who show that "scientists sought to capture living bodies in animated motion in order to establish precise measurements that could eventuate in scientific laws," and in so doing, "they at once performed research and created a representation of the thing being researched" (Banner and Ostherr). As science and representation entered the digital era, computer generated imagery became a fundamental vehicle for research into cellular (and smaller) forms of life (Kelty and Landecker; Curtis and Lue). The resulting feedback loops simultaneously made visualizations into evidence and made them function as rhetorical tools to persuade viewers of the validity of the evidence that the visualizations make manifest. This characteristic is shared by a range of computational technologies, within and beyond health care, and can be understood as part of a broader technological determinist epistemology, which attributes objectivity, neutrality, and therefore, truth to computational sources of information in deliberate contrast to the fallible subjectivity of human sources of evidence.

Data visualizations based on open-source Geographical Information Systems (GIS) have served a similar function as paradigmatic representations of Covid-19 around the world since the Johns Hopkins University (JHU) online interactive dashboard was first shared with the public on January 22, 2020, to visualize and track reported cases of the novel disease in real time. The site synthesizes and visualizes data collected from hundreds of sources, all documented in the JHU Github Readme page for the project (CSSE). Data sources include aggregators such as DXY (an online platform run by members of the Chinese medical community), the WHO, 1Point3Acres (a site run by a group of first-generation Chinese immigrants living in the United States), BNO News (a Dutch website that reports multinational data), the European Centre for Disease Prevention and Control, and Worldometer (Dong et al.). In addition, the JHU site gathers data from government health ministries around the world at the country/region or state/province level as well as from state, county, and city health departments across the United States. The data are synthesized and visually represented in the form of a dashboard built using the ArcGIS Hub Coronavirus Response template, an open-source data visualization tool created by the Environmental Systems Research Institute (Esri). The center of the site is a map visualizing cumulative case numbers worldwide, flanked by columns listing confirmed cases by country/region on one side and total deaths and total recovered on the other side of the map, with a graphical representation of the trend-lines below those tables. The world map can also be viewed by incidence rate, case-fatality ratio, global vaccinations, U.S. vaccinations, and U.S. testing rate.

While these representations appear to provide a thorough and comprehensive set of frameworks for "seeing" the pandemic, two fundamental questions remain: what do the data reveal, and what remains hidden? Even the creator of the dashboard, Ensheng Dong, a doctoral student in systems engineering at Johns Hopkins University, acknowledged a tension between what he called the "objectivity of numeric data" and the "subjectivity of data visualization" (Milner). For example, Dong explained that his decision to "display bright red dots over a stark, black background," was meant to "emphasize the alarming nature of the pandemic." In this scheme, larger dots meant higher Covid-19 caseloads in that region. "We're constantly adjusting the dot," Dong said. "We added a few other maps besides the cumulative and confirmed cases, such as active cases, to clearly communicate the data we were collecting and sharing. If more people in your country are recovering, you refer to that map. The dots are smaller, and you feel better" (Milner). The Johns Hopkins site was quickly followed by scores of others, 15 of which are listed and linked on the University of Minnesota Center for Infectious Disease Research and Policy website (University of Minnesota Center for Infectious Disease Research and Policy (CIDRAP)). There, site visitors can see data from early in the pandemic visualized in the form of maps showing high-speed rail and domestic flights into and out of Wuhan, China (Esri's StoryMaps Team), or a Sankey chart of numbers of people evacuated from Wuhan, China by citizenship (Robles). Many Covid-19 data visualizations use maps as their organizing principle, often built on the same ArcGIS tools used by Johns Hopkins, or other open-source GIS tools such as Geographic Map Open Objects Source Environment (GeoMOOSE 2020).

Dynamic cumulative data visualizations were also created, such as HealthMap's time-based map of Covid-19 incidence, depicted through an animated movie showing the appearance and expansion of colorful spheres representing the 71,503,614 confirmed Covid cases worldwide (as of June 23, 2021). The site also included a dashboard with a country list feature that allowed users to select a location, zoom in on the map, and observe the progress of the pandemic from a new vantage point, by pressing "play" again and watching for dots to appear in the new locale (HealthMap). The site creators described the time lapse animation as a "real-time visualization" designed with an interactive web application that automatically updated the results (Xu et al.). Data visualizations of transmission chains operationalized the logic of pandemic causality: by visually representing not only the incidence but also the evolution of contagion across a global map, the logic went, we could interrupt and contain the pandemic itself.

Data visualization of transmission chains was also central to an outbreak tracking tool, Go.Data (Ahmed et al.), developed for the World Health Organisation by the Global Outbreak and Response Network (GOARN) for use by community health workers, ministries of health, non-governmental organizations, United Nations agencies, and others during infectious disease outbreaks. Go.Data was deployed prior to the Covid-19 pandemic during the Ebola outbreaks in 2019 in Uganda (Sensasi and Edmond) and the Republic of Congo (Oka and Savage). The app collects case data, contact data, laboratory, and clinical data, and contact follow-up information, and a critically important feature is the visualization of disease transmission chains. As a WHO officer noted, "For epidemiologists, the visual representation of the transmission chain created by the Go.Data software is particularly valuable. It allows them to understand more easily and comprehensively how the disease spreads: which activities, environments and types of interaction are associated with high or low transmission rates. This means they can tailor the intervention to more quickly interrupt the spread" (Oka and Savage). This comment emphasizes the utility of data visualization as a tool for public health intervention that confers clarity on complex situations that can be otherwise difficult to interpret.

The widespread deployment of global maps of infection as a form of data visualization highlights a continuity with the centuries-old emphasis on national boundaries as barriers against the spread of disease in public health media (Ostherr, "How Do We See COVID-19?"). At the same time, these data-driven, frequently updated, and interactive geospatial dashboards enact a new mandate for real-time disease surveillance (Engelmann), in a real-time digital media world. These data visualizations have been embraced by health officials for their potential "to improve comprehension" by "enhancing the detection of patterns, and providing mechanisms for inference," yet researchers also point out the risk that these visualizations might mislead users, "due to misinterpretation or cognitive overload" (Carroll et al.). The ubiquitous presence of data visualizations in the Covid-19 pandemic conveys a visual impression of scientific mastery of the outbreak through data-driven documentation and global mapping. However, a recent review of the literature on the role of visual representation in shaping the effects of health communications finds that, "there are few evidence-based recommendations that can be made with confidence regarding communicating with visuals about infectious diseases because few studies have investigated visual influence in this particular context" (King and Lazard). Moreover, despite the extensive global sourcing of data to populate these visualizations, the fundamental flaws in the source data, due to inadequate and uneven access to testing worldwide, means that these representations present a seemingly complete visual containment of the pandemic – an impression of universal surveillance – that belies the gaps in the data and the unequal burden of suffering hidden in those gaps.

What remains invisible in these data visualizations? The racial and ethnic disparities in infection and mortality rates in the United States have been unevenly documented, resulting in the production of incomplete data-driven narratives. A study of access to Covid-19 testing sites across the state of Texas, for example, found that in many cities, testing was much more accessible in white communities than in communities of color (Martin). An effort by Verily (a health-focused Google company) to expand Covid testing among the state of California's "impoverished and underserved communities" was rejected by several counties months into the contract due to findings of data privacy infringements and complaints of racism in the distribution of testing sites (Pradhan and Gold). Other investigations found that in the early months of the pandemic, there was no reporting category for Native Americans, so cases in that community were marked as "other." As Abigail Echo-Hawk, chief research officer at Seattle Indian Health Board explained, "By including us in the 'other' category it effectively eliminates us in the data. If you eliminate us in the data, we don't exist. We don't exist for the allocation of resources" (Nagle). While reporting on these examples highlights the bias in the data, these gaps remain invisible in the visualizations themselves. Indeed, up to half of all Covid-19 case reports submitted to the Centers for Disease Control and Prevention in the year 2020 contained incomplete racial and ethnic demographic data, making accurate visualizations impossible to build on the basis of these data sets (Krieger et al.).

Digital contact tracing: mapping incomplete narratives

Accurate data visualizations depend on the availability of complete data, and in the Covid-19 pandemic, the most sought-after data were on the incidence of infections and deaths in a given locale. Yet, the accuracy of these data depended on the widespread availability of testing;

without testing, it was impossible to accurately document the existence of cases. As described above, one positive test result would produce one small dot on a map; 1,000 positive test results would create a larger dot. However, the quantification of Covid cases required integration of every case into the biomedical surveillance apparatus of reagents, swabs, tests, operations, logistics, collection of contact information, and communication of results, and access to these tools was not evenly distributed (Kaplan and Forman). Testing rates in the United States were significantly below the rates needed to contain or suppress the pandemic (Collins), and inaccurate diagnostic tests produced high false-negative rates (Woloshin et al.). In this context, one undocumented or inaccurate Covid-19 case (or 1,000) would produce no visible signal on the map.

While testing data can produce visual representation of the incidence of disease, contact tracing can make visible the linkages between instances of contagion – that is, it can provide a dynamic representation of contagion as it progresses in space and time, built on the principles of network visualization (Christakis and Fowler). The basic principles of contact tracing have not changed for decades and entail identifying, testing, and isolating those who are sick (or, in the case of Covid, those who test positive for the disease, even if they are asymptomatic). Then, the real work of contact tracing begins with interviewing confirmed or suspected Covid-19 cases, identifying the people who have been in close contact with the positive individual during the timeframe when they may have been infectious, and then connecting with contacts to encourage them to get tested and self-isolate. Public health officers routinely emphasize that throughout this process, the identity of patients and contacts is kept private, and contacts will not be informed of the source of their potential exposure (Harris Country Public Health).

Yet, from the earliest uses of disease surveillance, the tension between individual privacy and public health provoked concerns that vulnerable communities might be harmed rather then helped by reporting illness to authorities. In the United States, the first known instances of contact tracing date to the mid-18th century when tavern keepers in Rhode Island were required to report cases of infectious diseases such as cholera, yellow fever, and smallpox to local government officials (Fairchild et al. 1). Fears of intrusive monitoring were confirmed by the targeted and disproportionate surveillance of Black and immigrant communities suspected of harboring tuberculosis in the late-19th century (Roberts), and these concerns were reinforced by the emergence of a two-tiered system of contact tracing in association with venereal disease reporting in the early 20th century United States. Known as "veiled" reporting, individuals infected with syphilis who could afford to pay to be diagnosed by a private physician could be reported anonymously by numerical code; by contrast, "charitable patients," prostituted women, and the "destitute" were subject to exposure of personally-identifying information (Fairchild et al. 64–6). The consequences of and opposition to name-based reporting took on new significance in the early 1980s in the context of HIV/AIDS. Cases of housing and employment discrimination and social stigma against people with AIDS made clear the importance of confidential reporting, yet government institutions such as the Centers for Disease Control argued for the need to identify cases by name to conduct research and follow-up on this new and poorly understood disease (174–5). The consequences of gaps in the data, during the height of the AIDS crisis as during the height of the Covid pandemic, could be dire, as one HIV/AIDS advocate commented in the late 1980s: "If we create public health measures, which are doomed to scare people into avoiding public health departments, nobody gains, and the epidemic spreads" (Dembosky).

This brief history shows that concerns about privacy and misuse of data have been common features of public response to contact tracing efforts, whether due to stigma associated with sexually transmitted infections such as syphilis, fears of deportation among immigrant communities associated with tuberculosis, or threats of legal retaliations against gay men associated with HIV/AIDS during the 1980s, a time when homosexuality was still criminalized in much of the United States. The ongoing relevance of these concerns is demonstrated by a public health poster from Harris County Health Department that enumerated common worries in an attempt to increase public compliance with Covid-19 contact tracing. The poster, titled, "Contact Tracing Myths," posed the questions: "Can I get deported if I cooperate with a contact tracer? Will I lose custody of my children due to Covid-19? Do I have to pay for contact tracing? If I am a COVID-19 case contact, can I go to jail or be placed under house arrest? Are contact tracers able to locate and track people through phone apps or Bluetooth technology?" (Harris Country Public Health). As reflected in this series of concerns, fears about state surveillance and police power are interwoven with worries about citizenship status, familial displacement, and income insecurity, and the threat of technological surveillance, overlaid upon all of these concerns, compounded social resistance to contact tracing during Covid-19.

The datafication of the Covid-19 pandemic evidenced by the ubiquitous presence of data dashboards and digital mapping sites such as those discussed above shaped the rationale for developing and promoting digital contact tracing technology (DCTT), despite the lack of an evidence base demonstrating their accuracy and effectiveness in reducing the spread of disease (Ada Lovelace Institute; Kahn). The data-driven logic of pandemic management carried over from the wider trend in medicine that predated the pandemic and overdetermined the technocentric response. The question posed by governments and health officials around the world was not, "Is there a role for technology in contact tracing?" but rather, "How fast can we develop a technological solution to the problem of contact tracing?" Instead of addressing the human concerns around trust and privacy, especially in vulnerable communities that had suffered exploitation and abuse of power in the name of health surveillance, governments and technologists turned to digital tools because of their functional efficiency (Amann et al.). The vast scale of the pandemic made it difficult to imagine that human contact tracers could possibly keep up with the work load represented by the millions of cases worldwide.

The technocentric frame of the pandemic response made DCTT seem inevitable. An article published in the journal *Science* early in the pandemic (March 2020) summarized the logic: "Although SARS-CoV-2 is spreading too fast to be contained by manual contact tracing, it could be controlled if this process were faster, more efficient, and happened at scale. A contact-tracing app that builds a memory of proximity contacts and immediately notifies contacts of positive cases can achieve epidemic control if used by enough people" (Ferretti et al.). Early efforts by Google, Apple, and other technology companies emphasized a privacy-preserving approach based on local storage of data on smartphones, anonymized data exchange between phones using Bluetooth signals, and deidentification of information in the cloud. The retrospective view of these efforts may reveal them to be failures, as measured by population uptake rates (Kaptchuk et al.; Dong et al.; *The Lancet Digital Health*), accuracy of contact identification (Jaca et al.), successful protection of privacy (Ada Lovelace Institute), and effectiveness at reducing transmissions (Kucharski et al.; Braithwaite et al.). Yet, the sociotechnical dimensions of these apps are nonetheless worth examining as media that operationalize the data-driven logic of the pandemic response, thereby also revealing the consequences and limits of that approach.

The debate over DCTT in the Coronavirus pandemic may be best understood through comparison of centralized and decentralized data management methods in different apps. In the former model, data from a user's smartphone would be transmitted to a central repository, such as the National Health Service in the U.K., which would manage exposure notifications and follow-up, and also have access to the anonymized data for health surveillance and modeling (Hsu). The British government was ultimately forced to abandon this approach due to widely expressed privacy concerns, but the centralized approach was adopted in South Korea, Singapore, Vietnam, and China, among other locales, and was augmented by interlocking layers of additional surveillance such as smartphone scanning and social media mining, as well as forced compliance with Covid protocols (Dayaram; McCurry; Hsu; Lewis). Decentralized models, such as the Google-Apple Exposure Notification System (GAENS), foreground so-called "privacy protecting" phone-based data storage and phone-to-phone communication without an intermediary who could access the collected data in the system (Nield). Both models are vulnerable to technical failures such as misjudging distance or duration of exposure between phones, leading to false positives and false negatives that undermine the efficacy of the apps (Jaca et al.). Moreover, despite assurances to the contrary, the Google-Apple system was revealed to contain a significant privacy vulnerability that allowed personally identifiable information to be accessed by third parties (Ng). Additional contact tracing data breaches occurred in Pennsylvania (Bryan), California (Jercich), and Colorado (County), highlighting the elusiveness of truly anonymized data, as well as the value of personal health information to hackers and data brokers (Shachar).

In the locations where DCTT was used most effectively, personal privacy violations were integrated into the surveillance system by design. For example, a study of re-identification of DCTT users in South Korea found that inference of a patient's identity based on a travel log was readily accomplished with publicly available data showing the gender, age, home, and work locations of a patient (Jung et al.). Additional sensitive information such as hobbies, religion, and social relationships was also disclosed, and when combined with surveillance-camera footage, smartphone location data and credit card purchase records, these data enabled government agencies to "trace the recent movements of coronavirus patients and establish virus transmission chains" (Singer and Sang-Hun). While these techniques have been praised by some for their effectiveness in controlling the pandemic (Budd et al.), they have also given rise to fears of exposure to social shaming. Lee Su-young, a psychiatrist at Myongji Hospital in South Korea, observed, "[Some of my patients] were more afraid of being blamed than of dying of the virus" ("Coronavirus Privacy"). These concerns around mistrust and stigmatization for involvement in a viral transmission chain echoed those expressed in the context of contact tracing campaigns in Liberia during the Ebola outbreak there ("Liberia"), as well as those referenced above in the context of sexually transmitted diseases.

A review of ethical issues in the use of DCTT noted the value of human-to-human encounters in manual contact tracing, which provides "the opportunity to clarify misconceptions, address worries, and express sympathy and other important affects," in contrast to the limitations of DCTT, which "currently lacks a range of human capabilities and characteristics" (Kahn). Another review concluded, "Digital contact tracing with self-isolation probably reduces the number of secondary infections, but not as much as manual contact tracing with self-isolation" (Anglemyer et al.). The technical challenges were compounded by social concerns linked to the history of exploitative surveillance, which impacts both digital and manual contact tracing (Esmonde). Finally, the consequences of both counting and failing to count members of the most vulnerable communities pose significant challenges for DCTTs. As one scholar cautioned, "the gaps in our knowledge will be consequential and non-random, sabotaging our efforts to understand what's actually going on in the world and undermining our response" (Alkhatib).

Conclusion

The Covid-19 pandemic is an exemplary instance of data-driven healthcare. This technocentric frame resulted in high dependence on data tracking and visualizations to make sense of the evolving health situation worldwide. Deployment of DCTT as a tactic for responding to the problems revealed by the data visualizations extended the datacentric narration of the pandemic while obscuring the structuring absences of the invisible gaps in the data. This case study illuminates the appeal and seeming certainty of data during times of profound uncertainty, and reveals the cost to our most vulnerable communities of accepting interpretive frames that exclude them.

Works cited

Ada Lovelace Institute. *COVID-19 Rapid Evidence Review.* April 19, 2020, www.adalovelaceinstitute.org/evidence-review/covid-19-rapid-evidence-review-exit-through-the-app-store/.

Ahmed, Kamran, et al. "Novel Approach to Support Rapid Data Collection, Management, and Visualization during the COVID-19 Outbreak Response in the World Health Organization African Region: Development of a Data Summarization and Visualization Tool." *JMIR Public Health and Surveillance*, vol. 6, no. 4, Oct. 2020, p. e20355.

Alkhatib, Ali. "We Need to Talk about Digital Contact Tracing." *Interactions*, vol. 27, no. 4, Association for Computing Machinery, July 2020, pp. 84–9.

Amann, Julia, et al. "Digital Contact-Tracing during the Covid-19 Pandemic: An Analysis of Newspaper Coverage in Germany, Austria, and Switzerland." *PLOS ONE*, vol. 16, no. 2, Feb. 2021, p. e0246524.

Anglemyer, Andrew, et al. "Digital Contact Tracing Technologies in Epidemics: A Rapid Review." *Cochrane Database of Systematic Reviews*, no. 8. Chichester: John Wiley & Sons, Ltd, 2020.

Aung, Tricia, et al. "Leveraging Data Visualization to Improve the Use of Data for Global Health Decision-Making." *Journal of Global Health*, vol. 9, no. 2.

Banner, Olivia, and Kirsten Ostherr. "Design in Motion: Introducing Science/Animation." *Discourse*, vol. 37, no. 3. Detriot, MI: Wayne State University Press, 2015, pp. 175–92.

Beckman, Karen. "Animating Film Theory:" *Animating Film Theory*, edited by Karen Beckman. Durham, NC: Duke University Press, 2014, pp. 1–22.

Börner, Katy, et al. "Data Visualization Literacy: Definitions, Conceptual Frameworks, Exercises, and Assessments." *Proceedings of the National Academy of Sciences of the United States of America*, vol. 116, no. 6, February 2019, pp. 1857–64.

Braithwaite, Isobel, et al. "Automated and Partly Automated Contact Tracing: A Systematic Review to Inform the Control of COVID-19." *The Lancet Digital Health*, vol. 2, no. 11, Nov. 2020, pp. e607–21.

Bryan, Kristin L. "Lawsuit Filed in Federal Court Over Alleged Data Breach Concerning COVID Contact Tracing Information." *The National Law Review*, June 2, 2021, www.natlawreview.com/article/lawsuit-filed-federal-court-over-alleged-data-breach-concerning-covid-contact.

Budd, Jobie, et al. "Digital Technologies in the Public-Health Response to COVID-19." *Nature Medicine*, vol. 26, no. 8, August 2020, pp. 1183–92.

Carroll, Lauren N., et al. "Visualization and Analytics Tools for Infectious Disease Epidemiology: A Systematic Review." *Journal of Biomedical Informatics*, vol. 51, Oct. 2014, pp. 287–98.

Christakis, Nicholas A., and James H. Fowler. "Social Contagion Theory: Examining Dynamic Social Networks and Human Behavior." *Statistics in Medicine*, vol. 32, no. 4, Feb. 2013, p. 10.1002/sim.5408.

Christen, Oliver M., et al. "Dashboard Visualization of Information for Emergency Medical Services." *Studies in Health Technology and Informatics*, vol. 275, Nov. 2020, pp. 27–31.

Collins, Keith. "Is Your State Doing Enough Coronavirus Testing?" *The New York Times*, Nov. 13, 2020. *NYTimes.com*, www.nytimes.com/interactive/2020/us/coronavirus-testing.html.

Contreras, Sebastian, et al. "The Challenges of Containing SARS-CoV-2 via Test-Trace-and-Isolate." *Nature Communications*, vol. 12, no. 1, Jan. 2021, p. 378.

"Coronavirus Privacy: Are South Korea's Alerts Too Revealing?" *BBC News*, 5 March 2020, www.bbc.com/news/world-asia-51733145.

County, Pitkin. "Pitkin County – Notice of Data Privacy Incident." *PR Newswire*, January 14, 2021, www.prnewswire.com/news-releases/pitkin-county--notice-of-data-privacy-incident-301208971.html.

CSSE. *COVID-19 Data Repository by the Center for Systems Science and Engineering (CSSE) at Johns Hopkins University*. 2020. 2021. *GitHub*, https://github.com/CSSEGISandData/COVID-19.

Curtis, Scott, and Robert Lue. "Bridging Science, Art, and the History of Visualization: A Dialogue between Scott Curtis and Robert Lue." *Discourse*, vol. 37, no. 3, 2015, pp. 193–206.

Dayaram, Sareena. "Singapore's Coronavirus Playbook: How It Fought Back against the COVID-19 Pandemic." *CNET*, March 22, 2020,www.cnet.com/health/singapores-coronavirus-playbook-how-one-country-fought-back-against-covid19-epidemic/.

de Chadarevian, Soraya, and Nick Hopwood, editors. *Models: The Third Dimension of Science*. Redwood City, CA: Stanford University Press, 2004, www.sup.org/books/title/?id=1242.

Dembosky, April. "Tensions Around Contact Tracing During the AIDS Era Are Resurfacing With COVID-19." *KQED*, July 9, 2020, www.kqed.org/news/11828008/the-same-tensions-around-contact-tracing-during-the-aids-era-are-resurfacing-with-covid-19.

Dong, Ensheng, et al. "An Interactive Web-Based Dashboard to Track COVID-19 in Real Time." *The Lancet Infectious Diseases*, vol. 20, no. 5, May 2020, pp. 533–4.

Engelmann, Lukas. "#COVID19: The Spectacle of Real-Time Surveillance." *Somatosphere* (blog), March 6, 2020,http://somatosphere.net/forumpost/covid19-spectacle-surveillance/.

Esmonde, Katelyn. "For Contact Tracing to Work, Public Health Authorities Must Regain the Trust of Black Communities." *Vox*, June 2020, www.vox.com/first-person/2020/6/23/21299241/contact-tracing-covid-distrust-black-americans.

Esri. "COVID-19 GIS Hub." *Esri*, 2020. https://coronavirus-resources.esri.com/.

Esri's StoryMaps Team. "Mapping the COVID-19 Pandemic."*ArcGIS StoryMaps*, January 25, 2021, https://storymaps.arcgis.com/stories/4fdc0d03d3a34aa485de1fb0d2650ee0.

Fairchild, Amy L., et al. *Searching Eyes: Privacy, the State, and Disease Surveillance in America*. Oakland, CA: University of California Press, 2007.

Ferretti, Luca, et al. "Quantifying SARS-CoV-2 Transmission Suggests Epidemic Control with Digital Contact Tracing." *Science*, vol. 368, no. 6491, May 2020.

Gaycken, Oliver. "'A Living, Developing Egg Is Present before You': Animation, Scientific Visualization, Modeling." *Animating Film Theory*, edited by Karen Beckman. Durham, NC: Duke University Press, 2014, pp. 68–82.

Greene, Jeremy A. "Knowledge in Medias Res: Toward a Media History of Science, Medicine, and Technology." *History and Theory*, vol. 59, no. 4, 2020, pp. 48–66. Harris Country Public Health. *Contact Tracing*. 2020, https://publichealth.harriscountytx.gov/Resources/2019-Novel-Coronavirus/Contact-Tracing.

HealthMap. *Novel Coronavirus (COVID-19)*. 2020, www.healthmap.org/covid-19/.

Hsu, Jeremy. "Contact Tracing Apps Struggle to Be Both Effective and Private." *IEEE Spectrum: Technology, Engineering, and Science News*, Sept. 2020, https://spectrum.ieee.org/biomedical/devices/contact-tracing-apps-struggle-to-be-both-effective-and-private.

Jaca, Anelisa, et al. "Cochrane Corner: Digital Contact Tracing Technologies in Epidemics." *The Pan African Medical Journal*, vol. 37, no. Suppl 1, 2020, p. 8.

Jameson, J. Larry, and Dan L. Longo. "Precision Medicine – Personalized, Problematic, and Promising." *New England Journal of Medicine*, vol. 372, no. 23, June 2015, pp. 2229–34.

Jercich, Kat. "California Breach Highlights Contact Tracing Data Vulnerabilities." *Healthcare IT News*, March 19, 2021, www.healthcareitnews.com/news/california-breach-highlights-contact-tracing-data-vulnerabilities.

Jung, Gyuwon, et al. "Too Much Information: Assessing Privacy Risks of Contact Trace Data Disclosure on People With COVID-19 in South Korea." *Frontiers in Public Health*, vol. 8, Frontiers, 2020.

Kahn, Jeffrey. *Digital Contact Tracing for Pandemic Response: Ethics and Governance Guidance*. Baltimore, MD: Johns Hopkins University Press, 2020,

Kaplan, Edward H., and Howard P. Forman. "Logistics of Aggressive Community Screening for Coronavirus 2019."*JAMA Health Forum*, vol. 1, no. 5, May 2020, p. e200565.

Kaptchuk, Gabriel, et al. "How Good Is Good Enough for COVID19 Apps? The Influence of Benefits, Accuracy, and Privacy on Willingness to Adopt." *arXiv.org*, May 2020, http://arxiv.org/abs/2005.04343

Kelty, Christopher, and Hannah Landecker. "A Theory of Animation: Cells, L-Systems, and Film." *Grey Room*, vol. 17, Oct. 2004, pp. 30–63.

King, Andy J., and Allison J. Lazard. "Advancing Visual Health Communication Research to Improve Infodemic Response." *Health Communication*, vol. 35, no. 14, December 2020, pp. 1723–8.

Krieger, Nancy, et al. "US Racial and Ethnic Data for COVID-19 Cases: Still Missing in Action." *The Lancet*, vol. 396, no. 10261, Nov. 2020, p. e81.

Kucharski, Adam J., et al. "Effectiveness of Isolation, Testing, Contact Tracing, and Physical Distancing on Reducing Transmission of SARS-CoV-2 in Different Settings: A Mathematical Modelling Study." *The Lancet Infectious Diseases*, vol. 20, no. 10, October 2020, pp. 1151–60.

Landecker, Hannah. "Microcinematography and the History of Science and Film." *Isis*, vol. 97, no. 1, 2006, pp. 121–32.

Lewis, Dyani. "Why Many Countries Failed at COVID Contact-Tracing – but Some Got It Right." *Nature*, vol. 588, no. 7838, Dec. 2020, pp. 384–7.

"Liberia: Ebola Contact Tracing Lessons Inform COVID-19 Response." *UN News*, Apr. 2020, https://news.un.org/en/story/2020/04/1062582.

Martin, Rachel. "In Large Texas Cities, Access To Coronavirus Testing May Depend On Where You Live." *Morning Edition*, National Public Radio, May 27, 2020, www.npr.org/sections/health-shots/2020/05/27/862215848/across-texas-black-and-hispanic-neighborhoods-have-fewer-coronavirus-testing-sit.

Mayer-Schönberger, Viktor, and Kenneth Cukier. *Big Data: A Revolution That Will Transform How We Live, Work, and Think*. Boston, MA: Houghton Mifflin Harcourt, 2013.

McCurry, Justin. "Test, Trace, Contain: How South Korea Flattened Its Coronavirus Curve." *The Guardian*, April 23, 2020, www.theguardian.com/world/2020/apr/23/test-trace-contain-how-south-korea-flattened-its-coronavirus-curve.

Milner, Greg. "Creating the Dashboard for the Pandemic." *Esri*, August 26, 2020, www.esri.com/about/newsroom/arcuser/johns-hopkins-covid-19-dashboard/.

Nagle, Rebecca. "Native Americans Being Left out of US Coronavirus Data and Labelled as 'Other.'" *The Guardian*, April 24, 2020, www.theguardian.com/us-news/2020/apr/24/us-native-americans-left-out-coronavirus-data.

Ng, Alfred. "Google Promised Its Contact Tracing App Was Completely Private – But It Wasn't – The Markup." *The Markup*, April 27, 2021, https://themarkup.org/privacy/2021/04/27/google-promised-its-contact-tracing-app-was-completely-private-but-it-wasnt.

Nield, David. "How Covid-19 Contact Tracing Works on Your Phone." *Wired*, June 2020, www.wired.com/story/covid-19-contact-tracing-apple-google.

Oka, Saya, and Susannah Savage. "Speeding up Detection to Slow down Ebola: Smartphone App Is Game-Changer for Contact Tracing in Hotspots in the Democratic Republic of the Congo." *WHO Regional Office for Africa*, September 18, 2019, www.afro.who.int/news/speeding-detection-slow-down-ebola-smartphone-app-game-changer-contact-tracing-hotspots.

Ostherr, Kirsten. "Animating Informatics." *A Companion to Contemporary Documentary Film*, edited by Alexandra Juhasz and Alisa Lebow. Chichester: John Wiley & Sons, Ltd, 2015, pp. 280–97.

Ostherr, Kirsten. "How Do We See COVID – Visual Iconographies of Racial Contagion." *American Literature*, no. 8780923, Oct. 2020.

Pauwels, Luc. *Visual Cultures of Science: Rethinking Representational Practices in Knowledge Building and Science Communication*. Lebanon, NH: Dartmouth College Press/UPNE, 2006.

Pradhan, Jenny, and Rachana Gold. "Verily's COVID Testing Program Halted in San Francisco and Oakland." *Kaiser Health News*, October 26, 2020, https://khn.org/news/verilys-covid-testing-program-halted-in-san-francisco-and-oakland/.

Reiser, Stanley Joel. *Technological Medicine: The Changing World of Doctors and Patients*. Cambridge: Cambridge University Press, 2009.

Roberts, Samuel. *Infectious Fear: Politics, Disease, and the Health Effects of Segregation*. Chapel Hill, NC: University of North Carolina Press, 2009.

Robles, Pablo. "Coronavirus: The Disease Covid-19 Explained." *South China Morning Post*, February 7, 2020, http://bit.ly/2RgB7Ce.

SAS Institute Inc. *Data Visualization: What It Is and Why It Matters*. 2021, www.sas.com/en_us/insights/big-data/data-visualization.html.

Sensasi, Benjamin, and Mwebembezi Edmond. "WHO's Data Tool Improves Ebola Surveillance, Contact Tracing and Decision Making in Uganda." *WHO Regional Office for Africa*, July 26, 2019, www.afro.who.int/news/whos-data-tool-improves-ebola-surveillance-contact-tracing-and-decision-making-uganda.

Shachar, Carmel. "Protecting Privacy in Digital Contact Tracing for COVID-19: Avoiding a Regulatory Patchwork." *Health Affairs Blog*, May 19, 2020, www.healthaffairs.org/do/10.1377/hblog20200515.190582/full/.

Shah, Nigam H., and Jessica D. Tenenbaum. "The Coming Age of Data-Driven Medicine: Translational Bioinformatics' Next Frontier." *Journal of the American Medical Informatics Association*, vol. 19, no. e1, June 2012, pp. e2–4.

Shneiderman, Ben. "Inventing Discovery Tools: Combining Information Visualization with Data Mining." *Information Visualization*, vol. 1, no. 1, March 2002, pp. 5–12,

Singer, Natasha, and Choe Sang-Hun. "As Coronavirus Surveillance Escalates, Personal Privacy Plummets – The New York Times." *The New York Times*, March 23, 2020, www.nytimes.com/2020/03/23/technology/coronavirus-surveillance-tracking-privacy.html.

Strickland, Eliza. "An Official WHO Coronavirus App Will Be a 'Waze for COVID-19' – IEEE Spectrum." *IEEE Spectrum: Technology, Engineering, and Science News*, March 2020, https://spectrum.ieee.org/the-human-os/biomedical/devices/who-official-coronavirus-app-waze-covid19.

Tableau Software LLC. "Data Visualization Beginner's Guide: A Definition, Examples, and Learning Resources." *Tableau*, 2021, www.tableau.com/learn/articles/data-visualization.

The Lancet Digital Health. "Contact Tracing: Digital Health on the Frontline." *The Lancet Digital Health*, vol. 2, no. 11, November 2020, p. e561.

University of Minnesota Center for Infectious Disease Research and Policy (CIDRAP). "COVID-19 Maps & Visuals." *CIDRAP*, 2020, www.cidrap.umn.edu/covid-19/maps-visuals.

Woloshin, Steven, et al. "False Negative Tests for SARS-CoV-2 Infection – Challenges and Implications." *New England Journal of Medicine*, vol. 383, no. 6, Aug. 2020, p. e38.

Xu, Bo, et al. "Epidemiological Data from the COVID-19 Outbreak, Real-Time Case Information." *Scientific Data*, vol. 7, no. 1, March 2020, p. 106.

PART VIII

Social media

Our understanding of what constitutes health and disease, our notion of ourselves as well or sick beings, and our ability to share our stories of illness and impairment have been fundamentally and irrevocably impacted by social media. The final section of this book explores the mutable and complex relationship between people and platforms whether we are turning to the internet for information about a personal health concern, creating a collective of individuals and influencers around a chronic disease, or seeking a community to hear about a medical encounter.

In the first chapter, **"Paratext and medical authority in the world of the internet,"** Tod Chambers recounts an experience now common to most of us: turning to the internet for information about a worrisome symptom, the results of a medical test, or a recent diagnosis. What Chambers finds, as do we, is an extraordinary amount of information from a variety of sources, at times offering conflicting advice. Prior to the internet, we relied on gatekeepers to validate sources and determine reliability through author credentials, expert reviews, and trustworthy publishers, but Chambers wonders how do we judge what we read now?

In **"Chronic constellations: Instagrammatic aesthetics and crip time,"** Amanda Greene introduces us to the photography of Georgie Wileman whose unconventional self-portrait, rooted in her experience of endometriosis, was displayed at the National Portrait Gallery in 2017. Although the photograph is powerful on its own, its life beyond the gallery walls as it circulated on Instagram via the hashtag #ThisIsEndometriosis" makes it exceptional. Greene reads #ThisIsEndometriosis through a deliberate aesthetic, platform-specific, and disability-informed lens to illuminate how the campaign draws viewers into the temporal experience of the disease.

Finally, Caroline Wellbery explores what happens to stories of illness when the telling of them shifts from a private sphere to a public forum in **"Art spaces, performances, podcasts: community-building in a virtual age."** Publicly shared narratives disseminated through performances, podcasts, or videos can connect audiences, emphasize togetherness, and build community. However, for some individuals, the public virtual space can undermine the promise of authentic connection and become, instead, a source of alienation. She argues that it is the work of health humanities scholars and educators to highlight the advantages of sharing illness stories in the public sphere and to recognize those who are marginalized from and by it.

DOI: 10.4324/9781003007661-37

29

PARATEXT AND MEDICAL AUTHORITY IN THE WORLD OF THE INTERNET

Tod Chambers

Introduction

Following my yearly physical in the fall of last year, I received a disquieting message from my internist that my Prostate-Specific Antigen (PSA) test came back a bit high. He mentioned that they had just started using a new lab, but he thought it a good idea to repeat the test in three months. There has been some controversy concerning the routine use of PSA tests because elevated levels can be an indication of a number of medical conditions, a number of which are quite benign. As is often noted, the test's accuracy for indicating cancer is highly unreliable. The central concern has been that a high PSA may lead men to get unnecessary biopsies, a procedure that carries with it a number of potential risks. Raise the issue of PSA among a group of men, and it is not unusual to hear stories of infections following biopsies after their PSA level had gone up – with the final results being negative. In my particular case, the test three months later showed even higher results. I was then referred to a urologist, who examined me physically and had additional labs taken. The third PSA test came back with normal levels. The urologist I saw was cautious about what we should conclude from these tests and ordered a magnetic resonance imaging (MRI) scan to help with the diagnosis.

At this point I did what most people do when confronted with confusing information: I searched the internet, looking up PSA and the potential meanings of fluctuating levels. Not sufficiently literate to evaluate scientific information, I did not hazard a search through Medline or Google Scholar, resources that would provide a range of studies that require a degree of expertise to determine their relevance to my particular situation; instead, I clicked on Google, DuckDuckGo, and Bing. These general search engines produced what I suspect is not surprising to anyone, an extraordinary amount of information from a variety of sources. Some of these sources were related to websites associated with established medical institutions, such as the Mayo Clinic, MD Anderson Cancer Center, and the Cleveland Clinic. Other links sent me to entities that exist solely within the virtual world, but I had no means of independently determining their legitimacy. I had heard of some of these virtual entities, such as WebMD, but a large number popped up that I didn't recognize. Many of these links directed me to sites in which patients shared information about their medical experiences.

DOI: 10.4324/9781003007661-38

My situation is not unique; the development of the internet has resulted in an ongoing and continually evolving construction of determining authority for information. How, for example, would I have found reliable information about this condition if it had been discovered in my twenties, in the 1980s? I would have had been almost entirely dependent upon my physician – and possibly the experiences of friends and family. Maybe I would have gone to a library to look for information or a bookstore. If I had access to a research library at the time, I would have been able to obtain the most current information found in various medical journals, but such a journey without a medical Virgil could be as dangerous as simply leaving things to my imagination. Assuming that I could find a relatively recent book on the topic, how would I judge the validity of the information presented? Where I receive the information is an important aspect of the authority I would grant to a particular source of information, but other essential qualities also influence my evaluation.

Let us suppose that on my way to my public library I find, on the sidewalk, a heap of handwritten papers with detailed information about PSA tests and their indication for a cancer diagnosis. I pick up this pile, put it in my bag, and continue to the library where, with the help of a friendly librarian, I find a book on prostate cancer and its diagnosis written at my educational level. I take these two texts home and read them both. In looking through the two writings, I find that actually they say very similar things – but differ on important features concerning the validity of the PSA tests and their recommendations for further treatment. I assume that I, and most people, would consider these library books a more reliable source of information. But why?

Here we might realize that prior to the internet, our trust in sources was profoundly reliant on an entire series of gatekeepers both personal and textual that conveyed those sources' validity. These gatekeepers are important. Unlike my first text, the library book was not simply left on the ground; its presence in the library demonstrated that an array of knowledgeable individuals had decided the text was worth including in the library's collection. In such a situation, much of the task of determining reliability has been done for me (given my faith in public librarians not to simply take any text handed to them and stack it on the shelf). Librarians themselves lean on gatekeepers for help in this respect, though, as they cannot have the necessary expertise in every subject to determine which books to buy and include in circulation: for this, they turn to reviews in publications such as *Publisher's Weekly*, *Choice*, *The New York Times Book Review*, and *Kirkus Reviews*. A publisher's reputation may also serve as a prior form of gatekeeping. The publishers themselves pay additional gatekeepers in the form of external expert reviewers to judge the worth of the book proposal, including whether the author demonstrates the appropriate level of knowledge to write the book.

Simply stated, many gatekeepers must approve of a book before it appears on the shelf of my local library. I rely not only on the librarians for determining authority, for the book itself will persuade me of its authority through its title, publisher, associated texts, and author credentials. Literary critic Gérard Genette refers to these prior forms of ancillary materials as *paratexts*. These paratexts are key to the interpretive strategies we use when evaluating a new text, and they also influence our less conscious judgments. Lacking these paratexts, the loose packet of paper on PSA tests and treatment recommendations I found on the sidewalk – no matter how convincingly written – lack the ability to convince me of its authority over the book.

Intertextuality, transtextuality, and paratexts

To understand the nature of paratexts, we must first appreciate them as one type of textual relationship, that is, as a category of intertextuality. Intertextuality, as it has been used by literary scholars from Mikhail Bakhtin to Roland Barthes, does not merely refer to the specific influences of and allusions to particular prior texts but instead represents a more complex engagement of the necessary conditions for comprehension of a text. Most communication is only possible because we share prior texts – including texts of which we are not necessarily self-conscious. Theorists refer to the prior text as an *intertext*, "one or more texts which the reader must know in order to understand a work of literature in terms of its overall significance" (Riffaterre 56). It is for this reason that Barthes refers to these intertexts as always "already read: they are quotations without inverted commas" (160). While the school of New Criticism in the middle of the 20th century conceived of a literary artifact as an organic whole, whose meaning was corrupted when viewed in relation to any other cultural artifact (as, for instance, the author's biography), the notion of intertextuality raised by the post-structuralists in the later part of that century radically reconceived it as part of a "network" of texts, a network without beginning or end (Barthes 161). Michael Riffaterre notes that intertextuality includes not merely what was known prior to coming to the work but also extends to texts created afterward, which also can influence our understanding of that work. From this perspective, interpretation is always in some manner outside the author's control, dependent on prior texts (the already said) as well as on subsequent texts (the yet to be said). At times, however, intertextuality, especially in its most radical post-structuralist rendering, can seem an almost useless concept, leading critics to make vacuous statements concerning untraceable prior texts and criticizing anyone who cites particular intertexts as in some manner misunderstanding the entire concept (Culler 104).

It took a structuralist like Genette to clarify this post-structuralist intertextuality miasma. In three book-length studies of intertextuality – *Architext*, *Palimpsests*, and *Paratexts* – Genette creates a useful typology of the various ways in which a text is placed "in a relationship, whether obvious or concealed, with other texts" (*Palimpsests* 1). Such an approach to textuality permits Genette to establish what he calls an "open structuralism," in which structural features of texts should not be considered as Platonic eternal forms but rather as capable of evolving and changing over time. While Genette's typology provides a useful way to break down and understand the various relationships between texts, he decided to use the term intertextuality to mean only the explicit co-presence of a prior text; if I had quoted Genette's own words defining intertextuality in the prior sentence that itself would be an example of intertextuality. Genette uses the term *transtextuality* to mean ""all that sets the text in a relationship, whether obvious or concealed, with other texts" (*Palimpsests* 1). For Genette intertexuality is one form of transtextuality. Genette himself acknowledges the confusion he is causing by introducing the term transtextuality to mean what has been traditionally understood as intertextuality and limiting the meaning of intertextuality to a specific form of trantextuality. For this chapter, I will for the sake of clarity be using Genette's definitions.

Along with intertextuality, Genette discerns four other types of transtextual relationships: architextuality, metatextuality, hypertextuality, and paratextuality. Architextuality is his term for the manner in which a text fits within a broader system of classification, "the entire set of general or transcendent categories – types of discourse, modes of enunciation, literary genres – from which emerges each singular text" (*Palimpsests* 1). Metatextuality is when a text is a commentary on a prior text; this chapter could be viewed as an example of metatextuality since it includes commentary on Genette's work. Hypertextuality entails what Genette describes as "united text B (which I shall call the hypertext) to an earlier text A (I shall, of course, call it the hypotext, upon which it is grafted in a manner that is not that of commentary" (5). Paratexts are those explicit texts that are on the "threshold" of the text and frame the text for the reader. In physical texts, which were the sole subject of Genette's study, these included the title, author's name, any preface, and notes, as well as interviews with the author and external reviews. Genette describes paratexts as texts that act as transitional entities, existing both as part of the text and also as apart from the text. Dorothee Birke and Birte Christ argue that paratexts serve three functions (interpretive, commercial, and navigational) and that each of these is altered with the development of digital media (67–8).

For Genette, the most important functional quality of the paratext is the manner in which it attempts "to ensure for the text a destiny consistent with the author's purpose" (*Paratexts* 407). So if a novelist wants to ensure that her most recent work is not read as a piece of philosophy or sociology, she might use a paratext – in this case a subtitle – to designate the work "a novel." In the sphere of non-fiction writing, like presenting information about PSA tests, the paratext of the author's name is essential to the construction of authority: having a medical degree listed after the author's name on the cover of the book goes a long way in this regard. As already mentioned, Genette's discussion of paratexts was limited to the physical medium of the book, but, as Thomas Doherty reports, "media scholars quickly latched on to his peripheral vision to zoom in on the infestation of spin-offs and sidebars proliferating in the new digital environment" (Doherty). And with this shift came a need for rethinking paratexts in relation to media outside the physical book. I go into detail about this expanded definition of paratexts because the contrast between gathering information in the 1980s and gathering information in the late 20th and early 21st centuries is so dramatic. I still have a need for information, and I can still go to my library to find it – but consulting the internet as I did (and as I assume most people do) entails accepting that I have entered a form of media that lacks traditional gatekeepers and, often, their paratextual signifiers as well.

There are of course still gatekeepers for information on the internet. Before the rise of the search engines, such entities as Yahoo existed to provide a form of directory of sources; if I had gone to Yahoo in the 1990s, I would have been directed to such sources as "Prostate Help Association" with the description "publishes quarterly newsletter and information sheets on all aspects of prostate disease" and a link to the Prostate Center of South Florida's "On-Line library information about Prostate Diseases" ("Prostate Cancer"). Following the development of sophisticated search engines, Google most notably, Yahoo's authority was replaced with a sort of wisdom of the masses. Google does not rely on an explicit authority designating where one should search for information on prostate tests, for its algorithm rests instead on the number of links being made to a particular site. In this way, Google's searches are profoundly dependent on the internet's transtextuality, that is, not only the manner in which we go to websites to find information but also the manner in which the internet as part of its fundamental nature functions to connect texts together. As a medium the internet has been shaped to make explicit links to texts outside the current text. Of course, such a form of transtextuality has long been a part of print culture, most obvious in the practice of scholarly citations to other sources (Grafton). Yet the internet has greatly expanded transtextuality exponentially.

As Sérgio Tavares notes, the various paratexts within the internet, or what he refers to as "paramedia," create an entire host of different forms of paratextual relations, for, "[w]hile paratexts are analogical, delimiting, definitive, authoritative (created by the negotiation between an author, an editor, a sponsor) and static, paramedia is fluid, plural (it may come from the readership toward the authorship), posthuman (it may come from the interaction between authors, readers, and algorithms) and, ultimately, it's delimiting but dynamic (aggregating to [the] same container new texts produced with the same paratexts)" (27). To illustrate how these paramedia have changed the creation of authority – and, arguably, how they have deconstructed authority's more traditional markers – I will look at the paratexts, as well as interrelated forms of transtextuality, in the ongoing public debate surrounding vaccines.

The current controversy concerning vaccines is particularly good for my purposes, not because vaccine skepticism is new (see Hausman) but rather because its most recent manifestation arose and has gained a great deal of its currency through the internet. That said, however, this is not an essay on the vaccine debate – that is, I am not taking a position on the matter – but is rather an examination of how traditional sources of medical information in mainstream medical journals and websites compare to the anti-vaccine or vaccine-hesitant websites that have emerged in the 21st century. Because my analysis will be confined to independent websites, I am not considering third-party social networking websites such as Facebook, Twitter, and Instagram, where the presentation of material is constrained by the format and commercial interests of those hosting sites, meaning that the information creators do not strictly control the design elements.

The role of centrifugal and centripetal paratexts

Genette distinguishes between two types of paratexts: peritexts and epitexts. Peritexts are threshold texts that are a part of the text itself. Such peritexts can, and often do, change from one edition of a published text to another. Take, for example, a traditional text, the anthropologist Heidi Larson's (2020) book, *Stuck,* that examines how the rapid spread of rumor – primarily via the internet – has affected how parents make decisions about vaccinations. Larson's text is enfolded in a number of these texts that condition our reading. The first is the title itself, *Stuck*, with its subtitle, "How Vaccine Rumors Start – And Why They Don't Go Away," which signals to the reader that Larson's book is not only a provaccine book but also one that seeks to help us understand why people are hesitant. This title, along with the other texts around the book, are not necessarily the work of Larson alone but likely the result of a collaboration with the publisher, in this case Oxford University Press. (At times, the press will make peritextual choices for the author or overrule the desires of an author, but this is not the rule.) The back cover of Larson's book includes a number of blurbs that are, since this is a first edition, the result of the manuscript having been given to titular experts to provide positive and supportive quotations. For Larson's book, all three of the blurbs praising the book come from people at established universities. Their degrees – one an MD, one a PhD, and one an MD *and* PhD – lend additional authority to Larson's study. The inside cover of the book identifies Larson as a "Professor of Anthropology, Risk, and Decision Science and Director of the Vaccine Confidence Project at the London School of Hygiene & Tropical Medicine" and notes that she holds a position as "Clinical Professor of Health Metrics Sciences at the University of Washington" as well as having had prior positions at Clark and Harvard Universities. This biographical text contributes to the aura of authority that in turn influences how we approach and read her text. Larson holds positions at established academic institutions, and her book is acknowledged by other established academics as an important new study.

While peritexts are part of the text itself, Genette's second type of partatext, epitexts, comprises those texts that exist outside the text, such as reviews, interviews of the author, and letters of correspondence. Larson's book has been reviewed in the journal *Nature*. She has also been interviewed on the podcast "Social Science Bites" (Larson *Stuck*), and has given a TED talk on the thesis of the book as well. Another type of epitext, especially for non-fiction books, is the presence of prior publications; Larson has published on vaccine hesitancy in several scholarly articles targeted at academic audiences (Kostkova et al.).

As some of these epitexts exist solely in the digital world, we see how the two forms – traditional print and the electronic – have today become intimately entwined. I have a print version of Larson's book, but I could easily have an e-book version instead. Is there any difference between the paratexts of internet sources and those of the traditional print texts that were the subject of Genette's analysis? And if there is, does this difference also affect the authority of the communication? Giulio Lughi observes that:

> Traditionally, the concept of paratext implies – as a premise and in opposition – the existence of a text and the fact that this text is closed and autonomous. In the world of print there is a clear distinction (also as it relates to layout and type set) between the text and the paratextual elements: footnotes, comments, and reviews. In mass media there is a clear distinction between text (a film, for example) and trailer, or review, or behind the scenes. In digital media text uniformity falls apart, and the edges of the text are weakened: for instance, while surfing the net, the constant movement from one link to the next dissolves the sense of main text. (46)

According to some critics, this novel textual dynamic requires a new vocabulary. Birke and Christ, for example, write that the various hyperlinks embedded in e-books and the internet "forge[. . .] texts in ways that are unprecedented in printed books," and because of this, we urgently need "new concepts' so that we can "grasp the way in which links negotiate the text's position in a hyperlinked universe" (78).

In response to this need, Ellen McCracken (2013) advises replacing peritext and epitext with the notion of centripetal and centrifugal vectors. In digital media, she explains, centripetal paratexts are those that modify a reader's experience of the text. In this category, she includes such elements as "format, font changes, word searching, and other enhancements" (107). It seems clear that various paratextual features that serve a centripetal movement can prompt dramatic shifts in the reading experience; Niels Brugger lists some of these as being "the headline system, associated texts (fact boxes, interposed quotations/excerpts, etc.), single words or phrases (e.g. 'Read more'), lists (e.g. menus), 'kinetic' texts (e.g. an element that by mouse-over makes a hidden text visible), 'bread crumbs' that indicate the position of a web page on a website, header/footer, the title of the page shown on top of the browser window, and the URL" (86–7). These paratexts, according to Brugger, are necessary because various other texts would be ignored in electronic text as opposed to print text simply because they lack the physical qualities the print media uses to provide these directions to the reader, such as the manner holding a book allows one to know where in the book one is reading. A traditional academic book like Larson's has citations that are located at the bottom of the page, at the end of chapters, or at the end of the entire book. Readers coming across the superscripted reference notes within the text know where physically to look for these references; citations in electronic media may exist only when you click on a link that takes you to them.

Centrifugal vectors, for McCracken, are those links that pull one outside of the current text. She notes that in reading an e-book, you can "can easily engage with blogs, other readers' comments, or an author's web page without putting aside the e-device" (107). McCracken's focus on e-devices results in her being focused primarily on the centripetal in her analysis, with attention paid to the centrifugal mainly in terms of how it supports the commercial elements of a book. Since the focus of my analysis is internet writing, while the centripetal has a crucial role in the establishment of authority, the centrifugal also has a significant impact on the reception of the information conveyed.

Paratextual simulacrum

Larson's book is an example of an examination of the vaccine controversy in traditional print media. The importance of understanding the traditional manner in which paratexts function is that internet sources often adopt what could be termed *paratextual simulacrum*. This form of paratext essentially reproduces the print version of a text, creating a virtual representation that mimics the original physical form and, by doing so, also conveying the authority a reader gives to the earlier print genre. When one looks at the *Lancet* online essay, "Addressing the vaccine confidence gap," its paratextual simulacrum appropriates the paratexts of the physical *Lancet* journal. In the initial presentation of the article on the journal website, we find a simple text surrounded by key paratexts: there is a small icon image of the journal itself, and the distinctive typeface of the Lancet logo appears above the article. There is also the option to see the essay as a PDF, which creates a virtual representation of the essay as it would appear in the print version. Through the paratexts of icons and layout, the journal transfers its historical authority to the essays presented on its website.

The prior authority of the *Lancet* has special resonance in terms of the anti-vaccine movement, having issued one of the most notorious publications in the vaccine controversy. In 1998, Andrew Wakefield and others published a study in the *Lancet* in which it was claimed that there was a link between the MMR vaccine and colitis and autism spectrum disorders. After an investigation by Brian Deer, in which Wakefield was accused of both having conflicts of interests and including fraudulent data in his study, the journal formally retracted the essay in 2004. The essay, however, remains a part of the journal's publication history and is still available to read – although now it is labeled as "withdrawn" and in the PDF version has the word *withdrawn* in large scarlet font running diagonally across every page. This editorial paratext is a sign of shame for those who support vaccines but a banner of pride for others, specifically those who take it as evidence of a conspiracy by pharmaceutical companies to withdraw the essay for fear of economic repercussions (Boseley). Unlike physical copies of the essay, the digital copy allows a palimpsest paratext that conditions one's reading of it while at the same time preserves its presence in the digital universe.

Commercial paratext

One often used website for medical information is WebMD. A commercial site that began in the late 1990s, WebMD is, in general, a site for providing mainstream medical information. Searching it for information on the MMR vaccine, we find an entry that is supportive of the vaccine but which ends with a brief note that "over the years, some have suggested that the MMR vaccine is linked to autism spectrum disorder. The CDC stands firm that there's no evidence to support that idea. The benefits that the vaccine brings in disease prevention far outweigh any potential risks." Its discussion of the safety of the MMR vaccine also includes two paratextual advertisements above and to the side of the WebMD article. Both are advertisements for Shingrix, a vaccine for the prevention of shingles. McCracken, in her discussion of Amazon's Kindle, notes the presence of what she refers to as "commercial paratexts," advertisements for other Kindle books in the text, which she contends "embeds" commercial texts within the reading experience. Commercial paratexts also influence the reading of websites. In the WebMD example, anti-vaccine activists might use the commercial paratext on the MMR vaccine page to argue that Big Pharma is the primary reason that WebMD avoids endorsing criticism of the vaccine.

Compare the WebMD example to that of the anti-vaccine website, Safeminds. On that site, commercial paratexts are embedded in the website, but they are donation links for the organization itself. The homepage itself has three links to donations, one of which is under a section, "Support Us" (Donate, Join Us!, Contact Us) and another that is part of a grouped set of links labeled Learn More, Donate, and Advocacy. The difference between these two forms of commercial paratexts is that the mainstream medical website has commercial centrifugal paratexts, rhetorically indicating outside support and thus suggesting potential external influence; the anti-vaccine websites have centripetal paratexts that lead the reader inward to support and solidarity. The more traditional commercial paratexts in anti-vaccine websites incorporate books and documentaries that the organization sells as well as links to commercial websites that sell alternative medical treatments.

Celebrity transtextuality

One rhetorical strategy that anti-vaccine websites have effectively wielded is the power of association: creating a relationship with celebrities. In film studies, drawing upon Genette's study of transtextuality, Robert Stam, Robert Burgoyne, and Sandy Flitterman-Lewis suggest a form of textual relationship that exists between celebrities and their inclusion in films, by which the appearance of a celebrity can suggest a particular cultural milieu; they give as examples the French New Wave director François Truffaut's appearance in Steven Spielberg's *Close Encounters of the Third Kind* (1977) and Marshall McLuhan's appearance in Woody Allen's *Annie Hall* (1979). In both instances, the celebrity brings with them an association between the intellectual world they exist within and the film (207).

In a similar manner, the anti-vaccine advocacy organization Generation Rescue has had an extensive relationship with Jenny McCarthy, a model and popular radio host. Children's Health Defense has Robert F. Kennedy Jr. as its chair. Stam, Burgoyne, and Flitterman-Lewis also note a form of celebrity transtextuality they refer to as "genetic intertextuality," by which the children of movie stars carry with them the associations of their parents. Jamie Lee Curtis's role in the movie *Halloween* (Carpenter 1978) permits an echo with her mother's starring role in Alfred Hitchcock's *Psycho* (1960). Kennedy's endorsement of an anti-vaccine stance has particular rhetorical authority because of the genetic intertextuality of his family's political celebrity. This transtextual relationship between celebrity and anti-vaccine positions functions as a powerful aspect of the anti-vaccine movement's success with the public. Through their endorsements, a form of social charisma and thus authority becomes attached to the organization and its positions (Kylstra).

Rhetorical power of the pathography

One feature that clearly differentiates most anti-vaccine websites from mainstream medical ones is the presence of personal anecdotes. In "Story and Science," Ashley Shelby and Karen Ernst note the prevalence on anti-vaccine websites of personal medical horror stories stated as having a direct relationship to vaccines. Shelby and Ernst show how narratives that contain such themes as "dismissive doctors," "overnight autism," and healthy children suddenly becoming critically ill in turn " form a challenge to health care professionals, public health workers, and parents who vaccinate their children and are concerned about the rise in vaccine-preventable disease due in part to lower immunization rates" (1796). One of the key genres of the health humanities is the pathography – the patient's (or her caregiver's) narrative of illness – and many anti-vaccine websites weave pathographies into their articles. In some cases, this takes on the form of intertextuality, as in the direct quotation of parents' accounts. Another form is the paratextual narrative that resides either in a separate section or within the article's comment section.

Single anecdotes can have a potent persuasive effect, as Shelby and Ernst's observe, and I would add that each of these anecdotes exist within a particular architextuality as well. The fact that these narratives are in the plural, creating a recognizable subgenre of pathography, conveys its own rhetorical force. In other words, the accumulation of similar pathographies that Shelby and Ernst notes are not merely "anecdotes" but a genre of narrative, their persuasion constituted in part by the fact that they create a single cultural narrative: vaccinations cause illness and harm healthy children.

Centrifugal ecosystems

Above I quoted Lughi's contention that one of the ways in which paratexts shift in electronic media is because "the edges of the text are weakened" – because we move from one link to another, we do not experience discrete texts, and all the linked texts dissolve into one another. One might even argue that all of the internet is experienced as a single text, that all its texts are woven into each other in such a manner that they all become paratexts. Yet the ability to move from one text to another is, in fact, primarily dependent upon the author. In the WebMD article, "Antivaccine Web Sites Short on Science," Salynn Boyles writes that "The personal stories appearing on the antivaccination internet site Thinktwice.com are heartbreaking and terrifying. A mother blames routine immunizations for the death of one child and paralysis of another. Another mom is convinced the DPT vaccine caused her son's seizures and mental retardation" (Boyles). On the website, a number of paratextual links are part of the text itself. The words "immunizations" "seizures," and "mental retardation" all have hyperlinks to other articles in WebMD on this issue. The key text that Boyles is writing about, thinktwice.com, is, however, not linked, nor are there direct links to the stories cited. Boyles's article illustrates a major feature of websites that is not often noted: namely, that the author and the publisher of the website have control over its hyperlinks – and thus have some degree of control over what become an article's paratexts. WebMD is a centripetally focused website in that all of the paratexts reside within the domain of WebMD, even the biographies of the writers and reviewers which could easily have been links to external personal academic web pages or university websites. The only centrifugal paratexts are advertising.

Many academic websites offer looser constructions of this pattern. In discussing vaccine hesitancy, they will link to academic essays outside of themselves, such as those in the *Lancet* and *JAMA*, but like WebMD tend not to provide direct links to the actual subjects of their analysis: vaccine-hesitant organizations and their websites. This is not to suggest that anti-vaccine websites are more open than the academic sites, for they tend to limit their centrifugal paratexts to sites that support their perspective.

There is widespread concern that social media has created "echo chambers" in which the view of a particular perspective bounces back and forth, thus amplifying its authority without ever truly engaging in dialogue with an opposing perspective. Opposing positions exist as separate texts with paratextual links that generally provide additional support for their own authority. This is equally true of both sides of this debate.

Conclusion

This chapter has discussed the way transtexuality functions to create medical authority, both within mainstream and alternative perspectives on vaccines. As in print media, paratexts can influence how texts are read on the internet. In the vaccine debate, paratexts can increase or decrease the authority of the text. Paratextual links to pharmaceutical companies, I contend, reinforce the impression, rightly or not, that mainstream medicine has become beholden to commercial interests. Meanwhile, paratextual links to personal narratives and celebrity endorsements may explain why mainstream medicine has tended to discount the validity of parent's concerns over vaccines. The various gatekeeping in the paratextual centripetal and centrifugal also keeps both sides of the debate in separate rhetorical spheres.

I began this chapter by suggesting a thought experiment in which I needed medical information in the pre-internet era, and I compared the various paratextual elements that would lead me to trust a published book in a public library versus a group of loose-leaf papers found on the street. There is an element of the internet in which the presentation of information is now akin to the aftermath of an explosion: the library walls are down, and, in the blast tore many covers off its books. That loose pack of papers is now essentially indistinguishable from the other books. I am left without my traditional paratextual indicators and the paratexts that have replaced them no longer require the approval of traditional gatekeepers.

Works cited

Barthes, Roland. "From Work to Text." *Image, Music, Text*, translated by Stephen Heath, New York: Hill and Wang, 1988, pp. 155–64.

Birke, Dorothee, and Birte Christ. "Paratext and Digitized Narrative: Mapping the Field." *Narrative*, vol. 21, no.1, 2013, pp. 65–87.

Boseley, Sarah. "How Disgraced Anti-vaxxer Andrew Wakefield was Embraced by Trump's America." *The Guardian*, 2018. www.theguardian.com/society/2018/jul/18/how-disgraced-anti-vaxxer-andrew-wakefield-was-embraced-by-trumps-america.

Boyles, Salynne. "Antivaccine Web Sites Short on Science." *WebMD*. 2002. www.webmd.com/baby/news/20020625/antivaccine-web-sites-short-on-science#1. Accessed September 29, 2020.

Brugger, Niels. "The Website as Unit of Analysis?"*Northern Lights*, vol. 5, 2007, pp. 75–88.

Culler, Jonathan D. *The Pursuit of Signs: Semiotics, Literature, Deconstruction*. Ithaca, N.Y.: Cornell University Press, 1981.

Doherty, Thomas. "The Paratext's the Thing." *Chronicle of Higher Education*, January 6, 2014. www.chronicle.com/article/the-paratexts-the-thing/. Accessed August 23, 2020.

Genette, Gérard. *Palimpsests: Literature in the Second Degree*. Translated by Channa Newman and Claude Doubinsky. Lincoln, NE: University of Nebraska Press, 1997. Vol. 8 of *Stages*.

Genette, Gérard. *Paratexts: Thresholds of Interpretation*. Cambridge and New York: Cambridge University Press, 1997. Book 20 of *Literature, Culture, Theory*.

Grafton, Anthony. *The Footnote: A Curious History*. London: Faber and Faber, 2003.

Hausman, Bernice L. *Anti/vax. Reframing the Vaccination Controversy*. Ithaca, N.Y.: Cornell University Press, 2019.

Kostkova, Patty, Vino Mano, Heidi J. Larson, and William S. Schulz. 2017. "Who is Spreading Rumours about Vaccines? Influential Users Impact Modelling in Social Networks." *International Conference onDdigital Health*, 2017.

Kylstra, Carolyn. "Who Cares What Celebrities Think About Vaccines?"*New York Times*, August 23, 2019. www.nytimes.com/2019/08/23/opinion/anti-vaccine.html.

Larson, Heidi. "Heidi Larson on Vaccine Skepticism."*Social Science Bites*, edited by David Edmonds, Social Science Space, 2020,www.socialsciencespace.com/2020/09/heidi-larson-on-vaccine-skepticism/.

Larson, Heidi. *Stuck: How Vaccine Rumors Start – and Why They Don't Go Away*. New York: Oxford UniversityPress, 2020.

Lughi, Giulio. "Paratext between Time and Space in Digital Media." *The Politics of Ephemeral Digital Media: Permanence and Obsolescence in Paratexts*, edited by Sara Pesce and Paolo Noto. New York and Abingdon: Routledge, 2016, pp. 45–59.

McCracken, Ellen. 2013. "Expanding Genette's Epitext/Peritext Model for Transitional Electronic Literature: Centrifugal and Centripetal Vectors on Kindles and iPads." *Narrative*, vol. 21, no. 1, 2013, pp. 105–24.

"Prostate Cancer." Yahoo. 1997. https://web.archive.org/web/19970425032848/www7.yahoo.com/Health/Diseases_and_Conditions/Prostate_Cancer/. Accessed April 24, 2021.

Riffaterre, Michael. 1990. "Compulsory Reader Response: The Intertextual Drive." *Intertextuality: Theories and Practices*, edited by Michael Worton and Judith Still, Manchester, N.Y.: Manchester University Press, 1990, pp. 56–78.

Shelby, Ashley, and Karen Ernst. "Story and Science: How Providers and Parents can Utilize Storytelling to Combat Anti-vaccine Misinformation." *Human Vaccines & Immunotherapeutics,* vol. 9, no. 8, 2013, pp. 1795–1801.

Stam, Robert, Robert Burgoyne, and Sandy Flitterman-Lewis. *New Vocabularies in Film Semiotics: Structuralism, Post-structuralism and Beyond.* New York and Abingdon: Routledge, 1992.

Tavares, Sérgio. *Paramedia Threholds of the Social Text.* Vol. 332, *Jyväskylä Studies in Humanities.* Jyväskylä: University of Jyväskylä, 2017.

30
CHRONIC CONSTELLATIONS
Instagrammatic aesthetics and crip time

Amanda K. Greene

In 2017, Georgie Wileman's unconventional self-portrait, rooted in her own experience of endometriosis, was displayed at the National Portrait Gallery's Taylor Wessing Photographic Portrait Prize exhibition. This image ("2014-2017") was part of This is Endometriosis – a larger photographic undertaking, that Wileman describes as "a documentation of lives lived with endometriosis, a widely misunderstood disease that scars and destroys internal organs, causing extreme pain and irreparable damage." This project centers bodies and intimate, domestic spaces in strikingly vulnerable, desaturated photographs that illuminate how endometriosis sculpts the flesh and permeates the experience of everyday life. By capturing the feelings and practices of surviving what Lauren Berlant terms "crisis ordinariness," Wileman's photographic documentation immerses a viewer in "lives lived" with chronic illness, an uncomfortable temporality of prolonged trauma that eschews the linear progress (and promise) of curative time.

"2014-2017" draws a viewer into proximity with the scars on Wileman's pelvis, prompting readership of these physical traces left by endometriosis related surgery (Figure 30.1). The closely cropped image focuses attention on her bare flesh, while the placement of Wileman's hands and the dark clothes they pull away frame the white skin even more clearly. A series of thin black lines connect her scars, forming a simple, uneven geometric shape that stands out at the center of this carefully demarcated human canvas. Some of the scars are fresh while others barely visible; each is labeled with the year it was created and/or reopened. Bound together by these hand drawn marks, they become the basis of a new "constellation [...] of mistreatment and pain" (Wileman).

Although the photograph is powerful in its own right, its life beyond the gallery wall makes it more exceptional. In March 2019, the image became the foundation of a participatory social media campaign for endometriosis awareness month that the popular press (*Huffington Post, Forbes, Refinery 29, Vanity Fair Italy,* and more) widely covered that year. By circulating on Instagram via the hashtag #ThisIsEndometriosis, "2014-2017" encouraged others to share their stories of living with endometriosis by marking lines on their own skin, mapping out their own scars, and posting their own images with this same hashtag. Wileman deliberately catalyzed this movement through strategic social media outreach, contacting influencers and using her account to disseminate explanations of the campaign and instructions about how to participate:

DOI: 10.4324/9781003007661-39

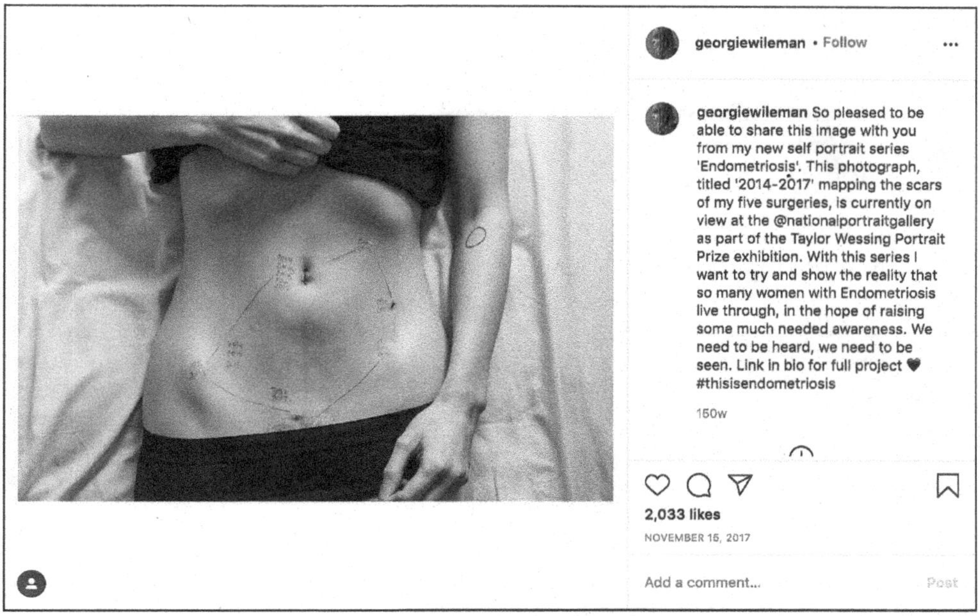

Figure 30.1 The post first sharing "2014-2017" on Wileman's Instagram account

> This campaign was born out of my photographic project by the same name [...]. By dating and connecting our scars, we are showing the true extent of endometriosis, and the ultimate failings of our healthcare systems [...] If you would like to participate in the project: 1. Date each scar (no matter how small) from an endometriosis related surgery with pen, with each year it was opened 2. Connect your scars with a single line 3. Take a picture of yourself on white sheets, using natural daylight 4. Post with the hashtag #thisisendometriosis and tag @georgiewileman.

The cultivation of this Instagrammatic afterlife is an artistic intervention in its own right, not a supplemental publicity stunt. Through this process, Wileman not only reached many more people than the original image or photographic series would have but also facilitated the co-creation of a new aesthetic assemblage online. As she reflects in one interview, this multi-authored portrait of lives lived with endometriosis exceeds the expressive potential of her own camera: "I knew I couldn't show the true extent of endometriosis alone. The repetition of the collective connected scars online is incredibly powerful, lines marking years of mistreatment and pain" (Wileman qtd. in Reid). This networked repetition of connected scars, themselves connected via hashtag, can be approached as its own arresting piece of digital, disability art.

In this chapter, I read #ThisIsEndometriosis through a deliberately aesthetic, platform specific, and disability-informed lens in order to illuminate how the campaign draws viewers into intimate contact with the temporal experience of endometriosis. I suggest that the unsettling power of the campaign is sustained by a number of tensions that emerge in or are heightened by its particular socially mediated context. For example, the insertion of a disability aesthetic into the familiar visual horizon of Instagrammism makes chronic pain beautiful and gaze worthy even as its subject appears incongruous with Instagram's typical positive, happy vibes. Furthermore, while time is central to the form and title of "2014-2017," the campaign's digital context intensifies this element; the constellated scars embed crip time within the platform's temporal norm of a continuous chronological scroll. These shapes become timelines tracking the repetitive cyclicality of chronic illness (and endometriosis in particular) and warped windows into the strange stasis of what Jasbir Puar labels "prognosis time" (sickness in waiting). The temporal paradigm embedded within the posts rips open the conventional linearity of curative time to make space for a range of illness narratives that "bend the clock" to the body's lived experience (Kafer).

By centering how the campaign's Instagrammatic context shapes crip time, this chapter extends work by Elena Gonzalez-Polledo and Jen Tarr, who compellingly argue that social media alters the forms of illness narratives by changing the kinds of temporal paradigms they operate under and the audiences they aim to reach. Chronic pain narratives on Tumblr, for example, "are structured in loops of recurrent improvement and flare up, and offer temporal structures that result from fragmented temporalities [...] profoundly reconfiguring understandings of the form and function of narrative in significant ways" (Gonzalez-Polledo and Tarr, 12). In the case of #ThisIsEndometriosis, new narratives emerge that rely on Instagrammatic cultures and affordances, but that also challenge the histories and ideals the platform's basic architecture supports.

The rest of the chapter begins by briefly introducing endometriosis and its place within a disability studies framework, before turning to the basic visual composition of the #ThisIsEndometriosis posts. Focusing on these images' disability aesthetic illuminates how the posts act on readers within the bounds of Instagram's own aesthetic norms in ways that make unsettled modes of crip time palpable. The campaign's temporalities come into focus even more clearly by considering the posts as *imagetexts*, attending to how written captions act in tension and dialogue with the visual content. My discussion emphasizes the importance of engaging with health and social media in meticulously medium-specific, platform-specific ways. When illness narratives occur on social media, this digital media ecosystem doesn't simply shape audiences or modes of distribution. Just as McLuhan's famous aphorism "the medium is the message" suggests, social media changes the nature of communication itself. Aesthetic forms and stories are never just "hosted" on platforms like Instagram but are fundamentally entangled in posting affordances, platform protocols, media cultures, and habitual modes of online readership.

Seeing endometriosis

Endometriosis, in physiological terms, is a chronic illness that occurs when tissue similar to the lining of the uterus grows outside of the uterus. This rogue tissue frequently causes pain and internal bleeding as endometrial tissue responds to cyclical hormonal fluctuations; it can also create adhesions that bind organs together and leave scars deep inside the body. While the condition has a diverse array of symptoms depending on exactly where in the body it manifests and what organs it impacts, the primary symptom of endometriosis is pain. In spite of the frequently disabling severity of this pain as well as the illness's prevalence (affecting approximately one in ten women during their reproductive years as well as many non-binary individuals), endometriosis remains an enigmatic illness with only limited treatment options. This is, in part, because many individuals' pain is often dismissed as a psychological issue or as an over-reaction to "normal" dysmenorrhea (Ballweg; Denny). As Cara E. Jones explains, "clinicians routinely dismiss endo as "bad periods." [...] Endo's reduction to "painful menses" has resulted in its normalization to the point of invisibility" (6). Representative of this tendency, a 2016 study of nurse attitudes toward endometriosis patients showed that "the nurses generally psychologized the health problems of women with endometriosis and attributed individual responsibility for their disease to them" (Bach et al.). Because of such stigma, 46 percent of endometriosis patients see five or more doctors before receiving their diagnosis (Ballweg; Cheong and Stones; European Endometriosis Alliance; Mihalyi et al.). Diagnosis, frequently and troublingly delayed, takes an average of eight years from the initial onset of symptoms (Rogers et al.; Adamson et al.).

One factor amplifying endometriosis's seemingly unseen/unseeable status, which is especially pertinent to the #ThisIsEndometriosis campaign, is the fact that a diagnosis can only be confirmed through laparoscopic surgery. Many women don't have access to this procedure because it is not covered by insurance or because doctors view it as an unnecessary risk that ultimately won't change their treatment plan. Consequently, the small scars left by laparoscopic surgeries become laden with meaning, signaling many individuals' first visible "proof" of their illness as well as bearing witness to this medically recognized moment. However, even this diagnostic event does not necessarily corroborate an individual's experience of the disease or ensure access to appropriate medical care. As Emma Wheelan writes: "Because pain severity does not correlate with observable extent of disease, patient and physician accounts of endometriosis may directly contradict one another. When the lived experience of illness is contradicted by a lack of objective confirmation, others (especially physicians) may doubt the reality of the experience" (957). Consequently, individuals diagnosed with endometriosis may still struggle be heard or to receive palliative procedures like regular excision surgeries.

Chronic pain is rarely at the center of disability studies conversations, partially because of the troubled status of pain and trauma in the field.[1] However, I align with the feminist work of scholars like Susan Wendell and Cara E. Jones by insisting that chronic illness, and endometriosis in particular, demands a disability studies lens. Jones asserts:

> We must understand endometriosis as a disability rather than a privately managed, female problem. When social beliefs delegitimize endo-as-disability, endometriosis is often presented as an obstacle for individuals to overcome through perseverance, effort, and informed decision-making, a trope disability theorists refer to as "the rhetoric of overcoming"
>
> *(Linton 2006, 228). (14)*

Understanding endometriosis as disability means attending to the ways this chronic illness shapes everyday experience and pushing against its co-optation by biocapitalist logics of overcoming and self-reliance. Just as endometriosis is entangled deep in the body's organs, it cannot be neatly extricated from the self as a concrete obstacle that an autonomous individual can bracket and fight against. Additionally, although pain is central to the experience of endometriosis, this illness and its impact on individuals' lives is much more than pain. A disability studies lens can therefore focalize the specific, holistic experience of endometriosis in ways that an approach rooted solely in pain communication cannot.

Disability, aesthetics

Although aesthetics is frequently laden with connotations of disinterested artistic judgment, disability aesthetics has its lineage in an embodied theoretical tradition represented by figures like Baumgarten who define aesthetics as "the science of sensuous cognition" (Baumgarten qtd. in Siebers 1). Tobin Siebers, who first proposed the concept of disability aesthetics, characterizes aesthetics as a deeply human activity that tracks what certain bodies feel in the presence of other bodies (whether those bodies be physical flesh, art objects, photographs of bodies, etc.).

Framed in this way, aesthetic interactions have profound implications for how bodies are "read" and apprehended on an everyday basis; they can fuel practices of "human disqualification" that reject otherness, or they can hold space for new forms of communication and understanding to emerge.

Disability aesthetics, as Siebers theorizes it, affirms that beauty is not confined to ideals of health, symmetry, and perfection:

> Disability aesthetics refuses to recognize the representation of the healthy body – and its definition of harmony, integrity, and beauty - as the sole determination of the aesthetic. Rather, disability aesthetics embraces beauty that seems by traditional standards to be broken, and yet it is not less beautiful, but more so as a result.
>
> *(3)*

Considering disability as beautiful is important because beauty can command attention, directly affecting the bodies of those who come into contact with it. As the "broken beauty" that Siebers describes reaches out to engage a viewer, it can prompt engagement with bodily textures and the histories mapped on the flesh as opposed to triggering revulsion or the flat sympathy that is all too common in popular imaging of disability. Ill, painful, and disabled bodies are not necessarily diminished or "enfreaked" by aestheticization; by contrast, aestheticization and beauty can hold these bodies and their feelings within the frame as real, concrete visual features that affect a viewer (Hevey 1997). At the same time, whereas perfectly symmetrical ideal bodies are so familiar they barely require readership and can be scrolled past without a second thought, disability generates what Ato Quayson terms "aesthetic nervousness." It short-circuits the "normal" order of things and incites a more intent, intense gaze.

Scars can be exemplary compositional features that help produce disability-grounded beauty because they themselves suddenly interrupt or short-circuit the expected shape of the body and texture of the flesh. As Petra Kuppers writes, "If skin renews itself constantly, producing the same in repetition, the scar is the place of the changed script: mountains are thrown up, the copy isn't quite right, crooked lines sneak over smooth surfaces" (1). Scars have been central in canonical disability studies such as Rosmarie Garland Thomson's reading of how model Matuschka's breast cancer photographs, with her bared mastectomy scar, elicit a viewer's look. Particularly when they appear on conventionally (white thin) beautiful female bodies, as is the case of Matuschka and many of the #ThisIsEndometriosis contributions, the contrast of the scar embedded in "ideal" bodily form produces a powerful and frequently sexualized allure.

In addition to commanding attention, scars also embed a temporal dimension within an image. A scar is "a palimpsest of different times, narratives, and patterns" that necessarily brings a temporal element into the aesthetic encounter (Kuppers 3). Whereas glossy smoothness is a "texture that signifies the willed erasure of its history," the uneven flesh of the scar haptically inscribes the body's histories (Sedgewick 14–15). It creates a connective friction that prolongs attention and locates the body in time: "the scar incites the look, invites the narrative, fuels the story, and anchors it back into (some version of) bodies, time, and space." The scar is an archive of experience that disrupts expectations of bodily form and amplifies disabled beauty; it reaches out and demands to be read.

It is important to foreground aesthetics in order to engage with #ThisIsEndometriosis as a distinctly Instagrammatic phenomenon. Although Instagram's "look" has shifted throughout its existence, the mode of stylized aesthetic communication it was founded on has remained its defining feature. As Lev Manovich succinctly summarizes: "if Google is an information retrieval service, Twitter is for news and links exchange, Facebook is for social communication, and Flickr is for image archiving, Instagram is for *aesthetic visual communication*" (41).

Disability aesthetics offers insight into how the campaign's graphic visual format came to gain traction and appreciation as 'beautiful' on a platform that has become synonymous with neat, filtered beauty. Usually, Instagram algorithmically filters out bodily imperfection both in individual photographs with easy application of automated retouching software that transforms skin into smooth impenetrable surface, and more generally in terms of the censorship of fat, nonbinary, and disabled bodies (Byström and Soda). Wileman's efforts were clearly essential to the campaign's popularity, but the images' aesthetic appeal amplified their influence by prompting them to be more widely shared, circulated, and algorithmically promoted.

#ThisIsEndometriosis's disability aesthetic is in artful dialogue with Instagram's own particular platform norms of beauty. While I don't want to dwell on exhaustively cataloging key components of Instagram's signature aesthetic, I will note a few trends that play a central role in a number of posts. In particular, features like minimalism, color and exposure filters, geometric lines, and "clean' white backgrounds are all common across the platform and feature heavily throughout the campaign. Indeed, a certain Instagram-friendly "look" is embedded in the instructions Wileman shares. Her initial directive doesn't just explain the basic premise of the campaign and describe how to draw the constellation of scars but also offers guidance on how to take the picture- specifying lighting, cropping, and background: "Take a picture of yourself on white sheets, using natural daylight." While not all of the posts conform to this standard a large majority do; furthermore, many are artistically composed and carefully processed.
One of the most "liked" posts in the campaign, created by artist @mabgraves, clearly showcases these Insta-friendly features and offers a clear example of how disability aesthetics converge with Instagrammism (Figure 30.2). The deliberately blurred focus, the use of filters or other retouching software to even the skin tone, and the clean white background are aesthetic choices that make the image amenable to Instagram's "natural" environment. The flowers and their pastel color schema also help integrate the visual quality of the image into something comfortably familiar. @mabgraves's positionality as a white small-bodied woman, the favored identity of the platform, further entrenches its integration. As a result, the image is not an aberration in

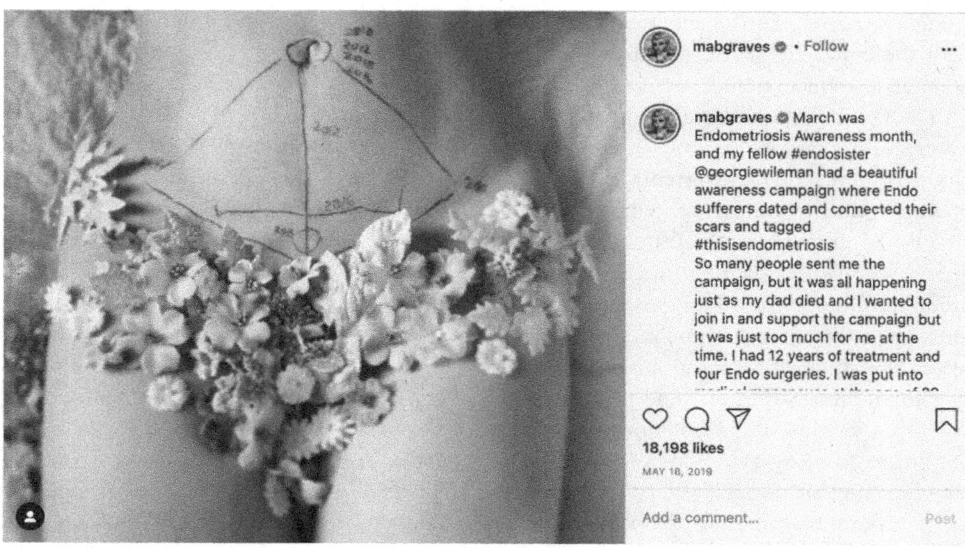

Figure 30.2 #ThisIsEndometriosis post by @mabgraves

the "eyes" of the algorithm (or of the algorithmically conditioned human user for that matter). The photograph is appealing on Instagram's own terms, but its disability aesthetic embeds a different kind of beauty within it, making it stand out as opposed to blending into the usual feed. The scars and lines on the body are transformed into an adornment, just like the flowers. They create an impression of fracturing form as the lines appear like dark cracks streaking across porcelain skin. Through these features the photographed body beckons to be appraised, read, seen. This aesthetic hybridity makes chronic pain beautiful. It encourages a prolonged gaze instead of evoking a shock or pity response or simply slipping past unseen.

Crip time(lines)

In some respects, @mabgraves's post is an outlier in the extent to which Instagrammism overwhelms the disability aesthetic. Notably, in contrast to the large majority of the other posts, this photograph buries "broken beauty" deep within the overt symmetry of the drawn marks. In Wileman's original image, the lines on her body do not coalesce into a neat diamond or another recognizable geometric form but forge their own awkward and shaky constellated shape. The aesthetic impact at the core of "2014-2017" as well as the majority of other contributions to the campaign comes from the striking yet simple asymmetry of the constellations and the visible scars that anchor them into the chronically ill body.

The #ThisIsEndometriosis images' disability aesthetic is rooted both in the actual scars left by surgery and in the asymmetrical cracks and folds that extend and connect them. Because endometriosis is an illness of invisible tangled tissues, these lines mimetically evoke the forms and patterns of pain radiating deep within the body. They materially evoke the adhesions that bind organs together deep within the body, constricting their movement. By bringing these forms to the visible surface of the body, individuals take back ownership of imaging their endometriosis, pushing back against the ultimate authority of the laparoscopic camera to officially define the illness's shape and severity. At the same time, the dark lines also act as an entryway or a frame embedded in the center of the photograph, reminiscent of the geometrically ripped screen in Lee Miller's surrealist "Portrait of Space" (1937). These misshapen frames that offer a single window into the experience off illness as it is warped by pain and illness clashes both with the circular view of the laparoscopic camera and with Instagram's signature, uniformly symmetrical square frames.

The constellations also challenge norms of self-presentation and readership on Instagram by creating a vision of time that contrasts with the one that the platform's continuous, chronological scroll inadvertently reifies. The hand drawn forms bring the already unsettled, uncomfortable palimpsestic temporality of the scar into an explicit reconfiguration of established histories and narrative arcs. Indeed, the series of dated scars connected by dark lines at the center of these images are themselves twisted "timelines" that starkly contrast models of linear forward progress. As opposed to an assumed, imagined, mythologized linear journey to the cure, the timelines present repetitive loops punctuated with layered moments of rupture and healing at the site of the scars. Cyclicality is relevant to many chronic illnesses that entail phases of relapse and recovery, but it is viscerally salient in the case of endometriosis given its physiological connection to cyclical hormonal shifts. The timeline moves into the future as it covers a range of years but also remains in stasis, stuck in place, circling the same terrain. Moreover, even though each scar is labelled with a concrete date (or dates) as in a conventional timeline, these nodes are not stabilizing or orienting points. They are palimpsestic punctures, moments of crisis where the script is suddenly changed but the story nevertheless continues on.

This unsettled temporality can be described as a form of crip time that permeates the everyday experience of living with endometriosis. As Alison Kafer defines it: "Crip time is flex time not just expanded but exploded [...] Rather than bend disabled bodies and minds to meet the clock, crip time bends the clock to meet disabled minds and bodies" (27). Crip time is both about changes in the fabric of the everyday and a radical reconsideration of the linear progress narratives that "curative imaginaries" offer. Curative imaginaries dominate discourse around illness in ways that reify the rhetoric of overcoming, placing burdens of healing and care on the individual patient. Such narratives simply cannot be lived in the case of a chronic illness that has only limited mitigating treatment options when pain pockmarks ordinariness. The multilayered meanings of the crooked constellations thrust a different temporal paradigm at the viewer that scaffolds struggles of care, diagnosis, recognition, and everyday survival.

Wileman's particular poetic evocation of the "constellation" reaffirms this crip temporality. Constellations have a cyclical quality changing their space in the sky over time, which reiterates the closed timeline the drawing evoke and mirrors the hormonal cycles of the illness. But the constellation also has philosophical significations that connect it to time as a disruptive force. Walter Benjamin famously drew on the constellation as a key figure of dialectics, writing, "It's not that what is past casts its light on what is present.... Rather, image is that wherein what has been comes together in a flash with the now to form a constellation. In other words, image is dialectics at a standstill" (462). While Benjamin is talking about historical progress narratives, curative narratives follow similarly problematic patterns; both insist on ableist vectors of continual improvement and compulsory capacity-building (Puar). Both delimit how future, past, and present can be understood in isolation and in relation to one another. The constellation that produces the flash rupturing history simultaneously explodes the clock and thrusts a viewer into crip time. The crip constellation is a rupture that doesn't nihilistically destroy time but short-circuits normative narratives.

Imagetextual illness

"Dialectics at a standstill" is not only present in the figure of the constellation but is also crystalized in the formal architecture of the Instagram post. The status of these Instagrammatic interventions as what W. J. T. Mitchell terms "imagetexts" is also key to their communicative power. Image and text each have different relationships to both reality and representation, which can create static, discomfort, and conflict when they are brought together. Yet, instead of being opposing, self-contained entities image and text are perpetually framing, interpellating, supplementing, and deconstructing one another in ways that make boundary lines nearly impossible to draw. As a result, meaningfully negotiating the spaces of imagetext becomes a dilemma of taking sides in a "choice between linguistic imperialism and defensive reflexes of the visual" (Mitchell 60). In other words, attributing more authority to the text as an "explainer" of the image or embracing the image as a "real" that words can only insufficiently annotate. The oscillation back and forth between these tendencies that the imagetext catalyzes establishes a dialectical relation that "opens up a space of intellectual struggle, historical investigation, and artistic/critical practice" (60). Engaging the complexities of the image-caption relationship is especially pertinent from a disability studies perspective given critical work by Georgia Kleege that affirms visual description as a creative crip practice that enhances the accessibility of visual culture as well as recent artistic-activist interventions in this area such as the "Activating Captions" project.

Instagram's interface often encourages the separation of image and text by hiding the written caption entirely. This prompts readers and posters alike to view the caption as inconsequential or superfluously doubling the image. These words, after all, may not even reach readers if the image doesn't first capture their curiosity. However, throughout #ThisIsEndometriosis, the majority of captions are lengthy, vulnerable personal narratives in which text and image hinge on one another and refigure one another's meanings. These textual accounts are not just explanations of the image that double its content but also narratives enabled and held by the space that the image creates. Buried stories are all too often not heard in the case of invisible illness, but the image's disability aesthetic solicits attention and offers an opportunity to remedy this silence, to make meaning without the onus of mending breakage.

Moreover, the line between text and image is not quite as clean as the square blocks and dividing frames of Instagram's interface would suggest. Because of the drawings and dates inscribed on the photographed body, text is already embedded within the image; at the same time, because of the caption's artistic affordances in terms of typography and emojis, the text is also defined by its visual presence. The uneasy dialectic between image and caption enables artistic/critical practice in which the representation of crip time is further complicated and negotiated. It holds a middle space for unique, uncomfortable stories in the caption that interact with the image in ways that multiply meaning and pathways into illness, pain, and disability experiences. The disability aesthetic of the photograph and the imagetextual form actively, dynamically annotate one another, enlivening the communicative power that exists between them, palpable as part of their constellated connection. In this dialogic relationship, they spur a cycle of rereading between one and the other.

When image and text are read together and in tension, the contours of crip time become more and more defined. Take this post (Figure 30.3) in which the textual caption explicitly references the image and hinges on its presence: "the days are dark as this picture feels... the pain of carrying around a body that doesn't want to serve me is as excruciating as the physical symptoms." This caption is a poetic description not of pain itself but of the routine experience of managing chronic pain and endometriosis. Word and image here mutually illustrate one another as the text refers back to the photograph as both a real index and a figurative encapsulation of affect. The image's aesthetic, in grayscale and against dark sheets, differs from Wileman's instructions, but, in dialogue with the text, it is viscerally impactful as a portrait of drowning in the dark sheets and "laying in a puddle of pain." Although there is an impulse to forward movement – scratching at the surface that perhaps evokes the accumulating tally of scars on her skin – her crip timeline is constrained by the repetition of the same thing. Yet she is not just drowning in this never-ending spiral of chronicity. Through its repetition, she is getting more and more "skilled" not at managing but simply occupying crisis ordinariness. The caption's typography draws attention to the visual dimension of the text as well. Without capitalization the sentences have no syntactic beginning and end. The periods neither shaping sentences nor creating resolution are nodes like the scars that briefly punctuate the ongoing circling of crip time. The periods also evoke the menstrual periods that cyclically erupt painful crisis into this unmoored temporal space as endometriosis symptoms flair in relation to this cycle: "all the time. every. single. day."

In the #ThisIsEndometriosis imagetexts, scars are often a place where narrative, flesh, and photography collide. These marks are frequently and directly mentioned in the captions as indexes of pain and illness. For example, one participant in the campaign begins with the simple assertion that "Every scar tells a story," and another proclaims: "These are my scars. These are my receipts for the pain I've gone through." Such rhetoric intertwines the captions with the scars by claiming the scars themselves as textual accounts of pain and illness written on the body. The captions and the drawn lines pull a reader into contact with these indexical marks while, at the same time, the scars' palimpsestic beauty holds space for more elaborate stories and figurative descriptions to enter the picture that go well beyond the surgical procedures themselves.

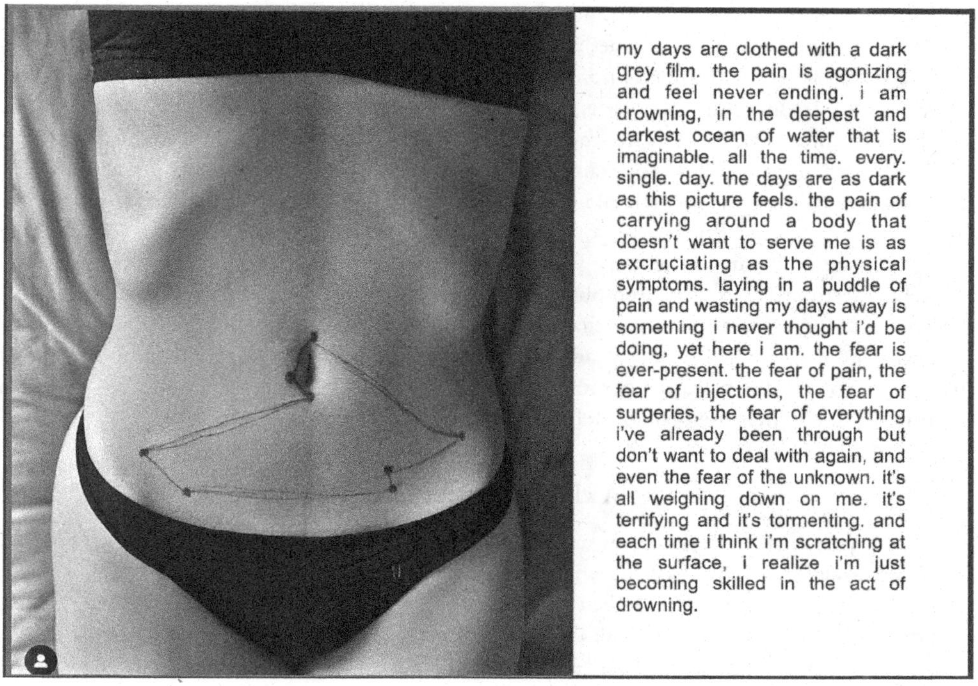

Figure 30.3 Image and text from a #ThisIsEndometriosis post

For example, in the following caption the author close reads her own scar as both a marker of wreckage and an embodiment of her resources for everyday survival:

> That incision – this scar – reminds me that I am alive. It reminds me that I have faced unseen challenges and overcome them even though, at the time, they fucking wrecked me. It reminds me that I have the strength to move forward through extreme amounts of discomfort to accomplish basic tasks like getting out of bed on my own, walking without a walker, or walking to a toilet. It reminds me that I have the resilience and the capacity to move forward in life and use all of the natural human disasters I experience as fuel.

"**That** incision – **this** scar" calls out the photograph and the scar as indexes of her experiences that anchor the words to the flesh. Likewise, the scar ("It") repetitively anchors the start of each sentence. However, the caption is not just about remembering past histories and affirming "this has been." It is also about occupying the present and the future. In addition to bearing witness to the moment when "that incision" was made, they are a "reminder" of being alive in the present and about the future possibilities of moving forward. Notably, though, moving forward is wrenched from curative time; it is not about getting out of the disaster zone but cultivating habits of everyday survival for when these "natural human disasters" inevitably cyclically return. The palimpsestic past offers map of the future that will be cyclically layered on top of it again and again.

One last feature of the captions that highlights the complexity of the imagetext and the production of crip time is the frequent inclusion of lists and numbers. These counts add new tallies to supplement the tallies left on the body by scarring, another palimpsest of punctuated marks breaking up the circling, repetitive timeline of chronic illness. For example: "2 surgeries 7 small scars 5 years of infertility 4 miscarriages 21 years of pain 10 doctors who didn't believe"; "4 surgeries, 14 incisions, 4 doctors, horrible drugs, infertility, excruciating pain, constant bloated belly, miscarriages."; "The scars The surgerys [sic.] The burns The tears The pain The bloat The exhaustion." These countable items are simultaneously points of crisis and cherished places where pain can be made legible to others. Numbers give form to the illness experience and index it, but lived experience constantly overflows their quantitative bounds. Just like the scars, they are only part of the story within the continuation and repetition of crisis ordinariness. Furthermore, these lists exemplify the impossibility of curative time. Although trials can be counted, there remains a sense that they are accumulated without end instead of moving toward closure. As one contributor affirms: "✨IT DOESN'T END✨." This is both a cry of frustration and an affirmation of chronic pain's crip time that connects the emoji stars/scars into their own simple imagetextual constellation within the caption.

A closing constellation

As this chapter draws to a close, it is worth remembering that #ThisIsEndometriosis is a multi-authored assemblage that hangs together through shared tropes and vocabularies as well as concrete Instagrammatic affordances like the # and @. Despite the richness of each individual post, the repetition and connection of all of these shapes, scars, experiences, and narratives fundamentally define the campaign. Every single post exists in relationship not just with the abstract idea of the campaign, Wilemen's original photograph, or the platform but is also entangled with particular visual and verbal rhetoric that collectively emerge out of the assemblage of connected posts. Each individual imagetext exists in a constellation of relationships – a node in the hashtag community and the larger campaign as opposed to a stand-alone site. Moreover, the campaign itself occupies its own kind of crip time. While it received the most attention and activity in 2019, there is no clearly bounded endpoint. It is still possible to add new images to the archive by following Wileman's instructions and deploying her hashtag. However, the campaign's timeline is also defined by cyclicality instead of simple linear accumulation given its imbrication in endometriosis awareness month, which means that every March triggers reposts of older images as well as a new influx of attention.

#ThisIsEndometriosis is a constellation in its own right, a rhizomatic narrative that joins multiple stories without collapsing them into the same thing. The radiating lines of the #'s visual form are constellated connectors that forge pathways between bodies and through time. Just like the drawn lines on the pelvis, though, these are not unifying figures that create a cohesive whole. #ThisIsEndometriosis draws participants in the campaign into dialogue but also opens up the conversation to a variety of other audiences and communities as additional hashtags and users are layered on top of them. Such socially mediated connections are usually thought in terms of networks, yet in the context of this campaign, these binding lines stand out instead as the scaffolding of new constellations.

As scholarship on health and social media moves forward, it is essential to embrace the ways platforms shape communicative form as opposed to merely approaching them as context, audience, or mode of circulation. Social media platforms are multimodal and dynamic phenomena that are intra-actively imbricated with individuals' expressive capacities, readership habits, and the body itself. Just as importantly, the rich communicative cultures that emerge in these spaces are invaluable resources that can aid in the development of new critical vocabularies. As Siebers writes, aesthetics is tool "by which [humans] imagine their feelings, forms, and futures in radically different ways, and by which they bestow upon these new feelings, forms, and futures real appearances in the world" (Siebers 3). Disability aesthetics and illness narratives on social media can offer visions of the emergent, dynamic social media ecosystems which they are entangled with that "short circuit" established figures and cut through normative filters. What profane illuminations might follow, for example, if we learn to look for constellations instead of remaining constrained by networks?

Note

1 This is stressed by both Kafer and Jones. For a longer meditation, see also Berger, James. "Trauma without disability, disability without trauma: A disciplinary divide." *JAC* (2004): 563–82.

Works cited

Activating Captions. April 6–June 8, 2021, ARGOS, Brussels.www.argosarts.org/event/activating-captions.

Adamson, G. David, Stephen Kennedy, and Lone Hummelshoj. "Creating Solutions in Endometriosis: Global Collaboration through the World Endometriosis Research Foundation." *Journal of Endometriosis*, vol. 2, no. 1, 2010, pp. 3–6.

Bach, Anne Mette, et al. "Practices and Attitudes Concerning Endometriosis among Nurses Specializing in Gynecology." *Global Qualitative Nursing Research*, vol. 3, 2016, 2333393616651351.

Ballweg, Mary Lou. "Blaming the Victim: The Psychologizing of Endometriosis." *Obstetrics and Gynecology Clinics*, vol. 24, no. 2, 1997, pp. 441–53.

Ballweg, Mary Lou. "Impact of Endometriosis on Women's Health: Comparative Historical Data Show that the Earlier the Onset, the more Severe the Disease." *Best Practice & Research Clinical Obstetrics & Gynaecologist*, vol.18, no. 2, 2004, pp. 201–18.

Benjamin, Walter. *The Arcades Project.* Cambridge, MA: Harvard University Press, 1999.

Berger, James. "Trauma without Disability, Disability without Trauma: A Disciplinary Divide." *Journal of Advanced Composition*, vol. 23, no. 3, 2004, pp. 563–82.

Byström, Arvida and Molly Soda (eds). *Pics or It Didn't Happen: Images Banned from Instagram.* Munich and London: Prestel, 2017.

Cheong, Ying, and R. William Stones. "Management of Chronic Pelvic Pain: Evidence from Randomised Controlled Trials." *The Obstetrician & Gynaecologist*, vol. 8, no.1, 2006, pp. 32–8.

Denny, Elaine."Women's Experience of Endometriosis." *Journal of Advanced Nursing*, vol. 46, no. 6, 2004, pp. 641–8.

European Endometriosis Alliance. "Endometriosis." 2006, www.endometriosis.org/news/general/historic-decision-for-womens-health-made-by-european-comission/.

Garland-Thomson, Rosemarie. *Staring: How We Look.* Oxford: Oxford University Press, 2009.

Gonzalez-Polledo, Elena, and Jen Tarr. "The Thing about Pain: The Remaking of Illness Narratives in Chronic Pain Expressions on Social Media." *New Media & Society*, vol. 18, no. 8, 2016, pp. 1455–72.

Hevey, David. "The Enfreakment of Photography." *The Disability Studies Reader*, edited by Lennard Davis. New York and Abingdon: Routledge, 1997, pp. 367–78.

Jones, Cara E. "The Pain of Endo Existence: Toward a Feminist Disability Studies Reading of Endometriosis." *Hypatia*, vol. 10, no. 10, 2016, pp. 1–18.

Kafer, Alison. *Feminist, Queer, Crip.* Bloomington, IN: Indiana University Press, 2013.

Kleege, Georgina."Audio Description Described: Current Standards, Future Innovations, Larger Implications." *Representations*, vol. 135, no. 1, 2016, pp. 89–101.

Küppers, Petra. *The Scar of Visibility: Medical Performances and Contemporary Art.* Chicago: University of Minnesota Press, 2007.

Linton, S. and L. J. Davis. *The Disability Studies Reader.* Milton Park: Taylor and Francis, 2006.

Manovich, Lev. "Subjects and Styles in Instagram Photography (Part 1)." *Instagram and Contemporary Image*, Instagram book, 2016.

Mihalyi, A., O. Gevaert, C. M. Kyama, P. Simsa, N. Pochet, F. De Smet et al. "Non-invasive Diagnosis of Endometriosis Based on a Combined Analysis of Six Plasma Biomarkers." *Human Reproduction*, vol. 25, 2010, pp. 654– 64.

Mitchell, William J. Thomas. "Word and Image." *Critical Terms for Art History,* edited by Robert S. Nelson and Richard Shiff, University of Chicago Press, 1996, pp. 51–62.

Puar, Jasbir K. *The Right to Maim: Debility, Capacity, Disability*. Durham, NC: Duke University Press, 2017.

Quayson, Ato. *Aesthetic Nervousness: Disability and the Crisis of Representation*. New York: Columbia University Press, 2007.

Reid, Madeline. "The Women Advocating for Endometriosis Awareness through Art."*Shift London,* March 14, 2019. www.shiftlondon.org/features/the-women-advocating-for-endometriosis-awareness-through-art/.

Rogers, Peter A.W., et al. "Priorities for Endometriosis Research: Recommendations from an International Consensus Workshop." *Reproductive Sciences*, vol. 16, no. 4, 2009, pp. 335–46.

Sedgwick, Eve Kosofsky, and Adam Frank. *Touching Feeling: Affect, Pedagogy, Performativity*. Durham, NC: Duke University Press, 2003.

Siebers, Tobin. *Disability Aesthetics*. Ann Arbor, MI: University of Michigan Press, 2010.

Pierre, Joshua St. "Living with Chronic Pain."*Journal of Critical Phenomenology*, vol. 3, no.2, 2020, pp. 30–2.

Wendell, Susan."Unhealthy Disabled: Treating Chronic Illnesses as Disabilities." *Hypatia,* vol. 16, no. 4, 2001, pp. 17–33.

Whelan, Emma. "'No one agrees except for those of us who have it': Endometriosis Patients as an Epistemological Community." *Sociology of Health & Illness*, vol. 29, no. 7, 2007, pp. 957–82.

Wileman, Georgie. "THIS IS ENDOMETRIOSIS." *Georgie Wileman*, www.georgiewileman.com/this-is-endometriosis-1.

31

ART SPACES, PERFORMANCES, PODCASTS

Community-building in a virtual age

Caroline Wellbery

Old stories, new platforms

The existential divide between individuals afflicted by illness and those who are as yet untouched is a fundamental yet perennially vexing problem for those reflecting on the human condition. For the health humanities, this divide – characterized by empathy on the one hand and emotional self-protection on the other – has long been framed in individual terms, separating the sick person from the well person.

This chapter explores what happens to stories of illness and medicine when their telling shifts from a private dyadic sphere to a public forum. Publicly shared illness narratives, disseminated live, in podcasts or videos, can enhance stories of illness or medical encounters by connecting an audience in real time, emphasizing collective togetherness. In particular, theatrical and spoken word performances have long been regarded as a way of building community by facilitating a shared experience. These works illustrate a spectrum of approaches through which narrators or performers explore illness identity in relation to the group. However, the performer can instead challenge the assembled community, undermining the collective experience by disrupting communal needs and expectations. Moreover, the community exists increasingly as an imaginary construct housed in cyberspace. For most of those who publicly share stories of illness and medicine, this is not a problem: on the contrary, they welcome these stories that blur genre boundaries and feature a constantly changing cast of listener-participants as democratizing. But health professionals should consider that for some, the public virtual sphere has undermined the promise or even possibility of authentic connection and has instead become a source of alienation. The health humanities can highlight the many advantages of narratives shared in the public sphere, while at the same time recognizing that there are those whom this cacophonous crowd has marginalized.

When it comes to grappling with the problem of suffering, the health humanities have privileged access. Stories of illness and death provide endless opportunity to study the manifestations and impacts of difficult experiences. That such a vast reservoir of stories exists is due in part to the obvious fact that illness and its consequences are experienced universally. In a digital world, which churns out fresh news faster than an assembly line, articles such as "I'm going to die. I might as well be cheerful about it" can still make headlines in the *New York Times* op ed pages, even when the essay's argument consists only of musings on the (yet healthy)

DOI: 10.4324/9781003007661-40

writer's resolve to die well (Piper). In the words of Heinrich Heine: "Es ist eine alte Geschichte, / Doch bleibt sie immer neu; / Und wem sie just passieret, / Dem bricht das Herz entzwei" (312). ("It's an old story, yet forever new, / when it happens to you / it's your heart that breaks in two.") Stories of illness and death are old as time yet always manage to feel surprising and brand new.

One facet of this newness is derived from the different cultural permutations through which we relate, as individuals, to collective experience. For example, Heine's verse in pointing to the gap between individual experience and the human experience at large reflects socio-politically on the emergence in the first half of the 19th century of an autonomous individual no longer subject to the pre-revolutionary hierarchies of the past. Increasingly, both the evolving self-efficacy of the individual and the vulnerability accompanying the loss of supportive institutions or communities have entered into our psychology to such an extent that we no longer recognize our individualizing perspectives on illness as anything but an intrinsic feature of our human nature.

One of the consequences of now saturated societal expectations of individual autonomy is our need to keep our vulnerabilities at bay, often at some cost and not only economically and physically but also to our psychological wholeness as well. In particular, we compartmentalize illness and death. Unless painful conditions become irreducibly personal and therefore unavoidable, as Heine's verse points out, they are easily walled off at arm's length in the form of an abstraction. Illness is "othered" through the protective mechanism of denial. As Freud is said to have written to his wife: "If one of us dies, I shall go to Paris." In order to prop up his psychological defenses, the speaker deflects his fear of death onto the very source of solace on which he ostensibly depends, in this case throwing his wife – and concomitantly, the serenity that comes with acceptance of one's mortality – under the bus.

In spite of these defenses, we cannot deny our biological fallibility. For this reason, illness narratives and other art forms play an important role in helping mediate between psychological defenses and the fears against which they protect. Engagement with the arts has often been described as a roundabout and therefore safe(r) way to deal with difficult emotions (Palmer 92; Gaufberg and Batalden 80). Artistic and narrative representations of illness create a cocooned environment providing vicarious access to afflicted individuals in close-knit relational settings who in some cases are shown actively seeking succor from individual others – for example, friends and family or a clinician. This allows the reader or viewer to participate intimately as well, with any expressions of pain leavened by the imaginary – or at least crafted – nature of the interaction. Whether the viewer projects himself standing in the attic shadows of Sir Luke Fildes' "The Doctor" (Fildes) or ghosts herself in as one of the visitors in "Last Days," Donald Hall's poetic chronicle of his wife Jane Kenyon's death (Hall), or feels herself buffeted in the chaos of Anne Boyer's powerful cancer narrative, "What cancer takes away," (Boyer) the experience arises in an atmosphere of interiority, of intimate presence, augmented by the personal nature of the recipient's private act of reading or examining a painting. This aesthetic of "as-if" intimacy plays an exemplary role in helping the recipient imagine, and therefore theoretically prepare, for his or her own illness experience.

Whereas the individual nature of such receptive encounters is mostly taken for granted, very little has been written in today's world of media-directed socialization about the role of the collective in mediating individual suffering, and in particular, about the ways in which the arts navigate the relationship between an individual illness experience and its public diffusion. For one thing, it might be useful to distinguish between the dyadic intimacy of, say, reading a book, from the communal experience of cybernetic immediacy. Illness narratives in their modern form have evolved into specific typologies, brilliantly captured in Arthur Frank's work (Frank);

other scholars, in a more modest format, have attempted to categorize physician-generated narratives in similar ways (Moniz et al.). What needs to be factored into these typologies is the narrative space in which they are performed. As oral and visual culture increasingly absorbs our attention, narrative *form* remains recognizably stable but narrative per*form*ance alters our reception of the story due to a growing emphasis on the immediacy of experience. Oral culture and "live" performance are not, of course, new. But internet culture, with its rapid-fire sound bites, Instagram and Twitter, with the facilitation of simultaneous commentary and real-time availability have foregrounded presence. Whether virtual or real, visual or aural, contemporary narrative art forms emphasize in-the-moment experiences. As the world contracts, however, we recognize that we are also part of a vast collective with which we have a less personal but more communal relationship. We are individuals, but increasingly we recognize ourselves also as part of a hive.

More than ever, access to technology has us wobbling between a sense of self and our role within diffuse, loosely defined communities, not just with respect to illness but in many aspects of our social and work-defined life. Our individual and collective existential states are not always, needless to say, congenial bedfellows. In our age of pandemics, cyberactivity, and globalization, we have more sharply come to see ourselves as one among many, indeed, among hundreds or hundreds of thousands; as, for example, when we face the realization that while certain persons suffering from Covid-19 die alone, even those solitary deaths coalesce into a phenomenon of collective namelessness. To be sure, a person with an isolating rare illness can find a supportive on-line gathering of likewise afflicted individuals. Yet in a parallel situation, a similarly suffering person may sink into isolation when, on social media, he finds himself contrasting his own diminished state with the artificial splendor of others' virtually represented lives.

As I intend to show, following up on Heine's verse, the arts offer a means to explore and expose the tension between individual and universally shared experiences, particularly in the context of stories about illness. At the same time, any interpretive effort must consider how internet-based technologies have transformed the arts; thus, reflecting on the medium as well as the message becomes an important part of understanding the arts' functional role relative to the stories they convey. Specifically, in just a handful of years, the arts have demonstrated a significant shift in the way in which they represent the vicarious experience of illness. Stories of illness no longer center around a private, dyadic engagement between solitary individuals, such as reading a book, but rather engage the public through a shared, collective experience.

Stories of medicine in the cyber-community: lessons from the academic podcast

Stories with a medical focus have lodged in an unprecedented number of new spaces, including stage performances on YouTube, blogs, on-line features in medical journals, virtual science pages, and even Instagram and Twitter. Indeed, this narrative take-over accelerated by the availability of virtual space has had medico-political consequences since cyberspace inevitably blurs the boundaries between news, invention, opinion, and fact. Personal "illness narratives" have become a subset of the broader representational phenomenon, "stories about medicine." Even medical scientists have begun to clamor for their own "narratives" to better reach wired – and therefore politicized – audiences, which in processing medical advice will now believe stories more than evidence (Meisel and Karlawish). The singular person's story has taken to the virtual stage to tell the pluralistic story of hospitals, organizations, and even of the public health system in general.

Many scientific journals now offer podcasts, yet another modality in which narrative and informational categories readily blur. Podcasts achieve what is sometimes called a narrative "voice" by structuring the presentation around a conversation. Scientific journals, such as the *Journal of the American Medical Association* (JAMA) and *Academic Medicine* have followed suit, adapting their content to podcasts and thus relaxing the stringent, depersonalized form of scientific writing. Instead of the passive voice and the disembodied "we" found, for example, in editorials not to mention clinical scholarship, podcasts feature individuals in conversation, presenting information in an active, apparently spontaneous exchange. The speakers blend objective content and subjective comment, capitalizing on a secret, homogenizing ingredient: the entertaining in-the-moment spontaneity of the event itself. This chattiness plays an important role in generating a sense of community among listeners. The bantering speakers, even in serious podcasts such as those produced by medical journals including JAMA's congenial conversations or *American Family Physician's AFP Podcast*, represent themselves to their listening audience as relatable figures. By chatting up their topics, the speakers engage in the same kind of talk as the ordinary listener might in her daily interaction, often featuring a collegial interchange between a well-prepared learner (the podcast host) and an authority (the expert).

No wonder then, that in one podcast from *Academic Medicine*, participants celebrate the derived sense of community as one of the many benefits of getting scientific information through podcasts ("The Role of Podcasts as Educational Tools"). *Academic Medicine*'s creation, in this instance of a "meta-podcast," in which listeners become the podcasters discussing podcasting, illustrates the fluidity of boundaries between speakers and listeners. The listeners newly minted as participant-performers explain how they experience that sense of fluidity: when they are listening to a podcast, they feel like they belong to a community of listeners. Their listening spills over into real-time interactions, for example, sparking conversations when, after hearing a podcast, they engage with their teachers and peers in clinical settings. Through these exchanges, learners discover that "...other people struggle with these things too... .thinking through these things in the same sort of way... is oddly reassuring and encouraging." (*Podcasts*, 11:46–11:58)

What is striking about the way this sense of community is generated is that it stands in stark contrast to the de facto isolation in which podcasts are actually heard. Health professionals, like many consumers of podcasts, will tune in particularly when they are engaging in a solitary activity, such as working out at the gym or driving to work. "Podcasts create a sense of connection between peers and faculty and even within a specialty. That [is] ironic given that people listen to podcasts generally by themselves, in a car, or exercising or in their house. It's kind of the one thing we do alone...and yet there is something about that listening experience that is shared..." (*Podcasts*, 13:58–14:19) Recruitment of the solitary individual into a communal sphere is one of the essential dynamics of podcasts, blogs, and other internet formats. Of note, the "social distancing'" that gave rise to a slew of viewing, listening and binge-watching recommendations during the Covid-19 crisis may not be such a radical break from an extant social structure in which many individuals have already found themselves alone or connected only to a limited circle. Virtual consumption of entertainment has long substituted for an extended community whose loss some decry as lacking in our society (Carney).

This dichotomous yet fluid position of networked individuals has drawn attention to the alone/together phenomenon. However virtual the world "out there," the listener is linked to a live event, and this live event generates a network of other listeners whose presence can be tracked, for example, by counting clicks and likely many other surveillance modalities or documented through tweets and posts. This sense of immediacy gives even the educational podcast – the most proper and sober instantiation of conversational togetherness – its power to connect the listener to a broader community: "they hear the host's voice and feel like they know them, they talk among themselves about what they hear on that podcast" (*Podcasts*, 14:22–14:31). The voice in the living room, in the car, or on the elliptical offers a reassuring sense of connection.

Communal art experiences foster resilience

In some ways, the nuances of the podcast-listening experience are not new. The arts have long been regarded as a way of building community by facilitating a shared experience. I would say that this is a fundamental motivation for the arts, which are rooted in participatory rituals (Dissanayake 182). The literal or symbolic act of gathering together applies even to reading, which has typically been thought of as a solitary activity cotemporaneous with the rise of the novel (Fischer) and manifesting as the lone act of curling up with a book. Reading communities no less than other groups of art consumers have – in addition to virtual offerings – relied on physical bodies in physical gatherings. Book clubs and public readings allow readers to connect with each other and meet authors. Movies also, though increasingly challenged to attract in-theater audiences even before the coronavirus closed movie houses, provide a sense of shared experience. A *Washington Post* headline during the corona crisis noted that "Without theaters, communal experience is missing" (May 16, 2020). The text elaborates: "When we laugh, cry, wince or gasp together, we are demonstrating that movies are a social medium. They need an audience to complete the circuit, close the feedback loop, make the meaning" (Hornaday). Even podcasts and other televised shows are often recorded in front of studio audiences – to replicate a sense of intimacy, some live performances have gone so far as to invite the audience to show up in pajamas (Vulture Festival).

Some artistic devices specifically incorporate the theme of creating community into their structure; the Greek chorus, an early example, was presumed to serve as a bridge between performance and audience (Calame). In Aeschylus' plays, such as *Agamemnon* and *The Eumenides*, the chorus is on stage, but like the audience, remains helpless to intervene; it is nonetheless in constant commentary, directing the emotional reactions of the audience. (One might recognize an analogous role for today's self-appointed commentators in social media). The point is not to change the grim course of action but to engage the viewer-participant and – even at the risk of disrupting the illusion enacted on stage – to bathe the audience in a sense that, however horribly, "we are all in this together."

Deliberately disrupting the performed illusion though self-conscious commentary may boost a participatory sense of community even more than lulling the audience into community through suspended disbelief. In a recent performance of *Timon of Athens*, servers strolled down the aisles prior to the start of the play, offering the audience Turkish delight on gilded trays – precisely the confection Timon's sycophantic guests are about to feast on in the first act (Higgins). By sharing this food, the audience becomes complicit in the world of the rich, self-indulgent elite portrayed on stage. Self-conscious acts like these wink at the audience, allowing viewers collectively to enjoy being in the know, even when this occurs at their own expense. That these kinds of disruptive acts can backfire (often deliberately) is well-known. As I will discuss below, disruptions can alienate the audience and even cause chaos, thus disbanding the community. The purpose of such disruptions is precisely to shake up the audience's sense of communal experience through the awakening jolt of discomfort (Aldama and Lindenberger). By challenging conventional assumptions about the art experience, the artwork explodes the illusory nature of the audience's claim to emotional or psychological protection within the safety of a communal space.

The arts' role in promoting communal experiences is not limited to performances: it can become visible even where the participating community is transient or vaguely defined. Museums are 'fixed spaces' for gathering but interesting in the fact that the viewing of displayed art is not a particularly collective experience. When a person walks through an exhibit, he finds himself jostling against others, vying for a vantage point, listening to audio explanations and being careful not to speak his thoughts too audibly to his companion because observations overheard risk falling into flat banalities or sounding pretentious. As Philip Kennicott, a prominent art critic, writes in advising museum-goers how to view art: "Imagine you have a magnetic repulsion to everyone else. Move toward empty space. Indulge in your misanthropy" (Kennicott).

No wonder then that artists such as Olafur Eliasson have sought ways of turning exhibited art into a collective experience, for example through his installation, "The Weather Report," which places viewers 'under one sun,' with many lying down uninstructed on the floor and viewing their collective reflections in the mirrored ceiling. As one commentator mused: "The location of this work, the Turbine Hall, gave a hum which when combined with viewing Eliasson's creation brought viewers to be a part of the place. It gave a sense of a close encounter" (publicdelivery.org /olafur- eliasson-the-weather-project/).

One of the most powerful thematizations of a unified museum-going collective is Icelandic artist's Ragnar Kjartansson's work, titled "The Visitors." In this video installation, he has assembled a band at a villa, assigning musicians separate rooms from which to perform their part. The viewer walks from screen to screen in a large exhibit space, watching one musician playing guitar in a bathtub, another singing from the library, another with his girlfriend in a bedroom. At the end of the hour-long performance, the musicians lay down their instruments, leaving their respective rooms to gather in front of the villa. The left-behind empty video-rooms in effect reroute the museum-goers. With no further musical action on the screens, the viewers too "abandon" the respective "rooms" they had been viewing and collectively turn to the one remaining active screen showing the outside of the villa where the musicians have gathered. Together, the museum-goers crowd in front of the screen as they watch the musicians descend from the porch into the surrounding greenery. The musicians have reconvened: so have the viewers, their collective gathering a kind of mimesis of the performers', assembling through a looking glass of the real world and the virtual world of a video respectively. While this work is available on YouTube (Kjartansson), this essential orchestration of the experience cannot be captured online, for obvious reasons.

As the previous examples suggest, artists' interest in community-building has grown. Artists may not succeed in creating actual communities, but they do at the very least raise awareness of community to highlight its absences. Kjartansson's project stands out because he uses the theme of video-conferencing technology to illustrate the simultaneity of separation and togetherness. This is, indeed, a defining feature of our interactions through the mediations of technology, as anyone isolated in the coronavirus pandemic quickly learned. For example, the creator of "The Nocturnists," a story-telling forum for and by healthcare professionals, recognized the importance of sharing stories as a way of creating a sense of community. After inviting listeners to send in accounts of their personal experiences, the editors brought listeners and hosts together on one platform, constructing through a series of linked vignettes the common storied experience that the pandemic had become (Silverman).

Illness performances

In today's high-stakes live (or 'live') performance environment, success often relies on confronting the audience, often with its own fallibilities, as exemplified by comedians such as

Dave Chapelle who rakes his listeners over the coals of their putative self-serving assumptions while rescuing them in the last minute with a comedic reprieve just in time before they burn (*Equanimity*). Illness narratives, however, are inherently less likely to rattle the cage of predictability than their socio-politically "edgy" counterparts and are, for that reason, potent mediators of community-building. Medicine hues to a certain traditionalism, such that even "chaos narratives," to borrow from the most torrid of Arthur Frank's categories, demand to be tamed. Inundated as we are with represented provocations and outrage, we nonetheless still expect medically-themed performances to encourage a sense of partnership and belonging, for example, through empathy – think Randy Pausch's 2007 "Last Lecture" (Pausch) in which he jokes about his fatal illness (pancreatic cancer) while speaking movingly about family, meaning, love and loss. When pitch-perfect, the performer/narrator holds the audience in a safe space free from alienation.

This is exactly what happens in Andrew Borowitz' performance of "An Unexpected Twist" in which he recounts his experience with a medical emergency, when he was hospitalized for a sigmoid volvulus (Borowitz). In this exceptionally crafted comedic performance, Borowitz demonstrates a keen awareness of the pitfalls that can potentially disrupt the compact between performer and audience. In addition to his performative skills that include self-commentary and well-timed pauses, he describes his experiences in Jonathan Swift-like fashion as though he were an astonished traveler in an alien world, thus inviting members of the audience to become allies, imagining themselves as potential patients navigating the maze of medical mumbo-jumbo. "… they have diverted my digestive tract elsewhere . . . Like when you've closed the upper roadway on the George Washington Bridge … later this nurse appears and her job in the hospital is to spread pro-ileostomy propaganda. I'm not kidding! She has a magazine called *The Phoenix* … a glossy magazine devoted to the ileostomy lifestyle -- who knew?" (Borowitz).

This wondrous journey, comprised of a concatenation of "routine" medical encounters reconceived as bizarre misadventures elicits the constant laughter of recognition, sealing the listeners' community cohesion. Borowitz 'has' the audience: at no point is it made to feel that alienation is a liability of its participation. Alienation occurs somewhere else: in the hospital's chaos and beyond the perimeters of the theatrical space.

These impacts on the public's response noticeably exceed older narrative forms, let's say for example the now near-extinct epistolary novel, which connected self and other in an intimate interpersonal space through the evocation of empathy. The intimacy of Baudelaire's call to the reader – 'mon semblable, mon frère' – gives way to a communal space. The satisfying story arc of Borowitz' tale (which ends with an awakened appreciation for all that surrounds him and for life's beautiful moments) relinquishes the privacy of the narrating persona to his audience. Intimacy is dispersed throughout the community; it 'belongs' to everyone. Storytelling as a public phenomenon may not do away with any single recipient's sense that she is somehow spoken to personally, but the performers' success is measured by an ability to control the recipients' collective identity. This identity can fold the individual into a comforting collective, but as I will next point out, can also highlight a crisis of alienation.

Disrupting community

For all the salubrious benefits of community-building, particularly through the communal sharing and performance of illness-narratives, it is important to recognize their role in eliding the ways in which the connections between performers and audience or amongst members of the audience are ultimately provisional. As the philosopher Jean-Luc Nancy (Nancy; Bernasconi) has argued, 'true communities' are a construct, a product of nostalgia, and in the final analysis, through exclusion of scape-goated others, a vehicle for discrimination and other divisions. This double-take, for example, is revealed in the performances of Martin O'Brien. A cystic fibrosis patient, he performs in the legacy of artist-provocateurs, such as Marina Abramovich. As a witness to one of his live performances, I experienced firsthand how a performer can crack the illusion of community and force the audience into the uncomfortable acknowledgment of its discriminatory views and internal divisions. This particular performance took place at a conference – audience members gathered directly subsequent to a champagne reception, still carrying flutes of champagne. Context is everything in setting the stage, literally and figuratively: the artist had selected an ugly, concrete surface near a dumpster for his outdoor performance space. He then proceeded to enact his experience of illness, half naked and crudely diapered, coughing up mucus, crawling across the rough pavement like a dog, and smearing himself with his secretions. Meanwhile some shocked on-lookers twirled their glasses and others slipped uncomfortably away.

My point here is not to dwell on the performance's specific details. O'Brien's performances have been documented on-line and analyzed many times. (Das; Wellbery; "Martin O'Brien"; "Until the last breath is breathed") I merely want to emphasize that his work falls within a genre of performances that aims to disrupt the covenant of community cohesion. The disruptive gesture cuts into the audience, slashes it into division – for example, by causing some people to leave. The general discomfort not only prevents the formation of participatory solidarity but also divides the audience from the performer. The performer's own alienation, for whom sickness is the underlying propellant – in the case of O'Brien but also other patient-performers in related circumstances – paradoxically requires the audience to reenact his separation from the expected societal norms. Should the viewer stay and acknowledge the suffering expressed in the performer's self-mutilation? Or should she, in removing herself, make explicit that the aesthetic experience is really only about satisfying the audience's wants and needs? O'Brien gives the audience an impossible choice – which is, one could say, his point. Just as Borowitz creates community in the moment, O'Brien destroys it.

However, these seemingly different approaches to the (dys)function of community represent two sides of the same coin. It might be tempting to assign ethical or even aesthetic values to the representations I have described. For example, one might want to say that Borowitz' community-building is a wholesome act, and O'Brien's disruptive performances are unwholesome. Or one might want to say that Borowitz' community is inauthentic, whereas O'Brien's dismantling of community exposes the painful costs of community coherence, such as the denial of suffering. The construction of cohesion and division are in fact integrally connected, manifesting as stories we tell ourselves about who we are as members of a community and about our identity as individuals.

So what does the shift toward public space, away from the dyadic intimacy between reader and narrator, mean? What conclusions can we draw from the shift toward a collective identity, often generated by social media, which nonetheless cannot obscure the absence of belonging at the margins of a constructed community? And finally, what implications does this technological shift have for the health humanities, in particular for its parsing of illness narratives? These are questions not readily answered. However, it is safe to say that the way in which narratives are consumed today through visual media and podcasts, along with the vast buzz of accompanying on-line commentary, has profoundly impacted our self-conception as individuals.

One central effect is that of an inherent paradox: we are more like others than we imagined, and also more anonymous than we imagined. As a commentator recently wrote in the *Washington Post*: "The problem is that everything is connected, and the problem is, despite all that, that we're not connected enough" (Roberts). The Covid-19 crisis has sharpened awareness of our conflicted relationship to our larger communities and beyond. It has caused us to reexamine everything from the way we share physical space with each other to our nationalistic tendencies. All of these conundrums point to the most profound affliction of our current human condition which in Western society has forced an outsized emphasis on individuals and independence: an incomplete ability to reconcile our existence as singular beings with our communal selves. This imperfect, hobbled union – along with the longing and disenchantment to which it gives rise – suggests that the dyad self/other noted when I began this chapter is not so separate from the dyad alone/together.

An important task of the health humanities, particularly in this brave new high-tech world, is to trace the paths that lead from the self to the other in its individual and collective forms. In this chapter, I have focused on the arts, and particularly narrative, as means of exploring these relationships, for example, how narratives have responded to and participated in creating the social realities of our current collective identity – together/alone. The health humanities, and their focus on the arts in particular are a strong source of potential wellness interventions that might boost community belonging (Fancourt and Steptoe), and diminish the individual's sense of separateness. We know from "social prescribing," for example, that such initiatives are possible (The Social Prescribing Network). At the same time, the health humanities as a source of critical analyses should continue to highlight the risks inherent in technologically constructed communities and to attend closely to the sounds of voices coming from the fissures within.

Works cited

Aldama, F. and H. Lindenberger. "Aesthetics of Discomfort: Conversations on Disquieting Art." Ann Arbor, MI: University of Michigan Press, 2016.

Bernasconi, Robert. "On Deconstructing Nostalgia for Community within the West: The Debate between Nancy and Blanchot." *Research in Phenomenology,* vol. 23, no. 1, 1993, pp. 3–21.

Borowitz, Andrew. "An Unexpected Twist." *YouTube*, uploaded by The Moth/World Science Festival, October 13, 2011, www.youtube.com/watch?v=4mvhjZ-ClLw. Accessed July 27, 2020.

Boyer, Anne. "What Cancer Takes Away." *The New Yorker*. April 8, 2019. www.newyorker.com/magazine/2019/04/15/what-cancer-takes-away. Accessed July 27, 2020.

Calame, Claude. "Performative Aspects of the Choral Voice in Greek Tragedy: Civic Identity in Performance." *Performance Culture and Athenian Democracy*, edited by Simon Goldhill and Robin Osborne. Cambridge, UK and New York, Cambridge University Press, 1999, pp. 125–54.

Carney, Timothy. *Alienated America*. New York: HarperCollins, 2019.

Das, Jareh. "On Curating Pain: The Sick Body in Martin O'Brien's *Taste of Flesh/Bite Me I'm Yours.*" *Leonardo*, vol. 49, no. 3, 2016, pp. 266–7.

Dissanayake, Ellen. *Art and Intimacy: How the Arts Began*. Seattle and London: University of Washington Press, 2000.

Equanimity, Performance by David Chapelle. Warner Theater, 2017. *Netflix*.

Fancourt, Daisy and Andrew Steptoe. "The Art of Life and Death: 14 Year Follow-up Analyses of Associations between Arts Engagement and Mortality in the English Longitudinal Study of Ageing." *BMJ*, vol. 367, no. 8227, 2019, p. l6377.

Fildes, Luke. "The Doctor." Tate Gallery. www.tate.org.uk/art/artworks/fildes-the-doctor-n01522. Accessed July 27, 2020.

Fischer, Steven Roger. *A History of Reading*. London: Reaktion Books, 2003.

Frank, Arthur. *The Wounded Storyteller: Body, Illness and Ethics*. Chicago, University of Chicago Press, 1995.

Gaufberg, Elizabeth and Maren Batalden. "The Third Thing in Medical Education." *The Clinical Teacher*, vol. 4, no. 2, 2007, pp. 78–81.

Hall, Donald. "Last Days." *Without*. Boston, MA: Houghton Mifflin, 1998, pp. 35–45.

Heine, Heinrich. "Ein Jüngling liebt ein Mädchen." *Das grosse deutsche Gedichtbuch,* edited by Karl Otto Conrady, Düsseldorf: Artemis & Winker, 1991, p. 312.

Higgins, Martin. "Review of Shakespeare and Middleton's *Timon of Athens* (directed by Simon Godwin for the Royal Shakespeare Company) at the Swan Theatre, Stratford-upon-Avon, December 8, 2018."

Shakespeare, vol. 15, no 2, 2019, pp. 203–5. Hornaday, Anne. "What is a Movie? With Theaters Shuttering, the Question gets Real." *The Washington Post*, March 20, 2020, www.washingtonpost.com/entertainment/what-is-a-movie-with-theaters-shuttering-the-question-gets-real/2020/03/18/930f16ec-6874-11ea-9923-57073adce27c_story.html. Accessed July 19, 2020.

Kennicott, Philip."How to View Art: Be Dead Serious About It, but Don't Expect Too Much." *The Washington Post,* October 7, 2014, www.washingtonpost.com/entertainment/museums/how-to-view-art-be-dead-serious-about-it-but-dont-expect-too-much/2014/10/01/28f7cdba-459a-11e4-b47c-f5889e061e5f_story.html. Accessed July 19, 2020.

Kjartansson, Ragnary. "The Visitors Complete Video." *YouTube,* www.youtube.com/watch?v=qOxG711lb0E. Accessed July 19, 2020.

"Martin O'Brien." ArtsAdmin, Toynbee Studios, www.artsadmin.co.uk/profiles/martin-o-brien/. Accessed July 27, 2020.

Meisel, Zachary F. and Jason Karlawish. "Narrative vs Evidence-Based Medicine – And, Not Or." *JAMA,* vol. 306, no. 24, 2011, pp. 2022–3.

Moniz, Tracy, Lorelei Lingard, and Chris Watling. "Stories Doctors Tell." *JAMA*, vol. 318, no. 2, 2017, pp. 124–5.

Nancy, Jean-Luc. "Coronavirus and Philosophers: M. Foucault, G. Agamben, J. L.Nancy, R. Esposito, S. Benvenuto, D. Dwivedi, S. Mohan, R. Ronchi, M. de Carolis." *European Journal of Psychoanalysis*, www.journal-psychoanalysis.eu/coronavirus-and-philosophers/. Accessed July 19, 2020.

"Olafur Eliasson's 'Weather Project' – Why did He Try to Recreate the Sun? "*Public Delivery,* publicdelivery.org/olafur-eliasson-the-weather-project/. Accessed July 19, 2020.

Palmer, P. J. "A Hidden Wholeness: The Journey toward an Undivided Life." San Francisco, CA: Jossey-Bass Publishers, 2004, pp. 92–3.

Pausch, Randy. *Last Lecture*. *YouTube*, uploaded by Carnegie Mellon University, December 20, 2007, www.youtube.com/watch?v=ji5_MqicxSo. Accessed July 27, 2020.

Piper, Mary. "I'm Going to Die. I Might as Well be Cheerful About It." *New York Times*, March 6, 2020, www.nytimes.com/2020/03/06/opinion/mortality-death. Accessed July 18, 2020.

Roberts, Molly. "We Did This to Ourselves." *The Washington Post*, April 8, 2020, www.washingtonpost.com/opinions/2020/04/08/we-made-this-disaster-ourselves/. Accessed July 27, 2020.

Silverman, Emily. "Stories from a Pandemic: Virus." *The Nocturnists*, April 14, 2020. http://thenocturnists.com/the-nocturnists-stories-from-a-pandemic. Accessed July 19, 2020.

Social Prescribing Network, The.www.socialprescribingnetwork.com/#:~:text=Social%20Prescribing%20is%20a%20means. Accessed August 27, 2020.

"The Role of Podcasts as Educational Tools in Medical Education." *Academic Medicine Podcast*, November 28, 2019, Burk-Rafel, Jesse (host), Trivedi, Shreya and Mason, Jess (podcasters) Riddell, Jeff (researcher). podcasts.apple.com/us/podcast/role-podcasts-as-educational-tools-in-medical-education/id1112697692?i=1000457114398. Accessed July 19, 2020.

"Until the Last Breath is Breathed." By Martin O'Brien. Tate Gallery. February 8, 2020. www.tate.org.uk/whats-on/tate-britain/performance/until-last-breath-breathed. Accessed July 27, 2020.

Vulture Festival: Complete line-up. "Playing House Pajama Bruch," March 16, 2017. www.vulture.com/2017/04/black-mirror-ansari-colbert-coming-to-vulture-festival.html. Accessed July 19, 2020.

Wellbery, Caroline. "The Pain Artist." Interacting with the Arts in Medicine. sites.google.com/a/georgetown.edu/mdarts/units/unit-3/section-1/essay-caroline-wellbery-the-pain-artist. Accessed July 27, 2020.

AFTERWORD

Audience construction and health care storytelling in the digital age

Joseph G. Turow

The fascinating range of studies in this book reflects the breadth and the importance of media storytelling about medicine and health care. The editors of this volume asked me to ruminate a bit on other avenues that scholars interested in stories about health care might take in view of the twists and turns of my own health- and non-health related research projects. To address their request, it's useful to explain why I turned to studying storytelling about health care, why I turned to what may seem a different direction entirely – marketers' constructions of audiences – and why what I have learned in that arena suggests new paths for exploring storytelling about health in the digital age.

My interest in television's storytelling about medicine beginning the 1980s had as its fundamental driver an interest in investigating the relation between the medium and institutional power. My understanding of an institution draws from anthropology: it is a complex of organizations, individuals, and other entities that exercise control over key areas of social life such as government, education, the military, and health care. It should be clear from these examples that institutions are by no means monolithic. To the contrary, the elements that comprise institutions are often at odds with one another as they jockey for material and symbolic resources that allow them to guide their sector of society in certain directions rather than others. The ability to accumulate such resources – for example, the newest machines, the best people, enough cash to accumulate them, and authority – adds up to the ability to build institutional power, including the ability to influence various media outlets (newspapers, magazines, television shows) and to tell stories to the various populations. Members of an institution can use various techniques to distribute self-serving media stories via those outlets. They can directly purchase advertising space and time to make their positions known; they can leverage public relations resources (for example, key people and companies) to affect the creation and framing of news narratives, and they can provide advisors to tellers of fictional stories who want to attract audiences by depicting an institution's activities in dramatic and/or comedic ways. None of these activities is likely to be straightforwardly successful. Media organizations have their own storytelling incentives and constraints as they deal with representatives from other institutions who want depictions that may not match the media practitioners' understanding of the considerations that should guide their portrayals. Those could include plot lines that they believe will interest audiences which key advertisers most want; procedures that take liberties with advisors' sense of accuracy to make the production efficient or tell a "good" story; themes

DOI: 10.4324/9781003007661-41

that please government authorities, sponsors, or advocacy groups; and, generally, approaches to settings, characters, and actions that have stood the test of ratings popularity over the years.

The investigation that resulted in my book, *Playing Doctor* (1989, 2010), picked up this logic. The fundamental aim was to gain insight into the cross-institutional processes that shaped changes and continuities in the depictions of an institution and its social power across the history of American television's prime time shows from the early 1950s through around 2010. I chose to track programs centering on the healthcare institutions because they have been a mainstay of the medium from its inception with tale-telling models dating back to prior decades of radio, movies, and books. My research involved viewing many hours of television series; reading thousands of pages of articles on the TV industry, medical industry, and general publications; and interviewing 122 Hollywood producers, directors, actors, scriptwriters, medical advisors, and network executives who worked over the years to create what all understood was a patterned prime-time approach – a "formula" – about health care. One point that was clear from the start was their narrow conception of health care. With few exceptions, the stories they told centered on physicians as the embodiment of the institutions (and for many years these were almost always male). The settings where the doctors practiced were almost always hospitals. Narrowing the institutional vista even more, the hospital work focused on acute rather than chronic problems, better to yield dramatic crescendos where life hung in the balance. Moreover, high tech specialized care was regular fare across programs from the early 1950s through the 2000s; the programs typically depicted health care as normatively unlimited where patients should (and often, because of heroic physicians) get the best, most advanced care without reflection on cost. In many ways, the "doctor show" formula presented a 1950s version of policymakers' understanding of health resources and medical power even while policymakers and others in the larger society were involved in roiling debates about the very elements that storytellers took for granted: that doctors should inevitably be captains of the healthcare ship, that hospitals are the best place for health care; that acute rather than chronic care is the largest social problem; and that issues around costs should be pushed to the side in favor of an emphasis on heroic actions.

In short, the story of television's interactions with health care was a tale of Hollywood's capture by dominant medical forces during one crucial period – starting in movies during the 1930s and continuing in TV through early 1960s. Those interactions cast a formula that kept the essential features of their institutional domination even as so many aspects of the real healthcare world were changing drastically. Such depictions, while championing the aims of physicians and the positions of acute-care specialists, may well have confused audiences who found themselves dealing angrily with healthcare norms that weren't following the fictional formula. As for the producers, writers, directors, and network executives who guided the stories, they worked to develop plots and characters in ways that would seem "realistic" even as they knew that they were furrowing a narrow terrain. They did it, they said, with an eye on the audience, reflected through ratings of hugely successful shows such as *ER* and *Gray's Anatomy*. Audiences, they believed, wanted to see the ultimate drama that could affect them and their loved ones: physicians and their professional helpmates grappling with patients' life and death even while those health professionals were struggling to hold their private lives together.

It's important to point out that conclusions about medical depictions and power from the first 50 years of television storytelling only set the stage for the presentations that producers and programmers will unfold over the next 50. That is because storytelling formulas are dynamic and dialectical. Media tale-tellers always face the ultimate risk of low audiences. In response, they continually negotiate tensions between continuity and change, between using tried and true setting, characters, and plot techniques that have traditionally drawn the desired crowds and choosing innovations that challenge past tropes to reflect the interests of hoped for audiences more directly. How daring they will be in the calculus of change over continuity will depend on various factors that involve personal, organizational, institutional, and societal factors. Another key theme emerged from my study of doctor-show storytelling as well as research on health-care public relations and other aspects of media production: the ways media creators construct their audiences is crucial as they justify their continuities and change in content. It became increasingly clear through my Hollywood work that all media audiences are industrial constructions. That is, the basic categories that organizations use to think about the people who are (or ought to be) targets of their programming are established in the relationships between the production organizations and their primary patrons – for example, the TV networks. The networks, in turn, interpret their preferred audience categories through their relationships with *their* patrons, the advertisers, who get their data from various qualitative and quantitative research programs (Nielsen and beyond). Fundamentally, it is the advertisers' understandings of American society and the people who count in that society that drive the ways production firms think of whom they have to reach. The central target may be eighteen to 34-year-old women, but that demographic may be colored by profiles of the likes and dislikes of viewer samples as well as stereotypes of medical show loyalists. These understandings inevitably trickle down to the producers, casting directors, and other creative types who form the programs and construct visions of society, including health care. Plot lines that succeeded ratings wise with this demographic may be used with slight variations across shows.

My awareness of the crucial (though often indirect) role that advertisers play in storytelling, including about health care, helped me as I embarked on a very different set of cross-institutional investigations that on the surface had little to do with the medical system. From the 1980s onward, I dived deeply into issues that lie at the intersection of marketing, digital media, and society. Propelled by a longstanding interest in the history and nature of advertising, I turned my attention to the profound changes that were taking place in the ad industry with the rise of digital technologies and particularly the launch of the commercial internet in the mid-1990s. (See, for example, Turow, 1995, 2006, 2011, 2017, and 2021.) My interest in storytelling has remained, but it has taken a very different slant. Rather than looking at the stories a sector of the media institution tells people in society about another institution, my explorations have centered on the ways the marketing sector uses media to tell people about themselves and their relation to others in the society. I have conducted research on the rise of target marketing, the development of personalization in the digital realm, the transformation of media planning and buying in the face of the internet, the ways in which stores try to track their customers in physical locations as they do online and in apps, and (most recently) the beginnings of voice profiling by marketers as they struggle to continually satisfy their needs for new, and allegedly more effective, forms of personalization. During my journeys, I have seen strong connections between various styles of personalization and prejudicial discrimination. Telling stories about people often means valuing some over others and treating them differently in the marketplace.

None of this may seem relevant to storytelling about health. Certainly, this area of my work doesn't intersect obviously with the writings in this volume. Yet I would argue that tracking the activities of marketers in the digital realm is a great way to notice new forms of health storytelling. Companies are using leading edge technologies to tell stories to and about their target audiences' bodies. The stories feature wellness and disease in the service of selling and, in that way, lay out norms and power over norms that aren't fundamentally different from the functions doctor shows play. Consider the Amazon Halo wrist band, which made it market debut in fall 2020. In the interest of "emotional health," it claims to tell you how you sound to your boss, mother, spouse, and others. The company assures device owners that it cannot use that information, but it is a proof of concept. Moreover, customer service centers are already using the voices of people who phone them to make decisions about which agents should handle, and try to upsell, individuals with certain emotions. Google, Amazon, and Spotify are also among the firms that have patents alleging an ability to use voice to improve their bottom lines by exploring their audience's bodies for usable data. One Amazon patent tells a story in a cartoon panel: a woman walks into her apartment and asks the Alexa assistant for a dinner recipe. The assistant picks up her speech irregularities that imply a cold ("based at least in part on an analysis of pitch, pulse, voicing, jittering, and/or harmonicity of a user's voice, as determined from processing the voice data"). From that conclusion, Alexa asks the woman if she wants chicken soup, and when she says no, offers to sell her cough drops with one-hour delivery. Note that Amazon owns a pharmacy, so it can exploit this kind of tale in various ways.

"Man, woman, birth, death, infinity." Intoned by the actor Sam Jaffe, the words began every episode of the hit doctor series, *Ben Casey*, that ran on ABC from 1961 to 1966. The writer James Moser understood that stories about birth and death – often through the lenses of caregivers – motivate so much of our civilization. Those stories take on many forms, including the ways that the storytellers tell stories about their audiences – which then lead to stories and other actions toward them. A new media-and-marketing world is rising that will have profound consequences for these stories as well as for the discriminatory options people have in their worlds. I invite you to join in understanding it.

Works cited

Turow, Joseph. *Playing Doctor: Television, Storytelling, and Medical Power*. New York, Oxford University Press, 1989.

Turow, Joseph. *Breaking Up America: Advertisers and the New Media World*. Chicago: University of Chicago Press, 1996.

Turow, Joseph. *Niche Envy: Marketing Discrimination in the Digital Age*. Cambridge, MA: MIT Press, 2006.

Turow, Joseph. *Playing Doctor*.1989. 2nd edition. Ann Arbor, MI: University of Michigan Press, 2010.

Turow, Joseph. *The Daily You: How the New Advertising Industry is Defining Your Industry and Your Worth*. New Haven and London: Yale University Press, 2011.

Turow, Joseph. *The Aisles Have Eyes: How Retailers Track Your Shopping, Strip Your Privacy, and Define Your Power*. New Haven and London: Yale University Press, 2017.

Turow, Joseph. *The Voice Catchers: How Marketers Listen In to Exploit Your Feelings, Your Privacy, and Your Wallet*. New Haven and London: Yale University Press, 2021.

INDEX